Cardiovascular Health and Disease in Women

PAMELA S. DOUGLAS, M.D.
Director, Noninvasive Cardiology
Cardiovascular Division
Beth Israel Hospital
Associate Professor of Medicine
Harvard Medical School
Boston, Massachusetts

W.B. SAUNDERS COMPANY
A Divison of Harcourt Brace & Company

Philadelphia   London   Toronto   Montreal   Sydney   Tokyo

W.B. SAUNDERS COMPANY
A Division of Harcourt Brace & Company

The Curtis Center
Independence Square West
Philadelphia, PA 19106

Library of Congress Cataloging-in-Publication Data

Cardiovascular health and disease in women/[edited by] Pamela S. Douglas.—1st ed.

p.   cm.

ISBN 0-7216-4567-4

1. Heart—Diseases—Sex factors.   2. Heart—Sex differences.   3. Women—Diseases.   I. Douglas, Pamela S. [DNLM: 1. Cardiovascular Diseases.   2. Women's Health.   WG 100 C26742]

RC682.C4 1993   616.1'2'0082—dc20

DNLM/DLC   92-48884

Cardiovascular Health and Disease in Women   ISBN 0-7216-4567-4

Copyright © 1993 by W.B. Saunders Company

All rights reserved. No part of this publication may be reproduced or transmitted in any form or by any means, electronic or mechanical, including photocopy, recording, or any information storage and retrieval system, without permission in writing from the publisher.

Printed in the United States of America

Last digit is the print number: 9   8   7   6   5   4   3   2   1

*To my parents, Rose and Josh Douglas,
for their enthusiastic support and encouragement
and, always, their love.*

Contributors

MICHAEL R. ADAMS, D.V.M.
Professor of Comparative Medicine, Bowman Gray School of Medicine, Wake Forest University, Winston-Salem, North Carolina
Clinical Implications of Animal Models of Gender Difference in Heart Disease

DIANE M. BECKER, Sc.D.
Associate Professor, The Johns Hopkins University School of Medicine, School of Hygiene and Public Health, Baltimore, Maryland; Attending Staff, The Johns Hopkins Hospital, Baltimore, Maryland
Smoking and Cardiovascular Disease

VERA BITTNER, M.D.
Assistant Professor of Medicine, Division of Cardiovascular Diseases, University of Alabama School of Medicine, Birmingham, Alabama
Hypertension

PETER BUTTRICK, M.D.
Associate Professor, Division of Cardiology, Montefiore Medical Center and Albert Einstein College of Medicine, Bronx, New York
Myocardial Function and Cardiomyopathy

THOMAS B. CLARKSON, D.V.M.
Professor and Chair, Department of Comparative Medicine and Director, Comparative Medicine Clinical Research Center, Bowman Gray School of Medicine, Wake Forest University, Winston-Salem, North Carolina
Clinical Implications of Animal Models of Gender Difference in Heart Disease

PATRICIA LENA COLE, M.D.
Assistant Professor of Medicine and Associate Dean for Student Affairs, Washington University School of Medicine, St. Louis, Missouri; Associate Physician and Director, Cardiac Catheterization Laboratory, Jewish Hospital At Washington University Medical Center, St. Louis, Missouri
Cardiovascular Physiology of Pregnancy

MICHAEL H. CRIQUI, M.D., M.P.H.
Professor, Department of Community and Family Medicine and Department of Medicine, University of California, San Diego School of Medicine, San Diego, California
Stroke and Peripheral Vascular Diseases

SUSAN M. CZAJKOWSKI, Ph.D.
Social Science Analyst, Behavioral Medicine Branch; National Heart, Lung, and Blood Institute, National Institutes of Health, Bethesda, Maryland
Psychosocial and Environmental Correlates of Heart Disease

RICHARD B. DEVEREUX, M.D.
Professor of Medicine, Cornell University Medical College, New York, New York; Director, Echocardiography Laboratory, The New York Hospital, New York, New York
Valvular Heart Disease

PAMELA S. DOUGLAS, M.D.
Director, Noninvasive Cardiology, Cardiovascular Division, Beth Israel Hospital; Associate Professor of Medicine, Harvard Medical School, Boston, Massachusetts
Coronary Heart Disease: Therapeutic Principles

KENNETH R. EPSTEIN, M.D.
Clinical Assistant Professor, Department of Medicine, Jefferson Medical College, Thomas Jefferson University, and Associate Director, Division of Internal Medicine, Department of Medicine, Jefferson Medical College, Thomas Jefferson University, Philadelphia, Pennsylvania; Attending Staff, Thomas Jefferson University Hospital, Philadelphia, Pennsylvania
The Female Patient

SUSAN B. EYSMANN, M.D.
Assistant Professor of Medicine, Northwestern University Medical School, Chicago, Illinois; Assistant Professor, Northwestern Memorial Hospital, Chicago, Illinois
Coronary Heart Disease: Therapeutic Principles

SYLVIA K. FIELDS, ED.D., R.N.
Senior Research Associate, Center for Research in Medical Education and Health Care, Jefferson Medical College, Thomas Jefferson University, Philadelphia, Pennsylvania
The Female Patient

LINDA P. FRIED, M.D., M.P.H.
Associate Professor, Medicine and Epidemiology, The Johns Hopkins University School of Medicine, Baltimore, Maryland; Active Staff, The Johns Hopkins Hospital, Baltimore, Maryland
Smoking and Cardiovascular Disease

MARK E. HANDS, M.D., B.S., F.R.A.C.P.
Consultant Cardiologist; Sir Charles Gairdner Hospital and St. John of God Cardiology, Perth, Western Australia, Australia
Pregnancy with Preexisting Heart Disease

SUZANNE G. HAYNES, PH.D.
Chief, Health Education Section, National Cancer Institute, Bethesda, Maryland
Psychosocial and Environmental Correlates of Heart Disease

KAREN B. JAMES, M.D.
Staff, Department of Cardiology, Section of Heart Failure and Transplantation, The Cleveland Clinic, Cleveland, Ohio
Heart Disease Arising During Pregnancy

MARC KLAPHOLZ, M.D.
Assistant Professor, Columbia College of Physicians and Surgeons, New York, New York; Assistant Attending, Medicine, St. Lukes Hospital, New York, New York
Myocardial Function and Cardiomyopathy

ROBERT D. LANGER, M.D., M.P.H.
Assistant Professor of Community and Family Medicine, Division of Epidemiology, University of California, Medical Center, San Diego, California; Attending Staff, Pomerado Hospital, Poway, California
Stroke and Peripheral Vascular Diseases

JOHN C. LaROSA, M.D.
Dean for Research, The George Washington University Medical Center, Washington, D.C.; Director, Lipid Research Clinic, Professor of Medicine and Health Care Sciences, The George Washington University, Washington, D.C.
Lipoproteins and Lipid Disorders

ROGERIO A. LOBO, M.D.
Professor of Obstetrics and Gynecology and Chief, Division of Reproductive Endocrinology and Infertility, University of Southern California School of Medicine, Los Angeles, California; Chief, Division of Reproductive Endocrinology and Infertility, Los Angeles County/University of Southern California Medical Center, Los Angeles, California
Hormones, Hormone Replacement Therapy, and Heart Disease

JOANN E. MANSON, M.D., Dr.P.H.
Assistant Professor of Medicine, Harvard Medical School, Boston, Massachusetts; Associate Physician, Brigham and Women's Hospital, Boston, Massachusetts
Carbohydrate Metabolism, Obesity and Diabetes

MARY L. O'TOOLE, Ph.D.
Associate Professor and Director, Human Performance Laboratory, Department of Orthopaedic Surgery, University of Tennessee, Memphis, Tennessee
Exercise and Physical Activity

SUZANNE OPARIL, M.D.
Professor of Medicine and Associate Professor of Physiology and Biophysics, University of Alabama School of Medicine, Birmingham, Alabama; Director, Vascular Biology and Hypertension Program, Division of Cardiovascular Diseases, and Attending Cardiologist, University Hospital, Birmingham, Alabama
Hypertension

PAUL M. RIDKER, M.D., M.P.H.
Instructor, Harvard Medical School, Boston, Massachusetts; Associate Physician, Division of Cardiology, Brigham and Women's Hospital, Boston, Massachusetts
Carbohydrate Metabolism, Obesity, and Diabetes

JOHN D. RUTHERFORD, M.B.Ch.B., F.R.A.C.P., F.A.C.C.
Professor of Medicine, The University of Texas, Southwestern Medical Center at Dallas, Gail Griffiths Hill Chair in Cardiology, Dallas, Texas
Pregnancy with Preexisting Heart Disease

MARIE A. SAVARD, M.D.
Clinical Associate Professor of Medicine, University of Pennsylvania School of Medicine, Philadelphia, Pennsylvania; Clinical Attending Physician, Pennsylvania Hospital and Presbyterian Hospital, Philadelphia, Pennsylvania
The Female Patient

ANGELA SPELSBERG, M.D., M.Sc.
Doctoral Student in Epidemiology, Harvard School of Public Health, Boston, Massachusetts
Carbohydrate Metabolism, Obesity, and Diabetes

MARTIN ST. JOHN SUTTON, M.B.B.S., F.A.C.C.
Consultant Cardiologist, The Royal Brompton National Heart and Lung Hospital, London, England
Cardiovascular Physiology of Pregnancy

JANICE D. WAGNER, D.V.M., Ph.D.
Assistant Professor of Comparative Medicine, Bowman Gray School of Medicine, Winston-Salem, North Carolina
Clinical Implications of Animal Models of Gender Difference in Heart Disease

BABETTE B. WEKSLER, M.D.
Professor of Medicine, Division of Hematology-Oncology, Cornell University Medical College, New York, New York; Attending Physician, The New York Hospital, New York, New York
Hemostasis and Thrombosis

NANETTE K. WENGER, M.D.
Professor of Medicine (Cardiology), Emory University School of Medicine, Atlanta, Georgia; Director, Cardiac Clinics, Grady Memorial Hospital, Atlanta, Georgia
Coronary Heart Disease: Diagnostic Decision Making

J. KOUDY WILLIAMS, D.V.M.
Assistant Professor, Department of Comparative Medicine, Bowman Gray School of Medicine, Wake Forest University, Winston-Salem, North Carolina
Clinical Implications of Animal Models of Gender Difference in Heart Disease

Preface

Recognition of women's health issues has become a battle cry for concerned citizens, for the press, and even for Congress. Heart disease is one of the areas in which knowledge is felt to be lacking, and patient care is thought to be adversely affected by that ignorance. Increasingly, clinicians and scientists are recognizing that many forms of heart disease are affected by gender. This recognition often begins with an appreciation of the clinical differences between men and women that exist in many areas, including the noninvasive diagnosis of coronary artery disease and the importance of hormonal status in the epidemiology of coronary heart disease—the list is long and is growing. It is a major goal of this text to enumerate and examine such differences. However, I believe that such an examination is just a beginning, albeit a substantial one. It is much more important to emphasize, as this text tries to do, current knowledge about the female heart itself rather than considering it only in comparison to that of the male heart. By casting the net so broadly, I hope to provide a more useful reference in the care of women patients (what to *do* with those differences) and a better understanding of the cardiovascular physiology of women, which, ultimately, must be achieved before attempting to explain the differences.

The contributions of epidemiology continue to be a mainstay of any review of heart disease in women. Clinical investigation has been slow to respond to the clues that population studies have provided, and basic science investigation has been even slower. It is hoped that this text, by providing current state-of-the-art reviews integrating epidemiology and clinical and basic knowledge, will stimulate additional work at all levels. The multi-authored format allows each topic to be considered by recognized experts in that area. Many of the contributing authors found the researching and writing of their chapters a challenging task. Often there were no prior reviews, or even primary papers, that addressed the topic directly. Many of the authors also confessed to learning a great deal from their research, attesting both to the depth of their efforts and to the need for and uniqueness of this text. I hope that each reader will similarly find new insight in its pages.

The book is divided into three sections. It begins with a chapter exploring the special frame of reference of the female patient and the unique aspects of the female patient-physician relationship. The section on clinical cardiovascular disease includes two very practically oriented chapters on coronary heart disease and goes on to consider hypertension, cardiomyopathy, vascular disease, and stroke. Inclusion of detailed information on these diseases, in addition to coronary disease, represents a particular strength. The next section explores risk factors for coronary disease, with a separate chapter for each of seven categories. In these chapters, a special effort has been made to integrate data from population studies identifying the importance of each risk factor; more basic information is then included on the mechanisms by which each may contribute to coronary heart disease in women. The last section includes three chapters on heart disease in pregnancy, an area in which expertise is all too often lost between the obstetrician and the cardiologist.

I wish to thank each of the authors for the enthusiasm with which they undertook their tasks and for the diligence, scholarship, and expertise with which they completed it. Each has added substantially to this book.

PAMELA S. DOUGLAS

Contents

SECTION 1
Introduction 1

CHAPTER 1
The Female Patient 3
SYLVIA K. FIELDS, Ed.D., R.N.
MARIE A. SAVARD, M.D.
KENNETH R. EPSTEIN, M.D.

SECTION 2
Clinical Cardiovascular Disease 23

CHAPTER 2
Coronary Heart Disease: Diagnostic Decision-Making 25
NANETTE K. WENGER, M.D.

CHAPTER 3
Coronary Heart Disease: Therapeutic Principles 43
SUSAN B. EYSMANN, M.D.
PAMELA S. DOUGLAS, M.D.

CHAPTER 4
Hypertension 63
VERA BITTNER, M.D.
SUZANNE OPARIL, M.D.

CHAPTER 5

Myocardial Function and Cardiomyopathy 105
MARC KLAPHOLZ M.D.
PETER BUTTRICK, M.D.

CHAPTER 6

Valvular Heart Disease 117
RICHARD B. DEVEREUX, M.D.

CHAPTER 7

Stroke and Peripheral Vascular Diseases 137
ROBERT D. LANGER, M.D., M.P.H.
MICHAEL H. CRIQUI, M.D., M.P.H.

SECTION 3

Coronary Heart Disease: Risk Factors and Their Clinical Modification 151

CHAPTER 8

Hormones, Hormone Replacement Therapy, and Heart Disease 153
ROGERIO A. LOBO, M.D.

CHAPTER 9

Lipoproteins and Lipid Disorders 175
JOHN C. LaROSA, M.D.

CHAPTER 10

Carbohydrate Metabolism, Obesity, and Diabetes 191
ANGELA SPELSBERG, M.D., M.Sc.
PAUL M. RIDKER, M.D., M.P.H.
JOANN E. MANSON, M.D., Dr.P.H.

CHAPTER 11

Smoking and Cardiovascular Disease 217
LINDA P. FRIED, M.D., M.P.H.
DIANE M. BECKER, Sc.D.

CHAPTER 12

Hemostasis and Thrombosis 231
BABETTE B. WEKSLER, M.D.

CHAPTER 13

Exercise and Physical Activity 253
MARY L. O'TOOLE, Ph.D.

CHAPTER **14**

Psychosocial and Environmental Correlates of Heart Disease 269
SUZANNE G. HAYNES, Ph.D.
SUSAN M. CZAJKOWSKI, Ph.D.

CHAPTER **15**

Clinical Implications of Animal Models of Gender Difference in Heart Disease 283
THOMAS B. CLARKSON, D.V.M.
MICHAEL R. ADAMS, D.V.M.
J. KOUDY WILLIAMS, D.V.M.
JANICE D. WAGNER, D.V.M., Ph.D.

SECTION **4**

Pregnancy and the Heart 303

CHAPTER **16**

Cardiovascular Physiology of Pregnancy 305
PATRICIA LENA COLE, M.D., F.A.C.C.
MARTIN ST. JOHN SUTTON, M.B.B.S., F.A.C.C.

CHAPTER **17**

Pregnancy with Preexisting Heart Disease 329
JOHN D. RUTHERFORD, M.B.Ch.B., F.R.A.C.P., F.A.C.C.
MARK E. HANDS, M.B., B.S., F.R.A.C.P.

CHAPTER **18**

Heart Disease Arising During Pregnancy 337
KAREN B. JAMES, M.D.

INDEX 361

SECTION 1

Introduction

CHAPTER 1

The Female Patient

SYLVIA K. FIELDS, Ed.D., R.N.
MARIE A. SAVARD, M.D.
KENNETH R. EPSTEIN, M.D.

Certain health problems are unique to women or affect women disproportionately, such as breast cancer, rheumatoid arthritis, and osteoporosis. However, cardiovascular disease (CVD), primarily coronary heart disease (CHD), continues to be the leading cause of death for both women and men in the United States (1) (Fig. 1–1). Death rates for CHD have been declining since the 1950s (2), probably due to advances in medical and surgical treatments as well as to life style changes (3), but they have not declined for women as rapidly as for men (Fig. 1–2). The considerable emphasis placed on the occurrence of CHD in men has resulted in an inclination to minimize its incidence and severity in women (4). Although myocardial infarction (MI) kills many women, CHD has not been considered a disease of women, either by physicians or by women themselves.

Until recently, most epidemiologic studies examining morbidity and mortality from CHD have focused largely on men, and therefore the conclusions drawn cannot be universally applied to women (5, 6). As a result of this significant gender gap in the research, women are being given conflicting advice by the media and by their physicians. We still do not have a clear picture of the long-term benefits and risks of postmenopausal hormone replacement therapy (HRT), low-dose aspirin, and vitamins such as beta-carotene and vitamin E in relation to primary and secondary prevention of cardiovascular disease (7). Meanwhile, most women are more concerned with the immediate risk of breast, uterine, and ovarian cancer than they are with the possibility of heart disease, which many women of all ages accept as a natural component of the aging process.

Gender differences have been identified in the risk factors, clinical picture, and prognosis of CHD. Although women generally utilize health services more frequently than men, they have less access to significant diagnostic and

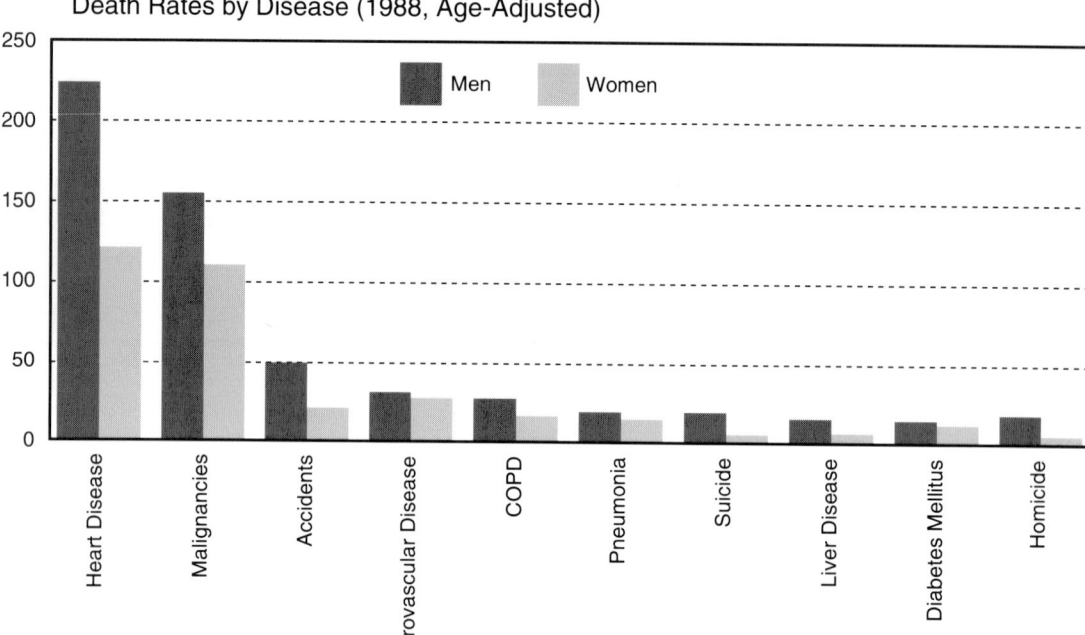

Figure 1–1. Death rates by disease (1988, age adjusted). (From United States Public Health Service, National Center for Health Statistics. *Vital Statistics of the United States, 1986.* Vol. II. *Mortality:* Part A. DHHS Pub. No. [PHS]89-1101. Washington, D.C., U.S. Government Printing Office, 1989.)

treatment modalities for cardiovascular disease (8). One reason may be that women and their physicians do not recognize the early signs of coronary artery disease, so that women are less likely to receive rigorous evaluation and invasive therapy when symptoms of CHD are present (9). The question of whether women receive differential care for acute MI compared with men has also been raised (10). At the same time, it is known that clinical trials of cardiovascular drugs have been conducted primarily in men, despite gender differences that may affect clinical decisions regarding drug therapy in women (11). Women may in fact rely too heavily on excessive medication or may be inappropriately treated with anxiolytics when other effective modalities are available (8).

For years women have been encouraged to have biannual Papanicolaou (Pap) smears, which ensure regular office visits beyond the childbearing years. More recently, the American Cancer Society has informed women through the media of their need for annual breast examinations, Pap smears, and periodic mammography. Unfortunately, this emphasis on regular gynecologic cancer screening, although critically important, has minimized the concern of both health care providers and patients about cardiovascular risk assessment and modification, as well as early diagnosis and treatment.

Many physicians have not fully developed their role as patient educator. Additionally, the physician-patient relationship is sometimes strained when the patient is a woman and the physician is a man (12). These factors may contribute to the poor adherence by women to medical recommendations for primary and secondary prevention of cardiovascular disease. Despite warnings, young women may still continue to smoke while taking birth control pills, and obesity, a significant CVD risk factor for women, is still a major problem for middle-aged and older women, especially black women (13). Women, who have been captive to "paternalistic" physician attitudes for years, are entitled not only to more information but also to the opportunity to be actively involved in their own care to enable them to make informed choices. (Although the objective of medicine is to reestablish the

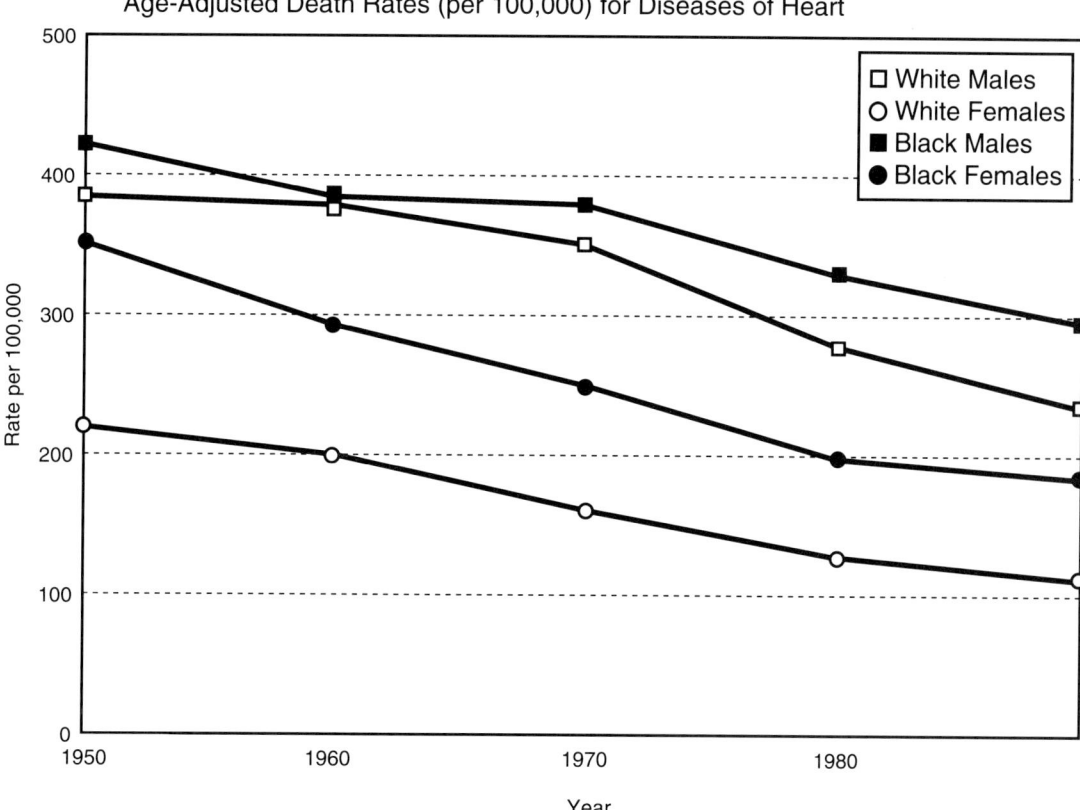

Figure 1–2. Age-adjusted death rates (per 100,000) for diseases of the heart. (From United States Public Health Service, National Center for Health Statistics. *Health, United States, 1988*. DHHS Pub. No. [PHS] 89-1232. Washington, D.C., U.S. Government Printing Office, 1989.)

patient's autonomy, paternalism refers to a medical decision intended to benefit the patient, yet made without the patient's full consent) (14).

Physicians, both generalists and cardiovascular specialists, have a monumental task ahead to help women of all ages understand that heart disease affects them as well as men and to ensure that women participate in primary and secondary prevention strategies as informed partners in clinical management decisions. Although this text thoroughly reviews the gender differences in pathophysiology, clinical presentation, risk factors, and treatment outcome for cardiovascular diseases, this chapter focuses on the unique medical risks, beliefs, and values each woman brings to the health care encounter. It explores how positive communication in the physician-patient relationship may influence clinical decision making, promote adherence to prevention and treatment programs, and ultimately improve the quality of life for women patients and their families.

GENDER DIFFERENCES IN MORBIDITY AND MORTALITY

Men and women have different patterns of morbidity and mortality. At every stage across the life span, women are biologically more advantaged and tend to live longer than men (15). Women's delayed onset of clinical coronary disease by 10 to 20 years may contribute to their longer life expectancy. However, of the 550,000 people who die each year of cardiovascular disease in the United States,

Table 1–1. CARDIOVASCULAR DISEASE IN THE U.S.: AN EPIDEMIOLOGIC OVERVIEW
(Death Rates [per 100,000] for Ischemic Heart Disease by Age, Race, and Sex: United States, 1986)

Age (yr)	Men		Women		Ratio[a]	
	White	*Black*	*White*	*Black*	*Men*	*Women*
35–44	35.8	56.1	7.1	17.6	1.6	2.5
45–54	154.3	183.5	35.5	80.4	1.2	2.3
55–64	450.1	457.0	147.8	252.3	1.0	1.7
65–74	1062.8	919.4	483.9	617.6	0.9	1.3
75–84	2472.7	1857.6	1503.0	1474.9	0.8	1.0
0–85+[b]	169.9	153.9	79.5	97.0	0.9	1.2

[a] Black-white.
[b] Age-adjusted by the direct method, standard: 1940 U.S. population.
National Center for Health Statistics. *Vital Statistics of the United States, 1986.* Vol. II. *Mortality.* Part A. DHHS Pub. No. (PHS) 89-1101. Washington, D.C., U.S. Public Health Service, 1989.

250,000 are women, and most die as a result of CHD (16). In white women aged 35 to 39 CHD is second only to breast cancer as a major cause of death. It is *the* major cause of death in black women aged 30 to 39. At all ages under 75, mortality for CHD is significantly higher for black women than for white women (17) (Table 1–1).

Although overall death rates for cardiovascular diseases have been declining over the past few decades, the extent to which this decline is due to improvements in medical care, including drug treatment and surgery, or to changes in life style continues to be debated. As much as 70% of the decline may be attributed to risk factor modification—i.e., control of cholesterol levels, cessation of cigarette smoking, and management of hypertension, especially in men (18). Death rates have not declined for women as rapidly as for men. Although some factors involved in this difference are clear, others still need to be confirmed.

There are many factors that are likely to affect health differently in women than in men. In addition to biologic factors, such as estrogen protection against atherosclerosis, there are psychologic, sociologic, economic, and environmental factors. Verbrugge has proposed five mutually exclusive reasons to account for sex differences in health (19):

1. Biological risks: the intrinsic differences between males and females based on their genes or hormones, which confer differential risks of morbidity.
2. Acquired risks: the risks of illness and injury encountered in work and leisure activities, lifestyle and health habits, psychological distress, and other aspects of a person's social milieu.
3. Psychosocial aspects of symptoms and care: how people perceive symptoms, assess their severity, and decide what to do to relieve or cure health problems, as well as their ability to take desired actions (illness behavior.)
4. Health-reporting behavior: how people talk about their symptoms to others, including interviewers.
5. Prior health care and caretakers: how therapeutic actions chosen by oneself or by a health professional influence the course of current diseases and the future onset of new diseases.

Of these five factors, two—biologic risks and, to a lesser degree, prior care—are considered by researchers to disfavor men with respect to health and longevity. Two others, psychosocial aspects and health-reporting behavior, are considered to improve women's morbidity experiences. Acquired risks are considered a mix: Some key life style behaviors such as smoking, alcohol consumption, and occupational hazards are more common in men, giving them higher long-term risks, but other life style behaviors, such as less strenuous recreational activity, obesity, emotional stresses, depression, and multiple role pressures, are thought to put women at higher risk.

Although past studies have explored these psychosocial and communication factors influencing health in women, many of the issues need to be reexamined in view of the social and economic changes that have taken place during the last few decades. Significant changes in women's social roles have occurred, which may affect cardiovascular as well as mental health. Fewer women today fill the single role of housewife. Many more women, including women with young children, are in the work force, in traditional (teaching, nursing) as well as formerly restricted occupations and professions such as medicine, business, and law

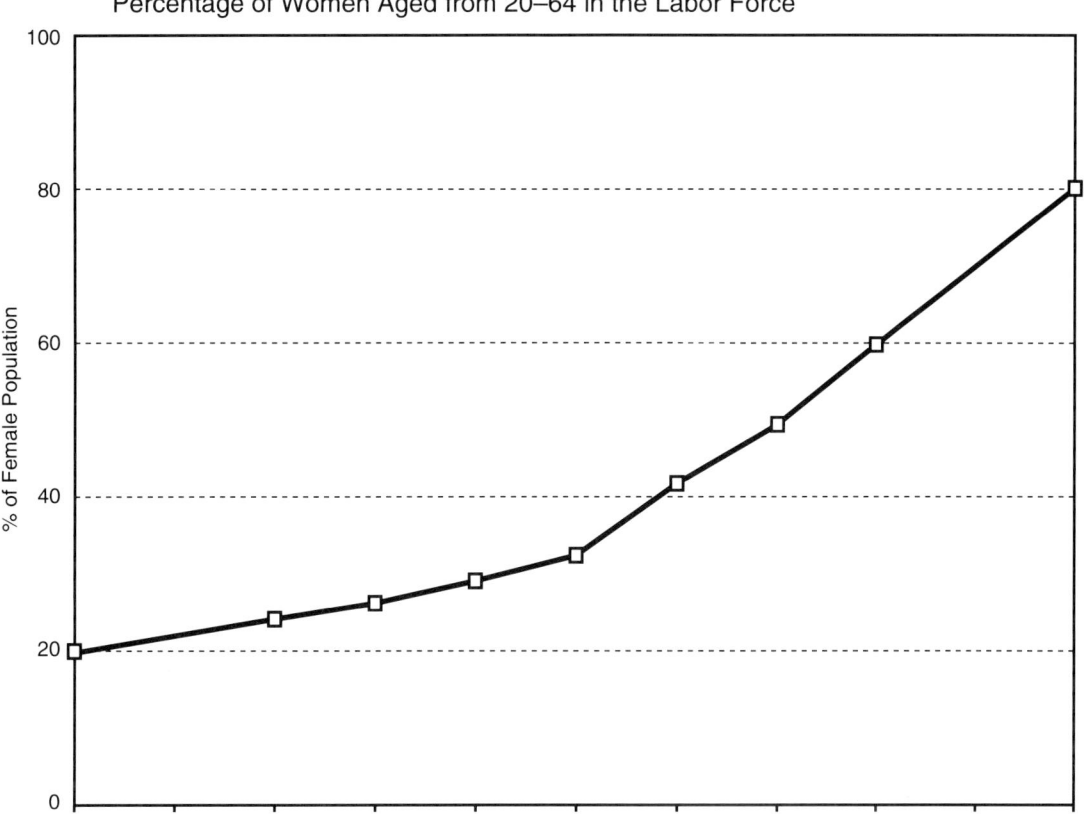

Figure 1-3. Percentage of women aged 20 to 64 in the labor force. Figures for the year 2000 are based on projections for women aged 25 to 64. (From Mathews, K. A. and Rodin, J. Women's changing work roles: Impact on health, family, and public policy. *Am Psychologist* 44:1391, 1989.)

(Fig. 1–3). Women may now be exposed to the same physical and emotional hazards of the work environment as men, but they are more often exposed to the pressures created by multiple roles and conflicting expectations. Studies in men have described the type A personality in ambitious workaholics as prone to MI, but generalizations to women cannot be made. However, increased substance abuse and work force participation by women have been implicated in shifting death rates due to cardiovascular disease (20). (New studies on stress as a risk factor for CHD in women are discussed in Chapter 14.)

Although many of the clinical features of CHD are similar in men and women, 30 years of observational data reported in the Framingham Study demonstrated significant gender differences (21). There are differences in the frequency and influence of certain risk factors, such as cholesterol levels, obesity, and cigarette smoking (see Chapters 9, 10, and 11). Men are more likely to be afflicted by acute illness, including sudden death. Women with clinically manifest coronary artery disease are usually older when they seek medical care, experience angina pectoris as the first symptom of their disease, and are more likely to have concomitant chronic diseases such as diabetes mellitus and arthritis. Because their disease is often more advanced when first acknowledged and treatment has been delayed, women experience more complications of the underlying pathology and have a poorer response to invasive therapy such as angioplasty and surgery (22). Women need a longer period for recuperation following MI or coronary artery bypass graft (CABG) surgery and tend to return to work less often than men (23). A recent sex-stratified analysis of functional disability of elderly long-term cardiac patients found that female survivors with angina were at greater

Table 1-2. MORBIDITY INDICATORS BY SEX AND SEX RATIOS IN THE UNITED STATES, 1987

Indicator	Females	Males	Sex Ratio (Female-male)
Restricted activity days			
Total days of disability (millions)	1,984	1,464	1.35
Days/person	16.1	12.7	1.28
Bed disability days			
Total days of disability (millions)	879	595	1.48
Days/person	7.1	5.2	1.36
Work loss days			
Total (millions)	304	299	1.02
Days/person	6.1	4.8	1.27
Hospital utilization rates			
Patients discharged per 1000 persons	159	116	1.37
Days of care per 1000 persons	968	860	1.20
Average stay (days)	6.1	6.9	0.88
Physician visits			
Total (millions)	765	523	1.46
Visits/person	6.2	4.5	1.38

From U.S. Bureau of the Census. *Statistical Analyses in the United States*, 1990. Washington, D.C., U.S. Government Printing Office, 1990.

risk for functional disability compared to men (24). Women are also less likely to engage in sexual activity following MI (25).

Some of the increased functional disability in women patients with CHD may be due to the fact that they are older and may be more socially isolated (26). The impact of social isolation on the quality of life for aging women, who usually outlive their male partners and often experience economic deprivation as a result, was recently described by Case and colleagues (27). The risk of a recurrent cardiac event (either a nonfatal reinfarction or cardiac death within 6 months following MI) was elevated for women living alone compared with men. Williams et al. provided evidence that the presence or absence of a spouse or confidant was the most important prognostic socioeconomic variable, independent of important medical prognostic factors, among medically treated patients with angiographically documented coronary disease (28). These findings have been supported by animal studies. Thomas Clarkson observed that social interactions favorably influenced high-density lipoprotein (HDL) cholesterol concentrations and the amount of atherosclerosis, whereas social isolation diminished the HDL and worsened atherosclerosis in female monkeys (29) (see Chapter 15).

Differences in Utilization of Health Care Services

Many gender-related differences exist in the use of health care services (30). Women constitute 52% of the population and account for about 70% of all health care interactions (31). Compared with men, women have more disability and access the health care system more often, even when controlling for pregnancy-related visits (32) (Table 1-2). Kessler and colleagues interviewed over 1600 health maintenance organization (HMO) patients to obtain data for their ongoing study of the relationship between personal and family characteristics and medical care utilization (33). Men made greater use of hospitals for their acute care, whereas women used more chronic disease custodial care services, both in institutions and in the home. There were also substantial sex differences in rates of office visits to physicians (33). Women are more likely than men to have a regular source of health care and a source of health information, according to the 1985 National Health Interview Survey (7). Eighty-three percent of women and 70% of men responded "yes" when asked, "Is there a particular clinic, health center, doctor's office, or other place that you go to if you are sick or need advice about your health?" (7).

Socioeconomic factors may hinder access to care with untoward effects for some groups of women, especially the elderly and minorities. When adjusted for age and the worse health status of the poor, persons below the poverty level have fewer physician visits (34). This is especially true of the elderly, among whom the poor have 25% fewer visits compared with persons above 200% of the poverty level. Likewise, adjusting for age and health status, blacks have fewer physician visits than whites (34). Among the elderly, blacks and the poor also are less likely to possess private insurance to supplement their Medicare health insurance coverage (35). Perhaps as a consequence of these disparities, blacks and those who live below the poverty level are less likely to receive preventive care services (36). These statistics are of particular concern in light of the fact that black women have one and a half times the death rate from heart disease as white women (37).

Bias in Clinical Decision Making

Although women utilize the health care system more frequently than men, recent studies indicate that they have less access than men to certain significant diagnostic and therapeutic interventions, especially those related to cardiovascular disease and organ transplantation (38). Ayanian and Epstein showed that in Massachusetts and Maryland women who were in the hospital for CHD were significantly less likely to undergo coronary angiography and revascularization, even among those men and women with confirmed MI (10). Tobin and colleagues noted an approximate 10:1 male-female ratio among patients referred for cardiac catheterization after an abnormal nuclear cardiac scan. Despite differences in reasons for referral for diagnostic testing, no sex differences were found in the use of antianginal drug treatment or in the distribution of types of angina (8). Women may not be receiving adequate attention to the signs and symptoms of cardiovascular disease and may be receiving too many medications when other options are available. Higher mortality rates for women than men following an initial heart attack and coronary bypass surgery support the premise that their disease is further advanced (39).

Women have long complained that physicians do not take them seriously and that their symptoms are interpreted as imaginary or "psychosomatic." In 1979, a research team investigated the way doctors responded to five medical complaints common in both men and women: chest pain, back pain, headache, dizziness, and fatigue. The investigators examined the extent of the work-up physicians ordered on patients with these complaints. The extent of the work-up is determined by the physician's assessment of the patient's complaint, how alarming the symptoms are, and how real the risk of serious disease appears. Investigators found that across the board "men received a more extensive work-up than women for all complaints studied." The researchers could not explain the difference on the medical facts alone and suggested that perhaps physicians did not take complaints as seriously when they came from women (40). In Tobin's study, even among patients with positive nuclear cardiac scans, women were much more often thought to have psychiatric or other noncardiac causes for their chest pain. Wolfe, Chairman of the AMA Women in Media Project, believes that since women come to see physicians more regularly, their complaints tend to be diluted: "When a man comes in the doctor feels there's really something going on or he wouldn't have come in" (41).

Despite differences in the way CVD may be manifest in women and men, which may affect the diagnostic and treatment indications in women, the question of possible gender bias in clinical decision making has challenged the medical profession. In a provocative editorial in the *New England Journal of Medicine* Healy stated, "being different from men has meant being second-class and less than equal for most of recorded time and throughout most of the world . . . . it is not surprising that women have all too often been treated less than equally in social relations, political endeavors, business, education, research, and health care" (42). Such a situation must negatively affect the care given and does a great disservice to female patients. In recognition of such bias, the Council on Ethical and Judicial Affairs of the AMA released a statement that "although various social, economic, and/or cultural factors may stimulate gender disparities in the provision of health care, the medical community cannot tolerate any discrepancy in the provision of care that is not based on appropriate biological or medical indications" (43).

Controversies Amid a Gender Gap in Medical Research

Despite the vast literature on the diagnosis and management of cardiovascular disease, a significant gender gap exists in the research. Many of the investigations have been conducted primarily with male subjects, and findings may not always apply to women (5). For example, clinical decisions about the selection and dose of drugs given to women with cardiovascular disease are often based on studies that were conducted primarily or exclusively on middle-aged men. Hormonal status, older age, and the lesser body mass of women, as well as other factors, may be significant contributors to the gender variability in concentration levels, effectiveness, side effects, and toxicity of many drugs (11).

As clinicians, researchers, and policymakers question whether CVD prevention efforts that were evaluated predominantly in men are generalizable to women, the broad spectrum of CVD in women is receiving increasing attention. For example, many recent studies (44, 45) suggest that estrogen use has a protective effect that appears to inhibit the development of atherosclerotic coronary lesions. However, no comprehensive randomized trial has yet been conducted, and women are receiving conflicting information. Some clinicians are recommending hormone replacement therapy for postmenopausal women to relieve menopausal symptoms as well as to prevent osteoporosis and cardiovascular disease for those at risk (46, 47). Others question this recommendation, with the result that many women are hesitant to risk possible long-term side effects (48).

Low-dose aspirin is another strategy that has been inadequately studied in women. Manson and colleagues, following studies and subsequent recommendations for aspirin therapy to prevent heart attack and stroke in men, noted a statistically significant reduction in the risk of a first myocardial infarction among women who took low-dose aspirin (one to six tablets per week) (49). However in one study a trend toward an increased risk of hemorrhagic stroke was present among women who reported taking larger doses. Aspirin now joins estrogen replacement therapy as a promising but incompletely evaluated primary and secondary prevention therapy in women (see Chapters 3 and 12).

Attempts to redress inattention to women as subjects of medical research and to document the relationship between risk factors, preventive therapies, and the major chronic conditions experienced by women are being initiated. The federal government is funding the largest community-based clinical intervention and prevention trial ever conducted, the Women's Health Initiative (WHI), a $500 million, 10-year study involving five of the National Institutes of Health. Diet, dietary supplements, and hormone therapy as prevention for cardiovascular disease, cancer, and osteoporosis will be examined in as many as 140,000 postmenopausal women. There has been criticism of the initiative from both men and women due to the complexity of the study, the difficulties in adhering to the severe fat-restricted diet required, and the possible side effects of the hormone replacement (50). However, some important issues related to the recruitment and retention of women in clinical trials are being addressed in this study, such as babysitting, transportation, and the participation of minorities and the elderly. The Women's Health Initiative will allow observational follow-up of a large cohort of women to better understand disease risk factors in this population. Without such controlled studies of these issues and universal guidelines for recommendations, women and their health providers are denied the opportunity to make informed decisions regarding their unique needs.

GENDER DIFFERENCES IN THE PERCEPTION OF HEALTH AND CARDIOVASCULAR DISEASE

Sex variances in morbidity and the use of medical care are at least in part a result of male and female differences in the way symptoms are perceived, evaluated, and acted upon. These differences are related to the way in which men and women come to define themselves as ill and are thought to occur as a result of childhood socialization as well as adult role expectations and obligations. Personality, attitudinal factors, and belief systems all contribute to the process. Three potential factors influence women's interest in health:

- Biologic events that focus attention on bodily changes and health matters
- Gender-related socialization, which may heighten a sense of vulnerability to illness
- Gender-specific role responsibilities.

Women place a greater value on health than men do, and, especially when they have children, they are generally more interested in health matters because they have greater responsibility for the family's health. The importance placed by women on wellness influences their symptom perception, approach to preventive strategies, and response to illness. The social acceptability of admitting illness, discussing symptoms, and seeking help also seems to differ for men and women. Men are socialized to be stoic and self-reliant, whereas women learn that it is acceptable to be dependent and seek help. Women tend to be more open and expressive than men in reporting their illnesses and in fact may express their illnesses more frequently (51). Because of menstruation, childbirth, lactation, and menopause, women learn to attend to bodily cues and changes. It has been suggested that some women may simply recognize and interpret changes and cues as symptoms more readily than men, therefore presenting for medical evaluation more often. Studies suggest that simply being more interested and concerned about health contributes to women's higher utilization rates of medical services for mild morbidities as well as those for which there is more discretion in defining illness and the need for care (52).

The Health-Belief Model

One of the most frequently cited social-psychological approaches designed to explain why healthy people take action to prevent illness is the Health Belief Model (53) (Fig. 1–4). This model is helpful in understanding why women may or may not choose to participate in cardiovascular health promotion and disease prevention recommendations. In the model human behavior is seen as being dependent upon two primary variables:

1. The value placed by a person upon a particular outcome.

2. The person's belief that a given action will result in that outcome.

According to this model the preventive action taken by an individual to avoid disease X is due to that particular individual's perception that he or she is personally susceptible to X and that the occurrence of the disease would have at least some severe personal implications. The assumption is that by taking a particular action, susceptibility will be reduced, or if the disease occurred, severity would be reduced. Although an individual may perceive that a given action may be effective in reducing the threat of disease, that action may not be taken if it is further defined as too expensive, too unpleasant or painful, too inconvenient, or perhaps too traumatic. Thus, the individual's subjective assessment of the health situation becomes a critical variable in the utilization of health services and may be more important than an objective medical diagnosis. Several studies show that there is no (sometimes even a negative) correlation between medical estimates of health and patient compliance (54). Common sense approaches do not necessarily match clinical approaches, and common sense often determines whether or not health services are sought (55). For women, it is clearly common sense to beware the threat of cancer, especially cancer of the reproductive system, which they believe has devastating effects, whereas they are less concerned about cardiovascular disease, which seems more remote and inevitable.

Women's Focus on Reproductive Health

Although women commonly use medical services more than men, they focus primarily on reproductive organ concerns rather than general health issues. Many women are more fearful of breast, ovarian, and uterine cancer than of cardiovascular disease, which is perceived to affect only the aged. Whereas one in nine women may develop breast cancer at any time during adult life, one in three women will eventually die from heart disease. The threat of breast cancer, however, looms over all women, and they feel vulnerable and power-

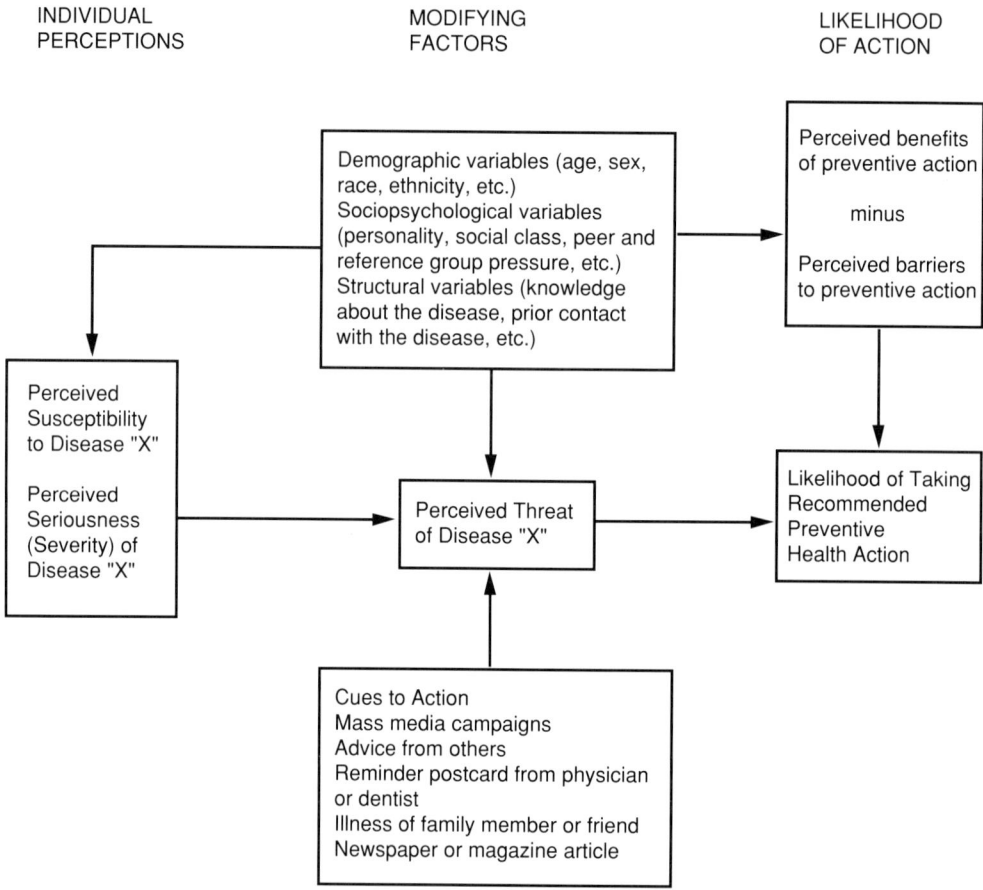

Figure 1–4. The health belief model and personal health behavior. (Modified from Becker M. H. [Ed.], *The Health Belief Model and Personal Health Behavior.* San Francisco, Society for Public Health Education, Inc., 1974.)

less to prevent it. All women are at risk for breast cancer, and regular screening cannot always prevent the disease or even detect it early enough in many instances. Not only is it an immediate life or death issue, it is one that significantly affects the feminine body image and sexuality and emphasises the vulnerability of women. Additionally, many women have the misconception that if they receive their annual Pap test and breast examination their general health is assured. Although early screening and treatment of risk factors for heart disease can clearly reduce the risks of atherosclerosis, the value of such screening in women is less widely appreciated and practiced.

The experience of chest pain has a different meaning for women than men and is contrary to previous explanations of why women seek health care more frequently than men. Angina in both young and elderly women may often escape both the patient's and the clinician's attention. Although the discovery of a breast lump or an abnormal mammogram is almost always viewed as a deviance, the development of angina, especially that with an atypical presentation, may not be interpreted as such. In a population in which a symptom is believed to be ubiquitous, the condition may be perceived as a normal state. This does not mean it is considered "good" but rather that it is thought to be natural and inevitable and thus to be ignored. The symptom therefore is simply not considered a deviation (56). Such is the case with angina in women, which may be perceived as natural by some elderly women. They may interpret the onset of exertional angina as normal fatigue and limit their physical activity as a result without complaint or request for an investigation. Some older women may fear being labeled a nuisance, a hypochondriac, or a "crabby old woman" and therefore may underreport their symptoms (57). The physician must therefore ask very clear and specific questions to elicit this history. The symptom of angina is often described not as a pain but just a discomfort that is limiting. Once the possibility of angina is considered, the patient may be unduly frightened by the immediate ordering of extensive tests without full explanation. When a patient does not knowingly present with angina, but it is suggested during the routine history, it is important that the physician communicate his or her concerns to the patient without triggering undue fear. On the other hand, if a patient presents with symptoms consistent with angina as a chief complaint, it is often easier to approach the work-up without misunderstanding.

Cardiovascular disease is often perceived as the natural way to end life in women's health belief system. "She died peacefully in her sleep" is a very acceptable explanation for the end of life at age 85 or 90. Despite the persistent pain of angina and the increasing number of drugs required for relief, the years of lessened energy and restricted activity, cancer is still perceived as a much greater threat. Preventive strategies for heart disease do not take precedence in the belief system of most women. Fear of a debilitating stroke may concern some older women, especially those who have cared for previously affected family members, but still the threat of cancer is perceived to be greater.

GENDER AND PATIENT-PHYSICIAN RELATIONSHIPS

Physicians' Attitudes Toward Women

There are many factors affecting the physician-patient relationship, including factors within the physician, the patient, and the health care system. For women patients there are special issues. Since the late nineteenth century, physicians have been held in high esteem by their patients. The physician's role was generally characterized as active and the patient's role dependent and passive—as a helping person and a person needing help. Women, as childbearers and childrearers who saw physicians far more frequently than men, accepted this paternalistic attitude. Until the social revolution of the 1960s and 1970s and the resulting women's health movement, this physician-patient relationship was not questioned (58).

Very little research has been conducted on the relationship between gender and doctor-patient relationships. A few studies suggest that physicians' interactions with patients are influenced by the patient's sex, ethnicity, social class, and nature of their complaints (59). Ehrenreich and other feminist writers infer that historical male dominance, not the sick role itself, promoted the dependence of women who sought medical help and the control of doctors over them (60). Physicians are accused of absorbing society's attitudes that demean women, reinforcing the idea that they are less competent (12). The conception that women are more emotionally unstable and volatile than men, are more likely to somaticize emotional upsets as physical problems, and are thus more inclined to have a higher prevalence of psychosomatic illness than men has persisted for many years. The assumption of a psychosomatic basis for women's complaints may be manifest by the prescription of psychoactive medications (antidepressants and tranquilizers), 70% of which are prescribed for women (61). Most of these drugs are prescribed by primary care physicians, not psychiatrists. The question of how many women seeking medical assistance today are provided with unnecessary pharmacologic therapy is not known. The handling of atypical chest pain associated with mitral valve prolapse is a case in point. Women with this condition need information and reassurance, not a prescription for antianxiety agents (see Chapter 6).

In approaching a physician for help, a woman brings not only a physical problem but also a social context, including relationships at work, in the family, and the wider community. Physical problems are inseparable from the wider social context. Women expect more than a physical diagnosis and drug treatment from their doctors. Often, however, the physician does not deal appropriately with their social concerns, specifically work-related problems, economic stress and insecurity, disturbed family life, demands of gender roles, sexuality, and anxiety about aging. Substance abuse, other self-destructive behaviors, and emotional instability, all of which are symptoms of underlying social concerns, are often dulled by medication and reassurances about the therapeutic benefits of behavioral change (62).

Patterns of Communication

The quality of communication between women and their physicians, who are predominantly male, has been widely criticized, and increasingly assertive female consumers of health care have pressed for change. As health promotion and disease prevention become more important components of health care in this country, the need for effective communication in educating patients about risk factors and influencing appropriate preventive behavior is increased.

Researchers have observed differences in communication patterns when the patient is a woman and the physician a man. Some studies have shown that female physicians interrupt their patients less often than male physicians, provide more verbalizations of empathy, and provide clearer explanations in response to patients' concerns (63). Wallen and colleagues analyzed 336 tape-recorded interactions between a stratified random sample of physicians and a sample of their patients and found that the sex of the patient affected the amount of information they received from male doctors (64). Female patients received the same number of spontaneous explanations as male patients, but although women asked more questions and in turn received more explanations, they were more often at a lower level of technicality.

For some patients there may be a therapeutic advantage to having a female physician. In 75 nonclinical studies of dyadic communication reviewed by Hall in 1978, more studies showed that female gender in the physician was an advantage in decoding nonverbal clues (65). In a family practice setting West (66) studied the distribution of interruptions in the medical interview. She found that patients interrupted female doctors as much as or more than the doctors interrupted them. Male doctors, however, interrupted their patients far more than they were interrupted by them (66).

Women and men will most likely select and continue with the practitioner who is sensitive to their special needs. As a result, many women are already selecting women obstetrician-gynecologists, nurse-midwives, family physicians, or nurse practitioners as their primary health provider and are seeking out female specialists who they believe will be more supportive. As more women enter the medical profession, the opportunity to select physicians by gender is increasing. However, the expectation that the caring behaviors of the profession will improve with the availability of more female physicians is speculative. It is difficult to prove, and there are still few empirical descriptions of the supposed differences in care (67). We do know that women have tended to choose specialties with high patient contact, such as pediatrics, obstetrics-gynecology, family practice, general internal medicine, and psychiatry. They also score higher on clinical ratings where the use of interpersonal and psychosocial factors are more evident (68, 69).

Patterns of physician-patient relationships have been changing as the physician's role has expanded from that of clinician to that of educator and manager as well (Table 1–3). Increasingly, physicians are entering into a partnership with their patients, a situation in which both parties receive more satisfaction than in the more traditional paternalistic approach. Ideally, each partner contributes to the relationship: the physician contributes knowledge about health and health care, and the patient contributes information about her own body and health history. Both partners can achieve their common goals when the relationship is based on mutual respect and nurtured through strong communication. The physician, however, must be both self-aware and attuned to the communications process (70).

Physicians and patients, regardless of gender, can modify their communication in simple ways. Waitzken recommends that physicians forego the traditional structured history format taught in medical school and let patients tell their stories with many fewer interruptions, cut-offs, and requests to return to the technical (62): "Patients should have the chance to tell their story in an open-ended way." Waitzken also recommends that patients be encouraged to take a more active role in questioning, challenging, and directing the flow of conversation. "Physicians should provide full explanations to patients, with information given in comprehensible terms without jargon, educating and supporting patients as they try to become more assertive consumers of health care." Unfortunately, current practice pressures point in the opposite direction. For example, standards of productivity (perhaps more prevalent in HMOs and prepaid group

Table 1–3. PHYSICIAN ROLES

Physician Factors	Clinician	Patient Educator	Resource Manager
Knowledge	• Knows biophysical and psychosocial factors in disease development • Knows associated risk factors • Knows levels of prevention for stages of disease • Knows appropriate diagnostic and therapeutic procedures	• Knows patient's cultural values and health belief system • Knows level of patient understanding of illness, the rationale for the management plan, expected outcomes, and potential economic and social problems • Knows effective methods to modify behavior and enhance compliance	• Knows economic, legal, and ethical ramifications of health behaviors and medical intervention • Knows efficient methods to coordinate care among disciplines • Knows available resources for patient • Knows methods for performing cost-benefit and cost-effective analysis
Skills	• Collects relevant history data • Performs manual skills appropriate to discipline • Interprets laboratory results appropriately • Makes early and accurate diagnosis • Recognizes risk factors in patient • Develops up-to-date therapeutic and rehabilitation plans • Monitors progress appropriately	• Applies principles of learning and reinforcement • Teaches effectively to ensure that patient and family understand rationale for management plan, expected outcomes, and potential problems • Encourages compliance with therapeutic plan	• Obtains essential data for decision analysis • Communicates effectively with other members of health care team • Uses human and other resources appropriately • Refers efficiently for consultation, diagnostic tests, procedures, and therapeutic intervention
Personal Qualities	• Approaches patient with sensitivity and compassion • Appreciates patient's uniqueness and lifestyle • Adheres to ethical and professional standards	• Considers individual differences in learning styles • Patiently reinforces learning for patient and family	• Facilitates team approach to develop and implement preventive and therapeutic plan • Involves patient and family in coordinated decisions

From Gonnella JS, Hojat M, Erdmann JB, Veloski JJ. What have we learned, and where do we go from here? In Gonnella JS, Hojat M, Erdmann JB, Veloski JJ (Eds), *Assessment Measures in Medical School, Residency, and Practice: The Connections. Acad Med* 68 (Suppl 2):79–87, 1993.

practices), often put constraints on extensive doctor-patient communication.

The Patient's Perspective

The physician-patient relationship can be enriched by inviting the patient's perspective (Table 1–4). Delbanco believes that improved health care will result from focusing on the needs and concerns of patients as they themselves define them (71). He suggests incorporating a Patient Review that addresses the preferences, values, and needs of each individual patient next to the organic review of systems in the traditional history format. Use of the Patient Review can encourage physicians to address the nontechnical aspects of care in a systematic way. (It is here that individual management decisions such as chronic medical therapy versus surgery for coronary disease could be discussed.) Comments by patients bring each dimension of the Patient Review into focus and point to its clinical importance during the assessment process as well as in evaluation of patient care outcomes.

"I feel very strongly that the patient has to participate. I mean, I have learned this. This is not a theoretical thing. I have learned that I have to be as involved in my care as the doctors."

"I ask for information when I don't have it immediately. I mean, if they are going to go poking inside my body, I want to know what they expect to find; and then if they find it, what they are going to do about it. I need information. That is my basic food."

"If they had told me what I could do, that would have been helpful. I've felt so vulnerable that I think I've been a little timid to do things. There wasn't much I could do, but I wasn't told what I

Table 1–4. ELEMENTS OF THE PATIENT'S REVIEW

Dimension of Care	Focus of Patient's Review
Respect for patient's values preferences, and expressed needs	What are the patient's short-term goals? What level of involvement does the patient want in decision making? What does she need, want, or expect from the health care system? What are her feelings about an advance directive?
Coordination and integration of care	Is care delivered by the range of providers effectively coordinated? Does the patient get consistent information from different clinicians?
Communication and education	Does the patient have the information she wants about her clinical status, diagnostic tests, and treatment options? Do the patient and her family know what they need to know to manage on their own to the extent that they are able to do so?
Physical comfort	Is pain alleviated as much as possible? Does the patient have the help she needs with bathing, eating, household chores, or other activities of daily living? Have remediable deficits in functional status been adequately addressed?
Emotional support and alleviation of fears and anxieties	Is the patient worried about his or her illness or its effect on the ability to care for one's self or one's dependents? What are the principal stresses in the patient's life? Is she worried about paying medical bills or about lost income due to illness? Does the patient have access to appropriate support networks to help with these worries?
Involvement of family and friends	Are family and friends appropriately included in planning and providing care? Do they have the support they need?
Continuity and transition	Do the patient and family understand medications to take, treatment regimens to follow, activities to pursue or to avoid, and danger signals to look out for? Are there clear plans for continuing care and treatment?

From Delbanco TL. Enriching the doctor-patient relationship by inviting the patient's perspective. *Ann Intern Med* 116:415, 1992, with permission.

could do, and it might have been encouraging" (71).

Although each professional functions in accordance with his or her own unique characteristics and patterns of behavior, effective communication channels may be fostered with the woman patient when certain general guidelines appropriate to all patient-physician interactions are considered. Only a few suggestions have been cited here, and readers are referred to several excellent texts on interviewing in the references at the end of this chapter.

CHANGING VIEW OF HEALTH AND DISEASE

Emphasis on Health Promotion and Disease Prevention

All medicine is changing. Although some of this change has been the result of the extension of medical knowledge and the perfection of techniques, much of it reflects increasing societal and individual health care expectations. Evidence from major clinical trials indicates that interventions to control risk factors, such as exercise, diet, and smoking cessation, have contributed to the reduction in risk and the resulting reduction in cardiovascular morbidity and mortality (3).

The very change in terminology from medical care to health care indicates a basic change in the concept of the role of the physician. Preventive care in addition to acute crisis care has become the objective. Today both men and women of all ages and all socioeconomic levels are more aware about health issues, more sophisticated in their questions, and more demanding of their caregivers, although men still may be underutilizing the system, and minorities and the poor have less access to preventive education and therapy. For the majority of Americans health promotion and disease prevention, especially against cardiovascular disease and cancer, are now prominent social concerns. Yet, although preventive services are regarded as fundamentally good health care, studies of physicians' preventive behavior have revealed that they are generally

Table 1–5. LEVELS OF PREVENTION IN CARDIOVASCULAR DISEASE

Primary Prevention	Secondary Prevention	Tertiary Prevention
Prepathogenesis	Period of pathogenesis	Period of pathogenesis
Health promotion Exercise Smoking cessation High-fiber, low-fat diet Weight control Diabetic control	*Early diagnosis* Stress testing Cholesterol screening	*Rehabilitation* Post-MI lifestyle changes (e.g., exercise, diet, smoking cessation) Medical therapy Aspirin therapy Revascularization
Specific protection Hormone replacement therapy Aspirin therapy	*Prompt treatment* *Disability limitation* Angioplasty CABG	

Adapted from Leavell HR, Clark EC (Eds), *Preventive Medicine for the Doctor in His Community,* 3rd ed. Toronto, McGraw Hill, 1965.

difficult to integrate into medical practice (72). Among practicing physicians treating CVD, preventive cardiology was identified regularly as one of the top ten self-expressed educational needs (73). Meanwhile, the medical profession has much to offer society at all levels of prevention of cardiovascular disease (Table 1–5).

Adherence to Preventive Regimens

In general, it is estimated that "patients may not follow short-term drug regimens anywhere from 15 to 90 percent of the time and only do so half the time for chronic conditions" (74). Among women who are prescribed hormone replacement therapy, 20–30% may never even get their prescription filled, in part because they are not convinced of the benefits and safety of the therapy (75). So, although time, effort, and expense are expended in the study of the effect of medications and other treatments for CHD in women, more attention needs to be devoted to whether or not women are willing and able to adhere to preventive and treatment regimens as recommended. The long-term regimens required to combat a chronic ailment and the particular problems of the populations with the highest risk of coronary disease combine to inhibit compliance.

It is particularly difficult to adhere to recommendations for life style changes. This is especially true in the absence of symptoms and when the benefit may be delayed. Women have not stopped smoking as readily as men despite known adverse health consequences, most likely because of a combination of factors, including fear of the rebound weight gain and more extreme addiction. In addition, recommendations for increased exercise have not been accepted by women as readily as by men, probably because sports have not been emphasized as much for them in earlier years.

Women with the highest risk of CHD are those who may find adherence to any regimen difficult (Table 1–6). Older women, black women (who are among the poorest members of our society), and women with stressful lives due to multiple roles are the least likely to have the social support, the family support, or the time and energy required to make even modest changes in their life styles. Initiating a regular exercise program may be difficult: A younger woman with children, home, and work duties may not have the time for exercise, and an elderly woman may feel too vulnerable to travel to an organized group or even to take a walk in her own neighborhood. In addition, cooking healthy foods may become a burden to a woman who also cooks for family members with no desire to follow a healthy diet. Finding the money for expensive prescriptions may not be a priority for a woman head-of-household who lacks visible symptoms of a major disease and is still able to function well.

Beyond life style and economic considerations, women, who are generally regarded as more intuitive than men, may be more perceptive of the attitudes of a physician who harbors some of society's prejudices toward women, blacks, and older people. As Zola states, "In reference to noncompliance, I am contending

Table 1–6. BARRIERS TO WOMEN'S ADHERENCE

Social	No support system or stable family situation
	Multiple roles (caregiver, worker, homemaker) resulting in lack of desire to make changes in life style (diet, exercise, etc.)
	Society's view of women (especially older women) as dependent and powerless may be internalized
	Fear of leaving home to travel to pharmacy or physician
Physical	Sensory loss, inability to remember, read, or hear directions; inability to keep schedule
	May feel well enough to function effectively
	May not have the stamina to shop for or cook healthful (nonconvenience) foods
Economic	May have little or no insurance coverage
	May lack resources to pay for expensive drug treatment
Psychological	Inability of physician to understand value system of patient
	Need for patient to be functional rather than cured
	Patient or family or friends may have received poor advice from physician
	More likely to pick up negative cues from physician (annoyance, lack of respect)
	Unsure of benefits of treatment
	Depression

that part of what patients are responding to when they do not cooperate is not the medical treatment but how they are treated, not how they regard their required medical regimen but how they themselves are regarded" (76).

Although the physician cannot address the many barriers to adherence for any given patient, there are strategies that can be used to encourage participation. For example, many women who are at risk for CHD, especially those with elevated low-density lipoprotein (LDL) cholesterol levels, have obesity as an accompanying problem. Other nutritional issues may be present including osteoporosis or gastrointestinal problems. In such circumstances, a trained nutritionist may be better prepared than a physician to provide time-consuming specific dietary education, guidance, and support. Ideally, a team approach in professional practice would include a full nutritional assessment and a therapeutic plan by a qualified nutritionist for each patient.

Of course, the physician's relationship with the patient certainly can have a powerful effect on the patient's adherence to primary and secondary preventive methods. As discussed in the section on the health belief model, a person's willingness to follow preventive recommendations is based on that individual's perception that the outcome to be prevented is one that she wants to avoid and that the recommended action really will help prevent the outcome. Therefore, the role of the physician in educating the patient about the importance of preventing the disease and the effectiveness of the recommended action is essential.

The first step in an effective education process is particularly important: The physician must identify the patient's knowledge, beliefs, and attitudes. Her social and cultural norms also must be understood. The patient then must be involved in selecting a plan of action that she is motivated to adhere to, thereby increasing her sense of efficacy and reinforcing the partnership between the patient and her physician. Effectively educating the patient also involves exploring the potential obstacles and ensuring that she is "buying into" the plan, because it is the patient's perception of a disease and the importance of prevention and therapy that correlates with compliance. However, because compliance is a multidimensional issue, it is also important to look beyond specific encounters to the political, economic, and social influences on a patient's decision to comply with preventive recommendations (77, 78). More studies that focus on the patient's experience and on the need for autonomy, control, and self-management are needed (79).

IMPLICATIONS FOR THE FUTURE

Although the threat of breast, ovarian, and uterine cancer is foremost in the minds of most women across the life cycle, many women today are better informed about health and disease and are demanding an emphasis on health promotion and disease prevention, including cardiovascular risk reduction. They need timely health information, supportive health professionals, preventive service, and appropriate technology. By attempting to learn what risks are significant and what diagnostic and treatment regimens are useful both for groups and for the individual woman patient, physicians have the opportunity to provide informed leadership and respond meaningfully to women's demands. This can only be accomplished through major clinical trials involving women and interpreting current studies in light of what is already known about women's special circumstances and concerns. Cardiovascular disease prevention in women poses a special challenge. Although screening for breast cancer with a physical examination and mammography gives immediate reassurance, the detection of risk factors for heart disease and their subsequent management can be easily ignored; for example, women have not reversed their smoking habits as quickly as men despite known adverse health consequences.

Women and their physicians need to form a partnership. With more medical research combined with increased participation on the part of women and their physicians who appreciate their special roles, responsibilities, interests, and values, the gap between knowledge and action can be bridged.

Acknowledgments

The authors wish to express their appreciation to Michelle Bolles, American Heart Association, and Diane Pohl, Jefferson Medical College, for their editorial assistance with this chapter.

References

1. U.S. Bureau of the Census. *Statistical Abstracts of the United States: 1990* (110th ed.). Washington, D.C., U.S. Bureau of the Census, 1990.
2. National Center for Health Statistics. Advance report of final mortality statistics, 1986. *Monthly Vital Statistics Report 37* (Suppl. 6).1–56, 1988.
3. Goldman L, Cook EF. The decline in ischemic heart disease mortality rates: An analysis of the comparative effects of medical interventions and changes in life style. *Ann Intern Med* 825:101–106, 1984.
4. Ibrahim MA. The changing health state of women. *Am J Public Hlth* 70:120–121, 1980.
5. Douglas P. Gender, cardiology and optimal medical care. *Circulation* 74:917–919, 1986.
6. Cotton P. Is there still too much extrapolation from data on middle-aged white men? *JAMA* 263:1049–1050, 1990.
7. U.S. Public Health Service. *Women's Health: Report of the Public Health Service Task Force on Women's Health Issues.* Washington, D.C., U.S. Department of Health and Human Services, 1985.
8. Tobin NJ, Wassertheir-Smoller S, Wexler JP, et al. Sex bias in considering coronary bypass surgery. *Ann Intern Med* 107:19–25, 1987.
9. Steingart RM, Packer M, Hamm P, et al. Sex differences in the management of coronary artery disease. *N Engl J Med* 325:226–230, 1991.
10. Ayanian JZ, Epstein AM. Differences in the use of procedures between women and men hospitalized for coronary heart disease. *N Engl J Med* 325:221–230, 1991.
11. Wenger N. Cardiovascular drugs: The urgent need for studies in women. *J Am Med Wom Assoc* 46:117–120, 1991.
12. Todd AD. *Intimate Adversaries: Cultural Conflict Between Doctors and Women Patients.* Philadelphia, University of Pennsylvania Press, 1989.
13. Kumanyika S, Adams-Campbell LL. Obesity, diet, and psychosocial factors contributing to cardiovascular disease in blacks. *Cardiovasc Clin* 21:47–73, 1991.
14. Pelligrino ED, Thomasma DC. *For the Patient's Good.* New York, Oxford University Press, 1988.
15. Strickland BR. Sex-related differences in health and illness. *Psychol Women Q* 12:381–399, 1988.
16. Eaker ED, Packard B, Wenger NK, et al. *Coronary Heart Disease in Women.* New York, Le Jaq Publishing, 1987.
17. Gillum R. Cardiovascular disease in the United States: An epidemiologic overview. *Cardiovasc Clin* 21:3–16, 1991.
18. Goldman L, Cook EF. The decline in ischemic heart disease mortality rates: An analysis of the comparative effects of medical interventions and changes in life style. *Ann Intern Med* 101:825, 1984.
19. Verbrugge LM. The twain meet: Empirical explanations of sex differences in health and mortality. *J Health Soc Behav* 30:282–304, 1989.
20. Rodin J, Ickovics JR. Women's health: Review and research agenda as we approach the 21st century. *Am Psychol* 45:1018–1034, 1990.
21. Lerner DJ, Kannel WB. Patterns of coronary heart disease morbidity and mortality in the sexes: A 26-year follow-up of the Framingham population. *Am Heart J* 111:383–390, 1986.
22. Dittrich H, Gilpin E, Nicod P, et al. Acute myocardial infarction in women: Influence of gender on mortality and prognostic variables. *Am J Cardiol* 62:1–7, 1988.
23. Chirikos TN, Nickel JL. Work disability from coronary heart disease in women. *Women Health* 9:55–74, 1984.
24. Sharpe PA, Clark NM, Janz NK. Differences in the impact and management of heart disease between older women and men. *Women Health* 17:25–43, 1991.
25. Papadopoulos C, Beaumont C, Shelley SI, et al. Myocardial Infarction and sexual activity of the female patient. *Arch Intern Med* 143:1528–1530, 1983.
26. Haurg MR, Folmar SJ. Longevity, gender and life quality. *Health Soc Behav* 27:332–345, 1986.
27. Case RB, Moss AJ, Case N, et al. Living alone after myocardial infarction. *JAMA* 267:515–519, 1992.
28. Williams RB, Barefoot JC, Califf RH, et al. Prognostic importance of social and economic resources among medically treated patients with angiographically documented coronary artery disease. *JAMA* 267:520–524, 1992.
29. Fanning O. Social interaction has a favorable effect on atherosclerosis in aging women. *Int Med World Rep* Jan. 1–14, 1992.
30. Hing E, Kovar MG, Rice D. *Sex Differences in Health and Use of Medical Care, United States, 1979.* Vital and Health Statistic, Series 3, No. 24. DHHS Pub. No. (PHS) 83–1048, 1979. Hyattsville, MD, National Center for Health Statistics, 1983.
31. Wallis LA, Klaus P. Toward improving women's health care. *J Am Med Wom Assoc* 45:219–221, 1990.
32. Wingard DL. The sex differential in morbidity, mor-

33. Kessler RC, Brown RL, Broman CL. Sex differences in psychiatric help-seeking: Evidence from four large scale surveys. *J Health Soc Behav* 22:49–64, 1981.
34. Kleinman JC, Gold M, Makuc D. Use of ambulatory medical care by the poor: Another look at equity. *Med Care* 19:1011–1128, 1981.
35. Rice T, McCall N. The extent of ownership and the characteristics of Medicare: Supplemental policies. *Inquiry* 22:188–200, 1985.
36. Woolhandler S, Himmelstein DU. Reverse targeting of preventive care due to lack of health insurance. *JAMA* 259:2872–2274, 1988.
37. National Center for Health Statistics. *Health, United States, 1988.* U.S. Public Health Service, DHHS Pub. No. (PHS) 89-1232. Washington, D.C., U.S. Government Printing Office, 1989.
38. Fiebach NH, Viscoli CM, Horwitz RI. Differences between women and men in survival after myocardial infarction—biology or methodology? *JAMA* 263:1092–1096, 1990.
39. Khan SS, Nessim S, Gray R, et al. Increased mortality of women in coronary artery bypass surgery: Evidence for referral bias. *Ann Intern Med* 112:561–567, 1990.
40. Armitagge KJ, Schneiderman LJ, Bass RA. Response of physicians to medical complaints in men and women. *JAMA* 241:2186–2187, 1979.
41. Wolfe C. Women confront second class care. *Health Week* 4 (Aug. 16–27):1, 1990.
42. Healy B. The Yentl syndrome. *N Engl J Med* 325:274–276, 1991.
43. Council on Ethical and Judicial Affairs, American Medical Association. Gender disparities in clinical decision making. *JAMA* 266:559–562, 1991.
44. Bush TL, Barrett-Connor E, Cowan LD, et al. Cardiovascular mortality and noncontraceptive use of estrogen in women: Results from the Lipid Research Clinics Program Follow-up Study. *Circulation* 75:1102–1109, 1987.
45. Stampfer MJ, Colditz GA, Willet WC, et al. Postmenopausal estrogen therapy and cardiovascular disease. Ten year follow-up from the nurses' health study. *N Engl J Med* 325:756–762, 1991.
46. Speroff L. Cardiovascular disease and postmenopausal hormone replacement therapy. *Endocrinologist* 1:49–55, 1991.
47. Mishell DR. Is routine use of estrogen indicated in postmenopausal women? *J Fam Prac* 29:406–416, 1989.
48. Begkvist L, Adami H-O, Persson I, et al. The risk of breast cancer after estrogen and estrogen-progestin replacement. *N Engl J Med* 321:293–297, 1990.
49. Manson JE, Stampfer MJ, Colditz GA, et al. A prospective study of aspirin use and primary prevention of cardiovascular disease in women. *JAMA* 266:521–527, 1991.
50. Cotton P. Women's health initiative leads way as research begins to fill gender gaps. *JAMA* 267:469–470, 1992.
51. Bernstein B, Kane R. Physicians' attitudes toward female patients. *Med Care* 19:600–608, 1981.
52. Hibbard JH, Pope CR. Another look at sex differences in the use of medical care: Illness orientation and the types of morbidities for which services are used. *Women Health* 11:21–36, 1986.
53. Becker M. The health belief model and personal health behavior: Introduction. *Health Education Monographs* 2:326–327, 1974.
54. Becker M, Maiman L. Sociobehavior determinants of compliance with health and medical care recommendations. *Med Care* 13:10–24, 1975.
55. Mechanic D, Volkart EH. Stress, illness behavior, and the sick role. *Am Soc Rev* 25:51–58, 1961.
56. Zola IK. Culture and symptoms-an analysis of patients' presenting complaints. *Am Soc Rev* 31:615–630, 1966.
57. Root MJ. Communication barriers between older women and physicians. Women and their health care providers; a matter of communication. *Pub Health Rep* Suppl. July-August:152–155, 1989.
58. Shorter E. *Bedside Manners: The Troubled History of Doctors and Patients.* New York, Simon and Shuster, 1985.
59. Corea G. *The Hidden Malpractice: How American Medicine Treats Women as Patients and Professionals.* New York, Morrow, 1977.
60. Ehrenreich B, English D. *For Her Own Good.* New York, Anchor, 1979.
61. Ogur B. Long day's journey into night: Women and prescription drug abuse. *Women Health* 11:99–115, 1986.
62. Waitzkin H. *The Politics of Medical Encounters: How Patients and Doctors Deal with Social Problems.* New Haven, Yale University Press, 1991.
63. Weisman CS. Communication between women and their health care providers: Research finding and unanswered questions. Women and their health care providers: A matter of communication. Proceedings of the National Conference on Women's Health, June 17–18, 1986. *Pub Health Rep* July-August, 1987, pp. 47–151.
64. Wallen J, Waitzkin H, Stoeckle JD. Physician stereotypes about female health and illness. *Women Health* 4:135, 1979.
65. Hall J. Gender effects in decoding non-verbal clues. *Psycho Bull* 83:8–45, 1978.
66. West C. *Routine Complications: Trouble with Talk Between Doctors and Patients.* Bloomington IN, Indiana University Press, 1984.
67. Stoeckle JD. *Encounters Between Patients and Doctors: An Anthology.* Cambridge, MIT Press, 1987.
68. Hojat M, Robeson MR, Veloski JJ. Gender comparisons in medical school and beyond: Two decades of longitudinal data. Presented at the 1992 Annual Meeting of the American Educational Research Association, San Francisco CA, April 1992.
69. Hojat M, Gonnella JS, Veloski JJ, et al. Differences in professional activities, perceptions of professional problems, and practice patterns between men and women graduates of Jefferson Medical College. *Acad Med* 65:755–756, 1990.
70. Bernstein L, Bernstein R. *Interviewing: A Guide for Health Professionals* (4th ed.). New York, Appleton and Lange, 1985.
71. Delbanco TL. Enriching the doctor-patient relationship by inviting the patient's perspective. *Ann Intern Med* 116:414–418, 1992.
72. Wechsler H, Levine S, Idelson RR, et al. The physicians role in health promotion—a survey of primary care practitioners. *N Engl J Med* 308:97–100, 1983.
73. Mann KV, Putnam RW. Physicians' perceptions of their role in cardiovascular risk reduction. *Prev Med* 18:45–58, 1989.

74. Hatem CJ, Lawrence RS. Improving compliance and health-promoting behavior. In Branch WT (ed): *Office Practice of Medicine,* 2nd ed. Philadelphia, WB Saunders, 1987, pp. 1075–1082.
75. Ravnikar VA. Compliance with hormone therapy. *Am J Obstet Gynecol* 156:1332–1334, 1987.
76. Zola IK. Structural constraints in the doctor-patient relationship: The case of noncompliance. In Eisenberg L, Kleinman A (eds): *The Relevance of Social Science for Medicine.* Boston, D. Reidel, 1981, pp. 241–252.
77. Kern DE. Patient compliance with medical advice. In Barker LR, Burton JR, Zieve PD (Eds.), *Principles of Ambulatory Medicine.* Baltimore, Williams & Wilkins, 1991, pp. 35–49.
78. Gerber KE, Nehemkis AM. Prologue: The dilemma of the chronically ill. In Gerber KE, Nehemkis AM (Eds.), *Compliance: The Dilemma of the Chronically Ill.* New York, Springer Verlag, 1986, pp. 3–11.
79. Roberson MHB. The meaning of compliance: Patient perspectives. *Qualitative Health Res* 2:7–26, 1992.

SECTION 2

Clinical Cardiovascular Disease

CHAPTER 2

Coronary Heart Disease: Diagnostic Decision Making

NANETTE K. WENGER, M.D.

That the morbidity and mortality from coronary heart disease, both in women and in men, constitute a major problem for our nation's public health is evident from 1987 U.S. statistics (Table 2–1), showing the substantial use of health care resources by both genders. However, despite the fact that coronary heart disease is the leading cause of mortality among U.S. women, accounting for about 250,000 deaths annually, the preponderance of information about the clinical recognition, manifestations, and prognosis of this disease is based on studies of populations consisting predominantly of men (1). Further, coronary heart disease is characteristically a disease of older women, in contrast to its occurrence in middle-aged and older men, for reasons as yet poorly understood.

This chapter highlights gender differences in the clinical syndromes and clinical outcomes of coronary heart disease as well as gender differences in diagnostic testing, all of which affect diagnostic decision making. Only as additional gender-specific data become available

Table 2–1. CORONARY HEART DISEASE: MORBIDITY AND MORTALITY, UNITED STATES 1987

	Women	Men
Population	125 million	118 million
Deaths	244,000	268,000
Hospitalizations	0.9 million	1.3 million
M.D. office visits	4.4 million	5.8 million
Prevalence	3.0 million	4.2 million
Health expenditures	$6 billion	$9 billion

will we be able to ascertain which components of the current traditional "male model" of coronary heart disease are applicable to both genders. However, even among women, clinical outcomes are less favorable in the less educated, unemployed, and economically disadvantaged subsets, as well as in those with social isolation or limited social support.

CLINICAL SYNDROMES AND CLINICAL OUTCOMES IN WOMEN

Prognostic data, based on natural history, for the various clinical subsets of coronary heart disease were readily derived from the early records compiled by the Framingham Heart Study, because only limited medical therapies were available for coronary heart disease and surgical treatment was still unknown. When contemporary data are examined for prognostic information about women and for prognostic gender differences, consideration must also be given to access to diagnostic procedures and to a variety of therapies; these features may be altered by physician decisions, patient decisions, and reimbursement issues, among others. Additional confounding prognostic variables include gender differences in response to the therapies selected, which in turn may be influenced by older age, by the comorbidity that is often a concomitant of aging, and by the need for urgent and emergency therapy in contrast to elective care. Societal perceptions of the risk of coronary heart disease for women may further influence access to care and thereby prognosis; these societal perceptions often continue to minimize the susceptibility of U.S. women to coronary heart disease and to its serious consequence, myocardial infarction.

Information about the clinical presentations and clinical outcomes of coronary heart disease according to gender, derived from the Framingham Study (2), reveals striking differences (Table 2–2). During 26 years of observation in the Framingham Heart Study, 60% of all coronary events occurred in men, with 40% occurring among a comparable number of women (2). The mean age at the initial clinical manifestation of coronary heart disease was 10 years older in women than in men, and at the occurrence of myocardial infarction it was an average of 20 years older. As a consequence of aging in the U.S. population, in which women have an average life expectancy 6 years longer than that of men, more women currently live into old age, when coronary heart disease is more likely to become manifest, and thus more deaths occur among elderly women than in elderly men. In 1988, cardiovascular deaths in the United States among women exceeded those in men (3), and both coronary morbidity and coronary mortality for women can be anticipated to increase with the progressive aging of our population, just cited, and the predominance of women in elderly populations. Although women tend to have a lower prevalence of most classic risk factors for coronary heart disease, differences in this risk profile are not adequate to explain the female disease pattern; better tolerance of coronary risk factors, when present, and protective hormonal and metabolic differences have been suggested (4). These suggestions highlight the importance of several potential

Table 2–2. MANIFESTATIONS OF CORONARY HEART DISEASE BY SEX IN SUBJECTS AGES 35 TO 84 YEARS: 26-YEAR FOLLOW-UP, FRAMINGHAM STUDY

Clinical Manifestations	% of Total Events		
	Men	*Women*	*Total*
Myocardial infarction	43	29	38
Sudden death	10	7	9
Angina pectoris			
Uncomplicated	26	47	34
With infarction	13	8	11
Coronary insufficiency			
(unstable angina)	8	9	8

From Lerner DJ, Kannel WB. Patterns of coronary heart disease morbidity and mortality in the sexes: A 26-year follow-up of the Framingham population. *Am Heart J* 111:383, 1986.

risk attributes unique to women: oral contraceptive use, pregnancy, hysterectomy, menopause, and postmenopausal hormonal replacement therapy, all of which warrant examination.

The occurrence of coronary heart disease is significantly more age-dependent among women (5), involving a 40-fold increase in coronary morbidity at ages 75 to 84 years compared with that at ages 35 to 44 years but lacking an abrupt change at menopausal age. As will be reemphasized later, it may be difficult to separate age and gender effects in women. Further, data about coronary disease in women were additionally curtailed by the virtual exclusion, until recent years, of elderly individuals of both genders from most clinical trials. Young women, however, experience an escalated coronary heart disease risk with premature menopause, whether natural or surgical, and after hysterectomy, both with and without oophorectomy; the underlying mechanism(s) require further elucidation (2). By age 75, coronary morbidity is comparable for men and women; potential explanatory factors include the development of more unfavorable coronary risk profiles, the effects of menopause, and the effects of aging. Although hypertension is less prevalent among younger women than among younger men, this pattern is reversed after about age 45. Diabetes mellitus is more prevalent among women than men and imparts a twofold greater risk of coronary heart disease in women than it does in men. Although women do not incur a perimenopausal decrease in high-density lipoprotein (HDL) cholesterol levels, both low-density lipoprotein (LDL) and total cholesterol levels increase prominently, to exceed those in men of comparable age. Elevated triglyceride levels are an independent risk factor in women and may be a better predictor of coronary heart disease than are LDL cholesterol levels.

Angina Pectoris

Angina pectoris, diagnosed solely on the basis of the clinical history, was described as the predominant initial presentation of coronary heart disease among women, occurring in 56% of the women in the Framingham Study compared with 43% of men. Women in the Framingham Study developed angina at least twice as often as they did myocardial infarction; and the incidence of angina has been described as double among black as compared with white cohorts of women (6). Additionally, the prognosis for Framingham Study women with angina was promulgated as being more favorable than that for men, with rare progression to myocardial infarction. Twenty-five percent of Framingham Study men with angina sustained myocardial infarction within the subsequent five years, twice the occurrence of myocardial infarction in women; in 86% of Framingham Study women, angina did not culminate in infarction (2). These early data from the Framingham Heart Study were interpreted by the clinical and research communities alike as indicating that angina was a benign problem among women and likely contributed to the lack of emphasis on coronary preventive strategies for women as well as to the exclusion of women from early research studies of prevention and therapies for coronary heart disease (7). Interpretation of angina as not constituting an adverse prognostic indicator in women ignored the observation that older women with angina in the Framingham Study, those aged 60 to 69 years, had an unfavorable outcome comparable to that of men with angina (8). These subset data remained largely unheeded and probably led to the limited attention paid to the problem of angina among women in clinical practice.

Subsequent data have challenged the diagnosis of angina pectoris as providing evidence of coronary atherosclerotic heart disease in women in the absence of confirmatory coronary arteriography (as was the case with the Framingham data). The major challenge to the unsubstantiated diagnosis of angina in women derived from reports of the Coronary Artery Surgery Study (CASS) Registry, published in the early 1980s. Among women and men with chest pain syndromes, referred by their treating physicians for coronary arteriography to evaluate suitability for coronary bypass surgery, 50% of women considered to have angina were found to have minimal or no obstruction of their epicardial coronary arteries at arteriography compared with 17% of men (9, 10). If such were the case in Framingham, and 50% of the Framingham women categorized as having angina indeed had no coronary heart disease, the rarity of progression of angina to myocardial infarction is not surprising. Noteworthy are the comparable coronary arteriographic data from the Cleveland Clinic, reported almost a decade earlier; only about 50% of premenopausal women considered to have angina had arteriographic confirmation of significant coronary atherosclerosis, whereas significant coronary disease was demonstrated in about 90% of older women (11, 12). Again, major age and gender interrelationships are evident, even among women with adverse coronary risk factor profiles (12, 13). Only with the widespread application of coronary arteriography was there general appreciation that many noncoronary chest pain syndromes in women can mimic angina pectoris. However, the "natural history" of women with arteriographically confirmed angina pectoris will never be known because medical and surgical therapies currently follow arteriographic confirmation of symptomatic coronary atherosclerotic obstruction.

Women with classic angina pectoris are described as having a high likelihood of coronary disease at coronary arteriography (14). Only about one-third of women with probable angina (or chest pain with some characteristics atypical for angina pectoris) have significant coronary disease at arteriography; and a trivial incidence of significant coronary disease is present at coronary arteriography in women with nonspecific chest pain syndromes (Table 2–3). Although the prognosis in the latter category appears favorable, it has yet to be delineated whether this problem preferentially affects women; the etiologic factor(s) remain uncertain and may be multiple.

Coronary artery spasm in the absence of fixed atherosclerotic coronary obstruction, so-called "variant angina," predominates in women (15, 16) and often occurs in younger women (17); the clinical course is typically benign (17). Variant angina in association with fixed atherosclerotic coronary obstruction appears to predominate in men (16, 18). Angina, presumed to be due to a decrease in coronary vasodilator reserve, again in the absence of coronary artery atherosclerotic obstruction, is also encountered more frequently in women and also entails a generally excellent prognosis (19). Myocardial ischemia due to abnormal coronary vasodilator reserve has been described in women with chest pain both typical and atypical for myocardial ischemia (19). Abnormalities of the resting electrocardiogram (ECG) may be present, coexisting hypertension is frequent, and myocardial perfusion abnormalities may be present on exercise radionuclide scintigraphy. Although a good symptomatic response to calcium-blocking drugs is common, some women have persisting chest pain. Microvascular endothelial dysfunction, abnormalities of coronary vascular resistance, and decreased coronary vasodilator reserve have been implicated as etiologic or contributory. The so-called syndrome X has also been associated with insulin resistance; with multisystem smooth muscle disorders that may result from endothelial, neural, or hormonal abnormalities; and with nonspecific cardiomyopathies. Abnormal visceral pain perception has also been described. Of concern is an unexplained deterioration of left ventricular function over time in a subset of these patients (20).

Myocardial Infarction

We will next examine the gender differences in prognostic information for myocardial infarction derived from the Framingham Heart Study. Myocardial infarction was less often the initial manifestation of nonfatal coronary disease in women in the Framingham Study (34% versus 50% in men). Nevertheless, when a myocardial infarction does occur as an initial event, the case fatality rates were higher in women, 39% versus 31% in men. In addition,

Table 2–3. PREVALENCE OF CORONARY ARTERY DISEASE AMONG WOMEN WITH CHEST PAIN AND NO PREVIOUS MYOCARDIAL INFARCTION

Study	Number of Women	Prevalence (%)			
		Total	Definite Angina	Probable Angina	Nonspecific Chest Pain
Chaitman et al. (71)	2810	26	72	36	6
Weiner et al. (72)	580	29	62	40	5
Guiteras Val et al. (76)	112	37	75	36	2
Hung et al. (77)	92	30	60	30	7

From Chaitman BR, Bourassa MG, Lam J, et al. Noninvasive diagnosis of coronary heart disease in women. In Eaker ED, Packard B, Wenger NK, et al. (Eds.), *Coronary Heart Disease in Women*. New York, Haymarket Doyma, 1987, p. 222.

a higher percentage of all coronary deaths in women occurred as the initial manifestation of myocardial infarction. Sixty-eight percent of all coronary heart disease deaths in the Framingham Study women constituted the initial manifestation of coronary disease compared with 49% among men (21). Age-related gender differences at both ends of the spectrum are noteworthy; young women (35 to 44 years) with myocardial infarction had an excessive mortality risk compared with men of similar age, and the case fatality rate of older women (aged 75 to 84 years) substantially exceeded that of their male counterparts (22).

Women in the Framingham Study also had an increased occurrence of unrecognized myocardial infarction, 35% versus 27% in men; about half of these episodes of unrecognized infarction in women were characterized as silent. These data are not surprising, given the increased incidence of silent or unrecognized infarction in elderly patients, particularly when it is complicated by diabetes or hypertension. But although silent infarction occurs more commonly in women, there is little information about the frequency or consequences of silent ischemia in women; this is an unmet need. For both women and men in the Framingham Study, silent myocardial infarction increased the subsequent likelihood of cardiac failure, stroke, and death.

Symptomatic myocardial infarction, in another study, had similar clinical presentations in women and men, with no gender differences evident in symptoms prior to infarction; half of the hospitalized women and men had no chest pain prior to infarction, and the rates for gender occurrence of antecedent stable and unstable angina were comparable (23).

Data from the Multicenter Investigation of Limitation of Infarct Size (MILIS) Study (24) suggest that non-Q wave myocardial infarction occurs more frequently in women; this has also been reported by others (25, 26). Contradictory data are offered by Marmor and associates (27), who described an equal occurrence of non-Q wave (subendocardial) infarction in both sexes, although in-hospital reinfarction predominated in women, 29% versus 12% in men; the latter was associated with an excess of hospital mortality for women, 23% versus 8% in men. Predominance of non-Q wave infarction correlates both with the better residual postinfarction ventricular function seen in women and with the increased likelihood of early reinfarction (24). Of note is that many patients with non-Q wave myocardial infarction were not included in a number of earlier epidemiologic studies, made prior to the availability of diagnostic cardiac serum enzyme tests, because they lacked the qualifying residual ECG abnormalities.

Conflicting data in regard to gender differences in postinfarction mortality (28) relate in part to the contributory effects of older age and the increased prevalence of diabetes, hypertension, and obesity among women, and in part reflect the question of whether acute in-hospital mortality, cumulative mortality, or longer-term mortality among survivors of hospitalization is addressed (22, 24, 29, 30). Not only was the initial outcome less favorable for women in the Framingham Study with infarction, but 1-year mortality was far greater. One-year mortality following symptomatic myocardial infarction in the Framingham Study was 45% for women and 10% for men (30). Forty percent of women, compared with 13% of men, had reinfarction during the first postinfarction year; women were more likely than men to have complicating stroke (12.7% versus 7.7%) and less likely to have postinfarction pericarditis than were men. That heart failure was reported as more common in women despite their better ventricular systolic function likely reflects ventricular diastolic dysfunction. However, among first-year survivors, men and women with symptomatic infarction had comparable 10-year mortality rates (39%), reinfarction rates (22%), and rates of development of cardiac failure (15%) (21). This less favorable hospital and first-year survival for women may be due to the average older age of women at the time of infarction or to increased occurrence of complications; as previously noted, complications often characterize non-Q wave infarction, in which, despite preserved ventricular function, the likelihood of reinfarction and associated adverse consequences is greater both during the acute hospitalization and in the early postinfarction months. These adverse outcomes for women following myocardial infarction contrast with the substantial survival advantage of Framingham Study women with angina pectoris compared with men (see earlier discussion). In the 1990s disparate outcome measures for angina and myocardial infarction and variable presentations in the spectrum of coronary atherosclerosis raise concern; in prior years there was less experience with extrapolation of epidemiologic data to clinical care, and these incongruities were largely unchallenged.

Thus, although women have lower mortality from coronary heart disease at a given age than men, this survival advantage is lost once coronary heart disease becomes clinically evident (22); the mortality of women with manifest coronary heart disease is equal to or greater than that of men (2). Based on Framingham Study data, the age-adjusted risk ratio for postinfarction coronary death was 6.0 in women and 4.2 in men (31). Diabetes was described in the Multicenter Postinfarction Study as an adverse prognostic factor independent of ejection fraction (32). Additional recent data regarding gender differences with myocardial infarction derive from the MILIS Study (24, 28). MILIS included 590 men (511 white and 79 black) and 226 women (163 white and 63 black). Women in MILIS had a better resting ventricular ejection fraction, both at hospital admission and at hospital discharge for myocardial infarction, despite their older age and greater prevalence of hypertension, diabetes, and family history of coronary disease; the higher ejection fraction was especially prominent among black women. Based on the male model of coronary disease, these women should have been anticipated to do well because of their preserved ventricular function. Nevertheless, the women in MILIS had a higher hospital mortality, 13% versus 7%, and a higher posthospital mortality for survivors, as well as more postinfarction angina and symptoms of heart failure. Black women had the highest in-hospital mortality from myocardial infarction when all other in-hospital characteristics of infarction were comparable for men and women. A contemporary report of coronary care unit data from Israel (33) described an age-adjusted hospital mortality of 23% for women compared with 16% for men; and the age-adjusted cumulative first-year mortality for women was almost 32% compared with 23% for men. Female gender in this report independently predicted increased mortality from myocardial infarction, and the presence of diabetes predicted mortality only for women. In a Swedish study, cessation of cigarette smoking improved survival among women with an initial episode of myocardial infarction (34); however, most trials of coronary risk reduction following myocardial infarction have included no or too few women to ascertain effects.

Thus, women are more likely than men to die early following myocardial infarction, and survivors have an increased rate of reinfarction, heart failure, and late deaths. Given this adverse outcome in women with myocardial infarction, what information is available regarding the influence of pharmacologic and other medical therapies on prognosis? Coronary thrombolytic therapy given in the early hours of a myocardial infarction is acknowledged to improve outcome in patients suitable for its use. In recent randomized studies of coronary thrombolysis that enrolled elderly patients, the survival benefit was greatest in older patients and was seen in both women and men (35); these data have not yet received appropriate clinical application in that the diagnosis of myocardial infarction in older women is less likely to trigger the use of thrombolytic drugs, even when eligibility criteria are met (36) (see Chapter 3). Despite the documented benefit of thrombolytic therapy for both genders (35), the gender ratio of death rates from myocardial infarction, both in-hospital and at 1 year, was unaffected by thrombolysis; mortality rates of women were double those of men, 29.8% versus 15.2%, at 1 year (37). Only two of the many drugs routinely used for myocardial infarction have been systematically compared for gender effect in reasonably sized clinical trials. Timolol (in the European studies) (38) and aspirin (in the International Study of Infarct Survival [ISIS] trial) (39) imparted equal gender benefits in limiting reinfarction. Gender comparison of the prognostic effect of vasodilator drugs is of particular interest; women have smaller coronary arteries and incur an excess of vasoreactive diseases (e.g., Raynaud's phenomenon, vasospastic angina), so that the theoretic benefit of vasodilator therapy requires validation. Women are also referred less frequently for exercise rehabilitation by their treating physicians despite evidence that women who participate in exercise training following infarction have functional improvement comparable to that of men (40).

Unequivocal myocardial infarction can occur in the absence of angiographically documented obstructive coronary lesions; coronary spasm, coronary thrombosis, thromboembolism with spontaneous clot lysis, and recanalization are among the postulated mechanisms, and oral contraceptive use has been suggested as etiologic (41) or contributory; these data, however, derive from studies of higher doses of oral contraceptives than those currently used.

A high incidence of postinfarction ventricular arrhythmias is described even in patients with patent coronary arteries (41), but their prognostic significance is uncertain. This phenomenon has occasionally been described in the postpartum period. It is unknown whether myocardial infarction, in the absence of coronary atherosclerotic obstruction, occurs excessively in women.

Cardiac Rupture. Cardiac rupture, both of the left ventricular free wall and of the ventricular septum, is more frequent among women (42, 43). Limited extent of coronary disease, lack of angiographic evidence of collateral circulation, and possible coronary spasm or thrombosis causing rapid coronary occlusion may predispose to cardiac rupture; older age, higher prevalence of hypertension, and preserved ventricular function also appear contributory (44).

Ventricular Arrhythmias. Although numerous studies of risk stratification following myocardial infarction identified ventricular arrhythmias, particularly complex forms of ventricular ectopy, as a prognostic factor for increased mortality, sex-specific differences were generally not examined, possibly because gender per se was not considered to impart a significant postinfarction risk. Puletti and coworkers (29) described a comparable postinfarction incidence of venticular arrhythmias with a comparable prognosis in women and in men.

Moss and associates (45) evaluated the impact of ventricular arrhythmias in the 194 women and 673 men enrolled in the Multicenter Postinfarction Research Trial. Whereas a decreased left ventricular ejection fraction (>30%) significantly increased the mortality risk for both men and women, frequent ventricular premature beats (≥1 per hour) and runs of ventricular premature beats (≥3 in a row) were independent adverse prognostic characteristics for postinfarction mortality for men but not for women. The distribution of frequent and repetitive ventricular ectopic beats was comparable among male and female patients. Reasons for the gender differences remain enigmatic, but the authors suggest that this feature may account for the lesser occurrence of sudden death among women. The women were older and had more hypertension and diabetes but less cigarette smoking than the men; these factors, as well as the influence of smaller heart size, neuroendocrine factors, lipid levels, and psychosocial features, require investigation. In particular, the lesser risk of postinfarction ventricular arrhythmia among women warrants confirmation in a larger cohort.

Among survivors of cardiac arrest known to have coronary disease, ventricular tachycardia or fibrillation was less frequently inducible at electrophysiologic study in women; the explanation for this gender difference remains elusive (46), but the observation is concordant with the reduced frequency of sudden death in women.

Ventricular Dysfunction. Ventricular function is generally better in women at any given age because of the discrepancy in age (10 to 20 years older) at which women develop overt coronary disease. In most large multicenter studies, left ventricular function has been the most powerful predictor of postinfarction morbidity and mortality; 5-year mortality as great as 85% is described with severe ischemic cardiomyopathy. The adverse effect of left ventricular dysfunction on morbidity and mortality appears similar for men and women (45). Left ventricular function, as measured by ejection fraction, is better in women than in men with documented coronary disease (10), possibly because of the better myocardial perfusion in elderly women, as documented by myocardial scintigraphy in at least one study (47). It may also reflect the greater likelihood that women have non-Q wave infarction, which is characterized by a lesser impairment of ventricular function. This advantage was lost by insulin-requiring diabetic women in the Framingham cohort, who exhibited a fivefold greater risk of heart failure compared with nondiabetic women; comparable data among men showed only a doubling of the heart failure risk with diabetes. Among insulin-dependent diabetic women (48), decreased myocardial compliance—related to hypertension, diabetes, or other factors—may accentuate transient ischemic ventricular diastolic dysfunction. Alternatively, greater restrictions of coronary blood flow, as with coronary spasm or thrombosis, may be operative. The relative frequency of systolic versus diastolic ventricular dysfunction in women is poorly defined, and both may underlie comparable symptoms of heart failure.

Although locations of infarct and regional wall motion abnormalities are comparable for men and women (10), left anterior descending coronary artery occlusion causing anterior myocardial infarction and consequent anterior wall motion abnormalities were described as predominating among young women using oral contraceptives (49). Even with comparable infarct size and history of prior infarction, women have a higher postinfarction left ventricular ejection fraction than is present among men (24); despite this lesser severity of left ventricular dysfunction, the postinfarction prognosis for women in one series was comparable to that for men (11). Data from the MILIS Study, in contrast, suggested a poorer postinfarction prognosis for women (24); despite their more favorable left ventricular ejection fraction both at admission and at hospital discharge, women had a greater 4-year postinfarction mortality, 36% compared with 21% among men; and black women had the highest postinfarction mortality, 48%. Women, particularly black women, also had an excess of postinfarction angina and congestive heart failure compared with men (24). Thus, the prognostic significance of ejection fraction appears to differ between men and women.

Increased occurrence of heart failure in the presence of preserved left ventricular systolic function implicates the mechanistic role of ventricular diastolic dysfunction, a common concomitant of older age and one postulated to relate to the increased prevalence of diabetes mellitus and hypertension among women (50). If diastolic dysfunction predominates among women with signs and symptoms of heart failure, therapeutic issues follow: are digitalis, diuretic, and vasodilator therapies associated with a more or less favorable outcome?

Adjustment of these postinfarction mortality data for known coronary risk factors and prognostic features (including ejection fraction) would result in a decreased mortality rate for women in general and for black women in particular. That ejection fraction was the determining factor demonstrates its prognostic importance in women following myocardial infarction. The importance of ejection fraction differs following coronary artery bypass graft (CABG) surgery, in which women have an adverse outcome not anticipated based on their preserved ventricular function. Despite better preoperative left ventricular function, lesser incidence of prior infarction, and less multivessel coronary artery disease (Table 2-4), features associated with favorable outcomes for men, women have a less favorable result following coronary artery bypass graft surgery (51–53) (see Chapter 3). Women in the Coronary Artery Surgery Study (CASS) (54) had a greater perioperative mortality, 4.5% versus 1.9% for men, and more congestive heart failure compared with men. The occurrence of heart failure in women despite a preserved ejection fraction suggests that impairment of ventricular diastolic function may be etiologic. Thus, preserved ventricular systolic function appears prognostically important for a favorable surgical outcome for men but not for women; female gender predicts perioperative CABG mortality better than does the severity of ventricular dysfunction or the severity of angina. Women surviving successful myocardial revascularization procedures have 5- and 10-year survival rates equal to or better than those of men, reflecting their better ventricular function. Preserved left ventricular systolic function is also a powerful predictor of favorable outcome for percutaneous transluminal coronary angioplasty (PTCA), but, again, only for men (55).

Psychosocial Features. Anxiety, depression, guilt feelings about illness, and sexual dysfunction are more common among women than men following infarction (50, 56); women's return to remunerative work is both less frequent and more delayed despite an early return to high-intensity household tasks (50). The potential contributions of increased severity or complications of infarction, older age at infarction, and differences in social support render interpretations complex. In the general population, three of four men 65 years of age and older are married and live with their wives, whereas three of five women of comparable age are without spouses. Further, the poverty rate for elderly women, about 19%, is the highest for any U.S. age group.

In most reports, women's attendance at exercise rehabilitation programs after a coronary event is lower and their dropout rates are greater (40). Is this related to emotional dysfunction or to lack of social support? Do women not like to exercise? Or are the scheduling, venue, program format, and exercise components of rehabilitation designed for the predominant population, middle-aged and working men, with little relevance for older women recovering from myocardial infarc-

Table 2-4. PREVALENCE OF MULTIVESSEL DISEASE,[a] LEFT MAIN CORONARY STENOSIS,[b] OR BOTH AMONG WOMEN WITH CHEST PAIN AND NO PREVIOUS MYOCARDIAL INFARCTION

Study	Number of Women	Prevalence (%)			
		Total	Definite Angina	Probable Angina	Nonspecific Chest Pain
Chaitman et al. (71)	2810	15	53	19	2
Weiner et al. (72)	580	16	39	22	0.8
Guiteras Val et al. (76)	112	12	29	4	0
Hung et al. (77)	92	16	44	8	3

[a] ≥70% stenosis.
[b] ≥50% stenosis.
From Chaitman BR, Bourassa MG, Lam J, et al. Noninvasive diagnosis of coronary heart disease in women. In Eaker ED, Packard B, Wenger NK, et al. (Eds.), *Coronary Heart Disease in Women*. New York, Haymarket Doyma, 1987, p. 222.

tion? Clearly, this problem warrants examination.

Silent Ischemia

Despite appreciation of the frequency and adverse prognostic significance (57) of this finding in patients with angina and myocardial infarction, gender differences in silent ischemia have not been examined. There is a compelling need to ascertain the incidence and impact of silent ischemia among women in view of their greater frequency of silent (unrecognized) myocardial infarction.

Unstable Angina

Several CABG surgical series describe a disproportionate number of women with unstable angina (51–53). This is also evident in the National Heart, Lung, and Blood Institute (NHLBI) PTCA Registry data (see later discussion). It remains uncertain whether this finding reflects a true preponderance of unstable angina among women or different indications and timing for referral for CABG and PTCA related to gender. Furthermore, although only a small percentage of patients with unstable angina have normal coronary arteries at coronary arteriography, this situation also occurs disproportionately among women (58).

Sudden Cardiac Death

Sudden cardiac death is relatively uncommon in women, accounting for less than 10 percent of coronary events in the Framingham Study population. Sudden death occurs about 20 years later in women than in men, presenting as a significant problem among women predominantly after age 65 to 74 years (2).

Sudden death constitutes a lesser proportion of all coronary deaths among women, 39% versus 50% for men. Among coronary deaths in the Framingham cohort, 37% were sudden in women versus 46% in men (21); sudden death as a sequel to overt coronary heart disease occurred in 5.3% of women versus 11.9% of men over a 10-year period. Although the Framingham Study data do not document a relationship between systolic blood pressure, cigarette smoking, or obesity and sudden death in women, other studies report the association of cigarette smoking with sudden cardiac death in women (59) as in men (60). Association of sudden death with a history of psychiatric illness and with alcohol consumption is also described for women (61).

ARE THERE GENDER-BASED DIFFERENCES IN ACCESS TO CARE (GENDER BIAS)?

A major concern in regard to diagnostic and therapeutic interventions and their effect on the well-being and prognosis of women relates to the issue of bias, or even inappropriate delay, in referral for myocardial revascularization. Earlier, this disparity possibly reflected a misperception of angina pectoris as a benign problem in women, but this is unlikely to be the case in the 1990s. In recent years a number of reports have documented gender-based differences in the use of diagnostic and therapeutic procedures for patients with suspected or defined coronary heart disease; this has raised questions as to whether CABG and PTCA are underused in women (or potentially used excessively for men). This concern is raised despite an almost doubled performance of coronary arteriography and a threefold increase in CABG for women during the 1980s. Caution is recommended in drawing conclusions from these data in the absence of information about advanced patient age and serious comorbidity because these may exert a substantial impact on clinical decisions made by patients and their physicians (7). Because this increased use of coronary arteriography and CABG surgery in women has not been correlated with clinical outcomes (as was the case for men), the resulting advantages or disadvantages remain unknown.

Any age-based restriction of care preferentially disadvantages women (62), given their predominant manifestations of clinical coronary heart disease at an advanced age. For example, in the early years of thrombolytic therapy for acute myocardial infarction, the 65-year age limit precluded consideration of most women, and even today coronary thrombolysis is described as underutilized in women (36) despite the documented benefit described above (35).

In one report of exercise radionuclide testing, physicians referred men for coronary arteriography 10 times more frequently than they did women when abnormal thallium exercise test results were reported (63); although these physicians asserted their disbelief that the chest pain of their women patients with abnormal test results was due to coronary heart disease, comparable antianginal medications were prescribed for men and women. Gender bias is suggested in consideration of patients for coronary arteriography, the performance of which appears as a substantial determinant in defining access to myocardial revascularization (63); yet results of noninvasive diagnostic tests typically determine referral for coronary arteriography, so that appropriate selection of these tests, incorporation of gender-based criteria for abnormality, and appropriate response to abnormal test results seem requisite. Coronary bypass surgery, when undertaken electively, based on abnormal findings at exercise testing that initiate referral for coronary arteriography, entails substantially less mortality than does urgent or emergency CABG in patients hospitalized for severe or unstable angina that is unresponsive to or poorly controlled with medical management; these data, however, derive from predominantly male populations. Yet clinicians considering referral of women with angina pectoris or myocardial infarction for CABG must weigh their less favorable surgical outcome; is myocardial revascularization the appropriate or desirable therapy, given the excess morbidity and mortality of women? Women patients must also consider these prognostic differences; women's risk of perioperative mortality following CABG is almost twice that of men.

Randomized clinical trial results are not available for women, for either PTCA or CABG surgery, so that outcomes are based on observational data; however, both CABG case report series (50–54, 64) and PTCA Registry and other data (55, 65, 66, 67) indicate substantial baseline differences by gender. This raises the issue of selection bias, i.e., differing criteria used to recommend CABG or PTCA for women and for men in the nonrandomized series from which these data were derived. It is also uncertain whether recent improvements in CABG surgery have altered the gender differences in success and in survival, as has occurred with PTCA. Detailed discussion of gender differences in medical and surgical revascularization is included in Chapter 3. To summarize, it has not been ascertained whether the excess mortality of women undergoing CABG is related to their referral at an older age with its potential increased incidence of comorbidity, including diabetes and hypertension, nor is it known whether smaller coronary arterial size is contributory or whether the pivotal issue in excess mortality is the performance of urgent or emergency surgery for severe and unstable preoperative angina pectoris. Is the scenario such that a trial of medical management is selected initially, and subsequent unsatisfactory responses result in referral for CABG at an older age and often on an urgent or emergency basis, with attendant greater mortality? Does this vicious circle in turn discourage clinicians from a more vigorous approach to the evaluation and treatment of chest pain syndromes in women (and is such an aggressive approach warranted)?

Hospital discharge records in Massachusetts and Maryland have documented a lesser use of invasive diagnostic and therapeutic procedures in women. Fifteen to twenty-eight percent more men than women hospitalized for coronary heart disease (including acute myocardial infarction) were referred for coronary arteriography; not surprisingly, a 27–45% greater performance of CABG was identified in men than in women (68). Further, use of the procedure for insured men exceeded that for uninsured men. Concordant data derive from the Survival and Ventricular Enlargement (SAVE) Study (69) and are based on patient information prior to the index infarction that occasioned admission to the SAVE Study because of major resultant damage to the myocardium (ejection fraction below 40%). Twice as many men as women (27% versus 15%) had prior coronary arteriography; this doubled use of the procedure for men contrasted with the greater functional disability due to anginal symptoms evident in women (based on standardized questionnaires). Only 50% of the women in SAVE reported no limitation of physical activity due to angina compared with 69% of the men. These data also define the limitations of medical management in averting functional disability in half of the women in this study. These limited data, however, support the need to evaluate the symptomatic burden in women undergoing traditional medical management as well as their likelihood of reinfarction and its adverse prognostic consequences. Twice as many men as women, 12% versus 6%, had had CABG prior to infarction; warranting attention is the fact that equal percentages of men and women who had had coronary arteriography were referred for CABG.

Outcome data regarding morbidity and mortality are required for interpretation of these differences in the use of procedures. The cause of these differences has not been ascertained. Were diagnostic or therapeutic procedures previously undertaken? Were they subsequently planned? What was the role of insurance reimbursement? Were differences related to physician decisions, and were they based on problems of comorbidity or other considerations? Or were these patient decisions, and what were the reasons for these decisions? Was there a relationship to patient expectations of care, to financial constraints, to social support? Gender differences are of interest, but *critical to ascertain* are differences between women with and without invasive management, both diagnostic and therapeutic, of their coronary heart disease (70).

DIAGNOSTIC TESTING FOR CORONARY HEART DISEASE IN WOMEN

An important and unmet need is the earlier recognition of coronary disease in women; yet elucidation of the etiology of chest pain in women poses a challenge. Because of the lower prevalence of coronary disease as well as of multivessel coronary disease in women than in men, except in the oldest age groups (71, 72), the predictive value of any symptom (e.g., chest pain) or of any noninvasive test is less in women than in men (73–75). These age-related differences among women were known as early as the 1970s, when coronary arteriographic data from the Cleveland Clinic (12) showed significant atherosclerotic obstruction in 50% of premenopausal women compared with about 90% of older women. Women also have a greater prevalence of noncoronary causes of chest pain, e.g., mitral valve prolapse, that may both mimic the pain of coronary heart disease and result in false-positive diagnostic tests; hormonal changes have also been implicated in the cause of false-positive ST-segment displacement.

Standard cardiovascular risk factors, however, may not be equally predictive of coronary heart disease in men and in women; based on Framingham Study data, vital capacity and HDL cholesterol levels appear as more powerful predictors of coronary heart disease in women than in men. However, at any level of cardiovascular risk, women have less morbidity than do men (2). Risk factor prevalence is greater among less well-educated women and in those with lower family income. Not yet addressed, as previously noted, are those risk factors unique to women: oral contraceptive use, pregnancy, hysterectomy, menopause, and postmenopausal hormone replacement therapy.

Clinical characteristics, including descriptors of the chest pain and coronary risk factors, as well as features of the resting electrocardiogram (ECG), may help in the selection of additional diagnostic procedures. In several coronary arteriographic series of women with chest pain syndromes but without prior infarction (71, 72, 76, 77), 60–75% of women whose pain was considered typical for angina had significant coronary disease; 29–53% had multivessel coronary disease. The prevalence of coronary disease was 30–40% among women with chest pain characterized as probable angina, and 4–22% had multivessel coronary disease. Only 2–7% of women with nonspecific chest pain symptoms had coronary disease, and virtually none had multivessel disease (14) (see Tables 2–3 and 2–4). Thus, a careful and detailed history offers useful information in excluding coronary disease if symptoms are nonspecific. Similarly, if results of exercise testing are normal, coronary disease is unlikely, but abnormal test results are likely to be false-positive tests. Particularly in older women, the clinical history should include the usual intensity of the physical activity of daily tasks because habitual low activity levels may lead to a false-negative suspicion for angina pectoris.

Exercise Testing: The Exercise ECG

Added contributors to the lower sensitivity of exercise testing among women, as already noted, include a higher prevalence of ECG changes with hyperventilation or position change, the frequently less severe multivessel coronary disease, a lesser likelihood of exercising to adequate intensity levels owing to comorbid illnesses or general deconditioning (more common not only in women in general but particularly at older ages when coronary disease is more likely [78]), and a higher prevalence of problems (e.g., mitral valve prolapse, left ventricular hypertrophy, or drug effects) that are characterized by repolarization changes on the exercise ECG that may mimic myocardial ischemia (79). As evidence of the importance of the severity of coronary obstruction, Hung and associates (77), described a 93% occurrence of abnormal exercise ECG results among women with multivessel coronary disease compared with 43% in women with single vessel disease or without significant coronary disease. Thus, the exercise ECG has a high likelihood of detecting severe multivessel coronary disease in women who exercise to adequate intensity.

Despite these limitations, carefully performed and analyzed exercise-based test procedures can help evaluate chest pain syndromes in women, and the value of a negative (normal) exercise ECG in women warrants emphasis. Because of their low prevalence of coronary disease, a negative test in women who are able to exercise to adequate intensity has a high specificity for the absence of significant coronary disease, comparable to the specificity described for men (72, 78). The exercise ECGs in men and women with normal resting ECGs in the CASS were of comparable specificity (72). Resting ST-T segment ECG abnormalities substantially lowered the exercise ECG specificity in both genders, but to a greater extent in women than in men; and women were significantly more likely to have resting ST-T segment ECG abnormalities (72). Thus, exercise test results, if normal, offer useful confirmation in excluding coronary disease, but abnormal test results are likely to be false-positive.

Exercise Radionuclide Studies

Exercise radionuclide perfusion studies are indicated for women with an abnormal resting ECG. Reports of *exercise thallium-201 scintigraphy* published to date have involved relatively small numbers of women (74, 77, 80, 81), but they describe high specificity for women (particularly when qualitative image analysis is used). Whether exercise single photon emission computed tomography (SPECT) thallium imaging increases the diagnostic accuracy for women (82) requires confirmation. Among 60 women with proximate coronary arteriography, Friedman and associates (83) described a sensitivity and specificity of exercise thallium scintigraphy of 75% and 97%, respectively; this contrasted with a sensitivity of exercise electrocardiography of 32% and a specificity of 41%. Comparable data can be collected from several other sources (74, 77), i.e., fewer false-positive tests (14). The lesser sensitivity of thallium scintigraphy in women likely reflects the decreased prevalence of multivessel disease in women (which is known to increase the test sensitivity in men). Interposition of breast tissue is recognized to cause false-positive perfusion defects in women by attenuating the radioactivity in thallium scintigraphy. Current radionuclide image interpretations consider gender differences; correction for fixed defects due to breast attenuation of the image can improve the test's predictive accuracy, rendering it comparable to that for men (81).

Gender-related data are not currently available for technetium-99m sestamibi imaging.

Exercise radionuclide ventriculography, by

contrast, is insensitive and has poor specificity for the diagnosis of coronary artery disease in women (84, 85); its use is *not* recommended. About 30% of women with normal coronary arteries fail to increase their ejection fraction with exercise, an increase that characteristically occurs in about 90% of their male counterparts (85, 86). Technetium-99m bloodtracer labeling is traditionally used.

Gender differences in the physiologic response to exercise appear to underlie the lack of value of exercise radionuclide ventriculography in women (using the male criterion of lack of increase in ejection fraction with exercise as suggesting coronary disease). Women have a smaller resting ventricular volume, a higher resting ejection fraction, and a smaller end-diastolic volume index than men; in response to exercise, women have a greater increase in the end-diastolic volume index and a lesser increase in ejection fraction than do men—responses that are not explained by differences in exercise capacity (87). By contrast, one report showed no gender difference in ventricular performance of normal but younger subjects in response to upright exercise (88); and another described similar manifestations of myocardial ischemia and ventricular dysfunction during exercise in men and in women with comparable coronary disease (89). The need for gender-based criteria for exercise radionuclide ventriculography remains controversial.

Peak exercise ejection fraction may provide a better indication of coronary disease in women than change in ejection fraction with exercise (90, 91). Peak exercise ejection fraction in the normal range appears to be better related to an excellent prognosis than change in ejection fraction with exercise.

Pharmacologic Radionuclide Perfusion Studies

Pharmacologic radionuclide perfusion studies (such as those using dipyridamole or adenosine thallium), of potential value in women who are unable to exercise or are unable to exercise to adequate intensity, must be examined for gender differences; a heart rate approximating 125 beats/minute or a rate-pressure product in excess of 17,000 to 20,000 is considered to provide reasonable risk stratification for men. Again, possible gender differences in vascular reactivity suggest the need for such analyses.

Exercise and Pharmacologic Echocardiography

Exercise echocardiography in a small series of women with a high prevalence of coronary disease (92) showed a high diagnostic sensitivity and specificity (86% for both); a postulated explanation is the preserved predictive accuracy of this procedure with single vessel disease. Development of new regional wall motion abnormalities with exercise is indicative of coronary disease. However, the high prevalence of coronary disease in this series, with about one-third of women having typical angina pectoris as well, possibly prejudiced the data favorably. Lack of radiation exposure is a favorable aspect of this procedure, as is the ability to identify other concomitant causes of chest pain, e.g., mitral valve prolapse. Impressively, in the 30% of women with equivocal exercise electrocardiograms and therefore nondiagnostic conventional exercise stress tests, exercise echocardiography had a predictive accuracy of 82%. Dipyridamole echocardiography in a population of women with a high prevalence of coronary disease also had high predictive value (93), better than that for the exercise ECG. These promising techniques warrant further validation.

Cardiac Fluoroscopy for Coronary Artery Calcification

Calcification of coronary atherosclerotic lesions at autopsy examination is more extensive in elderly women than in elderly men (80). Cardiac fluoroscopy to detect coronary calcification has been described (77) as having a sensitivity of 79% (similar to that of exercise testing) but a significantly higher specificity than exercise testing, 83%. In women with chest pain without prior infarction, coronary calcification was present in all those with multivessel coronary disease. Fluoroscopically detected calcium was present in both coronary arteries in 80% of women (77), whereas coronary calcification was absent in 88% of women with false-positive exercise ECGs (14). Comparable data have been reported by others (94, 95). Ghazzal and associates (96) considered fluoroscopy for coronary calcification an inexpensive, reliable indicator of coronary disease, particularly multivessel disease, in women older than 60 years with chest pain; the sensitivity and specificity among 106 consecutive women aged 34 to 87 years were 75% and 64%, respectively. Older age and increased number of diseased vessels increased the predictive value. Nevertheless, this inexpensive diagnostic test has not received widespread application.

Recommendations: Noninvasive Diagnostic Testing

Correction for the prevalence of coronary disease (pretest likelihood) and consideration of the variety of conditions tending to result in false-positive tests in women have been thought to result in comparable diagnostic value of exercise-based tests in men and women (72, 74).

Exercise electrocardiography appears cost-effective in the diagnostic evaluation of women with typical angina pectoris and a normal resting ECG, whereas for women with probable or atypical angina and abnormalities on the resting ECG, an enhanced diagnostic specificity is described with thallium exercise scintigraphy, cardiac fluoroscopy for coronary artery calcification, or both of these tests (14); their sensitivity is comparable to that of the exercise ECG. The very low pretest likelihood of coronary disease among women with nonspecific chest pain precludes any added clinical usefulness of most currently available noninvasive tests (14). Exercise radionuclide ventriculography does not add significantly to the diagnostic evaluation of women with any category of chest pain symptoms (14). Because of differences in the physiologic and ECG responses to exercise of women and men, gender-specific criteria may provide benefit, when they are available.

Use of clinical variables to estimate the likelihood of severe coronary disease (97) and sequential performance of noninvasive tests may improve the accuracy of the recognition and determination of severity of coronary disease among women with chest pain syndromes (14, 72, 74), allowing an appropriate selection of women for coronary arteriography. Logistic discriminant analysis of exercise variables, including exercise workload, peak exercise heart rate, and so on, may also improve the diagnostic value (98), as may use of gender-specific test criteria, but these concepts require validation in populations of women with both high and low prevalences of coronary disease before their merit can be determined.

Coronary Arteriography

In addition to its use in identifying the coronary pathoanatomy after abnormal results have been obtained at noninvasive testing, coronary arteriography should also be considered for use in elderly women and those at potential high risk of coronary disease with serious comorbid illness for whom noninvasive testing has proved unsatisfactory. This situation occurs not uncommonly during preoperative evaluation for noncardiac surgery.

SUMMARY: CLINICAL SYNDROMES AND CLINICAL OUTCOMES

Coronary heart disease is a serious problem among older U.S. women, accounting for about 28% of all fatalities. Preventive strategies must be implemented across the life span, although identification of anticipated benefits is hampered by the limited data base for so doing. The onset of coronary heart disease occurs consistently at an older age among women than among men. Gender differences in the incidence and age of onset of coronary atherosclerosis as well as in mortality from coronary heart disease remain largely unexplained. Although epidemiologic data suggest that angina pectoris is the predominant clinical presentation of coronary heart disease in women, and angina has been traditionally described as associated with a more favorable outcome in women than in men, coronary arteriographic data have documented that chest pain syndromes that mimic angina pectoris occur frequently in women in the absence of demonstrable coronary atherosclerotic obstruction. A more ominous prognosis is described for women than for men following myocardial infarction; the relative contributions to poorer outcome of gender, older age, and greater prevalence of diabetes and hypertension require elucidation. Although women sustain myocardial infarction as the presenting manifestation of coronary heart disease less frequently than do men, coronary events are more often fatal among women. Women are also more likely to have unrecognized infarction. Following infarction, although the age-adjusted risk ratio for coronary death is greater for women, they are less likely to die suddenly (31). Postinfarction left ventricular systolic function is better preserved among women despite an increased incidence of symptoms and signs of heart failure (probably diastolic dysfunction), especially among diabetic women; a lesser mortality risk from ventricular arrhythmias has also been suggested. Although the adverse prognosis of women following infarction remains inadequately explained because they incur increased early and late mortality and increased morbidity once myocardial infarction occurs, a major goal in the medical and surgical management of women with angina pectoris must be prevention of progression to myocardial infarction. The optimal approach to identifying women at high risk of a proximate coronary event has yet to be defined.

Prognostic data for many subsets of coronary atherosclerotic heart disease in the 1990s, in both women and men, appear to be related to the diagnostic and therapeutic interventions selected as well as to the timing of these interventions. Available data have challenged the applicability of the male model of coronary disease, which has been reasonably well studied in middle-aged men, to the population of older women with coronary heart disease seen in clinical practice. Prospectively derived information about the appropriate role of diagnostic and therapeutic procedures in the care of women both with chest pain syndromes and with defined coronary disease must be related to morbidity and mortality outcomes, so that optimal timing and utilization of invasive interventions can be defined.

References

1. Wenger NK. Coronary disease in women. *Annu Rev Med* 36:285, 1985.
2. Lerner DJ, Kannel WB. Patterns of coronary heart disease morbidity and mortality in the sexes: A 26-year follow-up of the Framingham population. *Am Heart J* 111:383, 1986.
3. American Heart Association. *1992 Heart and Stroke Facts.* Dallas, American Heart Association, 1991.
4. Oliver MF. What is the difference between women and men? (summary of closing comments). In Oliver MF, Vedin A, Wilhelmsson C (Eds.), *Myocardial Infarction in Women.* New York, Churchill Livingstone, 1986, p. 215.
5. Johansson S, Vedin A, Wilhelmsson C. Myocardial infarction in women. *Epidemiol Rev* 5:67, 1983.
6. Keil JE, Loadholt CB, Weinrich MC, et al. Incidence of coronary heart disease in blacks in Charleston, South Carolina. *Am Heart J* 108:779, 1984.
7. Wenger NK. Gender, coronary artery disease, and coronary bypass surgery. *Ann Intern Med* 112:557, 1990.
8. Kannel WB, Feinleib M. Natural history of angina pectoris in the Framingham Study. Prognosis and survival. *Am J Cardiol* 29:154, 1972.
9. The Principal Investigators of CASS and Their Associates. The National Heart, Lung, and Blood Institute Coronary Artery Surgery Study (CASS). *Circulation* 63 (Suppl. I):I-1, 1981.
10. Kennedy JW, Kllip T, Fisher LD, et al. The clinical spectrum of coronary artery disease and its surgical and medical management, 1974–1979. The Coronary Artery Surgery Study. *Circulation* 66 (Suppl. III):III-16, 1982.
11. Proudfit WL, Welch CC, Siqueira C, et al. Prognosis of 1000 young women studied by coronary angiography. *Circulation* 64:1185, 1981.
12. Welch CC, Proudfit WL, Sheldon WC. Coronary arteriographic findings in 1,000 women under age 50. *Am J Cardiol* 35:211, 1975.
13. Waters DD, Halphen C, Theroux P, et al. Coronary artery disease in young women: Clinical and angiographic features and correlation with risk factors. *Am J Cardiol* 42:41, 1978.
14. Chaitman BR, Bourassa MG, Lam J, et al. Noninvasive diagnosis of coronary heart disease in women. In Eaker ED, Packard B, Wenger NK, et al. (Eds.), *Coronary Heart Disease in Women.* New York, Haymarket Doyma, 1987, p. 222.
15. Selzer A, Langston M, Ruggeroli C, et al. Clinical syndrome of variant angina with normal coronary arteriogram. *N Engl J Med* 295:1343, 1976.
16. Pasternak RC, Hutter AM Jr, DeSanctis RW, et al. Variant angina. Clinical spectrum and results of medical and surgical therapy. *J Thorac Cardiovasc Surg* 78:614, 1979.
17. Scholl J-M, Veau P, Benacerraf A, et al. Long-term prognosis of medically treated patients with vasospastic angina and no fixed significant coronary atherosclerosis. *Am Heart J* 115:559, 1988
18. National Cooperative Study Group. Unstable angina pectoris: National Cooperative Study Group to compare surgical and medical therapy. III. Results in patients with S-T segment elevation during pain. *Am J Cardiol* 45:819, 1980.
19. Cannon RO III, Watson RM, Rosing DR, et al. Angina caused by reduced vasodilator reserve of the small coronary arteries. *J Am Coll Cardiol* 1:1359, 1983.
20. Cannon RO III, Camici PG, Epstein SE. Pathophysiological dilemma of syndrome X. *Circulation* 85:883, 1992.
21. Kannel WB, Abbott RD. Incidence and prognosis of myocardial infarction in women: The Framingham study. In Eaker ED, Packard B, Wenger NK, et al. (Eds.), *Coronary Heart Disease in Women.* New York, Haymarket Doyma, 1987, p. 208.
22. Johansson S, Ulvenstam G, Vedin A, et al. Sex differences in postinfarction prognosis and secondary risk factors. In Oliver MF, Vedin A, Wilhelmsson C (Eds.), *Myocardial Infarction in Women.* New York, Churchill Livingstone, 1986, p. 200.

23. Harper RW, Kennedy G, DeSanctis RW, et al. The incidence and pattern of angina prior to acute myocardial infarction: A study of 577 cases. *Am Heart J* 97:178, 1979.
24. Tofler GH, Stone PH, Muller JE, et al. Effects of gender and race on prognosis after myocardial infarction: Adverse prognosis for women, particularly black women. *J Am Coll Cardiol* 9:473, 1987.
25. Johansson S, Bergstrand R, Schlossman D, et al. Sex differences in cardioangiographic findings after myocardial infarction. *Eur Heart J* 5:374, 1984.
26. Pohjola S, Siltanen P, Romo M. Five-year survival of 728 patients after myocardial infarction. A community study. *Br Heart J* 43:176, 1980.
27. Marmor A, Geltman EM, Schechtman K, et al. Recurrent myocardial infarction: Clinical predictors and prognostic implications. *Circulation* 66:415, 1982.
28. Tofler GH, Stone PH, Muller JE, et al. Clinical manifestations of coronary heart disease in women. In Eaker ED, Packard B, Wenger NK, et al. (Eds.), *Coronary Heart Disease in Women*. New York, Haymarket Doyma, 1987, p. 215.
29. Puletti M, Sunseri L, Curione M, et al. Acute myocardial infarction: Sex-related differences in prognosis. *Am Heart J* 108:63, 1984.
30. Kannel WB, Sorlie P, McNamara PM. Prognosis after initial myocardial infarction: The Framingham Study. *Am J Cardiol* 44:53, 1979.
31. Waters DD. General discussion of Session III. In Eaker ED, Packard B, Wenger NK, et al. (Eds.), *Coronary Heart Disease in Women*. New York, Haymarket Doyma, 1987, p. 264.
32. Smith JW, Marcus FI, Serokman R, with the Multicenter Postinfarction Research Group. Prognosis of patients with diabetes mellitus after acute myocardial infarction. *Am J Cardiol* 54:718, 1984.
33. Greenland P, Reicher-Reiss H, Goldbourt U, et al. In-hospital and 1-year mortality in 1,524 women after myocardial infarction: Comparison with 4,315 men. *Circulation* 83:484, 1991.
34. Johansson S, Bergstrand R, Pennert K, et al. Cessation of smoking after myocardial infarction in women. Effects on mortality and reinfarctions. *Am J Epidemiol* 121:823, 1985.
35. Italian Group for the Study of Streptokinase in Myocardial Infarction (GISSI). Effectiveness of intravenous thrombolytic treatment in acute myocardial infarction. *Lancet* 1:397, 1986.
36. Maynard C, Althouse R, Cerqueira M, et al. Underutilization of thrombolytic therapy in eligible women with acute myocardial infarction. *Am J Cardiol* 68:529, 1991.
37. Gruppo Italiano per lo Studio della Streptochinasi nell'Infarto Miocardico (GISSI). Long-term effects of intravenous thrombolysis in acute myocardial infarction: Final report of the GISSI study. *Lancet* 2:871, 1987.
38. Pedersen TR. Six-year follow-up of the Norwegian Multicenter Study on timolol after acute myocardial infarction. *N Engl J Med* 313:1055, 1985.
39. ISIS-2 (Second International Study of Infarct Survival) Collaborative Group. Randomised trial of intravenous streptokinase, oral aspirin, both, or neither among 17,187 cases of suspected acute myocardial infarction: ISIS-2. *Lancet* 2:349, 1988.
40. Oldridge NB, LaSalle D, Jones NL, et al. Exercise rehabilitation of female patients with coronary artery disease. *Am Heart J* 100:755, 1980.
41. Engel HJ, Engel E, Lichtlen PR. Angiographic findings after myocardial infarction in women aged ≤50 years—role of oral contraceptives. In Oliver MF, Vedin A, Wilhelmsson C (Eds.), *Myocardial Infarction in Women*. New York, Churchill Livingstone, 1986, p. 173.
42. Vlodaver Z, Edwards JE. Rupture of ventricular septum or papillary muscle complicating myocardial infarction. *Circulation* 55:815, 1977.
43. Radford MJ, Johnson RA, Daggett WM Jr, et al. Ventricular septal rupture: A review of clinical and physiologic features and an analysis of survival. *Circulation* 64:545, 1981.
44. Naeim F, de la Maza LM, Robbins SL. Cardiac rupture during myocardial infarction. A review of 44 cases. *Circulation* 45:1231, 1972.
45. Moss AJ, Carleen E, and the Multicenter Postinfarction Research Group. Gender differences in the mortality risk associated with ventricular arrhythmias after myocardial infarction. In Eaker ED, Packard B, Wenger NK, et al. (Eds.), *Coronary Heart Disease in Women*. New York, Haymarket Doyma, 1987, p. 204.
46. Vaitkus PT, Kindwall KE, Miller JM, et al: Influence of gender on inducibility of ventricular arrhythmias in survivors of cardiac arrest with coronary artery disease. *Am J Cardiol* 67:537, 1991.
47. Boucek RJ, Romanelli R, Willis WH Jr, et al. Sex differences in obstructive coronary artery disease in patients 65 years of age or older with angina pectoris. *Circulation* 66:926, 1982.
48. Herman MV, Evans MD, Kay RH. Coronary heart disease and ventricular dysfunction in women. In Eaker ED, Packard B, Wenger NK, et al. (Eds.), *Coronary Heart Disease in Women*. New York, Haymarket Doyma, 1987, p. 198.
49. Mann JI, Vessey MP, Thorogood M, et al. Myocardial infarction in young women with special reference to oral contraceptive practice. *Br Med J* 2:241, 1975.
50. Fisher LD, Kennedy JW, Davis KB, et al. Association of sex, physical size, and operative mortality after coronary artery bypass in the Coronary Artery Surgery Study (CASS). *J Thorac Cardiovasc Surg* 84:334, 1982.
51. Loop FD, Golding LR, MacMillan JP, et al. Coronary artery surgery in women compared with men: Analyses of risks and long-term results. *J Am Coll Cardiol* 1:383, 1983.
52. Gardner TJ, Horneffer PJ, Gott VL, et al. Coronary artery bypass grafting in women. A ten-year perspective. *Ann Surg* 201:780, 1985.
53. Khan SS, Nessim S, Gray R, et al. Increased mortality of women in coronary artery bypass surgery: Evidence for referral bias. *Ann Intern Med* 112:561, 1990.
54. Kennedy JW, Kaiser GC, Fisher LD, et al. Clinical and angiographic predictors of operative mortality from the collaborative study in coronary artery surgery (CASS). *Circulation* 63:793, 1981.
55. Cowley MJ, Mullin SM, Kelsey SF, et al. Sex differences in early and long-term results of coronary angioplasty in the NHLBI PTCA Registry. *Circulation* 71:90, 1985.
56. Boogaard MAK, Briody ME. Comparison of the rehabilitation of men and women post-myocardial infarction. *J Cardiopulmonary Rehabil* 5:379, 1985.
57. Cohn PF. Silent myocardial ischemia. *Ann Intern Med* 109:312, 1988.
58. Alison HW, Russell RO Jr, Mantle JA, et al. Coro-

nary anatomy and arteriography in patients with unstable angina pectoris. *Am J Cardiol* 41:204, 1978.
59. Krueger DE, Ellenberg SS, Bloom S, et al. Risk factors for fatal heart attack in young women. *Am J Epidemiol* 113:357, 1981.
60. Spain DM, Siegel H, Bradess VA. Women smokers and sudden death: The relationship of cigarette smoking to coronary disease. *JAMA* 224:1005, 1973.
61. Talbott E, Kuller LH, Detre K, et al. Biologic and psychosocial risk factors of sudden death from coronary disease in white women. *Am J Cardiol* 39:858, 1977.
62. Jecker NS. Age-based rationing and women. *JAMA* 266:3012, 1991.
63. Tobin JN, Wassertheil-Smoller S, Wexler JP, et al. Sex bias in considering coronary bypass surgery. *Ann Intern Med* 107:19, 1987.
64. Stanton BA, Jenkins CD, Denlinger P, et al. Predictors of employment status after cardiac surgery. *JAMA* 249:907, 1983.
65. Savage MP, Goldberg S, Hirshfeld JW, et al. Clinical and angiographic determinants of primary coronary angioplasty success. *J Am Coll Cardiol* 17:22, 1991.
66. Holmes DR Jr, Holubkov R, Vlietstra RE, et al. Comparison of complications during percutaneous transluminal coronary angioplasty from 1977 to 1981 and from 1985 to 1986: The National Heart, Lung, and Blood Institute Percutaneous Transluminal Coronary Angioplasty Registry. *J Am Coll Cardiol* 12:1149, 1988.
67. Parisi AF, Folland ED, Hartigan P. A comparison of angioplasty with medical therapy in the treatment of single-vessel coronary artery disease. *N Engl J Med* 326:10, 1992.
68. Ayanian JZ, Epstein AM. Differences in the use of procedures between women and men hospitalized for coronary heart disease. *N Engl J Med* 325:221, 1991.
69. Steingart RM, Packer M, Hamm P, et al. Sex differences in the management of coronary artery disease. *N Engl J Med* 325:226, 1991.
70. Wenger NK. Coronary heart disease in women: An overview (myths, misperceptions, and missed opportunities). In Wenger NK, Speroff L, Packard B (Eds.), *Cardiovascular Health and Disease in Women* Greenwich, CT, LeJacq Communications, in press.
71. Chaitman BR, Bourassa MG, Davis K, et al. Angiographic prevalence of high-risk coronary artery disease in patient subsets (CASS). *Circulation* 64:360, 1981.
72. Weiner DA, Ryan TJ, McCabe CH, et al. Exercise stress testing. Correlations among history of angina, ST-segment response and prevalence of coronary-artery disease in the Coronary Artery Surgery Study (CASS). *N Engl J Med* 301:230, 1979.
73. Detry J-M R, Kapita BM, Cosyns J, et al. Diagnostic value of history and maximal exercise electrocardiography in men and women suspected of coronary heart disease. *Circulation* 56:756, 1977.
74. Melin JA, Wijns W, Vanbutsele RJ, et al. Alternative diagnostic strategies for coronary artery disease in women: Demonstration of the usefulness and efficiency of probability analysis. *Circulation* 71:535, 1985.
75. McCarthy DM, Sciacca RR, Blood DK, et al. Discriminant function analysis using thallium-201 scintiscans and exercise stress test variables to predict the presence and extent of coronary artery disease. *Am J Cardiol* 49:1917, 1982.
76. Guiteras Val P, Chaitman BR, Waters DD, et al. Diagnostic accuracy of exercise ECG lead systems in clinical subsets of women. *Circulation* 65:1465, 1982.
77. Hung J, Chaitman BR, Lam J, et al. Noninvasive diagnostic test choices for the evaluation of coronary artery disease in women: A multivariate comparison of cardiac fluoroscopy, exercise electrocardiography and exercise thallium myocardial perfusion scintigraphy. *J Am Coll Cardiol* 4:8, 1984.
78. Hlatky MA, Pryor DB, Harrell FE Jr, et al. Factors affecting sensitivity and specificity of exercise electrocardiography. Multivariable analysis. *Am J Med* 77:64, 1984.
79. Barolsky SM, Gilbert CA, Faruqui A, et al. Differences in electrocardiographic response to exercise of women and men: A non-Bayesian factor. *Circulation* 60:1021, 1979.
80. Sternby NH. Sex differences in atherosclerosis. In Oliver MF, Vedin A, Wilhelmsson C (Eds.), *Myocardial Infarction in Women*. New York, Churchill Livingstone, 1986, p. 166.
81. Goodgold HM, Rehder JG, Samuels LD, et al. Improved interpretation of exercise Tl-201 myocardial perfusion scintigraphy in women: Characterization of breast attenuation artifacts. *Radiology* 165:361, 1987.
82. Fintel DJ, Links JM, Brinker JA, et al. Improved diagnostic performance of exercise thallium-201 single photon emission computed tomography over planar imaging in the diagnosis of coronary artery disease: A receiver operating characteristic analysis. *J Am Coll Cardiol* 13:600, 1989.
83. Friedman TD, Greene AC, Iskandrian AS, et al. Exercise thallium-201 myocardial scintigraphy in women: Correlation with coronary arteriography. *Am J Cardiol* 49:1632, 1982.
84. Greenberg PS, Berge RD, Johnson KD, et al. The value and limitation of radionuclide angiography with stress in women. *Clin Cardiol* 6:312, 1983.
85. Higginbotham MB, Morris KG, Coleman RE, et al. Sex-related differences in the normal cardiac response to upright exercise. *Circulation* 70:357, 1984.
86. Gibbons RJ, Lee KL, Cobb F, et al. Ejection fraction response to exercise in patients with chest pain and normal coronary arteriograms. *Circulation* 64:952, 1981.
87. Hanley PC, Zinsmeister AR, Clements IP, et al. Gender-related differences in cardiac response to supine exercise assessed by radionuclide angiography. *J Am Coll Cardiol* 13:624, 1989.
88. Sullivan MJ, Cobb FR, Higginbotham MB. Stroke volume increases by similar mechanisms during upright exercise in normal men and women. *Am J Cardiol* 67:1405, 1991.
89. Hakki A-H, Iskandrian AS. Effect of gender on left ventricular function during exercise in patients with coronary artery disease. *Am Heart J* 111:543, 1986.
90. Gibbons RJ, Lee KL, Pryor D, et al. The use of radionuclide angiography in the diagnosis of coronary artery disease—a logistic regression analysis. *Circulation* 68:740, 1983.
91. Gibbons RJ, Fyke FE III, Clements IP, et al. Noninvasive identification of severe coronary artery disease using exercise radionuclide angiography. *J Am Coll Cardiol* 11:28, 1988.
92. Sawada SG, Ryan T, Fineberg NS, et al. Exercise echocardiographic detection of coronary artery disease in women. *J Am Coll Cardiol* 14:1440, 1989.
93. Masini M, Picano E, Lattanzi F, et al. High dose

dipyridamole-echocardiography test in women: Correlation with exercise-electrocardiography test and coronary arteriography. *J Am Coll Cardiol* 12:682, 1988.
94. Rifkin RD, Parisi AF, Folland E. Coronary calcification in the diagnosis of coronary artery disease. *Am J Cardiol* 44:141, 1979.
95. Hamby RI, Tabrah F, Wisoff BG, et al. Coronary artery calcification: Clinical implications and angiographic correlates. *Am Heart J* 87:565, 1974.
96. Ghazzal ZMB, Weintraub WS, Renwick G, et al. Calcification of the coronary arteries and the diagnosis of coronary heart disease in women. *Emory J Med* 5:9, 1991.
97. Hubbard BL, Gibbons RJ, Lapeyre AC III, et al. Identification of severe coronary artery disease using simple clinical parameters. *Arch Intern Med* 152:309, 1992.
98. Robert AR, Melin JA, Detry J-M R. Logistic discriminant analysis improves diagnostic accuracy of exercise testing for coronary artery disease in women. *Circulation* 83:1202, 1991.

CHAPTER 3

Coronary Heart Disease: Therapeutic Principles

SUSAN B. EYSMANN, M.D.
PAMELA S. DOUGLAS, M.D.

Coronary heart disease accounts for 250,000 deaths among women each year in the United States and is responsible for approximately one-third of all deaths in women. Despite the fact that heart disease is the leading cause of death among women and men, investigations into therapeutic interventions for coronary artery disease have been conducted almost exclusively in male populations. The U.S. Physician's Health Study demonstrating the benefits of prophylactic aspirin in decreasing the risk of myocardial infarction, the Veteran's Administration Cooperative Study and the European Coronary Surgery Study demonstrating the role of coronary artery bypass grafting in atherosclerotic coronary artery disease, and the Multiple Risk Factor Intervention Trial demonstrating the importance of risk factor modification are examples of major clinical studies with widespread influence on the management of patients with coronary artery disease that have not included women. Thus, there is a relative paucity of information on gender-specific responses to the treatment of coronary artery disease. Specifically, information for women patients regarding the primary prevention of ischemic heart disease, pharmacologic therapy for known coronary artery disease (secondary treatment), rehabilitation from ischemic heart disease, and the role of estrogen in the management of heart disease is greatly needed. The following discussion covers currently available data on the broad topics of primary prevention, secondary treatment, and medical management after myocardial infarction in women. With the exception of data on angioplasty and bypass surgery, for which gender-related differences in acute and long-term outcomes have been reported by several well-conducted trials, data on women appear to be lacking. Although much of the information learned from studies of male patients is germane, this chapter has attempted to highlight areas in which specific data are available for women, in which gender differences exist, and in which little information specific to women is known. If a given therapy for coronary artery disease has been excluded from this discussion, this does not imply that it is not effective but merely that its efficacy has not been well studied in this population.

CORONARY ARTERY DISEASE: PRIMARY PREVENTION

Many risk factors for coronary heart disease are shared by men and women including increased age, systemic hypertension, family history of premature coronary artery disease, sedentariness, cigarette smoking, plasma lipoprotein levels, diabetes mellitus, and obesity. Factors unique to women include oral contraceptive use, menopause, hysterectomy, and exogenous hormone use (1). Modification of one or more risk factors has been proposed as effective medical therapy in women as in men and will be discussed at length in subsequent chapters. However, few studies of risk factor modification have been performed in women using the clinical end point of cardiovascular disease or death.

In addition to known risk factor modification, prophylactic aspirin use represents a primary prevention for coronary heart disease. Whether aspirin has a reduced antithrombotic effect in women is controversial (2), with some laboratory studies (3–6), but not all (7–9), supporting the possibility. Aspirin has not been found to be equally efficacious in women and men in a variety of clinical settings. For example, the protective effects of aspirin against venous thromboembolism after total hip replacement (10) and against stroke or death in patients with threatened stroke (11) have been limited to men in some studies. Thus, data from men on the prevention of coronary heart disease with aspirin prophylaxis may not be generalizable to women (see Chapter 12 for further discussion).

The role of aspirin in the primary prevention of coronary heart disease in women has thus far been examined in several observational studies in which aspirin use was recorded historically. Results with this approach have been contradictory. In a cohort study of 8881 women and 5106 men in a retirement community in California, aspirin use reported historically was associated with an increased risk of ischemic heart disease in both men and women, and a reduced risk of acute myocardial infarction in men only (12). Aspirin use was evaluated only at the time of entry into the study, which had a 6.5-year follow-up period. In a smaller study of 3134 women without heart disease, stroke, systemic hypertension, or diabetes, the ratio of observed to expected deaths from coronary heart disease in women who reported using aspirin often was higher than that in women who never or seldom used aspirin (13). There are several possible interpretations of these data. Reported aspirin use may have caused the increased risk of ischemic heart disease, or, more likely, aspirin use could have been a marker for patients at greater risk of ischemic heart disease.

In contrast to these results, in the Nurses' Health Study, a 6-year observational study of over 87,000 healthy registered nurses 34 to 59 years of age, historically reported use of one to six aspirin tablets per week reduced the age-adjusted relative risk of a first myocardial infarction by 25% compared to nonusers (2). However, no risk reduction was observed in women who took more than seven aspirin per week. A primary prevention randomized trial of aspirin, the Women's Health Study, is now under way in women and is similar to those conducted in men.

Estrogen replacement therapy in postmenopausal women has not been completely examined but may be the most powerful form of primary prevention against coronary heart disease in women. A complete discussion of this topic can be found in Chapter 8.

SECONDARY TREATMENT OF CORONARY ARTERY DISEASE

Access to Care and Gender Bias

There is evidence that in clinical practice, coronary artery disease is less aggressively diagnosed and subsequently treated in women than in men. Although angina is the most common expression of coronary artery disease in women (14), fewer women than men with chest pain are referred for diagnostic studies. Tobin and colleagues have reported that after a positive nuclear exercise test, men were 10 times more likely than women to be referred for diagnostic cardiac catheterization but equally likely to be receiving antianginal drug therapy (15). Tobin and associates also found that women, even after similarly positive tests, were twice as likely as men to have their presenting symptoms attributed to somatic, psychiatric, or noncardiac causes. Such confusion about the diagnosis of coronary disease in women necessarily limits physicians' and patients' perceived effectiveness of antianginal therapy.

Steingart and colleagues found that women with postinfarction angina underwent cardiac catheterization only half as often as men and were twice as likely as men to be excluded from participation in the Survival and Ventricular Enlargement (SAVE) trial because cardiac catheterization was required for enrollment (16). Unequal access to diagnostic testing has most likely restricted the enrollment of women in clinical trials, thereby limiting the information available to guide treatment in female patients.

Gender differences in the application of therapeutic interventions are well documented. Khan et al., Loop et al., and the Coronary Artery Surgery Study (CASS) investigators have all found that women have been referred for coronary artery bypass graft (CABG) surgery later in the course of their disease than men (17–19). Women were frequently referred for bypass surgery with symptoms of unstable angina, heart failure, or cardiogenic shock, whereas men were more commonly referred for surgery after an abnormal exercise test. A report from the National Heart, Lung, and Blood Institute (NHLBI) coronary angioplasty registry showed similar differences between men and women referred for coronary angioplasty (20). Investigators from the Cleveland Clinic observed that women were more likely to have angina of increased frequency and severity than men referred for angioplasty. Furthermore, in the first 20 months after angioplasty, women reported features of typical angina more often and were hospitalized for chest pain more frequently (21% versus 13%, $p < .05$) than men but were referred for exercise testing less often (51% versus 60%, $p < .05$) despite prior angiographic documentation of coronary artery disease (21).

Steingart et al. determined that once women did undergo cardiac catheterization, they were as likely as men to be referred for coronary surgery (16). Healy has described these referral patterns for women as the Yentl syndrome at work: Once women have been shown to have coronary artery disease, they are then treated as men would be (22).

Sex-related differences in the prevalence of cardiovascular disease do not fully explain these gender-related differences in referral patterns for cardiac catheterization, angioplasty, and bypass surgery (16). It is possible that fewer women are referred for cardiac procedures because of concern about higher operative mortality rates in women undergoing coronary bypass surgery (18, 23–25). However, higher mortality rates may be the result of referral bias rather than its cause because women have more advanced disease at the time of referral. Alternatively, these referral pattern differences may suggest that men are over-referred for cardiac diagnostic and therapeutic procedures.

Drug Therapy

Antianginal Therapy. The mainstays of medical therapy for coronary heart disease include beta blockers, nitrates, and calcium antagonists. Such therapies may be equally effective in men and women, although few data regarding usefulness in women are available. The CASS, which included only 19% women, has not directly compared medical and surgical outcomes in women (26). Women in general have smaller coronary arteries in relation to their smaller body size (27), so that fluctuations in coronary tone may be of increased importance (28, 29). Therefore, nitrates and calcium antagonists may be preferred antianginal therapies in women; however, there are no clinical data available that examine this issue. Similarly, no large clinical trial has addressed the efficacy of any form of medical therapy for chronic stable angina in women.

Hormone Replacement Therapy. In addition to its use in preventing atherosclerosis, estrogen replacement therapy may also be a valuable treatment for women with known coronary artery disease. In a retrospective study of 2268 postmenopausal women undergoing coronary angiography, Sullivan et al. (30) reported that women who had received estrogen replacement had prolonged survival when coronary artery disease was present. Among women with mild to moderate coronary stenoses, 10-year survival was 85% in women who had never used estrogen compared to 95.6% in women who had ever used estrogen. In women with 70% coronary stenoses, survival was 60% among "never users" and 97% among "ever users." Estrogen use was found to have a significant independent effect on survival in women, but the effect was less in the absence of coronary artery disease. The potential of estrogen therapy in the management of coronary heart disease in women and the controversies which surround its efficacy and risks are further discussed in Chapter 8.

Management of Syndrome X. Syndrome X is a term coined to describe the patient presenting with chest pain and normal epicardial coronary arteries. The original report by Likoff et al. (31) in 1967 was a description of 15 women. Since then, many studies have described both women and men with the syndrome, although a female predominance has been generally accepted. Common aspects of the syndrome include atypical chest pain, demonstrable myocardial ischemia in only a subset of patients, inconsistent responses to conventional anti-ischemia therapy, and excellent long-term survival (32). Unfortunately, the exact etiology and therefore appropriate therapy have remained obscure, although several pathophysiologic characteristics of the syndrome have been examined. Some suggest that the syndrome represents a disorder of the microvascular circulation with reduced coronary vasodilator reserve (32). The demonstration of coexisting abnormal forearm hyperemic responses to ischemia (33), esophageal motility abnormalities (34), and abnormal bronchoconstrictor responses to methacholine inhalation (35) in some patients suggests a more generalized disorder of vascular and nonvascular smooth muscle function (32). Insulin resistance, lower pain thresholds, and deterioration in left ventricular function over time have all been reported in subgroups of these patients (32). In their recent review, Cannon et al. suggest that a primary disorder of smooth muscle itself or factors that regulate smooth muscle, including endothelial, neural, and hormonal factors, may eventually be uncovered (32). Given the female predominance of syndrome X, estrogen may be a regulatory factor worth close examination.

Cannon et al. (32) suggest beginning the management of patients with syndrome X with conventional anti-ischemic therapy, especially if there is evidence of inducible ischemia on stress testing. A trial of empirical therapy may be warranted in others. In all patients risk factor modification should be instituted (as discussed elsewhere in this text). In the absence of demonstrable ischemia, normal activity and exercise should be encouraged, and the routine use of narcotics, hospitalization, and repeat catheterizations after episodes of chest pain should be avoided.

Interventional Therapy

Acute Outcome. In data collected on 705 women and 2374 men in the NHLBI percutaneous transluminal coronary angioplasty (PTCA) registry through 1982, the initial years of clinical angioplasty application, significant gender differences were noted (20). At baseline, women were older, had a higher prevalence of severe angina and of unstable angina, had a longer duration of angina, and more frequently had a history of hypertension. Men more often had multivessel disease, prior bypass surgery, and an ejection fraction of less than 50%. Women undergoing PTCA had a lower clinical success rate (56% versus 62%), a lower angiographic success rate (60% versus 66%), and a higher in-hospital mortality rate (1.8% versus 0.7%) than men (Table 3–1). Multivariate analysis revealed female gender to be an independent correlate of reduced success with angioplasty in addition to prior CABG and age over 60 years. Compared with outcomes in men, unsuccessful results in women were more often due to failure to cannulate the artery and failure to cross the coronary lesion. Women's higher complication rates resulted from an increased incidence of coronary dissection, bradycardia, and hypotension. Despite increased in-hospital mortality in women, major complications as a whole (death plus nonfatal myocardial infarction plus emergency surgery) were no different in men and women. Mortality associated with emergency bypass surgery was much higher in women than in men (17.4% versus 3.2%), whereas

Table 3–1. PERCUTANEOUS TRANSLUMINAL CORONARY ANGIOPLASTY: GENDER DIFFERENCES IN BASELINE CHARACTERISTICS AND OUTCOME

	NHLBI PTCA Registry (20) (1977—9/1982)		Cleveland Clinic (21) (12/1980—12/1986)		Medical College of Virginia (38) (7/1979—8/1985)		Medical College of Virginia (38) (After 8/1985)	
	Women	Men	Women	Men	Women	Men	Women	Men
Baseline Characteristics								
Patients (N)	705	2374	969	2727	272	628	90	210
Mean age (yr)	56[a]	53	61	57				
Angina class 3 or 4 (%)	71[a]	61	51[c]	36				
Prior MI (%)	22.4	25.7	32	34				
Prior CABG (%)	5.5[b]	8.8	9[c]	15				
Clinical Results of PTCA								
Clinical success (%)	56.6[a]	62.3			82[a]	86	87	94
Angiographic success (%)	60.3[a]	66.2	93	93.5				
Procedural Difficulties								
Intimal tear (%)	16.5[b]	10.7	35[a]	30				
Complications								
Dissection (%)	5.8[b]	4.0	2.6	2.2				
Occlusion (%)	5.0	4.9	3.8	3.0				
Spasm (%)	4.7	4.1	0.5	0.2				
Death	1.8[a]	0.7	0.3	0.09	0	0.3	0	0
Nonfatal MI	4.7	5.1	2.0	0.8	2.9	3.8	3.3	1.4
Emergency CABG within 24 hr	6.5	6.6	3.8	2.3	6.3	4.8	3.3	1.4
Follow-up Clinical Events Post PTCA	in first 18 months		in first 20 months					
MI (%)	4.6	3.9	2.9	2.0				
Late CABG (%)	10.9	14.3	7.0	6.8				

[a] $p < .05$.
[b] $p < .01$.
[c] $p < .001$ women versus men.
NHLBI = National Heart, Lung, and Blood Institute, PTCA = percutaneous transluminal coronary angioplasty, MI = myocardial infarction, CABG = coronary artery bypass graft surgery.

mortality rates for elective CABG after failed PTCA were similar.

McEniery et al. (21), however, found equal success rates with angiographic angioplasty (both 93%) and emergency surgery (3.8% versus 3.2%) and similar death rates (0.3% versus 0.09%) in 969 women and 2727 men who underwent angioplasty from 1980 through 1986 at the Cleveland Clinic (see Table 3–1). However, during coronary angioplasty, women had significantly more procedural difficulties than men: more frequent ST-segment shifts during balloon inflation, more guiding catheter problems, more intimal tears at the PTCA site, and more problems with vascular access (21). In contrast to the NHLBI series, although the rate of all complications was slightly increased in women, the difference between the sexes was not statistically significant.

Ellis et al. (36) analyzed over 8000 PTCA procedures from the Emory experience between 1980 and 1986 and found that female gender, multivessel disease, and the presence of collaterals distal to the PTCA site independently predicted mortality after abrupt closure. Twelve of thirteen patients who died in connection with a cardiac complication were women.

To evaluate the effects of advancements in technology, refinements in technique, increasing operator experience, and higher-risk patients undergoing PTCA, Holmes and colleagues (37) compared results in the NHLBI PTCA registry through 1981 with procedures performed in 1985 and 1986. Despite overall reductions in complication rates, mortality, and improved success rates, female gender was again strongly correlated with increased in-hospital mortality in addition to advanced age, severe coronary disease, and poor left ventricular function. Cowley et al. (38) compared the results of acute angioplasty at the Medical College of Virginia prior to August 1985 with results after August 1985 in women (see Table

3–1). Clinical success improved from 82% to 87% in women and from 86% to 94% in men. Although clinical success prior to August 1985 was significantly different between the sexes, this difference was no longer significant in more recent years. Together, these studies suggest that with technologic advancements and increased operator experience, short-term angioplasty outcomes have improved in women.

More recently, the Cleveland Clinic has published preliminary data that, among patients who underwent coronary atherectomy, women had a higher complication rate than men (39). By multivariate analysis, female gender was a predictor of a major acute complication (emergency surgery or death) independent of age or presence of diabetes ($p < .03$). Preliminary studies with patients undergoing directional atherectomy and Palmaz-Schatz intracoronary stent placement at the Beth Israel Hospital have suggested that women have slightly lower success rates with the new device, equal major complication rates (emergency surgery, death, myocardial infarction), but more frequent minor complications (transfusion, vascular surgery, non-Q wave myocardial infarction) when compared with men (Fishman and Baime, personal communication).

It has been suggested that the early use of 3.0-mm PTCA balloons, which were sometimes oversized for women, predisposed women to abrupt closure with subsequent higher in-hospital mortality (40). Women's smaller body size and associated smaller caliber peripheral arteries make vascular access more complicated. The fact that more recent atherectomy and stent data confirm higher overall complication rates in women, however, suggests that other unknown factors predispose women to an increased risk of complications. Ellis and colleagues (36) have hypothesized that mortality from abrupt coronary artery closure is more likely to occur in women because they have a smaller intravascular volume and hence are less likely to adjust their volume status appropriately to cope with that physiologic stress. Additionally, they suggest that the smaller coronary arteries in women may contribute to the underestimation of the severity of coronary artery disease (40).

Long-Term Outcome and Restenosis. At a mean follow-up time of 18 months, the 305 women in the initial NHLBI study who underwent successful PTCA had similar symptomatic improvement (92% versus 90%), higher event-free survival (80% versus 69%), lower rates of repeat revascularization (18% versus 27%), and lower cumulative mortality (0.3% versus 2.2%, $p < .05$) than the 1092 men in the study (20). Angiographic restenosis was significantly more common in men (36% versus 22%) than in women.

McEniery et al., reporting on the Cleveland Clinic experience (21) at a mean follow-up of 6.9 months post PTCA, found that more women reported symptoms of angina pectoris responsive to nitroglycerin (27% versus 14%) and were hospitalized for chest pain (21% versus 13%) than men. However, occurrence rates for clinical events (myocardial infarction, repeat PTCA, and CABG) were similar at follow-up in women and men (15% versus 14%).

Holmes and colleagues' study comparing the early and late NHLBI experiences also reported lower restenosis rates in women compared to men (37). This finding has been observed in numerous additional studies (41–56). In a recent review of available data, Califf et al. concluded that the difference between restenosis rates in men and women was small (36% versus 28%) but highly significant (57, 58). However, two recent studies (59, 60) from the Cleveland Clinic failed to identify gender as a risk factor for restenosis post PTCA. In addition, in a careful meta-analysis that reviewed 212 published reports on angioplasty and selected 31 reports most likely to produce unbiased results, gender was not found to be significantly correlated with post-PTCA restenosis (61). In recent reports of predictors of restenosis following intracoronary stenting and directional atherectomy (62, 63), gender again was not found to be significant. These findings are consistent with the hypothesis that previously reported higher restenosis rates in men may have represented inadequate initial results in luminal reduction in the larger coronary arteries of men due to older angioplasty equipment (58). Most studies of restenosis are limited by incomplete angiographic follow-up, varying definitions of restenosis, and lack of multivariate analysis that corrects for confounding variables such as post-procedure luminal diameter. For all these reasons, at the present time the role of gender in the mechanism and rate of restenosis is uncertain.

In summary, although these data suggest that percutaneous interventions for coronary artery disease in women may yield higher in-

Table 3–2. OPERATIVE MORTALITY FOR MEN AND WOMEN AFTER CORONARY ARTERY BYPASS GRAFT SURGERY

Author and Affiliation	Study Period	Operative Mortality (%)		Relative Risk
		Men (n)	*Women (n)*	
Bolooki et al. (25) (U of Miami)	1969–1973	2.0 (51)	8.8 (34)	4.84
Tyras et al. (23) (St Louis U)	1970–1977	2.4 (1300)	3.7 (241)	1.58
Kennedy et al. (68) (CASS)	1975–1978	1.9 (5569)	4.5 (1061)	2.44
Douglas et al. (24) (Emory U)	1973–1979	1.0 (2663)	2.2 (492)	2.15
Killen et al. (69) (Mid-America Heart Inst)	1970–1976	0.9 (2243)	1.3 (385)	1.46
Loop et al. (18) (Cleveland Clinic)	1967–1981	1.3 (18,079)	2.9 (2445)	2.20
Hall et al. (70) (Texas Heart Inst)	1970–1981	2.6 (19,175)	5.3 (3109)	2.10
Laird-Meeter et al. (71) (Rotterdam)	1971–1980	1.0 (915)	2.4 (126)	2.46
Gardner et al. (72) (Johns Hopkins)	1974–1983	3.0 (2640)	7.4 (639)	2.57

The relative risk is the ratio of the mortality rate for women and the mortality rate for men.
n = number of patients; CASS = Coronary Artery Surgery Study.
From Davis KB. Coronary artery bypass graft surgery in women. In Eaker ED, Packard B, Wenger NK, et al. (Eds.), *Coronary Artery Disease in Women.* New York, Haymarket-Doyma, 1987, p. 249.

hospital mortality and procedural morbidity, few studies have adjusted these data for the baseline discrepancies in age and coronary artery size between men and women. The favorable long-term outcome in women post PTCA suggests that once the initial higher rate of complications is overcome, percutaneous interventions may be an excellent therapeutic option in women.

Coronary Artery Bypass Grafting

Preoperative Differences. Several studies have examined the preoperative characteristics of men and women who underwent coronary artery bypass surgery (18, 23, 24, 64). In general, the women were older and had more severe anginal symptoms and more unstable angina. Women were more likely to have had diabetes, hypertension, and congestive heart failure and were less likely to have had a myocardial infarction. Women were more likely to have had normal ventricular function and fewer diseased coronary arteries preoperatively, although the proportion of patients with left main coronary artery disease was similar for men and women. Thus, women had more significant clinical risk factors and less significant angiographic risk factors preoperatively.

Operative Mortality. Operative mortality following coronary artery bypass surgery has been extensively evaluated in men and women and has been consistently found to be higher in women (18, 23–25, 66–72). Table 3–2 consolidates the operative results of nine CABG studies (18, 23–25, 68–72) that have included women (73). When these data were combined, the relative risk of death in women post CABG compared to men was 2.19 (95% confidence interval 1.94 to 2.48) (73). This difference between men and women was present across all age ranges. However, elderly women (74–76) and women with significant left main coronary disease accompanied by an elevated left ventricular end-diastolic pressure (68) had a particularly high operative mortality. In one study, the surgical mortality for females with left main coronary artery disease was twice that for males (8% versus 4%, p = .02) (77).

In several studies, operative mortality has been adjusted for preoperative baseline differences between men and women. From a much larger cohort, Douglas et al. matched 412 pairs of men and women for age, preoperative angina classification, and number of diseased vessels and found that mortality was 2% in both groups (24). In contrast, Loop et al. also matched a subgroup of men and women for age, severity of angina, and number of diseased vessels and found that operative mortality remained higher for women (2.9% versus 1.4%) (18). However, when the authors adjusted for body surface area, gender was not an important risk factor for operative death. The CASS investigators also found that the mortality difference for men and women was primarily a result of difference in coronary artery size (19). When height, anginal classification, degree of heart failure, angiographic characteristics, and priority of operation were examined, gender did not predict operative mortality. Shorter patients, whether male or female, had higher operative mortality.

Two more recent studies have suggested that the discrepancy between mortality rates for men and women has decreased over time. Gardner et al. (72) observed that the operative mortality in women who underwent bypass surgery declined from 10.7% in 1975 to 2.4% in 1983. In 1983, unlike in 1975, men and women had comparable mortality rates. Miller et al. (78) reported on the Stanford experience from 1971 to 1975 and found that women had an increased operative mortality compared to men. However, from 1977 to 1979 gender was no longer a significant factor in operative mortality. In contrast, Cosgrove et al. (65) reported on the Cleveland Clinic CABG experience from 1970 to 1982 and found that female gender was a significant incremental risk factor for mortality in both early and late (1980–1982) periods.

Symptom Relief. Men have experienced greater relief from angina after CABG than women in several studies (18, 24, 25, 79), although these studies did not adjust for the preoperative discrepancy in frequency and severity of anginal symptoms in men and women. In their overall population, Douglas et al. found that 69% of men and 54% of women were asymptomatic at a mean follow-up of 21 months (24). In their overall populations, Loop et al. (18) and Johnson et al. (79) reported that 72% and 73%, respectively, of men and 61% and 61%, respectively, of women were symptom-free at 5 years. At 10 years of follow-up more men remained asymptomatic: 65% versus 57% (18) and 55% versus 41% (79). Symptom relief was not reported in any study for the smaller subgroups of male-female pairs matched for age, preoperative angina, and extent of coronary diasease.

Graft Patency. Regardless of variable follow-up intervals, studies have consistently found graft patency rates to be higher in men than in women (18, 23–25, 80). However, patients were restudied angiographically only when this was clinically indicated; thus, patency rates cannot be considered representative of the patency rate for all patients post CABG. Since women reported more frequent anginal symptoms post CABG (see earlier discussion), male and female patients who were restudied may not have been comparable. Despite these limitations, the data on both symptom relief and patency suggest that women had a lower rate of satisfactory revascularization than men.

Dipyridamole given preoperatively plus aspirin begun 7 hours postoperatively has been shown to reduce graft occlusions within 1 month of bypass surgery in women (81). Antiplatelet therapy reduced graft occlusions from 19% with placebo to 5% with therapy. Equivalent results have been found in men.

Long-Term Survival. There is no apparent difference in 5- and 10-year survival between the sexes after CABG. Table 3–3 summarizes five studies reporting these data (18, 23, 69, 70, 82). Five-year survival ranged from 90% to 94% for men and from 87% to 91% for women. Only Loop and colleagues' 5-year survival data (18) reached statistical significance between the sexes ($p < .05$). When operative mortality was excluded, there was no 5-year survival difference between men and women in Loop and colleagues' series. Eaker et al. (64) found no difference between the sexes at 6-year follow-up in the CASS registry. Furthermore, there were no differences between men and women in predictors of long-term survival.

Internal mammary artery grafts to the left anterior descending artery have been shown to improve long-term survival and reduce late cardiac events in men (83–85). Loop et al. found that women with internal mammary artery grafts had a 10-year actuarial survival of 82.7% compared to 71.3% in women with saphenous vein grafts only, although this difference was not statistically significant (83). Increased patency rates in internal mammary grafts compared to saphenous vein grafts have also been reported in women as in men (86).

In summary, although women have a higher surgical mortality and less favorable clinical response to CABG, their long-term prognosis is similar to that of men. Thus, these studies suggest that outcome after CABG may depend

Table 3-3. LONG-TERM SURVIVAL OF MEN AND WOMEN AFTER CORONARY ARTERY BYPASS GRAFT SURGERY

Author and Affiliation	Study Period	Sample Size (N)		5-Year Survival (%)		10-Year Survival (%)	
		Men	*Women*	*Men*	*Women*	*Men*	*Women*
Tyras et al. (23) (St Louis U)	1970–1977	1300	241	94	88	—	—
Killen et al. (69) (Mid-America Heart Inst)	1971–1976	—	385	—	90	—	75
Loop et al. (18) (Cleveland Clinic)	1973–1977	4448	552	93	91	—	—
	1971–1972	1809	191	—	—	78	79
Hall et al. (70) (Texas Heart Inst)	1970–1981	19,175	3109	90	87	70	69
Myers et al. (82) (CASS)	1974–1982	7607	1364	91	88	—	—

— = data not available; CASS = Coronary Artery Surgery Study.
From Davis KB. Coronary artery bypass graft surgery in women. In Eaker ED, Packard B, Wenger NK, et al. (Eds.), *Coronary Artery Disease in Women*. New York, Haymarket-Doyma, 1987, p. 249.

less on gender than on patient size (or coronary artery size) and preoperative risk factors such as age and functional class. Furthermore, unlike with interventional results, there has been little narrowing of the gender gap over time in the outcome of revascularization surgery.

Atherosclerosis Regression

The first report of regression of coronary atherosclerosis in women treated for hyperlipidemia was published in 1990. Forty-one women and 31 men with heterozygous familial hypercholesterolemia and baseline angiographic coronary lesions were randomized into control (diet counseling plus colestipol) and treatment groups (diet counseling plus combined drug regimens) (87). The reductions in low-density lipoprotein (LDL) (38% and 38%) and increases in high-density lipoprotein (HDL) (27% and 29%) cholesterol with treatment were comparable in both sexes. The average change in mean percentage area of stenosis in coronary lesions with treatment was significant in all 72 patients but was superior in women as compared with men, in whom significant regression was not documented (women: +1.07 in controls, indicating progression, versus −2.06 in the treatment group, indicating regression, p = .05; men: +0.41 in controls versus −0.88 in the treatment group, p = .42). This study suggests that the anticipated benefit of drug and diet therapy in the treatment of coronary atherosclerosis applies to women as well as men.

Ornish and colleagues (88) performed a prospective randomized controlled trial of multiple life style changes (low-fat vegetarian diet, moderate aerobic exercise, stress management training, smoking cessation, and group support) versus usual care for 1 year in patients with angiographically documented coronary atherosclerosis. Five of the forty-one subjects were women (one in the experimental group and four in the control group). All the women were postmenopausal, and none were taking supplemental estrogens. All five women showed angiographic regression of atherosclerosis after 1 year of study despite no or only moderate life style changes. In addition, the four women in the control group showed more angiographic regression than any of the male controls, even though some control men had made greater lifestyle changes.

These two small studies suggest that women may have a greater ability to undergo coronary atherosclerotic regression than men have. A great deal of further research is needed to substantiate these findings and investigate the potential mechanisms of gender-related differences.

Rehabilitation After Revascularization

After PTCA. Nothing is known about the potential benefit of prescribed exercise in women post angioplasty. Of all rehabilitative measures, only employment status post PTCA has been commented upon. In the Cleveland Clinic experience, women demonstrated a 28% drop in engagement in full- or part-time work after PTCA, whereas men showed a 13% rise (21). Although women were only 4 years older than men on average, more women than men retired. Fewer women than men reported symptomatic improvement with PTCA (89% versus 94%), but it is unlikely that this fully explains the much larger difference in employment status.

After CABG. Men and women partake in different physical activities after bypass surgery. Although women perform activities with higher energy requirements and resume household tasks sooner than men (89), men achieve higher physical activity levels one year after CABG than women (24). In part this result may be due to the greater number of men than of women enrolling in rehabilitation programs (90). In part it may be encouraged by the lack of data on the health benefits of exercise in women with coronary disease (see Chapter 13). No large randomized trial of exercise participation after CABG has looked at gender-specific differences. In a small study of 227 men (128 post myocardial infarction, 99 post CABG) and 37 women (27 post myocardial infarction, 10 post CABG) participating in a rehabilitation program in Ireland, women had a higher drop-out rate (18.9% versus 7.9%) and reduced attendance (77% versus 87%) compared to men (91). The authors suggested that reduced female compliance may have been due to heavier family commitments or to the belief that women perform sufficient exercise at home.

Return to work after cardiac surgery has been examined by gender in several studies (92–95). In Stanton and associates' prospective longitudinal study, 73% of CABG patients returned to work within 6 months after surgery, and there were no significant sex differences (95). Other studies have reported even lower reemployment rates for women, ranging from 16% to 61% (92–94).

MYOCARDIAL INFARCTION: THERAPEUTIC PRINCIPLES

Myocardial infarction is the leading cause of death in women in the United States, totaling more than 250,000 deaths among women annually. Studies vary as to whether the immediate and long-term prognosis of women is worse than that of men after myocardial infarction. Some have reported a more severe course in women (96–99), whereas others have suggested that the gender-related difference in prognosis is fully attributable to the older age of women and the greater prevalence of other diseases when they present with infarction (100, 101). However, a recent study of 5839 patients post myocardial infarction, 1524 of whom were women, revealed an increased age-adjusted in-hospital mortality (23.1% versus 15.7%) and increased cumulative 1-year age-adjusted mortality (31.8% versus 23.1%) in women compared with men (102). Adjusting for age, congestive heart failure, prior myocardial infarction, prolonged hypotension, lactate dehydrogenase level, Swan-Ganz catheter use, atrioventricular block, and infarct location by ECG, gender persisted as an independent predictor of mortality, with adjusted relative odds of death in women versus men of 1.72 (95% confidence interval 1.45 to 2.04). The study concluded that women's increased age did not fully account for their increased mortality. However, this and other studies of gender-related prognosis after myocardial infarction predate the widespread use of thrombolysis in the management of acute myocardial infarction.

Thrombolysis

Intravenous thrombolytic therapy has become the treatment of choice for acute myocardial infarction throughout the world, reducing mortality rates in both sexes. Preliminary studies have revealed no significant differences in the pharmacokinetics, utilization, or physiologic response to thrombolytic therapy in men and women (103). Furthermore, limited studies suggest that there are no gender differences in coronary artery patency rates or in reperfusion in response to thrombolytic therapies (103).

The clinical efficacy of thrombolytic therapies is based on reductions in mortality, morbidity, and future cardiac events through the salvage of left ventricular myocardium and the preservation of function. Men comprise the overwhelming majority of subjects in all the randomized trials of thrombolytic therapy. Nevertheless, gender differences in mortality have been examined in subgroup analyses. The Second International Study of Infarct Survival (ISIS-2) is the largest published trial of thrombolysis in patients with acute myocardial infarction, containing 3945 women and 13,125 men randomized to groups receiving intravenous streptokinase, oral aspirin, both, or neither (104). Both men and women benefited most from therapy with streptokinase and aspirin, showing a 45% reduction in mortality in men and a 31% reduction in women. Table 3–4 reviews the major thrombolysis trials that have reported mortality data by gender.

In GISSI-1 (Gruppo Italiano per lo Studio della Streptochinasi nell'Infarcto Miocardico), a study of over 11,000 patients with acute myocardial infarction randomized in open-label fashion to groups receiving intravenous streptokinase versus standard care, women who received streptokinase had reduced 21-day and 12-month mortalities compared to female controls (105). However, in-hospital and 1-year mortalities of both female treatment groups post myocardial infarction were double those of males. Overall, the relative reduction in mortality with streptokinase was similar for women and for men. On reviewing ISIS-2, GISSI-1, and several other smaller thrombolytic trials (Anglo-Scandinavian Study of Early Thrombolysis [ASSET], European Working Party, and Western Washington Trial) in Table 3–4, three striking patterns become apparent. First, thrombolytic therapy reduced mortality in patients with acute myocardial infarction in both men and women. Second, the mortality of women post myocardial infarction was higher than that of men in both the placebo and thrombolytic groups. Third, GISSI excluded, these randomized trials have shown a relatively lower reduction in mortality in women compared to men.

If the pharmacokinetics and reperfusion efficacy of thrombolytic agents are similar in men and women, how can we explain why women do not benefit as much from thrombolysis as men? One hypothesis is that the older age of women presenting with myocardial infarction contributes to their relatively lower reduction in mortality post thrombolysis. Data from GISSI-2, a randomized trial comparing streptokinase (SK) alone, SK + heparin, tissue plasminogen activator (tPA) alone, and tPA + heparin, do not support this theory. Mortality for the 2482 women and 9899 men in GISSI-2 is reported in Table 3–5 by age and sex (110). For both women and men, mortality increased with increasing age. However, at every age, even at ages less than 50 years, women had a higher mortality than men.

A second hypothesis is that women have reduced myocardial salvage resulting in less effective preservation of myocardial function. Alternatively, women may have a higher rate of recurrent cardiac events post thrombolysis. No large clinical trial has published data on gender-specific differences in recovery of left ventricular function or recurrent cardiac event

Table 3–4. MORTALITY BY GENDER IN THROMBOLYSIS TRIALS

Study		N	Mortality (Thrombolysis)		Mortality (Control Group)		Reduction in Mortality (Thrombolysis)	
ISIS-2 (104)			SK + ASA		Placebo			
	Women:	3945	Women:	12.2%	Women:	17.5%	Women:	31%
	Men:	13,125	Men:	6.7%	Men:	12.0%	Men:	45%
GISSI-1 (105)			SK		Standard care			
	Women:	2313	Women:	18.5%	Women:	22.6%	Women:	19%
	Men:	9398	Men:	8.8%	Men:	10.6%	Men:	17%
GISSI-1–12-Month			SK		Standard care			
Follow-up (106)	Women:	2310	Women:	28.3%	Women:	31.3%	Women:	10%
	Men:	9386	Men:	14.5%	Men:	16.0%	Men:	10%
ASSET (107)			rtPA + heparin		Placebo + heparin			
	Women:	1151	Women:	8.6%	Women:	10.9%	Women:	21%
	Men:	3854	Men:	6.8%	Men:	9.4%	Men:	28%
European			SK		Heparin			
Working Party	Women:	133	Women:	20.3%	Women:	26.6%	Women:	24%
(108)	Men:	597	Men:	18.1%	Men:	26.2%	Men:	31%
WWT–12-Month			SK		Standard care			
Follow-up (109)	Women:	59	Women:	13.3%	Women:	21.0%	Women:	37%
	Men:	309	Men:	7.5%	Men:	13.4%	Men:	44%

ISIS = International Study of Infarct Survival, GISSI = Gruppo Italiano per lo Studio della Streptochinasi nell'Infarcto Miocardico, ASSET = Anglo-Scandinavian Study of Early Thrombolysis, WWT = Western Washington Trial, SK = streptokinase, ASA = aspirin, rtPA = reverse tissue plasminogen activator.

Table 3–5. GISSI-2: MORTALITY (%) BY AGE AND SEX

Age (years)	Male	Female
<40	1.7	4.2
41–50	2.5	4.7
51–60	4.0	5.4
61–70	7.6	11.2
71–80	15.0	22.4
>80	26.7	35.7

GISSI = Gruppo Italiano per lo Studio della Streptochi-nasi nell'Infarcto Miocardico.

From Fresco LC, Franzosi MG, Magglioni AP, et al. The GISSI-2 trial: Premises, results, epidemiological (and other) implications. *Clin Cardiol* 8:32–36, 1990. Copyrighted and reprinted with the permission of Clinical Cardiology Publishing Co., Inc. and/or the Foundation for Advances in Medicine and Science.

despite noting the gender-specific differences in mortality.

A third hypothesis is that women have a higher complication rate post thrombolysis than men. Across most studies, the risk of intracranial bleeding and stroke in selected patients receiving thrombolysis is 1% or less (111). In a review of the Thrombolysis and Angioplasty after Myocardial Infarction (TAMI) trials (112), female gender was not an independent predictor of in-hospital mortality. Nevertheless, the authors stressed the overall poor clinical outcome of elderly women compared with all other patients enrolled, an outcome that was independent of infarct vessel patency and subsequent angioplasty success rate (Table 3–6). Major bleeding (in 43%) and transfusions (in 61%) were significantly increased in women.

Hemorrhagic events in the Thrombolysis in Myocardial Infarction (TIMI) trial have also been examined by gender. Among patients who received a 100-mg dose of reverse tissue plasminogen activator (r-tPA) and were randomized to the conservative strategy, 5.9% of women versus 3.8% of men had a major hemorrhagic event (intracranial hemorrhage, cardiac tamponade, hemoglobin drop greater than 5.0 g/L, or death due to exsanguination), and 22.1% of women versus 10.8% of men had a major or minor hemorrhagic event (113). These differences are postulated to be partly related to smaller body size in women, who therefore received relatively more drug. Further investigation is needed regarding gender-specific, weight-determined, and age-determined dosage modifications of thrombolytic agents. In a circumstance unique to women, there are no published data regarding the bleeding risks of thrombolytic therapy in menstruating women who present with myocardial infarction. TAMI investigators did not withhold therapy in this group, a decision sanctioned by gynecologic colleagues, believing that potentially refractory uterine bleeding could be controlled (111).

Finally, although Table 3–4 reveals lower relative reductions in mortality with thrombolysis in women compared to those seen in men, absolute reductions appear to be similar. For example, in ISIS-2, thrombolysis reduced mortality from 17.5% to 12.2% in women, a 5.3% reduction, and from 12.0% to 6.7% in men, a 5.3% reduction. In ASSET, women's mortality fell 2.3% and men's 2.6% in absolute terms. Thus, the relatively lower reduction in benefit in women may be more a function of their high underlying mortality with myocardial infarction and less a failure of thrombolysis.

In most of the trials of thrombolytic therapy, an upper age limit of 70 or 75 years has been used. Because women suffering from acute myocardial infarction are an average of 10 years older than men (114), this may explain the relative paucity of women studied in thrombolytic trials. However, investigators of the Western Washington r-tPA trial examined the role of gender in receiving treatment after eligibility for thrombolytic therapy was established and found that only 55% of eligible women received r-tPA compared with 78% of eligible men (115). Mean age was the same for eligible women and men who were not treated. The utilization of cardiac catheterization, PTCA, and bypass surgery was not significantly different in men and women. Possible reasons for this difference in the utilization of thrombolysis were not discussed. Further assessment of gender bias in the decision to use thrombolytic agents must be evaluated if we are to offer the best care to women with evolving myocardial infarctions and if we are to improve our understanding of gender-related differences in the morbidity and mortality of women and men following thrombolysis.

Drug Therapy After Myocardial Infarction

Beta Blockers. The Beta Blocker Heart Attack Trial (BHAT) randomized 3235 men and 602 women post myocardial infarction to

Table 3-6. HIGH-RISK PROFILE OF ELDERLY WOMEN IN THE THROMBOLYSIS AND ANGIOPLASTY IN MYOCARDIAL INFARCTION (TAMI) TRIALS

	Women Aged ≥65 Years (%) (n = 49)	All Other Patients (%) (n = 659)	p Value
Death	22	6	.0001
Infarct-related artery patency (90 min)	81	70	.113
PTCA success	81	80	.92
Major bleeding[a]	43	17	.0001
Transfusion ≥2 U	61	27	.0001

[a]Intracranial or retroperitoneal hemorrhage or observed blood loss estimated at ≥2 units. PTCA = coronary angioplasty.

From Topol EJ, Califf RM, George BS, et al. Insights derived from the thrombolysis and angioplasty in myocardial infarction (TAMI) trials. J Am Coll Cardiol 12:24A–31A, 1988.

groups receiving propranolol (180 to 240 mg/day) or placebo from 1977 through 1981 (116, 117). Women were older, more often had hypertension and diabetes, and had higher cholesterol levels than men (118). Propranolol treatment resulted in equivalent reductions in overall mortality (39% in women versus 24% in men, p = ns) and nonfatal myocardial infarctions (48% in women versus 9% in men, p = ns) in both men and women. In the propranolol-treated group, side effects were reported with equal frequency in men and women after adjustment for the frequency of side effects in the placebo group (118).

In the Timolol Myocardial Infarction Study (119), patients who had survived an acute myocardial infarction were randomized to timolol (193 women and 752 men) or to placebo (207 women and 732 men). Timolol therapy resulted in equivalent reductions in mortality in women (41%) and men (35%). Nonfatal reinfarction was also significantly reduced in both sexes (28% in women and 31% in men).

Aspirin. The Aspirin in Myocardial Infarction Study (AMIS) was a clinical trial of aspirin 1 g/day versus placebo in men and women who had survived a myocardial infarction (120, 121). Treatment was started from 2 months to 5 years after the qualifying myocardial infarction. Women were older, had higher systolic blood pressures, and had higher cholesterol levels at baseline than men (118). More women had a history of heart failure and were taking digoxin, diuretics, or nitrates than men and thus were sicker at baseline (118). No significant survival benefit was found with aspirin administration in either sex. In aspirin users, side effects were reported with equal frequency in mean and women, although side effects in the placebo group were reported more frequently in women (118). Compliance with the medication regimen was achieved by similar proportions of men and women, 71.6% and 69.4%, respectively (118). Several other double-blind, randomized trials of aspirin for the secondary prevention of coronary events have included small numbers of women but have not demonstrated a statistically significant survival benefit (122–124). Data on women, however, were not reported separately.

Although AMIS was a large study that randomized 4524 men and 503 women, the finding of no survival advantage with aspirin after myocardial infarction has not been characteristic of other trials (125). In ISIS-2, aspirin alone reduced vascular mortality by 23% and also reduced reinfarction and stroke rates significantly (104). In a review of 25 randomized trials of antiplatelet treatment, vascular mortality was reduced by 15% in patients with transient ischemic attack, stroke, unstable angina, or myocardial infarction (126). Since data on men and women, however, were not reported separately, these studies are difficult to interpret.

Angiotensin-Converting Enzyme (ACE) Inhibitors. No data currently exist on the benefits of ACE inhibitors post myocardial infarction in women. However, the Survival and Ventricular Enlargement (SAVE) study has randomized 390 women and 1841 men following myocardial infarction to ACE inhibitors or placebo (127). Early results have yet to be published.

Heparin. No gender-related differences in the response to anticoagulants are known.

Angiography and Revascularization After Myocardial Infarction

To determine whether there was a gender difference in the selection of patients for diagnostic and therapeutic cardiovascular procedures early after myocardial infarction, Krumholz et al. examined all 1350 men and 1123 women discharged from the Beth Israel Hospital during the years 1984 to 1990 with a strictly defined diagnosis of acute myocardial infarction (128). Women had coronary angiography during their hospitalization less frequently than men (22% versus 34%, odds ratio .55), but age-adjusted rates were similar (odds ratio .91). After cardiac catheterization, women were as likely as men to be referred for angioplasty but were less likely than men to be referred for CABG. However, after controlling for age and coronary disease severity, the difference in CABG rates was of borderline statistical significance (odds ratio .65). These results also support Healy's (22) contention that once women have been shown to have coronary artery disease, they are treated "as men would be." However, these results differ from those of two other studies that evaluated the rates of invasive cardiac procedures in women and men with myocardial infarction. Ayanian and Epstein (129) and investigators from the SAVE study (16) reported that men were more likely than women to have an invasive cardiac procedure after myocardial infarction. The patient populations, the clinical practice setting, the criteria used to define myocardial infarction, and the methods used to identify and exclude patients in these three studies were not altogether comparable, which may explain the differences in results.

Few studies have looked for gender-related differences in the role of primary angioplasty versus thrombolysis in patients with an acute myocardial infarction, even though older women may have more bleeding complications with thrombolysis than men (112). However, several studies have investigated gender-related differences in mortality with primary PTCA and PTCA after thrombolysis. Stack and colleagues reported the results in 216 consecutive patients, including 45 women, who had acute myocardial infarction treated under a protocol of intravenous streptokinase followed by emergency PTCA. Independent predictors of in-hospital mortality were cardiogenic shock, older age, lower ejection fraction, and female sex (130). Kahn et al. (131) reported on 169 women and 445 men with acute myocardial infarction who underwent primary angioplasty without antecedent thrombolytic therapy. Multivariate predictors of late mortality (32 months follow-up), but not early mortality, included female gender. Several studies have examined the predictors of success for coronary angioplasty performed for acute myocardial infarction and have found gender did not predict procedural success (132), artery patency (132), or early in-hospital mortality (133, 134).

Rehabilitation After Myocardial Infarction

In a recent meta-analysis of 22 randomized trials of rehabilitation with exercise after myocardial infarction, O'Connor et al. (135) reported that only four studies (136–139) suitable for inclusion in the analysis included women. Thus, women constituted only 3% of randomized subjects, precluding any separate analysis or conclusions. However, even for men, the efficacy of physical exercise as a secondary prevention measure has not been fully proved despite two large meta-analyses (135, 140).

One study suggests that the paucity of women enrolled in cardiac rehabilitation programs may be secondary to the increased number of comorbid conditions in women that preclude their participation in exercise testing (141). In this Canadian study, 5 of 323 women were considered clinically and physiologically eligible after myocardial infarction for the rehabilitation program. Seventy-one percent of women were excluded because of age greater than 65 years, and women were excluded more often for cardiac, medical, or psychiatric reasons than men. Available evidence also suggests higher dropout rates in formal rehabilitation programs for women than for men (91, 142, 143), and greater work disability in women 24 months after myocardial infarction (144).

SUMMARY

Risk factor modification, hormone replacement therapy, and aspirin administration may be effective forms of primary prevention and secondary management of coronary heart disease in women. Little information is available regarding gender-specific responses to antianginal medications in the management of coronary heart disease. Limited studies suggest that there may be great potential for atherosclerotic regression in women who undertake cholesterol-lowering therapy and life style changes.

Women do not appear to have equal access to diagnostic and therapeutic modalities for coronary disease compared to men. Women are referred for coronary revascularization later in the course of their disease, which may contribute to their increased in-hospital mortality after coronary angioplasty and CABG. Despite less favorable short-term outcomes after coronary angioplasty, which may, however, be improving in recent years, women have equal if not higher event-free survivals. Outcome after CABG has not improved and appears to depend less on gender than on coronary size and preoperative risk factors.

Prognosis after myocardial infarction is probably significantly worse in women independent of age, although this is not a universal finding. Thrombolysis reduces mortality in women with acute myocardial infarction; however, there is a relatively smaller reduction in mortality in women compared to men despite limited evidence suggesting that patency rates are similar in men and women. Women over 65 may be particularly at risk for hemorrhagic events with thrombolysis in the absence of gender-, weight-, and age-determined dosages. Although beta blockers have been shown to improve survival in women after myocardial infarction, insufficient numbers of women have been enrolled in postinfarction therapeutic and rehabilitation trials. Thus, the benefits of aspirin and exercise prescriptions remain unproved in women at the present time.

The growing body of literature suggests that gender is one of the important clinical variables that should be considered when primary and secondary medical therapy and coronary revascularization for coronary artery disease are examined.

References

1. Eaker ED, Packard B, Wenger NK, et al. Coronary artery disease in women. *Am J Cardiol* 61:641–644, 1988.
2. Manson JE, Stampfer MJ, Colditz GA, et al. A prospective study of aspirin use and primary prevention of cardiovascular disease in women. *JAMA* 266:521–527, 1991.
3. Spranger M, Aspey BS, Harrison MJG. Sex difference in antithrombotic effect of aspirin. *Stroke* 20:34–37, 1989.
4. Escolar G, Bastida E, Garrido M, et al. Sex-related differences in the effects of aspirin on the interaction of platelets with subendothelium. *Thromb Res* 44:837–847, 1986.
5. Kelton JG, Hirsch J, Carter CJ, et al. Sex differences in the antithrombotic effect of aspirin. *Blood* 52:1073–1076, 1978.
6. Philpot VB, Lippton HC, Kadowitz PJ. Effect of aspirin on serum thrombin time and bleeding time. *Prostaglandins Leukot Med* 19:123–130, 1958.
7. Husted SE, Pederson AK, Peterson T, et al. Systemic availability of acetylsalicylic acid in normal men and women and its effect on in vitro platelet aggregability. *Eur J Clin Pharmacol* 24:679–682, 1983.
8. Ho PC, Triggs EJ, Bourne DWA, et al. The effects of age and sex on the disposition of acetylsalicylic acid and its metabolites. *Br J Clin Pharmacol* 19:675–684, 1985.
9. Patrignani P, Filabozzi P, Patrono C. Selective cumulative inhibition of platelet thromboxane production by low-dose aspirin in healthy subjects. *J Clin Invest* 69:1366–1372, 1982.
10. Harris WH, Salzman EW, Athanasoulis CA, et al. Aspirin prophylaxis of venous thromboembolism after total hip replacement. *N Engl J Med* 297:1246–1249, 1977.
11. The Canadian Cooperative Study Group. A randomized trial of aspirin and sulfinpyrazone in threatened stroke. *N Engl J Med* 299:53–59, 1978.
12. Paganini-Hill A, Chao A, Ross RK, et al. Aspirin use and chronic diseases: a cohort study of the elderly. *Br Med J* 299:1247–1250, 1989.
13. Hammond EC, Garfinkel L. Aspirin and coronary heart disease: Findings of a prospective study. *Br Med J* 2:269–271, 1975.
14. Kannel WB, Abbott RD. Incidence and prognosis of myocardial infarction in women: The Framingham Study. In Eaker ED, Packard B, Wenger NK, et al. (Eds.), *Coronary Artery Disease in Women*. New York, Haymarket-Doyma, 1987, pp. 208–214.
15. Tobin JN, Wassertheil-Smoller S, Wexler JP, et al. Sex bias in considering coronary bypass surgery. *Ann Intern Med* 107:19–25, 1987.
16. Steingart RM, Packer M, Hamm P, et al. Sex differences in the management of coronary artery disease. *N Engl J Med* 325:226–230, 1991.
17. Khan SS, Nessim S, Gray R, et al. Increased mortality of women in coronary artery bypass surgery: Evidence for referral bias. *Ann Intern Med* 112:561–567, 1990.
18. Loop FS, Golding LR, MacMillan JP, et al. Coronary artery surgery in women compared with men: Analysis of risks and long-term results. *J Am Coll Cardiol* 4:383–390, 1983.
19. Fisher LD, Kennedy JW, Davis KB, et al. Association of sex, physical size, and operative mortality after coronary artery surgery (CASS). *J Thorac Cardiovasc Surg* 84:334–341, 1982.
20. Cowley MJ, Mullin SM, Kelsey SF, et al. Sex differences in early and long-term results of coronary angioplasty in the NHLBI PTCA registry. *Circulation* 71:90–97, 1985.
21. McEniery PT, Hollman J, Knezinek V, et al. Com-

parative safety and efficacy of percutaneous transluminal coronary angioplasty in men and in women. *Cathet Cardiovasc Diagn* 13:364–371, 1987.
22. Healy B. The Yentl syndrome. *N Engl J Med* 325:274–276, 1991.
23. Tyras DH, Barner HB, Kaiser GC, et al. Myocardial revascularization in women. *Ann Thorac Surg* 25:449–453, 1978.
24. Douglas JS, King SB, Jones EL, et al. Reduced efficacy of coronary bypass artery in women. *Circulation* 64(Suppl. 2):11–16, 1981.
25. Bolooki H, Vargas A, Green R, et al. Results of direct coronary artery surgery in women. *J Thorac Cardiovasc Surg* 69:271–277, 1975.
26. Douglas P. Gender, cardiology and optimal medical care. *Circulation* 74:917–919, 1986.
27. James TN. Anatomy of the coronary arteries in health and disease. *Circulation* 32:1020–1029, 1965.
28. Du X-J, Dart AM, Riemersma RA, et al. Sex differences in presynaptic adrenergic inhibition of norepinephrine release during normoxia and ischemia in the rat heart. *Circ Res* 68:827–835, 1991.
29. Hutter AM. Coronary artery disease in women: Medical management. In Eaker ED, Packard B, Wenger NK, et al. (Eds.), *Coronary Disease in Women.* New York, Haymarket-Doyma, 1987, pp. 229–232.
30. Sullivan JM, VanderZwaag R, Hughes JP, et al. Estrogen replacement and coronary artery disease. Effect on survival in postmenopausal women. *Arch Intern Med* 150:2557–2562, 1990.
31. Likoff W, Segal BL, Kasparian H. Paradox of normal selective coronary arteriograms in patients considered to have unmistakable coronary heart disease. *N Engl J Med* 276:1063–1066, 1967.
32. Cannon RO III, Camici PG, Epstein SE. Pathophysiological dilemma of syndrome X. *Circulation* 85:883–889, 1992.
33. Sax FL, Cannon RO, Hanson C, et al. Impaired forearm vasodilator reserve in patients with microvascular angina: Evidence of a generalized disorder of vascular function? *N Engl J Med* 317:1366–1370, 1987.
34. Cannon RO, Cattau EL, Yakshe PN, et al. Coronary flow reserve, esophageal motility and chest pain in patients with angiographically normal coronary arteries. *Am J Med* 82:217–222, 1990.
35. Cannon RO, Peden DB, Berkebile C, et al. Airways hyperresponsiveness in patients with microvascular angina: Evidence for a diffuse disorder of smooth muscle responsiveness. *Circulation* 82:2011–2017, 1990.
36. Ellis SG, Roubin GS, King SB III, et al. In-hospital cardiac mortality after acute closure after coronary angioplasty: Analysis of risk factors from 8,207 procedures. *J Am Coll Cardiol* 11:211–216, 1988.
37. Holmes DR Jr, Holubkov R, Vliestra RE, et al. Comparison of complications during percutaneous transluminal coronary angioplasty from 1977 to 1981 and from 1985 to 1986: The National Heart, Lung and Blood Institute Percutaneous Transluminal Coronary Angioplasty Registry. *J Am Coll Cardiol* 12:1149–1155, 1988.
38. Cowley MJ, Kelsey SF, Costigan TM, et al. Percutaneous transluminal coronary angioplastin women: Gender differences in outcome. In Eaker ED, Packard B, Wenger NK, et al. (Eds.), *Coronary Artery Disease in Women.* New York, Haymarket-Doyma, 1987, pp. 251–256.
39. Casale PN, Whitlow PL, Franco I, et al. Women have a higher major complication rate with new devices for percutaneous revascularization. *J Am Coll Cardiol* 19:94A, 1992.
40. Ellis SG. Elective coronary angioplasty: Techniques and complications. In Topol EJ (Ed.), *Textbook of Interventional Cardiology.* Philadelphia, WB Saunders, 1990, pp. 199–222.
41. Levine S, Ewels CJ, Rosing DR, et al. Coronary angioplasty: Clinical and angiographic follow-up. *Am J Cardiol* 55:673–676, 1985.
42. Vandormael MG, Deligonul K, Kern MJ, et al. Multilesion coronary angioplasty: Clinical and angiographic follow-up. *J Am Coll Cardiol* 10:246–252, 1987.
43. deFeyter PJ, Suryapranata H, Serruys PW, et al. Coronary angioplasty for unstable angina: Immediate and late results in 200 consecutive patients with identification of risk factors for unfavorable early and late outcome. *J Am Coll Cardiol* 12:324–333, 1988.
44. Lambert M, Bonan R, Cote G, et al. Multiple coronary angioplasty: A model to discriminate systemic and procedural factors related to restenosis. *J Am Coll Cardiol* 12:310–314, 1988.
45. Guiteras VP, Bourassa MG, David PR, et al. Restenosis after successful percutaneous transluminal coronary angioplasty: The Montreal Heart Institute experience. *Am J Cardiol* 60:50B–55B, 1987.
46. Myler RK, Topol EK, Shaw RE, et al. Multiple vessel coronary angioplasty: Classification, results, and patterns of restenosis in 494 consecutive patients. *Cathet Cardiovasc Diagn* 13:1–15, 1987.
47. Fleck E, Regitz V, Lehnert A, et al. Restenosis after balloon dilatation of coronary stenosis: Multivariate analysis of potential risk factors. *Eur Heart J* 9:15–18, 1988.
48. Leimgruber PP, Roubin GS, Hollman J, et al. Restenosis after successful coronary angioplasty in patients with single-vessel disease. *Circulation* 73:710–717, 1986.
49. Mata LA, Bosch X, David PR, et al. Clinical and angiographic assessment 6 months after double vessel percutaneous coronary angioplasty. *J Am Coll Cardiol* 6:1239–1244, 1985.
50. Rapold HJ, David PR, Guiteras Val P, et al. Restenosis and its determination in first and repeat coronary angioplasty. *Eur Heart J* 8:575–586, 1987.
51. Ellis SG, Roubin GS, King SB III, et al. Importance of stenosis morphology in the estimation of restenosis risk after elective percutaneous transluminal coronary angioplasty. *Am J Cardiol* 63:30–34, 1989.
52. Kober G, Scherer D, Koch R, et al. Criteria for primary success and long-term results. Analysis of 152 consecutive transluminal coronary angioplasties. In Kaltenbach M, Gruntzig A, Rentrop K, Bussman W-D (Eds.), *Transluminal Coronary Angioplasty and Intracoronary Thrombolysis.* Berlin, Springer-Verlag, 1982, pp. 95–101.
53. Galan KM, Hollman JL. Recurrence of stenoses after coronary angioplasty. *Heart Lung* 15:585–587, 1986.
54. DiSciascio G, Vetrovec GW, Cowley MJ, et al. Early and late outcome of percutaneous transluminal coronary angioplasty for subacute and chronic total coronary occlusion. *Am Heart J* 111:833–839, 1986.
55. Meier B, King SB III, Gruentzig AR, et al. Repeat

coronary angioplasty. *J Am Coll Cardiol* 4:463–466, 1984.
56. Hirshfeld JW Jr, Schwartz J, Jugo R, et al. A multivariate model for predicting the risk of restenosis after PTCA (abstr). *Circulation* 78(Suppl II):II-289, 1988.
57. Califf RM, Ohman M, Frid DJ, et al. Restenosis: The clinical issues. In Topol EJ (Ed.), *Textbook of Interventional Cardiology*. Philadelphia, WB Saunders, 1990, pp. 363–394.
58. Califf RM, Fortin DF, Frid DJ, et al. Restenosis after coronary angioplasty: An overview. *J Am Coll Cardiol* 17:2B-13B, 1991.
59. Hollman B, Badhwar K, Beck GJ, et al. Risk factors for recurrent stenosis following successful coronary angioplasty. *Clev Clin J Med* 56:517–523, 1989.
60. Arora RR, Konrad K, Badhwar K, et al. Restenosis after transluminal coronary angioplasty: A risk factor analysis. *Cathet Cardiovasc Diagn* 19:17–22, 1990.
61. Bobbio M, Detrano R, Colombo A, et al. Restenosis rate after percutaneous transluminal coronary angioplasty: A literature overview. *J Invas Cardiol* 3:214–224, 1991.
62. Carrozza JP Jr, Kuntz RE, Levine MJ, et al. Angiographic and clinical outcome of intracoronary stenting: Acute and long-term results from a large single-center experience. *J Am Coll Cardiol* 20:328–337, 1992.
63. Fishman RF, Kuntz RE, Carrozza JP Jr, et al. Long term results of directional coronary atherectomy: Predictors of restenosis. *J Am Coll Cardiol* 20:1109–1110, 1992.
64. Eaker ED, Kronmal R, Kennedy JW, et al. Comparison of the long-term, postsurgical survival of women and men in the Coronary Artery Surgery Study (CASS). *Am Heart J* 117:71–81, 1989.
65. Cosgrove DM, Loop FD, Lytle BW, et al. Primary myocardial revascularization. *J Thorac Cardiovasc Surg* 88:673–684, 1984.
66. Khan SS. Why women have a significantly higher bypass surgery mortality rate. *Cardiology Board Review* 8:54–67, 1991.
67. Richardson JV, Cyrus RJ. Reduced efficacy of coronary artery bypass grafting in women. *Ann Thorac Surg* 42:S16–S21, 1986.
68. Kennedy JW, Kaiser GC, Fisher LD, et al. Multivariate discriminant analysis of the clinical and angiographic predictors of operative mortality from the Collaborative Study in Coronary Artery Surgery (CASS). *J Thorac Cardiovasc Surg* 80:876–887, 1980.
69. Killen DA, Reed WA, Arnold M, et al. Coronary artery bypass in women: Long-term survival. *Ann Thorac Surg* 34:559–563, 1982.
70. Hall RJ, Elayda MA, Gray A, et al. Coronary artery bypass: Long-term follow-up of 22,284 consecutive patients. *Circulation* 68(Suppl. II):II20–II25, 1983.
71. Laird-Meeter K, Penn OC, Haalebos MM, et al. Survival in 1,041 patients with consecutive aortocoronary bypass operations. *Eur Heart J* 5:35–42, 1984.
72. Gardner TJ, Horneffer PJ, Gott VL, et al. Coronary artery bypass grafting in women. *Ann Surg* 201:780–784, 1985.
73. Davis KB. Coronary artery bypass graft surgery in women. In Eaker ED, Packard B, Wenger NK, et al (Eds.), *Coronary Artery Disease in Women*. New York, Haymarket-Doyma, 1987, pp. 247–250.
74. Loop FD, Lytle BW, Cosgrove DM, et al. Coronary artery bypass graft surgery in the elderly. Indications and outcome. *Clev Clin J Med* 55:23–34, 1988.
75. Gersh BJ, Kronmal RA, Schaff HV, et al. Long-term (5-year) results of coronary bypass surgery in patients 65 years old or older: A report from the Coronary Artery Surgery Study. *Circulation* 68(Suppl. II):II190–II199, 1983.
76. Jeffrey DL, Vijayanagar RR, Bognolo DA, et al. Results of coronary bypass surgery in elderly women. *Ann Thorac Surg* 42:550–553, 1986.
77. Chaitman BR, Rogers WJ, David K, et al. Operative risk factors inj patients with left main coronary-artery disease. *N Engl J Med* 303:953–957, 1980.
78. Miller DC, Stinson EB, Oyer PE, et al. Discriminant analysis of the changing risks of coronary artery operations: 1971–1979. *J Thorac Cardiovasc Surg* 85:197–213, 1983.
79. Johnson WD, Kayser KL, Pedraza PM. Angina pectoris and coronary bypass surgery: Patterns of prevalence and recurrences in 3,105 consecutive patients followed up to 11 years. *Am Heart J* 108:1190–1197, 1984.
80. Golding LR, Groves LK. Results of coronary surgery in women. *Cleve Clin Q* 43:113–115, 1976.
81. Chesebro JH, Clement IP, Fuster V et al. A platelet-inhibitor-drug trial in coronary-artery bypass operations. Benefit of perioperative dipyridamole and aspirin therapy on early postoperative vein-graft patency. *N Engl J Med* 307:73–78, 1982.
82. Myers WO, Davis K, Foster ED, et al. Surgical survival in the Coronary Artery Surgery Study CASS registry. *Ann Thorac Surg* 40:245–260, 1985.
83. Loop FD, Lytle BW, Cosgrove DM, et al. Influence of the internal-mammary-artery graft on 10-year survival and other cardiac events. *N Engl J Med* 314:1–6, 1986.
84. Grondin CM, Campeau L, Lesperance J, et al. Comparison of late changes in internal mammary artery and saphenous vein grafts in two consecutive series of patients 10 years after operation. *Circulation* 70 (Suppl. I):1208–1212, 1984.
85. Lytle BW, Loop FD, Cosgrove DM, et al. Long-term (5 to 12 years) serial studies of internal mammary artery and saphenous vein coronary bypass grafts. *J Thorac Cardiovasc Surg* 89:248–258, 1985.
86. Loop FD, Irarrazaval MJ, Breede JJ, et al. Internal mammary artery graft for ischemic heart disease. *Am J Cardiol* 39:516–522, 1977.
87. Kane JP, Malloy MJ, Ports TA, et al. Regression of coronary atherosclerosis during treatment of familial hypercholesterolemia with combined drug regimens. *JAMA* 264:3007–3012, 1990.
88. Ornish D, Brown SE, Scherwitz LW, et al. Can lifestyle changes reverse coronary heart disease? *Lancet* 336:129–133, 1990.
89. Boogard MAK, Brody ME. Comparison of the rehabilitation of men and women post-myocardial infarction. *J Cardiopul Rehab* 5:379–384, 1985.
90. Parchert MA, Creason N. The role of nursing in the rehabilitation of women. *J Cardiovasc Nurs* 3:57–64, 1983.
91. O'Callaghan WG, Teo KK, O'Riordan J, et al. Comparative response of male and female patients with coronary artery disease to exercise rehabilitation. *Eur Heart J* 5:649–651, 1984.
92. Hemenway D, Sherman H, Mudge GH, et al. Comparative costs versus symptomatic and employment

benefits of medical and surgical treatment of stable angina pectoris. *Med Care* 23:133–141, 1985.
93. Almeida D, Bradford JM, Wenger NK, et al. Return to work after coronary bypass surgery. *Circulation* 68 (Suppl. 2):II205–II213, 1983.
94. Stanton BA, Zyzanski SJ, Jenkins CD, et al. Recovery after major heart surgery: Medical, psychological, and work out-comes. In Becker R, Katz J, Polonius M-J, et al. (Eds.), *Psychopathological and Neurological Dysfunction Following Open-Heart Surgery*. Berlin, Springer-Verlag, 1982, pp. 217–226.
95. Stanton BA, Jenkins CD, Denlinger P, et al. Predictors of employment status after cardiac surgery. *JAMA* 249:907–911, 1983.
96. Kannel WB, Sorlie P, McNamara PM. Prognosis after myocardial infarction: The Framingham Study. *Am J Cardiol* 44:53–59, 1979.
97. Henning R, Lundman T. The Swedish Cooperative CCU Study. Part I: A description of the early stage. *Acta Med Scand* 586 (Suppl.):27–29, 1975.
98. Puletti M, Sunseri L, Curione M, et al. Acute myocardial infarction: Sex-related differences in prognosis. *Am Heart J* 108:63–66, 1984.
99. Tofler G, Stone P, Muller J, et al. Effect of gender and race on prognosis after myocardial infarction: Adverse prognosis for women, particularly black women. *J Am Coll Cardiol* 9:473–482, 1987.
100. Peter T, Harper R, Luxton M, et al. Acute myocardial infarction in women. *Med J Aust* 1:189–191, 1978.
101. Dittrich H, Gilpin E, Nicod P, et al. Acute myocardial infarction in women: Influence of gender on mortality and prognostic variables. *Am J Cardiol* 62:1–7, 1988.
102. Greenland P, Reicher-Reiss H, Goldbourt U, et al. In-hospital and 1-year mortality in 1,524 women after myocardial infarction. *Circulation* 83:484–491, 1991.
103. Becker RC. Coronary thrombolysis in women. *Cardiovasc Disease Women* 77 (Suppl. 2):110–123, 1990.
104. ISIS-2 Collaborative Group. Randomized trial of intravenous streptokinase, oral aspirin, both, or neither among 17,187 cases of suspected acute myocardial infarction: ISIS-2. *Lancet* 1:349–360, 1988.
105. Gruppo Italiano per lo Studio Della Streptochinasi Nell'Infarto Miocardico (GISSI). Effectiveness of intravenous thrombolytic treatment in acute myocardial infarction. *Lancet* 1:397–402, 1986.
106. Gruppo Italiano per lo Studio Della Streptochinasi Nell'Infarto Miocardico (GISSI). Long-term effects of intravenous thrombolysis in acute myocardial infarction: Final report of the GISSI study. *Lancet* 2:871–874, 1987.
107. Anglo-Scandinavian Study of Early Thrombolysis (ASSET). Trial of tissue plasminogen activator for mortality reduction in acute myocardial infarction. *Lancet* 2:525–530, 1988.
108. European Working Party. Streptokinase in recent myocardial infarction: A controlled multicentre trial. *Br Med J* 3:325–331, 1971.
109. Kennedy JW, Martin GV, Davis KB, et al. The Western Washington intravenous streptokinase in acute myocardial infarction. *Circulation* 77:345–352, 1988.
110. Fresco C, Franzosi MG, Maggioni AP, et al. The GISSI-2 trial: Premises, results, epidemiological (and other) implications. *Clin Cardiol* 8:32–36, 1990.
111. Topol EJ. Thrombolytic intervention. In Topol EJ (Ed.), *Textbook of Interventional Cardiology*. Philadelphia, WB Saunders, 1990, p. 94
112. Topol EJ, Califf RM, George BS, et al. Insights derived from the thrombolysis and angioplasty in myocardial infarction (TAMI) trials. *J Am Coll Cardiol* 12:24A–31A, 1988.
113. Bovill EG, Terrin ML, Stump DC, et al. Hemorrhagic events during therapy with recombinant tissue-type plasminogen activator, heparin, and aspirin for acute myocardial infarction. *Ann Intern Med* 115:256–265, 1991.
114. Lerner DJ, Kannel WB. Patterns of coronary heart disease morbidity and mortality in the sexes. A 26-year follow-up of the Framingham population. *Am Heart J* 111:383–390, 1986.
115. Maynard C, Althouse R, Cerqueira M, et al. Under-utilization of thrombolytic therapy in eligible women with acute myocardial infarction. *Am J Cardiol* 68:529–530, 1991.
116. β-Blocker Heart Trial Research Group. A randomized trial of propranolol in patients with acute myocardial infarction. I. Mortality results. *JAMA* 247:1707–1714, 1982.
117. β-Blocker Heart Trial Research Group. A randomized trial of propranolol in patients with acute myocardial infarction. II. Morbidity results. *JAMA* 250:2814–2819, 1983.
118. Furberg CD, Friedman LM, MacMahon SW. Women as participants in trial of the primary and secondary prevention of cardiovascular disease: Part II. Secondary prevention: The beta-blocker heart attack trial and the aspirin myocardial infarction study. In Eaker ED, Packard B, Wenger NK, et al. (Eds.), *Coronary Artery Disease in Women*. New York, Haymarket-Doyma, 1987, pp. 241–246.
119. Rodda BE. The Timolol Myocardial Infarction Study: An evaluation of selected variables. *Circulation* 677:I101–I106, 1983.
120. The Aspirin Myocardial Infarction Study Research Group. The aspirin myocardial infarction study. Final results. *Circulation* 62 (Suppl 5):V79–V84, 1980.
121. The Aspirin Myocardial Infarction Study Research Group. A randomized, controlled trial of aspirin in persons recovered from myocardial infarction. *JAMA* 243:661–669, 1980.
122. Elwood PC, Sweetnam PM. Aspirin and secondary mortality after myocardial infarction. *Lancet* 2:1313–1315, 1979.
123. Breddin K, Loew D, Lechner K, et al. Secondary prevention of myocardial infarction. Comparison of acetylsalicylic acid, phenprocoumon and placebo. A multicenter two-year prospective study. *Thromb Haemost* 41:225–236, 1979.
124. Persantine-Aspirin Reinfarction Study Research Group. Persantine and aspirin in coronary heart disease. *Circulation* 62:449–461, 1980.
125. Hennekens CH, Buring JE, Sandercock P, et al. Aspirin and other antiplatelet agents in the secondary and primary prevention of cardiovascular disease. *Circulation* 80:749–756, 1989.
126. Antiplatelet Trialists' Collaboration. Secondary prevention of vascular disease by prolonged antiplatelet treatment. *Br Med J* 296:320–331, 1988.
127. Moyé LA, Pfeffer MA, Braunwald E. Rationale, design and baseline characteristics of the survival and ventricular enlargement trials. *Am J Cardiol* 68:70D–79D, 1991.
128. Krumholz H, Douglas PS, Lauer MS, et al. Selection

of patients for coronary angiography and coronary revascularization early after myocardial infarction: Is there evidence for a gender difference in the use of procedures? *Ann Intern Med* 116:785–790, 1992.
129. Ayanian JZ, Epstein AM. Differences in the use of procedures between woman and men hospitalized for coronary heart disease. *N Engl J Med* 325:221–225, 1991.
130. Stack RS, O'Connor CM, Mark DB, et al. Coronary perfusion during acute myocardial infarction with a combined therapy of coronary angiography and high-dose intravenous streptokinase. *Circulation* 77:151–161, 1988.
131. Kahn JK, O'Keefe JH Jr, Rutherford BD, et al. Timing and mechanism of in-hospital and late death after primary coronary angioplasty during acute myocardial infarction. *Am J Cardiol* 66:1045–1048, 1990.
132. Ellis SG, Topol EJ, Gallison L, et al. Predictors of success for coronary angioplasty performed for acute myocardial infarction. *J Am Coll Cardiol* 12:1407–1415, 1988.
133. Kahn JK, Rutherford BD, McConahay DR, et al. Results of primary angioplasty for acute myocardial infarction in patients with multivessel coronary artery disease. *J Am Coll Cardiol* 16:1089–1096, 1990.
134. Brodie BR, Weintraub RA, Stuckey TD, et al. Outcomes of direct coronary angioplasty for acute myocardial infarction in candidates and non-candidates for thrombolytic therapy. *Am J Cardiol* 67:7–12, 1991.
135. O'Connor GT, Buring JE, Yusuf S, et al. An overview of randomized trials of rehabilitation with exercise after myocardial infarction. *Circulation* 80:234–244, 1989.
136. Sanne H. Exercise tolerance and physical training of non-selected patients after myocardial infarction. *Acta Med Scand* (Suppl. 551):1–124, 1973.
137. Wilhelmsen L, Sanne H, Elmfeldt D, et al. A controlled trial of physical training after myocardial infarction. Effects on risk factors, nonfatal reinfarction, and death. *Prev Med* 4:491–508, 1975.
138. Marra S, Paolillo V, Spadaccini F, et al. Long-term follow-up after a controlled randomized post-myocardial infarction rehabilitation programme: Effects on morbidity and mortality. *Eur Heart J* 6:656–663, 1985.
139. Palatsi I. Feasibility of physical training after myocardial infarction and its effect on return to work, morbidity and mortality. *Acta Med Scand* (Suppl. 599):4–84, 1976.
140. May GS, Eberlein KA, Furberg CD, et al. Secondary prevention after myocardial infarction: A review of long-term trials. *Prog Cardiovasc Dis* 24:331–352, 1982.
141. Walling A, Tremblay GJL, Jobin J, et al. Evaluating the rehabilitation potential of a large population of postmyocardial infarction patients: Adverse prognosis for women. *J Cardiopulmonary Rehabil* 8:99–106, 1988.
142. Murdaugh C: Coronary artery disease in women. *J Cardiovasc Nurs* 4:35–50, 1990.
143. Oldridge NB, LaSalle D, Jones NL. Exercise rehabilitation of female patients with coronary heart disease. *Am Heart J* 100:755–757, 1980.
144. Chirikos TN, Nickel JL. Work disability from coronary heart disease in women. *Women Health* 9:55–74, 1984.

CHAPTER 4

Hypertension

VERA BITTNER, M.D.
SUZANNE OPARIL, M.D.

EPIDEMIOLOGY OF HYPERTENSION

It is estimated that over 62 million Americans aged 6 and older have high blood pressure; 46% do not know they have it, and 67% are not on therapy (1). Prevalence increases with age, is higher in blacks than in whites, and is higher in men than in women overall (1). Risk of vascular complications rises with increasing levels of systolic and diastolic blood pressure without a clear threshold (2). The definition of hypertension is thus somewhat arbitrary. Table 4–1 details the classification scheme recommended by the 1988 Report of the Joint National Committee on Detection, Evaluation, and Treatment of High Blood Pressure (3).

Hypertension in Women in the United States

Data on the prevalence of hypertension in women are derived from national surveys (4, 5), longitudinal follow-up studies (6), and screenings for clinical trials (7, 8). In the National Health and Nutrition Examination Survey II (NHANES II), 16,204 persons aged 6 to 74 years were examined between 1976 and 1980 (4). Mean systolic blood pressures rose with age in both sexes and in blacks and whites (Fig. 4–1A). Mean diastolic blood pressures also increased with age but decreased slightly in the oldest age groups (Fig. 4–1B). Mean diastolic blood pressure was higher in adult men than in women at all ages; mean systolic blood pressure was higher in men until age 54 but was higher in women in the oldest age group. Black men and women in the 35- to 74-year-old age group had higher mean diastolic pressures than their white counterparts; mean systolic pressures were higher in black men than in white men between the ages of 35 and 64 and higher in black women than white women between the ages of 35 and 74. In NHANES II, hypertension was defined as systolic blood pressure ≥ 160 mmHg or diastolic blood pressure ≥ 95 mmHg or current use of antihypertensive drugs. Hypertension was present in 21.2% of white men, 20% of white

Table 4–1. CLASSIFICATION OF BLOOD PRESSURE IN ADULTS AGED 18 YEARS OR OLDER

	Range (mmHg)	Category
Diastolic BP	< 85	Normal BP
	85–89	High normal BP
	90–104	Mild hypertension
	105–114	Moderate hypertension
	≥ 115	Severe hypertension
Systolic BP (if diastolic BP is < 90 mmHg)	< 140	Normal BP
	140–159	Borderline isolated systolic hypertension
	≥ 160	Isolated systolic hypertension

BP = blood pressure
Classification based on the average of two or more readings on two or more occasions
From U.S. Public Health Service, National Institutes of Health. *The 1988 Report of the Joint National Committee on Detection, Evaluation, and Treatment of High Blood Pressure.* (NIH Publication No. 88-1088. Washington, D.C., U.S. Department of Health and Human Services, 1988.)

women, 28.3% of black men, and 39.8% of black women. The prevalence of elevated blood pressure increased with age among white men and women and among black women; in black men, elevated blood pressure was less common in the oldest age group than in 55- to 64-year-olds.

Prevalence data for hypertension from the NHANES I Epidemiologic Follow-up Study (5), stratified by age, race, and sex, are shown in Figure 4–2. Prevalence rates rise with age in all race and sex groups. Hypertension is more common in black men and women than in white men and women in most age groups. In younger age groups, men have more hypertension than women, whereas women older than 64 years are more likely to be hypertensive than men in the same age group. This "crossover," seen in this and other cross-sectional studies, is not apparent in the 30-year longitudinal data from the Framingham study (6). Mean systolic blood pressure in older women approached that of older men but did not exceed it; mean diastolic blood pressure was lower in women at all ages and declined in both sexes after age 65.

The Community Hypertension Evaluation Clinic (CHEC) Program screened 1 million Americans between 1973 and 1975 (7). White women had the lowest prevalence of diastolic hypertension (> 90 mmHg) in all age groups (223.1/1000). Diastolic hypertension was most common in black men (307.1/1000) and black women (297.9/1000); white men had an intermediate rate (269.7/1000). The racial differences in prevalence of severe diastolic hypertension (≥ 110 mmHg) were even more striking. White women again had the lowest rate (21.6/1000); white men had a slightly higher rate (26.6/1000), and both black men (57.2/1000) and black women (55.2/1000) had markedly higher rates. Mean systolic pressures rose with age in all subgroups and were higher in men than in women until age 50 for blacks and age 65 for whites. Mean diastolic pressures were higher in men than in women at all ages and, in contrast to mean systolic pressure, reached a plateau after age 60. Women of both races were less likely to have undiagnosed hypertension, and their blood pressures tended to be better controlled than those in men.

The Hypertension Detection and Follow-up Program (HDFP) Cooperative Group (8) screened 158,906 persons aged 30 to 69 in 14 communities between 1973 and 1974. Hypertension (diastolic blood pressure ≥ 95 mmHg) was more prevalent in men than in women of both races: 28.1% of black men, 23.1% of black women, 13.5% of white men, and 8.4% of white women were hypertensive. The prevalence ratio between black and white women was 2.1 among persons with mild hypertension (diastolic blood pressure 95 to 104 mmHg), 3.7 among moderate hypertensives (diastolic blood pressure 105 to 114 mmHg), and 7.1 among persons with severe hypertension (diastolic blood pressures ≥ 115 mmHg). As in the CHEC program, women of both races were more likely than men to be diagnosed, to be treated, and to have their blood pressure controlled.

Isolated systolic hypertension (ISH) (see Table 4–1) becomes increasingly common after age 50 and is more prevalent in women than in men (9). It is estimated that more than 3 million persons in the United States have ISH. As summarized by Silagy and MacNeil (9), prevalence rates have varied widely from study to study. In Framingham, for example, 14% of men and 23% of women over age 65 had ISH; in those older than 75, the respective prevalence rates were 25% for men and 30% for women. ISH rates as low as 3.1% among white women in an elderly retirement community in California and as high as 38.9%

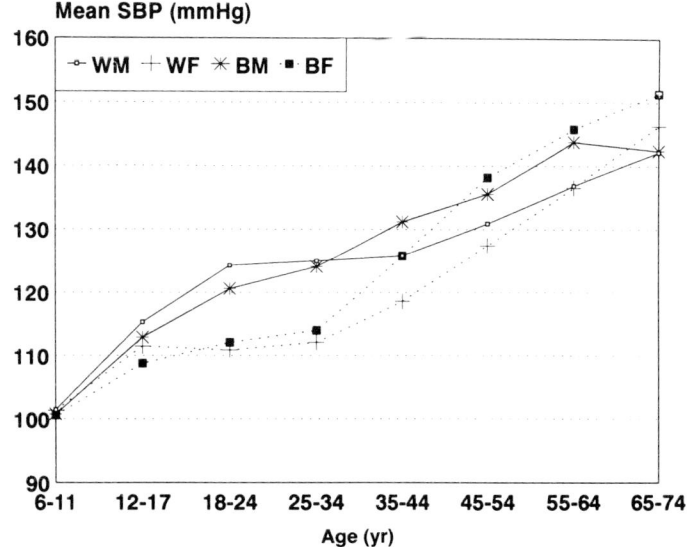

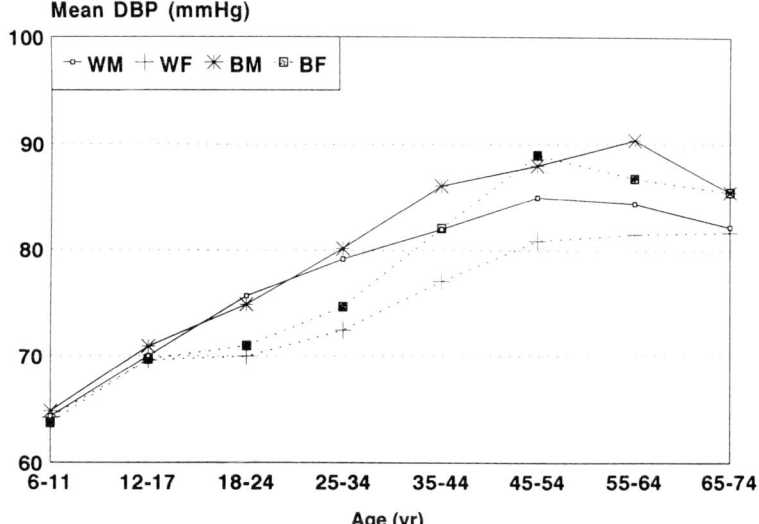

Figure 4–1. Blood pressure changes with age. A, Mean systolic blood pressure (SBP) with age. B, Mean diastolic blood pressure with age. Mean systolic blood pressures rise with age in both sexes and in blacks and whites (A). Mean diastolic blood pressures also increase with age but decrease slightly in the oldest age groups (B). Mean diastolic blood pressure is higher in adult men than in women at all ages; mean systolic blood pressure is higher in men until age 54 but is higher in women in the oldest age group. Black men and women in the 35- to 74-year-old age group have higher mean diastolic pressures than their white counterparts; mean systolic pressures are higher in black men (BM) than in white men (WM) between the ages of 35 and 64 and higher in black women (BF) than in white women (WF) between the ages of 35 and 74. (Data from Rowland M, Roberts J. Blood pressure levels and hypertension in persons ages 6–74 years: United States, 1976–1980. NCHS Advance Data from Vital and Health Statistics 84, 1982.)

among black women in the 1960 to 1962 National Health Examination Survey (NHES) have been reported.

The influence of menopause on blood pressure is controversial. Longitudinal studies from Framingham (10), Allegheny County (11), and the Netherlands (12) did not document any rise in blood pressure with menopause. In the last study, there was even an inverse relationship between systolic blood pressure and years since menopause. In contrast, cross-sectional studies by Staessen and associates (13) and Weiss (14) found significantly higher systolic and diastolic blood pressures in postmenopausal women. Staessen and colleagues (13) reported a fourfold higher prevalence of hypertension in postmenopausal compared to premenopausal women (40% vs 10%, p < .001). After adjusting for age and body mass index, postmenopausal women were still more than twice as likely to have hypertension than premenopausal women. The discrepant results remain unexplained.

Gender-specific incidence rates for hypertension are available from the NHANES I Epidemiologic Follow-up Study (Fig. 4–3) (5). Incidence rates of hypertension over an average follow-up of 9.5 years rose with age in both races and sexes and were higher in blacks than in whites. White men between the ages

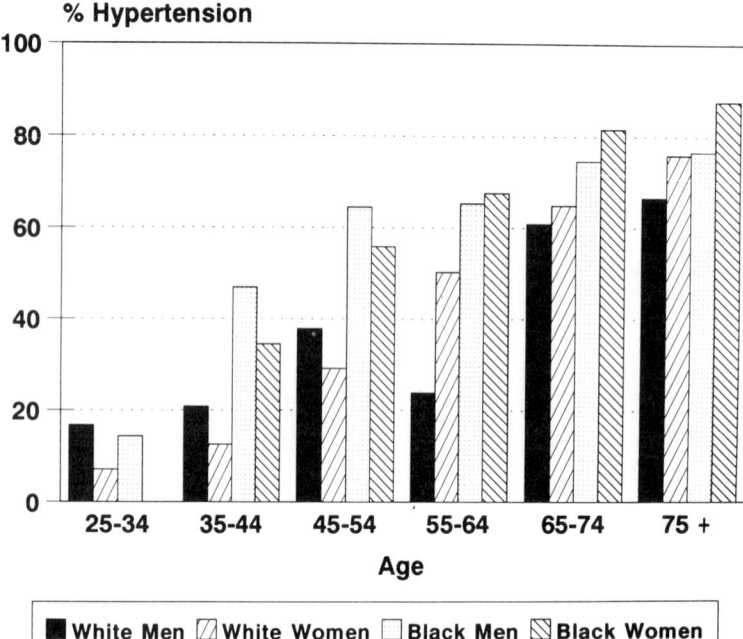

Figure 4–2. Prevalence of hypertension stratified by age, race, and sex. Prevalence rates rise with age in all race and sex groups. Hypertension is more common in black men and women than in white men and women in most age groups. In the younger age groups, men are more likely to be hypertensive than women, whereas women older than 64 years are more likely to be hypertensive than men in the same age group. (Data from Cornoni-Huntley J, LaCroix AZ, Havlik RJ. Race and sex differentials in the impact of hypertension in the United States. The National Health and Nutrition Examination Survey I Epidemiologic Follow-up Study. *Arch Intern Med* 149:780–788, 1989.)

of 25 and 54 had higher incidence rates than white women in the same age group; above age 55, the incidence rate was slightly higher in the women. Black men had a higher incidence rate than black women in the 35- to 54-year-old age group, while black women in the younger and older age groups were more likely to develop hypertension.

Hypertension in Women in Other Countries

In the early 1980s the WHO Monica Project was initiated in 27 countries (Australia, New Zealand, Canada, United States, Israel, China, Japan, and many European countries) to assess the relationship between trends in coronary and cerebrovascular disease and risk factor prevalence in the population. Results from the initial cross-sectional survey are now available (15). Subjects consist of a representative probability sample of 35- to 64-year-old men and women with a minimum sample size of 200 persons per sex, 10-year age group, and site. Large variations in blood pressure distribution and proportion of hypertensives were apparent in both genders. Median systolic blood pressures in women ranged from 118 to 141 mmHg; median diastolic blood pressures, from 72 to 89 mmHg. Age-adjusted prevalence rates of hypertension (BP > 159/94 mmHg or treatment with antihypertensives) in women ranged from 40.5% in the German Democratic Republic to 12.6% in Glostrup, Denmark (Fig. 4–4).

Nissinen et al. (16) reviewed survey data on hypertension in developing countries from 25 studies carried out in the 1970s and 1980s. Blood pressure was higher in older age groups and among men. The difference between the sexes was greatest in younger age groups in most countries. Among women, the prevalence of hypertension was lowest in Ethiopia (2–3%) and highest among urban Zulus (25% in 31- to 40-year-olds and 41% in 41- to 50-year-olds). In general, hypertension prevalence rates parallelled affluence, with the poorest countries having the lowest prevalence.

Secular Trends

Trends in blood pressure levels and hypertension prevalence can be assessed by comparing the results from the National Health Examination Surveys performed in the 1960s (NHES I to III), NHANES I and IA performed between 1971 and 1975, and NHANES II performed between 1976 and 1980 (4). Mean systolic blood pressure levels in 1976 to 1980 were lower than in 1971 to 1975 and in 1960

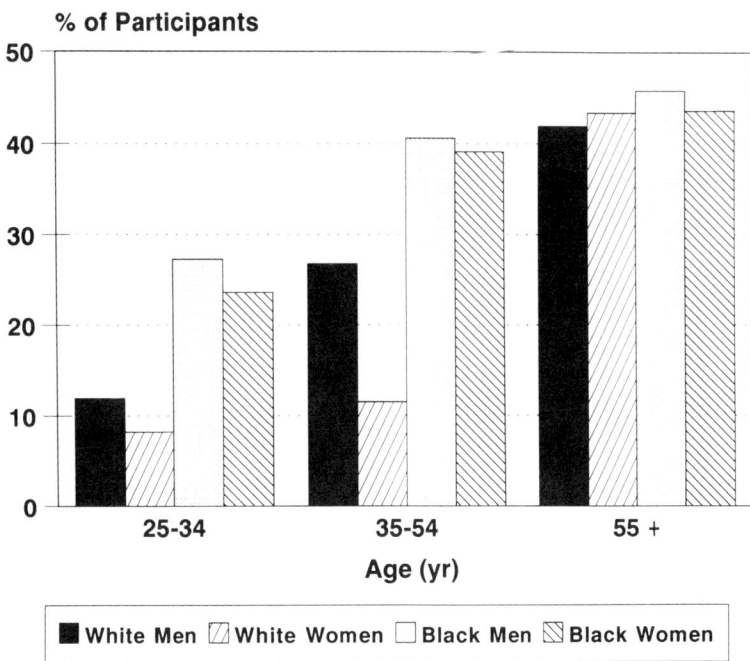

Figure 4–3. Incidence of hypertension. Incidence rates of hypertension rise with age in both races and sexes and are higher in blacks than in whites. White men between the ages of 25 and 54 have a higher incidence than white women in the same age group; above age 55, the incidence is slightly higher in women. Black men have a higher incidence than black women in the 35- to 54-year-old age group, whereas black women are more likely to develop hypertension in the younger and older age groups. (Data from Cornoni-Huntley J, LaCroix AZ, Havlik RJ. Race and sex differentials in the impact of hypertension in the United States. The National Health and Nutrition Examination Survey I Epidemiologic Follow-up Study. *Arch Intern Med* 149:780–788, 1989.)

to 1962, but mean diastolic blood pressure levels in 1976 to 1980 were similar to those in 1960 to 1962 in all four sex and racial groups. The age-adjusted prevalence rate of elevated blood pressure decreased from 17.7% to 14.5% between 1960 to 1962 and 1976 to 1980; the decrease was statistically significant in black men and women and in white women but did not reach significance in white men. The prevalence of hypertension, defined as blood pressure elevation or treatment for hypertension, has not changed significantly since 1960 to 1962, except for an increase among white men from 16.3% in 1960 to 1962 to 21.4% and 21.2% in the later studies. In the three surveys, prevalence rates of hypertension among white women were 20.4%, 19.6%, and 20% and among black women, 39.8%, 35.5%, and 39.8%, respectively.

More recent data on secular trends of blood pressure are available from the Minnesota Heart Surveys performed in a predominantly (96%) white population of 25- to 74-year-olds in 1980 to 1982 and 1985 to 1987 (17). Mean systolic blood pressures declined in women of all ages; the decline was most pronounced (4 to 5 mmHg) in those over age 55. Mean systolic blood pressure in men was unchanged. Mean diastolic blood pressures declined by approximately 1 mmHg in both sexes; the decline was observed in all age groups except 45- to 54-year-old men. Age-adjusted prevalence rates for hypertension decreased slightly from 21.8% to 18.7% in women and from 24.4% to 22.1% in men; neither decline reached statistical significance. More women were aware of their hypertension and adequately controlled with therapy in the second survey; this increase in awareness and treatment was not observed in men.

Surveys among black men and women in Minnesota were performed in 1973 to 1974 (n = 554) and in 1985 (n = 998) (18). Mean systolic blood pressure decreased in men from 135 mmHg to 129 mmHg and in women from 128 mmHg to 123 mmHg. The declines were most pronounced in the older age groups. Mean diastolic blood pressure decreased in men from 83 mmHg to 81 mmHg but did not change in women. The prevalence of hypertension (blood pressure elevation or treatment for hypertension) increased significantly in women from 25% to 38% ($p < .01$) but not in men (32% to 37%, p = NS). This increase in prevalence of hypertension in women is unexplained.

Economic Impact

The cost of hypertensive disease in the United States in 1992 is estimated at $14.8

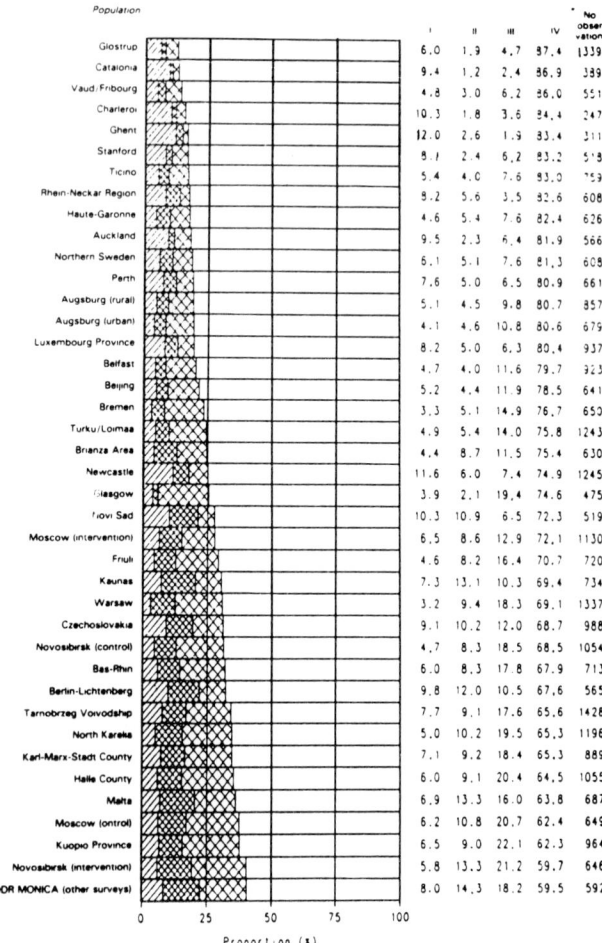

Figure 4–4. Prevalence of hypertension in 27 countries of the WHO Monica Project. The percentage of subjects in each of four blood pressure categories is shown:

Category I: systolic blood pressure (SBP) < 160 mmHg, diastolic blood pressure (DBP) < 95 mmHg on therapy for hypertension;
Category II: SBP > 159 mmHg, DBP > 94 mmHg on therapy for hypertension;
Category III: SBP > 159 mmHg, DBP > 94 mmHg with no therapy;
Category IV: SBP < 160 mmHg, DBP < 95 mmHg with no therapy.

Prevalence of hypertension (categories I to III) among women ranges from 40.5% in the German Democratic Republic (labeled DDR MONICA) to 12.6% in Glostrup, Denmark. (From The WHO Monica Project. Geographical variation in the major risk factors of coronary heart disease in men and women aged 35–64 years. *World Health Statistics Quarterly* 41:115–140, 1988.)

billion (1): $4.4 billion for hospital and nursing home services, $5.1 billion for physician and nursing services, $3 billion for drugs, and $2.3 billion in lost productivity. In 1980, per capita cost was lowest for uncomplicated hypertension but more than tripled when hypertension was associated with cardiovascular disease, renal disease, or diabetes mellitus (19). Although there were no significant age, gender, or race differences in overall expenditures for care, expenditures were higher in women for treatment of hypertension, whereas in men more resources were used for treatment of cardiovascular complications, e.g., cardiovascular surgery (19). Costs of screening for and treatment of hypertension are higher in women than in men when expressed as cost per quality-adjusted life-year (QUALY) saved, where QUALY is a measure of life expectancy corrected for morbidity (20, 21).

PATHOPHYSIOLOGY OF HYPERTENSION

Pathogenesis of Essential Hypertension

In more than 95% of cases of human hypertension, the cause of elevated blood pressure cannot be identified. These individuals have "essential" hypertension. Essential hypertension represents a collection of genetically based diseases or syndromes with a number of underlying inherited biochemical abnormalities. Many of the pathologic features of essential hypertension are compensatory mechanisms that offset a primary abnormality. Factors that have been implicated in the genesis of essential hypertension include increased sympathetic nervous system activity, increased or "inappropriate" renin secretion, overproduction of an unidentified Na^+ retaining hormone, chronic high Na^+ intake, inadequate dietary intakes of K^+ and Ca^{2+}, deficiencies of vasodilators such as prostacyclin, atrial natriuretic peptide and endothelium-derived relaxing factor (nitric oxide), excesses of vasoconstrictors such as angiotensin II, endothelin, and thromboxane, congenital abnormalities of the resistance vessels, diabetes mellitus, insulin resistance, obesity, increased activity of vascular growth factors, and altered cell ion transport (22).

Genetic Factors

The genetically mediated mechanisms by which blood pressure is controlled are diverse, interrelated, and incompletely understood. Epidemiologic and genetic segregation studies strongly suggest that hypertension is inherited as a polygenic disease, but the genes involved have not yet been identified. One strategy that has been used to search for hypertension-related genes utilizes the techniques of gene mapping and reverse genetics (23, 24). The principle of reverse genetics is that genes can be localized by linkage analysis and then cloned based on their chromosomal position (24). This approach has been successful for a variety of human diseases inherited in a simple Mendelian fashion (25–27). The reverse genetic approach is highly problematic for human diseases with polygenic or quantitative inheritance (28), however, since unambiguous identification of the disease phenotype and definition of a homogeneous population for study may be difficult or impossible (29). One solution to this problem is to utilize animal models for genetic dissection of complex traits in order to identify genes that can be studied in human populations. The ability to cross inbred strains eliminates the problem of genetic heterogeneity, and use of a sufficient number of animals can give the statistical power to detect genes affecting a quantitative trait. Recently, linkage studies in crosses between the stroke-prone spontaneously hypertensive rat (SHR-SP, a substrain of the most extensively studied rodent model of essential hypertension) and the normotensive Wistar-Kyoto (WKY) strain have led to the localization of a gene, Bp1 or BP/SP-1, that contributes significantly to blood pressure variation, and particularly to NaCl-sensitive hypertension, in the F_2 generation (29–31). This gene maps to rat chromosome 10 and is clearly linked to angiotensin-converting enzyme (ACE), a key enzyme in the renin-angiotensin system and a target of antihypertensive therapy. Comparison of the human and rat genetic maps indicates that this gene could reside on human chromosome 17q in a region that also contains the ACE gene (32). More complete mapping of the rat genome and investigation of other rodent models of NaCl-sensitive hypertension are needed to evaluate the significance of this finding. More importantly, this linkage has yet to be tested in humans.

A second approach that has been used to search for hypertension-related genes is the candidate gene approach, in which a gene that may be involved in blood pressure regulation is identified and cloned, a polymorphism is identified in the gene, and linkage of that polymorphism to blood pressure is investigated over several generations. This approach has been used to demonstrate that the renin gene or a closely linked gene is partially responsible for the development of NaCl-sensitive hypertension in the Dahl-S strain of rat (33). In contrast, in the spontaneously hypertensive rat (SHR) and SHR-SP strains, linkage analysis did not reveal an unequivocal relationship between the renin gene and hypertension (34, 35). Linkage analysis has recently been used to test the Na^+-H^+ antiporter as a candidate gene in human hypertension (36). Linkage of the Na^+-H^+ antiporter to hypertension was excluded because the number of Na^+-H^+ antiporter alleles shared between siblings in a population of 93 hypertensive sibling pairs was not greater than random. From this, the authors concluded that an abnormality in the gene for the Na^+-H^+ antiporter rarely, if ever, contributes to the pathogenesis of essential hypertension. This does not rule out an abnormality in the control of Na^+-H^+ antiporter gene transcription or in an interacting system. No other candidate gene has been clearly linked to essential hypertension in humans, but a specific genetic cause has recently been found for a rare form of inherited hypertension, glucocorticoid-remediable aldosteronism (37).

Thus, the tools of molecular biology provide, for the first time, the means of defining the genetic basis of the hypertensive diseases. Once a specific set of blood pressure-regulating genes is identified, genetic markers that permit early detection of individuals at risk for developing hypertension will be available. This will provide the basis for designing rational and targeted preventive and therapeutic strategies.

Renal Sodium Handling

A defect in the excretion of NaCl and water is central to the pathogenesis of systemic hypertension (38). The normal kidney responds to increments in perfusion pressure by increasing NaCl and water excretion, thus reducing intravascular volume and restoring blood pressure to normal levels. Hemodynamic, neural, and humoral factors participate in the control of volume and blood pressure homeostasis by regulating renal Na^+ handling. In hypertensive subjects this relationship is perturbed in such a way that higher perfusion pressures are needed to produce a natriuresis, favoring the maintenance of hypertension. A variety of neurohumoral factors, intrinsic and extrinsic to the kidney, influence the relationship between perfusion pressure and Na^+ excretion. In addition, a kidney subjected to elevated blood pressure over time develops structural changes that limit its ability to excrete Na^+ and water in response to increases in pressure. Kidneys altered in this fashion, when transplanted into a normotensive recipient, cause that individual to become hypertensive. This phenomenon has been demonstrated in several rodent models (39) and in human essential hypertension (40). Thus, the kidney contributes to the development of hypertension by controlling fluid and electrolyte homeostasis. Further study is needed to determine whether the kidney plays a causative or permissive role in the pathogenesis of hypertension and to define the cellular and molecular mechanisms by which altered renal function elevates blood pressure.

Autonomic Function

The autonomic nervous system is involved in the initiation and maintenance of essential hypertension. In patients with early hypertension, there is evidence of diminished resting parasympathetic inhibition and enhanced sympathetic stimulation of the cardiovascular system (39). These patients have elevated plasma renin and norepinephrine levels and enhanced vascular responses to stress as a consequence of their increased sympathetic activity. The efferent pathways through which increased sympathetic nervous system activity leads to sustained hypertension include enhanced vascular reactivity to the sympathetic neurotransmitter noradrenaline and stimulation of renal Na^+ and fluid retention through the renal nerves. In this way the two major pathophysiologic mechanisms of hypertension are related.

Patients with essential hypertension have an exaggerated pressor response to stress and an exaggerated depressor response to relaxation (22). Blood pressure falls during meditation and other states of relaxation and rises during isometric exercise and the stress of mental arithmetic to a greater extent in these patients than in normotensive control subjects. The impressive fall in blood pressure that is frequently seen when a hypertensive patient is removed from his home environment and brought into the hospital suggests that environmental stress exacerbates hypertension. The increased prevalence of hypertension in urban populations compared to rural groups and the occurrence of age-related rises in blood pressure in societies with changing value systems but not in those with a stable social structure provide evidence of a psychogenic contribution to essential hypertension. Stress presumably mediates its pressor effect through the sympathetic nervous system (22).

Hemodynamics

Cardiac output is elevated early in the course of essential hypertension and may cause secondary increases in peripheral vascular resistance that are responsible for maintaining the hypertension (22). This concept of total body autoregulation has been used to explain the adaptation of resistance vessels to increases in cardiac output. According to this theory, systemic resistance vessels respond to an increased cardiac output and increased intravascular volume by constricting in order to reduce tissue blood flow to normal (38). Patients with essential hypertension of recent onset gener-

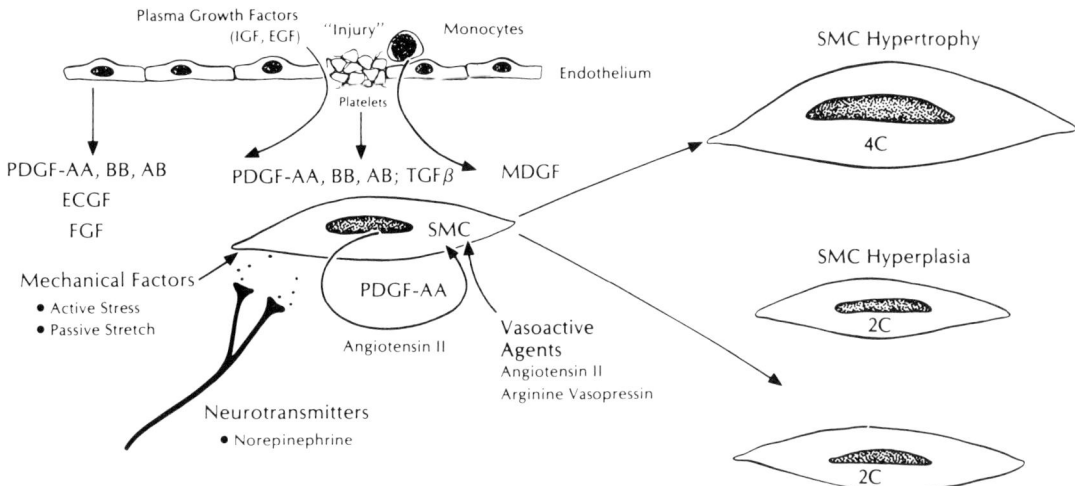

Figure 4–5. Factors that may play a role in growth regulation of smooth muscle cells under normal conditions and after vascular injury. The growth response of the smooth muscle cell may be hypertrophy or hyperplasia. Endothelial injury may influence the growth of smooth muscle cells owing to (1) increased influx of plasma growth factors such as insulinlike growth factor I (IGF) into the vessel wall through denuded vessel segments; (2) increased endothelial macromolecular permeability; (3) release of growth factors from platelets (e.g., platelet-derived growth factors [PDGF-AA, BB, AB], transforming growth factor β [TGFβ]) or monocytes (e.g., macrophage-derived growth factor [MDGF]) at sites of injury; or (4) increased production of growth factors by endothelial cells (e.g., PDGF-AA, BB, and AB; endothelial-derived growth factor [ECGF]) or smooth muscle cells themselves as a response to the injury. Other factors that may influence the growth of smooth muscle cells in the absence of vessel injury include norepinephrine and other neurotransmitters, mechanical factors, and contractile agonists from circulating blood or endothelial cells, or generated by smooth muscle cells themselves. (From Owens GK. Control of hypertrophic versus hyperplastic growth of vascular smooth muscle cells. *Am J Physiol* 257:H1755–H1765, 1989.)

ally show a pattern of increased cardiac output (about 15% greater than normotensive control levels), tachycardia, and venoconstriction, with normal or even low peripheral vascular resistance at rest (41). In contrast, patients with longstanding established hypertension usually have normal cardiac output and increased peripheral vascular resistance. Longitudinal studies of untreated hypertensive patients have documented a fall in cardiac output, due mainly to a decrease in stroke volume, and an increase in total peripheral resistance over time (42, 43). These observations are compatible with the notion that increases in cardiac output initiate essential hypertension and that changes in peripheral vascular resistance occur later and are more important in maintaining the blood pressure elevation.

Growth Factors, Oncogenes, and Cardiovascular Hypertrophy

Hypertrophy of the heart and blood vessels, whether primary or secondary to increases in blood pressure and hence vessel wall tension, plays an important role in the pathogenesis of hypertension. The myogenic responses to elevations in blood pressure and flow are characterized by vasoconstriction, increased Ca^{2+} influx into vascular smooth muscle cells, and, over the long term, increased myocyte growth. The resultant vascular hypertrophy tends to reduce blood flow to the tissues and to elevate intravascular pressure. Some of the stimuli to growth of vascular smooth muscle cells are illustrated in Figure 4–5. The growth factors have contractile effects on vascular smooth muscle cells and trigger many of the same cellular signaling events that are activated by vasoconstrictor agents such as norepinephrine, angiotensin II, and endothelin. Conversely, many of the endogenous vasoconstrictors stimulate vascular smooth muscle cell growth via receptor-mediated mechanisms. Of the endogenous vasoconstrictors, angiotensin II is a particularly important autocrine and paracrine regulator of cardiovascular hypertrophy. Blood vessel walls contain an active renin-angiotensin system (44), and inhibition of vascular angiotensin II production with angiotensin-converting enzyme inhibitors prevents or reverses vascular hypertrophy more effectively than treatment with other antihypertensive agents that have equipotent blood pressure-lowering effects (39, 45). Further, ACE inhibitors may prevent restenosis following angioplasty, suggesting that angiotensin II may participate in the vascular remodeling characteristic of the atherosclerotic process (46).

Contractile agonists, growth factors, mechanical stretching of blood vessels, and shear stress imposed on the endothelium by blood flow share cellular signaling effects that stimulate vascular growth (39). Many of these stimuli activate phospholipase C, which hydrolyzes phosphatidylinositol biphosphate to generate inositol triphosphate and diacylglycerol. The former mobilizes Ca^{2+} from intracellular stores; the latter modulates Ca^{2+}-sensitive protein kinase C, which activates Na^+/H^+ exchange and alkalinizes the cell. Cellular alkalinization is associated with both vasoconstriction and growth or division. Alternate signaling events, including cyclic AMP production, have also been described.

Proto-oncogenes, including c-fos, c-myc, and c-jun, that are induced in association with these signaling events render the cells competent to replicate their DNA in response to growth factors (47). Whether the protein products of these competence genes are responsible for vascular growth is uncertain. The regulation of vascular growth in hypertension is an area of active investigation and may give rise to new approaches, including gene therapy, to antihypertensive treatment.

Cardiac hypertrophy resulting from the actions of the above growth factors and neurohumoral and physical stimuli is an important concomitant of hypertension, mainly because it predisposes to congestive heart failure. The development of both cardiac hypertrophy and heart failure in persons with hypertension exhibits a sexually dimorphic pattern. A past medical history of hypertension is common among individuals with congestive heart failure; the risk of developing heart failure increases in parallel with the level of arterial pressure in both sexes, but women are less likely to develop heart failure than men with the same level of arterial pressure (48). Normotensive women have a smaller left ventricular mass than men by echocardiographic criteria (49), and the prevalence of left ventricular hypertrophy by echocardiographic criteria is consistently lower in women than in men when a single cut-off value for normal blood pressure is applied to both sexes (50, 51). Compared to men with the same level of arterial pressure, women have smaller left ventricular dimensions and enhanced left ventricular performance; the sex difference in left ventricular structure is more pronounced in premenopausal women and tends to disappear after the menopause (52). The sexually dimorphic pattern of cardiac adaptation in hypertension appears to reflect, at least in part, the effects of sex hormones on the heart. Androgens exert a trophic influence on the myocardium: sex differences in heart size in animal models can be abolished by orchidectomy and restored by testosterone replacement (53–55). Further, there are specific estrogen receptors in cardiac muscle (56) through which endogenous estrogens may exert a positive inotropic effect in premenopausal women, giving rise to enhanced left ventricular performance (52). These sex differences in cardiac adaptation may be a major pathophysiologic mechanism accounting for the lower risk of congestive heart failure and other cardiovascular morbidity and mortality in premenopausal women than in age-matched men with essential hypertension.

Insulin Resistance

Insulin resistance, defined as a reduction in whole-body disposal of glucose in response to exogenous insulin, has been described in essential hypertension (22). Whole-body insulin-induced glucose uptake and nonoxidative glucose disposal (glycogen synthesis and glycolysis) are markedly reduced and plasma insulin levels are elevated, presumably as a compensatory mechanism, in insulin-resistant subjects. Several mechanisms have been hypothesized to explain the relationship between hyperinsulinemia and blood pressure: (1) Insulin induces renal Na^+ retention by increasing Na^+ reabsorption in the distal nephron and possibly in the proximal nephron as well (57). Thus, hyperinsulinemia could elevate blood pressure by expanding plasma and extracellular fluid volume. (2) Hyperinsulinemia in the presence of normal blood glucose levels increases sympathetic nervous system activity, which can in turn elevate blood pressure (39). (3) Insulin is a potent stimulus for receptor-mediated growth of vascular endothelial and smooth muscle cells (58), thus leading to increased peripheral vascular resistance and blood pressure. (4) Insulin, by altering plasma free fatty acid levels, modulates Na^+-K^+-ATPase activity, thus altering cellular cation transport in a manner that could increase peripheral vascular tone and blood pressure (39).

Hyperinsulinemia has been shown in large prospective studies to be predictive of the development of atherosclerotic cardiovascular disease in male subjects (59–61). Further, hyperinsulinemia is associated with hypertension (62), obesity, and glucose intolerance (the GOH conditions) and with dyslipoproteinemia, the principal risk factors for atherosclerotic cardiovascular disease (63). Recently, the Israel Study of Glucose Intolerance, Obesity and Hypertension (the Israel GOH Study) showed that hyperinsulinemia was not associated with atherosclerotic cardiovascular disease in women or in men free of the GOH conditions (63). Findings are similar in the Australian Study (61), and the Paris Prospective Study (59). In the Israel GOH Study, all excess cardiovascular disease risk associated with the male sex was confined to hyperinsulinemic individuals with at least one of the GOH conditions. The pathophysiologic mechanisms relating male sex, insulin (or insulin resistance), and accelerated atherosclerosis remain to be elucidated.

Interventions that reduce insulin resistance, such as weight loss, diets low in carbohydrates and high in unsaturated fats, and aerobic exercise, also reduce blood pressure, supporting the concept that essential hypertension is an insulin-resistant state (22). Further study is needed to elucidate the relationships between hypertension, insulin resistance, and two related syndromes, obesity and glucose intolerance.

ANIMAL MODELS OF HYPERTENSION

Rodents have been used extensively in the study of hypertension. A variety of genetically hypertensive lines of rats have been developed over the past 35 years and have been used to study both the pathophysiology and the molecular genetics of hypertension (29, 64, 65). A sexually dimorphic pattern in the development of hypertension has been observed in these rodent models: Blood pressure levels are higher in males than in females (66–68). In the DEA/2J and CBA strains of mice, the male develops higher blood pressure than the age-matched female (68). In the Dahl NaCl-sensitive (Dahl-S) rat, the SHR of the Okamoto strain, and the desoxycorticosterone acetate (DOCA)-NaCl hypertensive rat, hypertension develops more rapidly and becomes more severe in the male than in the female (69–73).

There is abundant evidence that gonadectomy alters the natural history of hypertension in these models. Gonadectomy at an early age (30 days) retards the development of hypertension in both male and female SHR (70). Neonatally androgenized female SHR exhibit a pattern of blood pressure similar to that of the male during maturation (66), whereas neonatally castrated male SHR exhibit the pattern typical of intact females. Further, even late (17 weeks of age) gonadectomy of SHR significantly decreases the rate of rise of blood pressure in both sexes (74). The data of Ganten et al. (73) show that both surgical castration at 18 days of age and chemical castration with the androgen receptor antagonists cyproterone (which does not elevate circulating testosterone levels) and flutamide (which leads to a feedback elevation of gonadotrophic hormones and plasma testosterone) at 10 days of age attenuate the development of hypertension in male stroke-prone SHR. These treatments had no effect on blood pressure in male stroke-prone SHR with established hypertension (25 weeks old). These data suggest that testosterone contributes to the development of hypertension in young male SHR but not to the maintenance of established hypertension in the mature animal. Similarly, the subsequent development of DOCA-NaCl hypertension is attenuated in male rats gonadectomized at an early (3 weeks) age (75), probably owing to decreased pressor responsiveness to endogenous vasopressin (72).

Our laboratory has tested the effects of castration and gonadal hormone replacement in young male and female SHR on the subsequent development of hypertension and on the neurohumoral mechanisms that participate in this process (55). We observed that intact male and female SHR showed a progressive increase in blood pressure with growth: males attained systolic blood pressure levels of 244 ± 6 mmHg, and females reached 205 ± 3 mmHg at 22 weeks of age (Fig. 4–6). Orchidectomy at age 4 weeks significantly attenuated the blood pressure elevation in the male (195 ± 4 mmHg at age 22 weeks), but ovariectomy at age 4 weeks had no effect on the development of hypertension in the female. The pattern of development of hypertension in orchidectom-

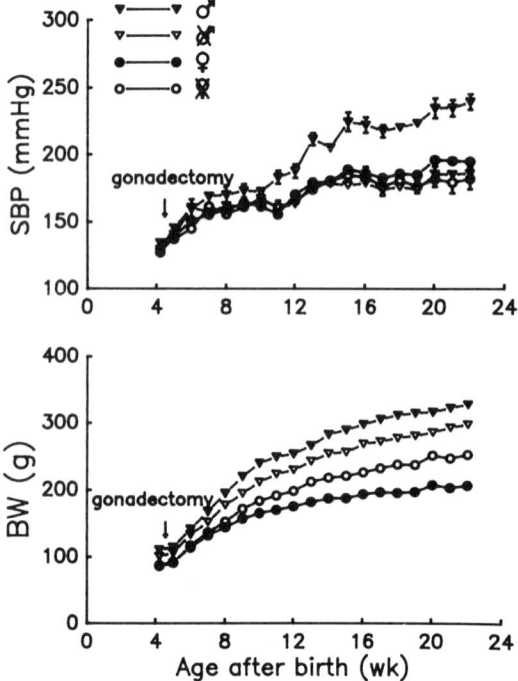

Figure 4–6. Effects of gonadectomy on systolic blood pressure (SBP) and body weight (BW) in male and female spontaneously hypertensive rats (SHR). Results represent means ± standard error of the mean (SE) values for groups of eight to nine animals measured individually. (From Chen YF, Meng QC. Sexual dimorphism of blood pressure in spontaneously hypertensive rats is androgen dependent. *Life Sci* 48:85–96, 1991.)

in sympathetic fibers innervating the rat vas deferens (81), raising the possibility that similar mechanisms could operate at noradrenergic nerve terminals on resistance vessels and in the brain. Autoradiographic studies with [^{3}H] dihydrotestosterone have demonstrated labeling of nuclei in rat spinal cord and brain regions involved in cardiovascular control, including the area postrema, dorsal motor nucleus of the vagus, nucleus ambiguus, A5 neuronal group, raphe nuclei, central gray of the midbrain, basal hypothalamus, periventricular nucleus, preoptic region, bed nucleus of the stria terminalis, dorsolateral septum, and amygdala (82). Thus, it has been hypothesized that testosterone may influence the synthesis or release (or both) of neurotransmitters or neuromodulators in the hypothalamus and caudal medulla that have cardiovascular effects. Dihydrotestosterone and catecholamines are

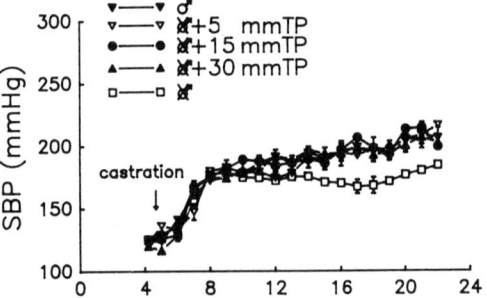

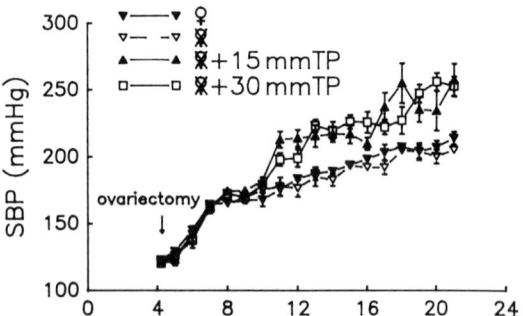

Figure 4–7. *Top,* Effects of orchidectomy and testosterone replacement on systolic blood pressure (SBP) in male spontaneously hypertensive rats (SHR). Results represent means ± standard error of the mean (SE) values for groups of six animals measured individually. *Bottom,* Effects of ovariectomy and testosterone administration on systolic blood pressure (SBP) in female SHR. Results represent means ± SE values for groups of seven animals measured individually. (From Chen YF, Meng QC. Sexual dimorphism of blood pressure in spontaneously hypertensive rats is androgen dependent. *Life Sci* 48:85–96, 1991.)

ized males was the same as that in intact and ovariectomized females (see Fig. 4–6). Administration of testosterone propionate to gonadectomized rats of both sexes conferred a male pattern of blood pressure development (Fig. 4–7). Thus, the sexually dimorphic pattern of hypertension in the SHR is dependent on androgens rather than estrogens.

Testosterone interacts with a variety of neurohumoral systems that are involved in the control of blood pressure and volume homeostasis (76). One mechanism that has been proposed to explain the effects of testosterone on blood pressure in the SHR is enhanced sympathetic nervous system activity (55, 77). Sympathetic tone is markedly increased during the developmental phase of hypertension in male SHR (78–80) but returns toward normotensive control levels in the established phase of hypertension. Sympathetic neural function has not been carefully studied in female or castrated male SHR during the developmental phase of hypertension. Testosterone modulates norepinephrine storage and release co-localized in 50–80% of catecholaminergic neurons in the pons and dorsolateral corner of the fourth ventricle, adjacent to the nucleus olivaris superior, in the locus coeruleus, arcuate nucleus, periventricular nucleus, and the region of the lateral lemniscus (83), suggesting that testosterone may influence blood pressure via effects on catecholaminergic pathways in the brain.

Our laboratory has shown that stores of norepinephrine in the posterior hypothalamic region are significantly greater in intact male rats and testosterone-treated rats of both sexes than in intact or ovariectomized females (55). The posterior hypothalamic area is a sympathoexcitatory region: Electrical stimulation of discrete neuronal groups in this area increases arterial pressure, heart rate, and vascular resistance (84–87), and this effect is greater in SHR than in normotensive WKY control rats (85, 86). Even prior to the onset of hypertension, the noradrenergic innervation of the posterior hypothalamic area is greater in male SHR than in normotensive male rats (88). This finding, together with previous observations that testosterone stimulates the development of noradrenergic neurons in the hypothalamus (89), suggests that exposure to androgen at a young age in SHR of either sex may accelerate the differentiation of the noradrenergic system in this brain region. Thus, it is possible that intact male and testosterone-treated gonadectomized SHR of both sexes may have increased androgen-dependent sympathetic outflow during the developmental phase of hypertension and that this may contribute to the increased blood pressure seen in the male of this strain. Further study is needed to test this hypothesis.

The distribution of estrogen-binding sites (90, 91) and the extent of co-localization of estrogen and catecholamines (83) in rat brain are similar to the patterns described for testosterone. In addition, co-localization of dopamine and estradiol has been described in the arcuate and periventricular nuclei, and co-localization of serotonin and estradiol has been observed in the raphe nuclei (83). Thus, estrogen, like testosterone, may influence blood pressure via effects on catecholaminergic pathways in brain. Studies in female SHR are needed to test this hypothesis.

Evidence from a number of laboratories indicates that androgens stimulate renin-angiotensin system activity. Submandibular gland renin activity decreases after castration and increases following testosterone treatment, as well as during puberty, in male mice (92–96). Dihydrotestosterone treatment of female NMRI two-renin-gene mice results in an increase in renin mRNA concentration in the submandibular gland, adrenal gland, and brain, and a decrease in renin mRNA concentration in the kidney (96). Testosterone treatment of male WKY rats castrated as weanlings and normal adult female WKY rats causes significant increases in renal angiotensinogen mRNA levels (97). Further, in the transgenic rat line TGR (mRen2)-27 that expresses an extra (DAB mouse Ren2) renin gene, blood pressure is ~ 100 mmHg higher in adult males than in adult females (98). This suggests that testosterone-driven overexpression of the mouse renin gene may contribute to the exaggerated (male greater than female) sexual dimorphism of hypertension in this transgenic rat strain (76).

To test the hypothesis that androgens participate in the development of hypertension in the SHR through effects on expression of the renin or angiotensinogen genes, our laboratory examined renin and angiotensinogen gene expression in kidney and liver of male and female SHR that were gonadectomized or sham-operated at 4 weeks of age (77). Subgroups of gonadectomized rats of both sexes were supplemented with exogenous testosterone propionate. Plasma renin activity was significantly higher in intact male rats than in intact females 18 weeks after gonadectomy; orchidectomy was associated with significant decreases in plasma renin levels, while testosterone treatment resulted in significant increases in plasma renin activity in both sexes (female greater than male) (Fig. 4–8). This finding is consistent with the hypothesis that the androgen-dependent development of hypertension in SHR may be related to activation of the renin-angiotensin system.

Renal and hepatic angiotensinogen mRNA levels are androgen dependent in both sexes: they decrease following gonadectomy and increase following testosterone replacement (Fig. 4–9). Thus, androgens can be added to the list of hormones and local modulators, including estrogen, insulin, glucocorticoids, angiotensin II, volume depletion, and dietary NaCl restriction (99–102), that regulate angiotensinogen synthesis and release. The liver is the major source of plasma angiotensinogen and contains the highest concentrations of angiotensinogen mRNA transcripts of any organ. Therefore, enhanced hepatic angiotensinogen

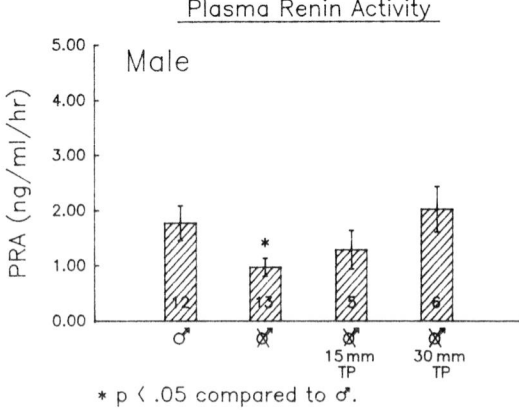

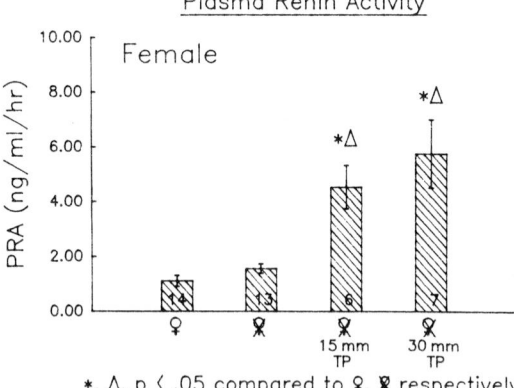

Figure 4–8. Effects of gonadectomy and testosterone administration on plasma renin activity in male and female spontaneously hypertensive rats (SHR). Results represent means ± standard error of the mean (SE). Numbers in each column represent the number of animals per group; 15 mm and 30 mm indicate the length of Silastic capsules; TP = testosterone propionate, ♂̸ = gonadectomized male, ♀̸ = gonadectomized female. (From Chen YF, Naftilan AJ, Oparil S. Androgen dependent angiotensinogen and renin mRNA expression in hypertensive rats. *Hypertension* 19:456–463, 1992.)

production stimulated by either endogenous or exogenous testosterone could contribute to the elevation in plasma renin activity observed in intact male and testosterone-replaced SHR.

Estrogens also stimulate hepatic angiotensinogen synthesis by enhancing gene transcription (103, 104). An estrogen response element has recently been identified in the 5′ flanking region of the human (105) and rat (106) angiotensinogen genes. Despite the marked stimulatory effect of estrogens on hepatic angiotensinogen synthesis, which results in increased circulating angiotensinogen levels, blood pressure elevations are unusual in pregnant subjects and in subjects receiving exogenous estrogen. The reason for this is unknown but may be related to feedback inhibition of renin release by increased circulating angiotensin II levels or to estrogen-induced down regulation of angiotensin II receptor density in a variety of tissues, including adrenal cortex and pituitary gland (107).

In contrast to angiotensinogen, renal renin mRNA levels were androgen dependent in female SHR only: They decreased following ovariectomy and increased to male levels following testosterone replacement (77). Neither castration nor testosterone replacement altered renal renin mRNA levels in male SHR. The latter finding is consistent with previous reports in normotensive mice and rats. Mouse renal renin levels are similar in both sexes, and neither castration of adult male mice nor administration of androgen to adult female

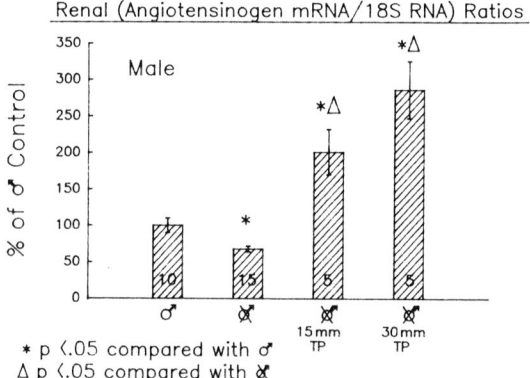

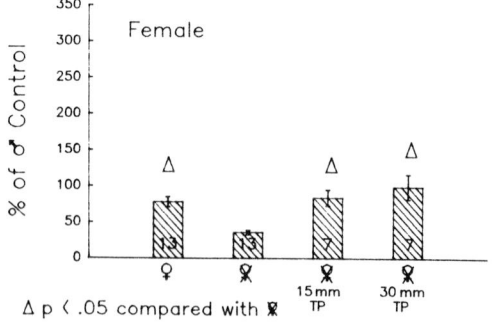

Figure 4–9. Effects of gonadectomy and testosterone administration on renal angiotensinogen mRNA to 18S ribosomal RNA ratios in male and female spontaneously hypertensive rats (SHR). Results represent means ± standard error of the mean (SE). Numbers in each column represent the number of animals per group. TP = testosterone propionate, ♂̸ = gonadectomized male, ♀̸ = gonadectomized female. (From Chen YF, Naftilan AJ, Oparil S. Androgen dependent angiotensinogen and renin mRNA expression in hypertensive rats. *Hypertension* 19:456–463, 1992.)

mice has a significant stimulatory effect on renal renin activity or mRNA levels (96, 108). Further, mouse renal renin levels and renin mRNA levels remain stable throughout ontogeny in both sexes (95). In contrast, renin expression in the submaxillary gland, testis, adrenal gland, and brain of the mouse are androgen dependent (96, 108). The mechanisms of this tissue-specific differential regulation of renin gene expression in response to androgens remain to be elucidated.

Despite the unresponsiveness of renal renin mRNA to androgen, a sexual dimorphism (male higher) of active plasma renin has been found in SHR (current study) and of inactive plasma renin in Wistar rats (109), in mouse strains with one or two renin genes (110), and, although less pronounced, in humans (111). In male mice and rats, inactive plasma renin originates mainly from the kidney (109–111). Thus, renin release appears to increase in response to testosterone in the absence of increased renal renin mRNA concentrations. This lack of correlation between plasma renin activity and renal renin mRNA confirms the observations of Pratt et al. that Na$^+$ restriction significantly increases plasma renin concentration without affecting renal renin mRNA levels in male SHR and WKY rats (100). Although testosterone-induced increases in renal size may have been at least partially responsible for the observed enhancement in plasma renin activity in intact male and testosterone-supplemented SHR in our study (77), it is clear that regulation of plasma renin activity occurs at the post-transcriptional level in response to a number of stimuli in other models.

Thus, the androgen-dependent increment in blood pressure seen in intact male or testosterone-replaced SHR of either sex appears to be, at least in part, related to activation of the renin-angiotensin system. Unpublished data from the laboratory of Berecek indicate that lifetime treatment with the angiotensin-converting enzyme inhibitor captopril abolishes the sexual dimorphism of hypertension in SHR, lending further support to this concept.

Sex hormone-dependent alterations in endothelial function may contribute to the increased severity of hypertension in male subjects and the apparent vasoprotection seen in females with elevated endogenous estrogen levels. The endothelium of male rats has reduced smooth muscle relaxing (vasodilator releasing) potency compared to that of female rats (112). Estrogen treatment enhances endothelium-dependent relaxation of rabbit femoral arteries in response to acetylcholine (113), and chronic estrogen replacement therapy in ovariectomized cynomolgus monkeys reverses the paradoxical constriction of the coronary arteries in response to intracoronary infusion of acetylcholine (114). Estrogen does not alter coronary vasodilator responses to nitroglycerine or plasma lipid levels, blood pressure, heart rate, or resting coronary artery diameter in this model. Further, acute intravenous administration of estrogen (ethinyl estradiol) produces the same effect in atherosclerotic coronary arteries of surgically postmenopausal cynomolgus monkeys that consumed an atherogenic diet for 18 months (115). Taken together, these findings suggest that estrogen facilitates endothelium-dependent dilation of blood vessels, probably by increasing the release of or response to endothelium-derived relaxing factor and possibly by inhibiting the release of or response to constrictor factor(s) (114). The role of these mechanisms in the pathogenesis of hypertension is currently the subject of intense investigation.

Estrogen and progesterone receptors have been described in arterial endothelial and smooth muscle cells of several mammalian species (116, 117). Treatment of ovariectomized baboons with estradiol results in redistribution of aortic intracellular estrogen receptors from the cytoplasmic fraction to the nuclear fraction and in increased cytoplasmic concentrations of progesterone receptors (117), implicating these sex steroids in the regulation of arterial cell function. Estrogen treatment also results in reductions in lipoprotein-induced aortic smooth muscle proliferation (118), inhibition of intimal proliferation associated with mechanical endothelial injury (119–121), reduced cholesterol ester influx and hydrolysis (122), inhibition of platelet aggregation (123), and increased prostacyclin production (124). Thus, vascular estrogen receptors appear to be physiologically functional and elevations in circulating endogenous estrogen levels may influence the growth and functional characteristics of vascular endothelial or smooth muscle cells (114). These cellular mechanisms may account for the vasoprotective effect of estrogens and the vascular complications of hypertension that are observed in female subjects.

HYPERTENSION AS A RISK FACTOR

It has been known since the 1920s that hypertension is associated with premature

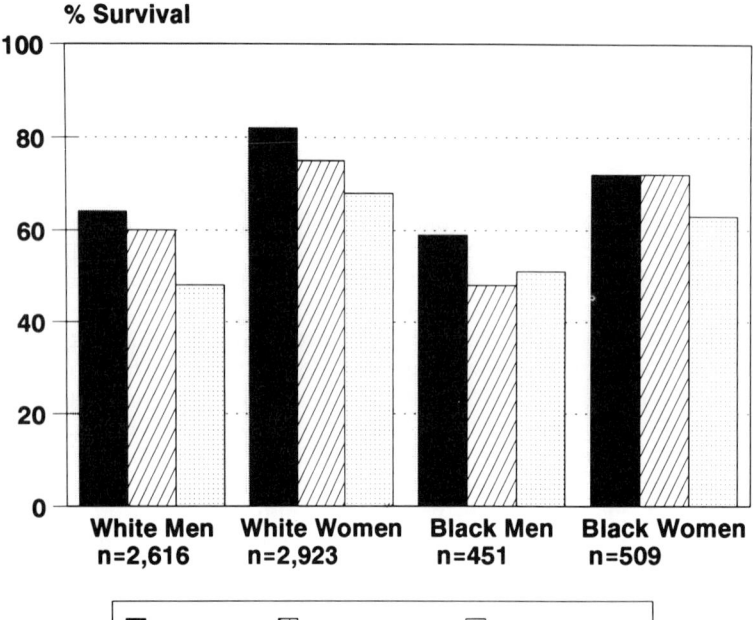

Figure 4–10. Twelve-year survival rates in persons ≥ 50 years old in the NHANES I Epidemiologic Follow-up Study (5). Survival rates were decreased among hypertensives in all race-sex subgroups. The decrease in survival was statistically significant among whites but did not reach statistical significance among blacks due to the small sample size.

death in both genders (125,126). Morbidity due to hypertension occurs either predominantly as a direct consequence of the elevated intravascular pressure (e.g., in congestive heart failure, aortic dissection, renal insufficiency, and hemorrhagic stroke) or via acceleration of atherosclerosis (coronary heart disease, claudication, atherothrombotic stroke). In this section, we will discuss the available data from observational studies relating blood pressure to mortality and cardiovascular morbidity in women. The impact of antihypertensive therapy on some of these end points is addressed in the section, Clinical Trials of Antihypertensive Therapy.

Mortality

Deubner et al. (127) examined 10-year survival rates in 2033 individuals (aged 40 to 69 at entry into the study in 1960 to 1962) in Evans County, Georgia, by sex, race, age, and blood pressure levels. Survival rates were consistently lower in those who had a systolic blood pressure above 139 mmHg or a diastolic blood pressure above 94 mmHg. The hypertension attributable risk for systolic and diastolic hypertension was lower in white women than in black women or in men of both races. For both systolic and diastolic hypertension, the population-attributable fraction (the proportion of deaths due to hypertension in relation to overall mortality rate) in each subgroup was highest for black women (0.61 for systolic hypertension, 0.47 for diastolic hypertension). White women had fractions of 0.42 for systolic hypertension, similar to that of men of both races, and 0.15 for diastolic hypertension, the lowest among all four gender-racial groups.

More recent data are available from the NHANES I Epidemiologic Follow-up Study (5) (Fig. 4–10). The survival analysis included 2616 white men, 2923 white women, 451 black men, and 509 black women. Twelve-year survival rates for persons aged 50 and older in all racial-gender subgroups were lower in individuals with hypertension than in persons with normal blood pressure. This decrease in survival was statistically significant among whites but not among blacks owing to the smaller sample size.

Thus, hypertension is a significant risk factor for excess mortality in both sexes. Systolic hypertension is an important predictor of mortality in both black and white women, whereas diastolic hypertension appears to have a much greater impact on mortality in black women.

Congestive Heart Failure

The Framingham Study provides the best available data about the impact of hypertension on the subsequent incidence of congestive heart failure in women (128). During 30 years of follow-up of 5070 men and women, 85 women in the 35- to 64-year-old age group and 144 women in the 65- to 94-year-old age group developed heart failure. Women with a systolic pressure of > 180 mmHg were six to seven times more likely to develop heart failure in both age groups than those persons with systolic blood pressures of < 120 mmHg. The relative risk in men was comparable to that of women in the younger age group but lower (relative risk 2.2) in the older age group. An even more striking increase in relative risk of developing heart failure was apparent when women with and without left ventricular hypertrophy were compared (relative risk of 17 in the younger and 6.7 in the older age group). Overall, it is estimated that 55% of patients with congestive heart failure in this Framingham cohort had a history of hypertension and that one-third of cases of congestive heart failure could be attributed directly to hypertension (129). Although more subject to bias, recent data from clinical trials suggest that hypertension may be less important as an etiologic factor of heart failure in the 1980s. For example, approximately 40% of individuals in the Studies of Left Ventricular Dysfunction (SOLVD) Registry had hypertension, but only 7% of patients were classified as having heart failure on that basis (unpublished data). Increasing mortality rates from heart failure, especially in older individuals and despite more effective antihypertensive therapy, suggest that treatment of hypertension may significantly postpone but not entirely prevent the development of heart failure (129).

Renal Failure

The causal relationship between severe accelerated or malignant hypertension and renal failure and the efficacy of antihypertensive therapy in preventing acute renal failure in this setting are well established (130, 131). The data relating renal insufficiency and mild to moderate hypertension are less extensive (130–135). Associations between blood pressure level and progression of renal dysfunction were reported by Lindemann et al. (132) and Klahr (133) in patients with mean systolic pressures of 107 mmHg and 100 mmHg, respectively. Data from the Hypertension, Detection and Follow-up Program are consistent with these observations (134): Patients with the highest blood pressure values at entry also had the highest creatinine levels, and the decline of renal function over the course of treatment was most pronounced in those with the highest diastolic pressures. Patients in the Stepped Care group tended to have smaller rises in serum creatinine than those in Referred Care.

One of the larger observational studies with gender-specific data is that of Tierney et al. (135), who retrospectively analyzed renal function in 6880 patients with hypertension followed for a mean of 5.2 years in the General Medicine Clinic at the University of Indiana. The mean age was 55.8 years; 70% were women and 72% were black. Hypertension was mild with a mean enrollment blood pressure of 150/92 mmHg and a mean blood pressure of 142/86 mmHg during therapy. Renal insufficiency, defined as a creatinine of ≥ 2 mg/dL, developed in 18.1% of patients during follow-up. White females had an incidence of 11.9% and black females an incidence of 18%. The incidence in white and black men was 15.1% and 25%, respectively. Heart failure, age, diabetes, mean systolic blood pressure during treatment, male gender, and black race were highly statistically significant, independent predictors of the development of renal dysfunction by multivariate analysis.

Hypertension is the most common underlying illness in patients undergoing dialysis (132), and the incidence is increasing (130). Reports from end-stage renal disease registries (136, 137) indicate that the incidence of hypertensive end-stage renal disease in all age groups is lower in white and black females than in white and black males, respectively. The differences between the two genders tend to diminish with advancing age. Black women have markedly higher rates than white women in all age strata (odds ratios of 4 to 9). These racial differences are partially but not entirely explained by the earlier onset of hypertension, increased severity of blood pressure, and lower socioeconomic status in black women than in white women.

Coronary Heart Disease

The relationship between hypertension and atherosclerosis is complex. Elevated blood pressure results in altered arterial structure and function and abnormal flow patterns, but hypertension alone is not sufficient to induce atherosclerosis (138). However, hypertension in the presence of other risk factors, particularly hypercholesterolemia, clearly accelerates the progression of atherosclerosis (139). In western societies, hypertension and hypercholesterolemia frequently coexist. Among participants of NHANES II, for example, 40% of persons with hypertension had blood cholesterol levels of ≥ 240 mg/dL and 46% of those with blood cholesterol levels of ≥ 240 mg/dL had hypertension (140). Persons with hypertension and dyslipidemia often have glucose intolerance and upper body obesity. This constellation of risk factors, variously referred to as syndrome X (141), the deadly quartet (142), or familial dyslipidemic hypertension (143), confers a markedly increased risk of coronary heart disease.

Kannel et al. (144), reporting 14-year follow-up data from the Framingham cohort, showed that hypertension was a powerful independent predictor of coronary heart disease in both sexes. The relationship between blood pressure and development of coronary heart disease was graded with no threshold in risk at lower blood pressure levels. Systolic blood pressure was a better predictor of risk than diastolic blood pressure, especially in older age groups and in women. In women, systolic blood pressure was the second (to age) most powerful predictor of coronary heart disease; in men, systolic blood pressure ranked fourth behind age, serum cholesterol, and cigarettes smoked. Stokes et al. (128) extended these observations to 30 years of follow-up. The relationship between systolic blood pressure and coronary heart disease incidence was again significant in both sexes in univariate and multivariate analyses. The strength of the relationship varied with age. Below age 65, the risk of coronary heart disease at a systolic blood pressure of above 180 mmHg compared to a systolic blood pressure of 120 mmHg was higher in women (fivefold increase) than in men (threefold increase); in older individuals, the risk was higher in men (fivefold increase) than in women (threefold increase). Left ventricular hypertrophy was an independent contributor to coronary heart disease risk in both sexes, especially in the older age group.

In the Walnut Creek Contraceptive Study (145), 16,759 women between the ages of 18 and 54 were followed for up to 7 years. Hypertension was an independent risk factor for myocardial infarction, resulting in a threefold increase in risk by multivariate analysis. In the Rochester Coronary Heart Disease Project (146), hypertension was a significant risk factor for coronary heart disease events (myocardial infarction and sudden death) among 40- to 59-year-old women who were followed for up to 23 years. Assuming a causal relationship between hypertension and coronary heart disease events, the authors estimated that hypertension accounted for 45% of myocardial infarctions and sudden deaths in this cohort.

Data on the relationship between hypertension and coronary heart disease in black women are limited. Tyroler et al. (147) reported coronary heart disease (angina pectoris, myocardial infarction, and sudden death) incidence over 87 months of follow-up for participants in the Evans County Study. Incidence of coronary heart disease was higher in men than in women and higher among white men than among black men. Rates for white and black women were similar. Relative risks of coronary heart disease were computed for systolic blood pressure of > 160 mmHg versus < 140 mmHg and for diastolic blood pressure of > 95 mmHg versus < 90 mmHg. Higher systolic blood pressure was associated with increased coronary heart disease risk among white men and women and among black men (relative risks of 1.8, 2.5, and 4.4, respectively), but not among black women. Similarly, higher diastolic blood pressure was associated with an increased risk of coronary heart disease in white men and women and in black men (relative risks of 1.8, 2.1, and 2.1, respectively), but not in black women. In the Charleston Heart Study (148), predictors of coronary heart disease incidence and mortality were determined. Among black women, the most predictive variables for fatal and nonfatal coronary heart disease were low education, systolic blood pressure, and diabetes; systolic blood pressure, diabetes, and cigarette smoking were most predictive in black men. The risk of dying from coronary heart disease during 25 years of follow-up was increased twofold in black women with systolic blood pressure of ≥ 150 mmHg and over threefold in black men with hypertension.

MacMahon et al. (149) pooled data from nine epidemiologic studies to assess the relationship between diastolic blood pressure and coronary heart disease. Three of the nine studies (Chicago Heart Association, Lipid Research Clinics Prevalence Study, and Framingham Study) included women. Thus, 14,611 women and 403,732 men were entered in the analysis. The relative risk of coronary heart disease increased in log-linear fashion with increasing quintiles of diastolic blood pressure. After adjustment for age, blood cholesterol level, and smoking, a 7.5-mmHg difference in usual diastolic blood pressure was associated with a 29% difference in coronary heart disease risk. The magnitude of the effect was similar in men and women.

The relationship between hypertension and severity of angiographic coronary disease is less clear. There was no relationship between angiographic coronary disease ($\geq 70\%$ stenosis in a coronary artery) and a history of hypertension in a case-control study of 415 middle-aged (mean age 51) women (150), whereas a history of hypertension was a significant risk factor for coronary stenosis among 933 women (mean age approximately 60 years) undergoing angiography in the Milwaukee Cardiovascular Data Registry (151). Neither study tried to correlate the severity of hypertension with the extent of coronary disease.

Stroke

Atherothrombotic brain infarction accounts for nearly two-thirds of stroke cases; cerebral embolization occurs in 5–14% of cases, and intraparenchymal and subarachnoid hemorrhage in 14–20% of strokes. The incidence of stroke is about 30% higher in men than in women and is higher in blacks than whites. Hypertension is strongly related to atherothrombotic and hemorrhagic stroke and is considered the dominant predisposing factor for stroke (152).

Kannel et al. analyzed the relationship between blood pressure and stroke among participants in the Framingham Study who had been followed for 14 years (153). The risk of stroke was proportional to the systolic and diastolic blood pressure levels in both sexes without a risk threshold. Risk gradients were similar for systolic and diastolic blood pressure. After 30 years of follow-up, systolic hypertension was the most important risk factor for stroke in both sexes (128). Compared to individuals with a systolic blood pressure of < 120 mmHg, 35- to 64-year-old men with a systolic blood pressure of > 180 mmHg had an eightfold higher risk of stroke, and 35- to 64-year-old women with this systolic pressure had a fivefold increase in risk; among individuals between 65 and 94 years, the respective increases in risk were 3.25-fold in men and fourfold in women. Left ventricular hypertrophy on electrocardiography (ECG) was an even more powerful predictor of stroke than hypertension. Men with left ventricular hypertrophy had a 12-fold higher risk of stroke between the ages of 35 and 64 years and a 10-fold higher risk over age 65; in women, risk was increased by a factor of 3.2 in the younger age group and by a factor of 5.25 in the older age group.

Folsom et al. (154) recruited a cohort of 41,837 women (55 to 69 years of age) from a random sample of all women listed on the 1985 Iowa driver's license list (response rate 42.7%) and followed these individuals for 2 years. Data on risk factors and medical conditions were obtained by mail survey. Hypertension was an independent predictor of stroke in a multivariate model, increasing stroke risk by twofold. In a group of elderly men and women (aged 65 to 84 years; 1056 men, 1053 women) followed for 9 years by Khaw et al. (155), systolic blood pressure was significantly higher in men and women who experienced a stroke during the follow-up period (147 versus 156 mmHg for men, 145 versus 156 mmHg for women; $p < .05$). A 20-mmHg higher systolic blood pressure was associated with a 20% increase in risk of stroke in this elderly population (relative risk 1.2; 95% confidence limits 1–1.5); this increase in risk was statistically significant in men but not in women.

Pooling data from nine epidemiologic studies, including three studies with women subjects, MacMahon et al. (149) estimated that a 7.5-mmHg difference in usual diastolic blood pressure was associated with a 46% difference in risk of stroke in both sexes.

Several studies have evaluated the relationship between blood pressure and cerebral atherosclerosis as determined by angiography or noninvasive imaging of the carotid arteries (156–164) in men and women. In the Italian Multicenter Study of Reversible Cerebral Ischemic Attacks (156), the relationship between blood pressure and the presence, extent, and severity of cerebral vessel atherosclerosis by angiography was studied in 462 patients (340 men, 122 women) with a clinical diagnosis of reversible ischemic attacks. Age ranged from 20 to 70 years; 170 patients (38.3%) had a history of hypertension. Angiograms were normal in 96 patients (37 women, 59 men) and abnormal in 366 patients (85 women, 281 men). The presence of angiographic lesions was associated with age in both sexes, with hypercholesterolemia in men and with a history of hypertension in women. Individuals with a history of hypertension were more likely to have longer cerebral ischemic attacks (> 24 hr) than persons without such a history, were more likely to have diffuse (intra- and extracranial) atherosclerosis, and had more severe disease angiographically. After adjusting for age and sex, systolic blood pressure was found to be the best predictor of extent and severity of extracranial atherosclerosis in this group of patients but did not predict intracranial atherosclerosis (157).

Whisnant et al. (158) analyzed risk factors among 752 patients (457 men, 295 women) with angiography-proven carotid atherosclerosis. After adjustment for age and sex, smoking, hypertension, diabetes, and current systolic blood pressure were independent predictors of extracranial carotid artery disease. In a subgroup of 240 patients (148 men, 92 women) who also had lipoprotein analyses (159), smoking, hypertension, age, and low-density lipoprotein (LDL) cholesterol were significant predictors of carotid artery atherosclerosis. A sex-specific analysis is not available in either report. Schneidau and colleagues (160) performed serial intravenous digital subtraction angiography in 209 patients and found significantly higher systolic and diastolic blood pressures at follow-up in patients who showed angiographic progression of disease over the 2-year follow-up period; progression was not related to baseline blood pressure.

The prevalence of carotid atherosclerosis by ultrasound evaluation and its relation to risk factors were assessed in 517 healthy French women between the ages of 45 and 54 years who volunteered for a health check-up (161). Nearly one-third of women had intimal medial thickening and 8.7% had atheromatous plaques. Multiple regression analysis revealed that age, smoking, HDL cholesterol, LDL cholesterol (or apoprotein B), and systolic (or diastolic) blood pressure were independently related to the severity of carotid atherosclerosis. There were no associations between carotid disease and blood glucose, body mass index, and several hematologic variables.

Crouse and colleagues (162) correlated risk factors and extent of extracranial carotid atherosclerosis as measured by B-mode ultrasonography in 376 patients (182 men, 194 women) hospitalized for coronary angiography. Hypertension was a significant risk factor for extracranial carotid atherosclerosis in patients with and without coronary artery disease. A history of hypertension was also a significant risk factor for extracranial atherosclerosis in 183 men and 199 women studied with carotid ultrasound by Rubens et al. (163). The severity of extracranial carotid artery obstruction as determined by Doppler pulsed wave ultrasound was positively correlated with systolic blood pressure in a group of elderly stroke patients (n = 118; 66 men, 52 women) (164). Gender-specific analyses are not available for the last three studies.

Hypertension is a powerful independent predictor of stroke in women and, based on limited available data, is also associated with the extent of extracranial carotid atherosclerosis. The relationship between blood pressure and intracranial cerebral atherosclerosis in women remains unclear.

Peripheral Vascular Disease

Data on the relationship between peripheral vascular disease and hypertension in women are limited. In the Framingham Study 30-year Follow-Up (165), systolic hypertension was the second (to smoking) strongest risk factor for intermittent claudication in both sexes. Blood glucose and total cholesterol ranked third and fourth. Criqui and colleagues (166, 167) determined the prevalence of and predictors for large vessel arterial disease in a group of 338 women and 275 men previously studied under a Lipid Research Clinics protocol. Subjects ranged in age from 38 to 82 years with a mean age of 66 years. Intermittent claudication was present in 2.2% of men and in 1.7% of women; the prevalence of large vessel arterial disease by noninvasive vascular testing was fivefold higher in both sexes. Claudication and large vessel arterial disease documented by noninvasive testing became more common with increasing age in both genders. Systolic blood pressure was the only significant predictor of large vessel peripheral arterial disease among women; among men, independent predictors included smoking, systolic blood pressure, and hyperglycemia; body mass index and decreased HDL levels were of borderline significance. Hypertension was also a significant predictor of peripheral arterial disease in a very elderly group of patients (mean age 82 ± 8 years) reported by Aronow and colleagues (168). Peripheral arterial disease was 1.7 times more prevalent in men and 1.5 times more prevalent in women in hypertension. Boissier et al. (169) studied 659 men and 330 women consecutively referred to angiologists in southern France for claudication or rest ischemia of the lower limbs. Among men, 87.5% were smokers, whereas only 19.4% of the women smoked. Women presented on average 8 years later than men (64 versus 72 years old) and had a higher prevalence of hypertension (52.4% versus 32.1%) and of diabetes (32.1% versus 17.6%). Hypertension prevalence among both men and women was several-fold higher than in the general population of the region. All apparent sex differences in risk factors disappeared after adjustment for smoking, as did the difference in age of presentation. The authors concluded that the effects of smoking, hypertension, and diabetes on the development of peripheral vascular disease do not differ between men and women. All studies cited above included predominantly white individuals—similar data in black women are not available.

CLINICAL TRIALS OF ANTIHYPERTENSIVE THERAPY

In the 1960s, three studies in middle-aged individuals with severe hypertension (170–172) were reported. The two smaller studies included more than 50% women (171, 172). These three trials demonstrated consistent reductions in stroke, congestive heart failure, aortic dissection, and hypertensive nephropathy and retinopathy. Effects of treatment on mortality could not be evaluated because there were too few deaths during the short follow-up periods.

During the last 30 years several large multicenter trials have been undertaken in patients with mild, moderate, and severe diastolic and systolic hypertension (173–192). The trials differ significantly in type and intensity of pharmacologic therapy, inclusion and exclusion criteria, and study end points. Except for the study by the Veterans Administration Cooperative Study Group on Anti-hypertensive Agents (173), the Multiple Risk Factor Intervention Trial (174), and the Oslo Study (175), all trials included both men and women. In addition to reporting overall morbidity and mortality statistics, some studies have attempted to analyze data in women separately (177–178, 180–183, 187–189, 191). However, none of these trials included enough women to analyze gender subgroups convincingly. Not surprisingly, these subgroup analyses have yielded variable results regarding the risk-benefit ratio of pharmacologic treatment of hypertension in women, particularly in white women. In this section, we will briefly review in chronologic order the design and results of the hypertension trials that have included women subjects (Table 4–2).

U.S. Public Health Service Trial

The U.S. Public Health Service Trial (176) was a double-blind placebo-controlled study in 389 subjects (78 women) ≤ 55 years old (mean age approximately 44 years) with diastolic blood pressures of between 90 and 114 mmHg. Only 28% of the subjects were nonwhite. Most individuals (79%) had diastolic blood pressures of between 90 and 105 mmHg. On entry, none of the subjects had evidence of major end-organ damage due to hypertension; 41% had previously been on blood pressure medication. Patients in the active treatment group received chlorothiazide and reserpine, which resulted in a mean 16-mmHg decrease in systolic and a mean 10-mmHg decrease in diastolic blood pressure at 6 months with sustained responses throughout the 7-year follow-up period. Women of both races had the best response. Dropout rates were high in both the active treatment group and the placebo group (33.2% and 34.7%, respectively). Major end points (death, fatal and nonfatal myocardial infarction, and stroke) were rare and equally distributed among the two treatment groups (eight events in the active group, nine events in the placebo group). Treatment benefits were evident only when morbid events (new ECG changes, radiologic cardiomegaly, and treatment failure) were analyzed. There was a 60% reduction in these morbid events in the active treatment group. Events were not analyzed by gender.

Hypertension Detection and Follow-up Program (HDFP)

The HDFP study (177–183) had a unique design in that it compared community-based management of diastolic hypertension (referred care, RC) with a more intensive, fixed-

Table 4–2. CLINICAL TRIALS IN HYPERTENSION IN WOMEN

Study (yr published)	No. of Women	Age (yr)	Entry BP (mmHg)	Follow-Up (yr)	Therapy	Results in Women
U.S. Public Health Service Trial (1977)[176]	78	≤ 55	DBP 90–114	6.5–9	CTZ + RES	No change in mortality; morbid events −60%
HDFP (1979–1988)[177-183]	5039	30–69	DBP ≥ 90	Reports at 5, 6, 7 and 8.3 yr	CLTD	Mortality −16.9%; significant decrease in BF at 5 yr; significant in WF at 6.7 and 8.3 yr
Australian Therapeutic Trial (1980)[184-185]	1257	30–69	DBP 95–109	4	CTZ	Trial end points −30% (p = NS)
EWPHE (1985)[186-187]	588	mean 72	DBP 90–119	4.7	HCTZ + TMTR	CV mortality −18% (p = NS)
Coope et al. (1986)[188]	273	60–79	SBP ≥ 170 or DBP ≥ 105	4.4	BDFZ +/or ATEN + others	No change in mortality; CVA −35%
MRC (1985)[189]	8306	35–64	DBP 90–109	5.5	BDFZ or PROP	Higher mortality in women in treated group
SHEP (1991)[191]	2690	>60	SBP 160–219 DBP <90	4.5	CLTD +/− ATEN	CVA −36% overall; benefits in WF, WM, BF, but not BM
STOP Hypertension (1992)[192]	1025	70–84	SBP > 180 + DBP ≥ 90; or DBP > 105	2.08	Multiple	Trial end points −40%; no sex-specific data

ATEN = atenolol; BDFZ = bendrofluazide; BF = black female; BM = black male; CLTD = chlorthalidone; CTZ = chlorothiazide; CV = cardiovascular; CVA = stroke; DBP = diastolic blood pressure; HCTZ = hydrochlorothiazide; HDFP = Hypertension Detection and Follow-up Program; MRC = Medical Research Council; PROP = propranolol; RES = reserpine; SBR = systolic blood pressure; SHEP = Systolic Hypertension in the Elderly Program; TMTR = triamterene; WF = white female; WM = white male.

protocol study clinic-based approach (stepped care, SC). The SC protocol used chlorthalidone alone or in combination with reserpine, hydralazine, guanethidine, or other antihypertensive agents if needed. There was no placebo group. Out of 10,940 subjects aged 30 to 69 years, 1344 black and 1185 white women were assigned to the SC arm; 1354 black and 1156 white women were placed in the RC arm.

Mortality. After 5 years of follow-up, there was a 16.9% reduction in all-cause mortality in the SC group (women and men combined), which increased to 18% at 6.7 years. At 8.3 years (including a 2-year post-trial period), the reduction in mortality was 15%.

There were significant differences in response according to gender and race at the 5-year follow-up point. White women had better blood pressure control in the RC group compared to black women and to both black and white men, resulting in a correspondingly lower mortality rate. Compared to this low risk RC group, white women in the SC group had a statistically nonsignificant increase of 2.1% in all-cause mortality at 5 years, whereas black women in the SC group (who had more left ventricular hypertrophy by ECG [180], more cardiomegaly by chest radiograph [180], and probably a longer duration of hypertension) experienced a 27.8% reduction in all-cause mortality compared to their RC counterparts.

Schnall et al. (181) separately analyzed 5-year mortality in white women with diastolic blood pressures of greater than 105 mmHg on entry into HDFP. There were 272 women in the SC group and 234 women in the RC group. Mortality was 2.7 times higher in the SC women than in the RC women (9.19% versus 3.42%, p < .007). The difference was more pronounced in those with diastolic blood pressures of greater than 115 mmHg than in those with diastolic blood pressures of between 105 and 114 mmHg (272% excess mortality versus 124% excess mortality, p = NS). In contrast, mortality in white SC women with diastolic blood pressure of below 105 mmHg was lower than that in white RC women with mild diastolic hypertension (3.61% versus 5.09%). The authors speculated that excessive reduction of blood pressure could have been detrimental in white women with moderate to severe hypertension. Unfortunately, this hypothesis cannot be tested, since data on average blood pressure reduction stratified by sex and severity of diastolic hypertension at entry into HDFP have not been published. Adverse effects of medication cannot be ruled out.

When the follow-up was extended to 6.7 years (182), the apparent adverse effect of SC on white women was no longer present. White SC women had a 22% lower mortality than white women in the RC group, and black SC women had a 15% reduction. The survival advantage persisted in all race and sex groups to the 8.3-year follow-up point, with higher relative reductions in mortality in blacks than in whites. With longer follow-up, the relative benefits of the SC regimen seemed to increase for younger subjects and decrease for older subjects, although the absolute reduction in deaths in the older age group remained higher. A separate analysis of mortality in white women with moderate to severe diastolic hypertension is not available for the extended follow-up time points.

Morbidity. Total stroke rates were lower in all race-gender subgroups in the SC arm at 5 years. After adjusting for age and entry diastolic blood pressure, white women in the SC group experienced a 30.4% reduction in fatal and nonfatal strokes and black women had a 45.5% reduction. The relative reduction in stroke rates was highest (50%) in those without prior end organ damage and without pretrial antihypertensive therapy.

The 5-year incidence of fatal coronary heart disease and nonfatal myocardial infarction was 16.3% lower in the entire SC group compared to the entire RC group (8.7/100 versus 10.4/100 events). Women in the SC group experienced a 15.2% reduction compared to women in the RC group. Blacks in the SC group had a 13.2% lower incidence of fatal and nonfatal coronary events than their RC counterparts. Data stratified by race and sex are not available. The 5-year incidence of angina pectoris as determined by Rose questionnaire was generally lower in the SC group than in the RC group (6.4% versus 8.95%; p < 0.01; 28% reduction in favor of SC). This reduction was seen in all subgroups except in white SC women, who reported more angina than white women in the RC group, although the difference is reported to be "small."

Improvement in cardiomegaly and regression of left ventricular hypertrophy by ECG criteria were most pronounced in black women in the SC group; white women in the SC group showed favorable trends for both outcomes.

Australian Therapeutic Trial in Mild Hypertension

The Australian Trial (184) was a randomized, placebo-controlled study involving 3427 white individuals (1257 women) 30 to 69 years old with a diastolic blood pressure of > 95 mmHg but < 110 mmHg and systolic blood pressure of < 200 mmHg who did not have any preexisting cardiovascular disease. Pharmacologic therapy in the active treatment group consisted of chlorothiazide and, if necessary, a second-line (propranolol, alpha-methyldopa, pindolol) and a third-line agent (hydralazine, clonidine) to achieve an initial diastolic blood pressure of < 90 mmHg and to further decrease the diastolic pressure to < 80 mmHg at the 2-year point. Both fatal (all-cause mortality, cardiovascular mortality) and nonfatal end points (stroke, transient ischemic attack, myocardial infarction, other ischemic heart disease, heart failure, aortic dissection, retinopathy, encephalopathy, renal insufficiency) were analyzed after 4 years of follow-up. By intention to treat analysis, there were significant reductions in cardiovascular deaths and in the combined category "all trial endpoints" in the active treatment group (57.7% and 19.6%, respectively). There was no difference in ischemic heart disease (98 versus 109 events in active and placebo groups, respectively), but cerebrovascular events were reduced significantly (17 versus 31 events, p < .025). A significant reduction in cumulative all-cause mortality in the active treatment group was apparent when only patients adhering to the trial regimen were analyzed.

In both treatment groups, men had higher event rates than women. The relative reduction in trial end points was 26% in men (67 versus 91 events) and 30% in women (24 versus 36 events), but only the former was statistically significant by standard testing. Using a Cox proportional hazards model, the authors showed in a subsequent paper (185) that the benefit in women was statistically significant by univariate and multivariate analysis. The treatment benefit was particularly apparent in older women smokers.

Study by the European Working Party (EWP)

The European Working Party (186, 187) studied 840 subjects (70% women) with a mean age of 72 years who had diastolic pressures of 90 to 119 mmHg and systolic pressures of 160 to 239 mmHg in a double-blind randomized design comparing hydrochlorothiazide/triamterene (if necessary supplemented with alpha-methyldopa) and placebo with a mean follow-up of 4.7 years. Mortality analysis was by intention to treat. All-cause mortality was not changed by therapy, but cardiovascular mortality decreased by 27% (p = 0.037) due to a significant decrease in cardiac mortality (−38%, p = .036) and a statistically nonsignificant decrease in cerebrovascular mortality (−32%).

When analysis was restricted to the randomized portion of the trial, changes in all-cause mortality remained insignificant, but there were significant reductions in cardiovascular (−38%), cardiac (−47%), and stroke (−43%) mortality as well as in fatal myocardial infarction (−60%). Nonfatal stroke and study-terminating events were also reduced significantly.

Events were analyzed by gender. Women had an 18% (p = NS) reduction in cardiovascular mortality, whereas men had a statistically significant 47% reduction. Both men and women had a significant 44% reduction in cardiovascular study-terminating events. Multivariate Cox proportional hazards analysis suggested that the effect of therapy was not gender dependent but that there was an age dependence in that individuals over 80 years of age did not seem to benefit from treatment. Since 90% of the 155 individuals over age 80 were women, this may partially explain the lesser treatment effect on cardiovascular mortality in women.

Randomized Trial of Treatment of Hypertension in Elderly Patients in Primary Care

This randomized, general practice–based, British multicenter study (188) enrolled 884 patients, 273 (30.8%) women and 611 (69.2%) men, of between 60 and 79 years of age and followed these individuals for a mean of 4.4 years (range 1–10 years). Antihypertensive therapy consisted of atenolol or bendrofluazide, and, if blood pressure was inadequately controlled (i.e., > 170/105 mmHg), other agents were added. Untreated controls were followed according to the same protocol as patients on therapy but did not receive any placebo tablets. Data were analyzed on an "intention to treat" basis. Blood pressure was consistently lower in the treatment group, but even at the eighth year of the study, only 62% of treated patients were at goal pressure compared to 31% of controls. There was no difference in overall mortality, but fatal strokes were reduced by 70% and all (fatal and nonfatal) strokes by 42% in the treated group with a similar magnitude of benefit in the 60- to 69-year-old and 70- to 79-year-old subgroups. There were no significant differences in fatal coronary events or other cardiovascular end points. Women experienced a 35% reduction in all strokes compared to a 47% reduction in men; neither gender subgroup result reached statistical significance due to limited sample sizes.

Medical Research Council (MRC) Trial

The MRC trial (189) was a single-blind, general practice–based British trial involving 17,354 patients (8306 women) aged 35 to 64 years with diastolic blood pressures of between 90 and 105 mmHg and systolic blood pressures of < 200 mmHg. Patients with recent cardiovascular events, heart failure, angina, and diabetes mellitus were excluded. Patients were randomized to receive either active treatment (bendrofluazide or propranolol with or without additional alpha-methyldopa) or placebo and were followed for 5.5 years. Diastolic blood pressure was approximately 5 mmHg lower in the active treatment group than in the placebo group; only 70% of individuals in the active treatment group achieved the diastolic blood pressure goal of ≤ 90 mmHg, whereas 40% achieved this level in the placebo group. There were no statistically significant differences in all-cause mortality or coronary events between groups, although the trends favored the active treatment group. There were significant reductions in stroke rate (−46%) and incidence of all cardiovascular events (-18%) in the active treatment group compared to the placebo group. Gender subgroups were analyzed posthoc. The effects of the active treatment regimen on all-cause mortality were significantly different in men versus women. Men in the active treatment group experienced a reduction from 8.2 to 7.1 deaths per 1000 person years, whereas women in the active treatment group had a higher mortality rate than in the placebo group (4.4 versus 3.5 deaths per 1000 person years). There were no gender differences in the other trial endpoints.

Systolic Hypertension in the Elderly Program (SHEP)

In 1991, the final mortality results of the SHEP trial (190, 191) were reported. SHEP was a randomized double-blind placebo-controlled trial in 4736 elderly (> 60 years old) individuals (2690 women; 440 black, 2250 white) with a 4.5-year follow-up period that assessed the effects of treatment of isolated systolic hypertension (diastolic blood pressure < 90 mmHg; systolic blood pressure 160–219 mmHg) using chlorthalidone with or without low-dose atenolol. The prevalence of cardiovascular and cerebrovascular disease at entry was low. The goal of therapy was to lower systolic blood pressure to < 160 mmHg in those with baseline BP of > 180 mmHg and to lower systolic blood pressure by 20 mmHg in those with systolic pressures of between 160 and 179 mmHg. These goals were achieved in 70% of patients in the active treatment group and in 44% of those in the placebo group (by year 5, 44% of placebo patients were on antihypertensive therapy). The primary end point of the study was the combined incidence of fatal and nonfatal stroke; multiple secondary end points relating to cardiovascular morbidity and mortality, and quality of life measures were also assessed. Overall stroke rate was reduced by 36%, with lower incidence rates in all age groups and all blood pressure levels. Gender analysis showed favorable effects in black women (7 versus 21 events), white women (48 versus 64 events), and white men (39 versus 64 events) but not in black men (9 versus 8 events). Analysis of secondary cardiovascular end points revealed significant reductions in fatal plus nonfatal coronary heart disease events (relative risk [RR] 0.73; 95% confidence intervals [CI]: 0.57,0.94) and fatal plus nonfatal cardiovascular events (RR 0.68; 95% CI: 0.58,0.79) as well as favorable trends in all-cause mortality, total cardiovascular deaths, and total coronary heart disease deaths. Gender-specific data for these secondary end points are not available.

Swedish Trial in Old Patients with Hypertension (STOP-Hypertension)

The STOP-Hypertension study (192) was a prospective randomized double-blind trial of antihypertensive therapy in 1627 elderly patients (63% women) who were between 70 and 84 years old at entry and had either systolic pressures of > 180 mmHg with diastolic pressures of ≥ 90 mmHg or diastolic pressures of > 105 mmHg regardless of systolic blood pressure. Individuals with isolated systolic hypertension, severe systolic (> 230 mmHg) or diastolic hypertension (> 120 mmHg), orthostatic hypotension, and recent (within the last 12 months) myocardial infarction or stroke were excluded. Treatment consisted of either atenolol (50 mg), hydrochlorothiazide plus amiloride (25/2.5 mg), metoprolol (100 mg), pindolol (5 mg), or a combination of diuretic and beta-blocker. Two-thirds of actively treated patients received combination therapy. The study was terminated by the Safety Committee after a mean follow-up time of 25 months. During treatment, the mean difference in systolic and diastolic pressures between actively treated patients and placebo-treated patients was 19.5–8.1 mmHg. The combined incidence of fatal and nonfatal stroke, fatal and nonfatal myocardial infarction, and other cardiovascular death (the primary study end point) was significantly lower in actively treated individuals compared to placebo-treated patients (RR 0.6; 95% CI: 0.43,0.85). Further, the incidence of fatal plus nonfatal stroke and all-cause mortality were also significantly lower in patients on antihypertensive therapy (RR for the latter 0.57; 95% CI: 0.37,0.87). Secondary end points such as congestive heart failure, uncontrolled hypertension, transient ischemic attacks, and angina pectoris were also less frequent in actively treated patients (40 events versus 132 events, $p < .001$). The beneficial effects of antihypertensive therapy were evident at all ages studied. A gender-specific analysis was not performed.

Pooled Results

MacMahon and colleagues (193) pooled the gender-specific results of the HDFP and MRC trials. Compared to men in the respective control groups, the 6639 women in the control groups of these two trials had a 46% lower mortality rate (3.1% versus 5.8%) and 23% fewer fatal and nonfatal strokes (1% versus 1.3%). Further, women in the control group of the MRC trial had 80% fewer nonfatal and fatal coronary events than men in the control group (0.8% versus 4.4%). The likelihood of detecting statistically significant treatment effects in women is thus reduced.

In the pooled analysis there was a nonsignificant 4% decrease in overall mortality in treated women (95% CI: -20% to $+16\%$), a result that was not significantly different from that obtained in men (17% reduction; 95% CI: -27% to -4%). The incidence of fatal and nonfatal stroke was significantly reduced in treated women (43% reduction; 95% CI: -57% to -23%), a benefit similar to that seen in treated men (37% reduction; 95% CI: -51% to -19%). Coronary event rates were not pooled because of different end point definitions in the two studies.

In summary, most multicenter trials of antihypertensive therapy have shown treatment benefits in women as well as men, although the magnitude of benefit tended to be lower in women and reached statistical significance only in the extended follow-up report of HDFP and in the Australian study. Event rates in black women were higher than in white women, and treatment benefits were more pronounced. The apparent adverse effects on mortality in white women seen in the MRC trial and in white women with moderate to severe diastolic hypertension in the HDFP study remain unexplained and should be explored by future research. In contrast to the apparent lack of mortality benefit in the very elderly in the EWP study, significant stroke reductions in all age groups and in both sexes were seen in SHEP and suggest that a moderate reduction in systolic blood pressure by low-dose pharmacologic therapy is beneficial even in advanced age. The importance of antihypertensive therapy in the elderly is further underscored by the recently published STOP-Hypertension Study, which included predominantly elderly women and showed striking benefits in cardiovascular end points and all-cause mortality.

MANAGEMENT OF HYPERTENSION IN WOMEN

Diagnostic Work-Up

Except for the forms of hypertension unique to women, those related to pregnancy and oral contraceptive pill ingestion, the diagnosis and treatment of hypertension do not differ between the sexes. The initial evaluation of the hypertensive patient should determine baseline arterial blood pressure, assess the degree of target-organ damage, screen for secondary causes of hypertension, identify other cardiovascular risk factors, and characterize the patient (race, age, lifestyle, concomitant illnesses) to facilitate choice of therapy (22, 194). The accurate and reproducible measurement of blood pressure by the cuff technique is the most critical part of the diagnostic evaluation. The procedures and choice of equipment for blood pressure measurement should conform to the American Heart Association's Recommendations for Human Blood Pressure Determination by Sphygmomanometers (194, 195) and/or the American Society of Hypertension's Recommendations for Routine Blood Pressure Measurement by Indirect Sphygmomanometry (196). Blood pressure should be taken after the patient has been seated comfortably for at least 5 minutes with his or her arm bared, supported, and positioned at heart level. The patient should not have smoked or ingested caffeine within 30 to 40 minutes prior to measurement because nicotine and caffeine can produce significant transient elevations in blood pressure (194). Constriction of the upper arm by a rolled sleeve should be avoided because it distorts the blood pressure measurement. Two or three measurements should be taken at each visit, with at least 2 minutes between readings. Proper cuff size is critical to accurate blood pressure measurement. Falsely elevated readings can be obtained when the bladder is too short, and the error is magnified if the cuff is too narrow. Mercury manometers are preferred, but aneroid manometers can be used if they are standardized frequently against a mercury manometer. In nonpregnant individuals, the diastolic reading is taken when Korotkoff sounds disappear (Korotkoff phase V). The diagnosis of hypertension in adults is made when the average of two or more diastolic blood pressure measurements on at least two subsequent visits is 90

Table 4–3. ESSENTIAL COMPONENTS IN DIAGNOSIS OF HYPERTENSION

Medical History
- Family history of high blood pressure, diabetes mellitus, dyslipidemia, and premature cardiovascular disease
- History of oral contraceptive use
- Pregnancy history
- History and symptoms of cardiovascular, cerebrovascular, and renal disease, and diabetes mellitus
- Other cardiovascular risk factors (including obesity, smoking, and dyslipidemia)
- Known duration and levels of elevated blood pressure
- History of weight gain, leisure-time physical activities, sodium intake, and alcohol use
- Results and side effects of previous antihypertensive therapy
- Symptoms suggesting secondary hypertension
- Psychosocial and environmental factors (e.g., family situation, employment status and working conditions, educational level) that may influence blood pressure control
- Use of medications that either raise blood pressure or interfere with the effectiveness of antihypertensive drugs, including corticosteroids, nonsteroidal anti-inflammatory agents, nasal decongestants and other cold remedies, appetite suppressants, cyclosporine, tricyclic antidepressants, and monoamine oxidase inhibitors

Physical Examination
- Two or more blood pressure measurements separated by 1 or 2 minutes with the patient either supine or seated, and after standing for at least 2 minutes

---

mmHg or higher, or when the average of multiple systolic blood pressure readings on two or more subsequent visits is consistently greater than 140 mmHg. Once hypertension is diagnosed, the need for antihypertensive treatment should be assessed, and, when indicated, diagnostic evaluation for secondary causes of hypertension should be undertaken. In view of the rarity ($< 5\%$ of the adult hypertensive population) of secondary causes of hypertension and the high cost and significant risk of elaborate diagnostic studies, the routine pretreatment work-up should be limited to defining the severity of the hypertension and identifying target organ damage and associated cardiovascular risk factors. Since many patients with secondary hypertension are potentially curable, a careful history and physical examination should be performed to exclude treatable secondary causes. Essential components of the medical history and physical examination are summarized in Table 4–3 (194).

The initial laboratory evaluation can be restricted to tests generally performed as part of a routine medical checkup: hematocrit, urinalysis to exclude proteinuria and hematuria suggestive of renal disease, creatinine or blood urea nitrogen levels to assess renal function, serum K^+ levels, chest film to assess heart size and rule out aortic coarctation, and electrocardiogram. Other tests that can be obtained as part of most automated blood chemistry batteries, such as the blood glucose, serum cholesterol (total and high-density lipoprotein), triglyceride, and uric acid levels, are helpful in assessing other cardiovascular risk factors and can be used as a baseline for monitoring the effects of antihypertensive treatment. Serial electrocardiograms and echocardiograms may be useful in assessing the effects of hypertension and antihypertensive treatment on the heart.

Nonpharmacologic Treatment

The goal of antihypertensive therapy is to reduce overall cardiovascular risk and cardiovascular morbidity and mortality. The decision to initiate therapy is governed by the extent of blood pressure elevation and the presence or absence of target organ damage, additional cardiovascular risk factors, or both. Antihypertensive treatment is indicated in patients with diastolic blood pressure measurements of 95 mmHg or higher and in those with lesser elevations (90 to 94 mmHg) who are at high risk of developing cardiovascular morbidity or mortality. The high-risk group includes patients with target-organ damage, diabetes mellitus, or other major risk factors for coronary artery disease. The initial goal of therapy is to lower diastolic blood pressure to levels below 90 mm Hg with minimal adverse effects. An effort should be made to correct other cardiovascular risk factors in all hypertensive patients.

Lifestyle modifications, particularly dietary changes, are the foundation of both the prevention and the treatment of hypertension (194, 197–200). These measures are effective in lowering the blood pressure of many people who follow them and may also reduce other cardiovascular risk factors. Although the ability of lifestyle modification to reduce cardiovascular morbidity or mortality in hypertensive subjects has not been conclusively documented, these interventions offer multiple benefits at little cost and with negligible risk. Even when not adequate to control hypertension, they may reduce the doses of antihypertensive medications needed to lower blood pressure to the normal range (201). Lifestyle modification is particularly important for hypertensive patients who have additional cardiovascular risk factors, such as dyslipidemia or diabetes (140).

Weight Reduction. There is a direct relationship between body weight and resting blood pressure, and epidemiologic studies have consistently shown that overweight individuals are at increased risk of developing hypertension and cardiovascular disease. Weight loss is closely correlated with blood pressure reduction and is potentially the most efficacious of all nonpharmacologic measures in the treatment of hypertension. Weight loss has been shown conclusively to reduce blood pressure in a large proportion of hypertensive individuals who are more than 10% above ideal weight (202). A reduction in blood pressure usually occurs early during a weight loss program, often with as small a weight loss as 10 pounds (203). Weight reduction in overweight hypertensive subjects enhances the blood pressure lowering effect of concurrent antihypertensive agents and may significantly reduce concomitant cardiovascular risk factors. Therefore, all hypertensive patients who are above their ideal weight should initially be placed on an individualized weight reduction program involving caloric restriction and increased caloric expenditure by regular physical activity. In obese patients with mild hypertension, blood pressure control may be attempted with weight loss in conjunction with other lifestyle modifications prior to initiating pharmacologic therapy. Even if pharmacologic therapy is needed, the weight loss program should continue to be vigorously pursued (194).

Alcohol Restriction. Excessive alcohol intake elevates blood pressure and can cause resistance to antihypertensive therapy (194, 204). A detailed history of current alcohol consumption should be elicited, and hypertensive patients who consume alcoholic beverages should be counseled to limit their daily intake to 1 ounce of ethanol (2 ounces of 100 proof whiskey, 8 ounces of wine, or 24 ounces of beer). Alcohol intake in excess of these amounts is associated with an increased prevalence of hypertension (205). Although significant hypertension may develop during withdrawal from heavy alcohol consumption, the pressor effect of alcohol disappears within a few days after alcohol consumption is reduced (206).

Exercise. Regular exercise produces moderate reductions in blood pressure in patients with mild to moderate hypertension (207), and exercise may also enhance functional health status and reduce the risk of all-cause and cardiovascular disease mortality (208). Sedentary and unfit normotensive individuals have a 20–50% increased risk of developing hypertension during follow-up compared to their more active and fit peers. Effective lowering of blood pressure may be achieved with only moderate physical activity (40–60% of VO_{2max}); for most sedentary patients, an activity such as 30 to 45 minutes of brisk walking daily will be beneficial. Most patients with uncomplicated hypertension can be safely encouraged to increase their level of physical activity without an extensive medical or physical fitness evaluation (209).

Dietary Sodium Restriction. The blood pressure response to dietary sodium chloride (NaCl) restriction in patients with essential hypertension is heterogeneous; individuals vary greatly in their pressor responsiveness to dietary NaCl supplementation and their depressor responsiveness to NaCl restriction (NaCl sensitivity) (210). The prevalence of NaCl sensitivity is higher in blacks, older people, and patients with higher levels of blood pressure. Moderate dietary NaCl restriction (to 100 mEq Na^+, 6 g NaCl or 2.3 Na^+/day) can be recommended to all hypertensive patients, realizing that blood pressure will be controlled in only a subset of these. In patients who still require pharmacologic therapy, medication requirements may be decreased. Moderate NaCl restriction can be achieved by the simple and tolerable measures of not adding NaCl to food during preparation or at the table and avoiding processed foods containing NaCl as the preservative. NaCl substitutes in which Na^+ is replaced with K^+ are useful in hypertensive patients with normal renal function. Patients should be instructed to avoid concomitant decreases in Ca^{2+} and K^+ intake.

Dietary Potassium Supplementation. Epidemiologic studies have demonstrated an inverse relationship between dietary K^+ intake and blood pressure (211), and dietary K^+ supplementation is associated with small reductions in blood pressure (212) and with reduced antihypertensive medication requirements. The antihypertensive effect of K^+ supplementation appears to be related to concomitant Na^+ intake in that the higher the Na^+ intake, the more effective K^+ supplementation is in reducing blood pressure. Hypertensive patients should maintain adequate K^+ intake ($\sim$ 100 mEq/day) by eating fresh fruits and vegetables, in particular potato skins and low-fat dairy products and, if necessary, by use of K^+ supplements.

Dietary Calcium Supplementation. Epidemiologic studies have also demonstrated an inverse relationship between dietary Ca^{2+} intake and blood pressure (213). Further, a low Ca^{2+} intake may enhance the pressor effects of a high NaCl intake (214). Clinical studies of the antihypertensive effects of Ca^{2+} supplementation have produced mixed results: Only 40–45% of hypertensive patients given oral Ca^{2+} supplementation (1 g elemental Ca^{2+}/day) show significant reductions in blood pressure. Patients with NaCl-sensitive essential hypertension who are ingesting a high-NaCl diet appear to be sensitive to the antihypertensive effects of dietary Ca^{2+}; those with NaCl-resistant hypertension are not. Early data suggest that patients with NaCl-sensitive essential hypertension may benefit from maintaining at least 1000 mg/day Ca^{2+} intake either through the diet or with supplements. Maintenance of Ca^{2+} intake at these levels may also be beneficial for other reasons, such as the prevention of osteoporosis and gastrointestinal malignancy. The latter indications are particularly important to female patients.

Dietary Magnesium Supplementation. Epidemiologic evidence suggests that there is an inverse association between dietary magnesium and blood pressure (215). However, there is no convincing evidence that increasing magnesium intake is effective in lowering blood pressure in hypertensive subjects.

Other Dietary Modifications. Although restriction of saturated fat intake and increasing the ratio of unsaturated to saturated fats in the diet are useful in lowering total cardiovascular risk (140, 216), these dietary interventions have minimal effects on blood pressure (217). The reported efficacy of omega–3 fatty acids in lowering blood pressure (218) is achieved at such high and poorly tolerated doses that this intervention is not recommended for the treatment of hypertension. Similarly, no consistent effects on blood pressure have been achieved by varying proportions of carbohydrate or protein in the diet or by increasing consumption of garlic or onion (194).

Smoking Cessation and Caffeine Restriction. Caffeine and nicotine raise blood pressure acutely, but neither cigarette smokers nor coffee drinkers have an increased incidence of sustained hypertension. Further, there is no evidence that quitting smoking or caffeine products benefits blood pressure control. Patients should be advised to avoid cigarettes and caffeine-containing beverages immediately prior to having their blood pressure checked, but in the absence of excessive sensitivity to caffeine, no limitation of consumption of caffeine-containing beverages is indicated in hypertensive subjects. Because of the high incidence of associated malignancy and accelerated cardiovascular disease, smoking cessation should be strongly urged in all patients (194).

Relaxation-Stress Reduction. Relaxation and stress management produce only modest blood pressure lowering even in highly motivated patients. Therefore, although these techniques may have beneficial side effects, including decreased anxiety and an improved sense of well-being, they have limited clinical application in the treatment of hypertension (198, 219).

Recommendations for Lifestyle Modification in Patients with Essential Hypertension. Lifestyle modification should be encouraged in all hypertensive patients, either as definitive treatment or as an adjunct to drug therapy (22). Therapy should be tailored to the individual characteristics of each patient (e.g., weight reduction and exercise for the overweight patient and moderation in alcohol consumption for the heavy drinker). A reasonable general approach for all patients includes (1) reduction of dietary NaCl and increases in dietary Ca^{2+} and K^+, (2) weight loss for the overweight patient, (3) regular exercise, (4) moderation of alcohol consumption, and (5) smoking cessation and reduction in dietary saturated fat for overall cardiovascular health. This approach has been shown to produce significant sustained reductions in blood pressure while reducing overall cardiovascular risk.

Pharmacologic Therapy

Pharmacologic treatment of hypertension clearly is effective in lowering blood pressure and reducing cardiovascular morbidity and mortality (220, 221). Specific current treatment strategies and therapeutic recommendations are made in the 1992 Report of the Joint National Committee on the Detection, Evaluation and Treatment of High Blood Pressure (194). Several long-term large clinical trials of antihypertensive treatment that have included both men and women have shown no differences in blood pressure response or outcome between the sexes (222). Thus, currently available data do not support a systematically different approach to the management of hypertension in women, but further study is warranted (194, 223). Further, it should be remembered that no antihypertensive drug has been shown to be safe for the fetus in the first trimester of pregnancy (224), so women of reproductive potential who are receiving these agents should be given specific counseling about contraception and family planning. They should be advised to consult their physician as soon as they become aware that they are pregnant. Finally, some antihypertensive agents are poorly tolerated in women because of their adverse effects, e.g., minoxidil and hirsutism.

Hypertension Associated with Oral Contraceptives

Most women taking oral contraceptives experience a small but detectable increase in blood pressure (225); a small percentage experience the onset of frank hypertension that resolves with withdrawal of oral contraceptive therapy. Hypertension is two to three times more common in women taking oral contraceptive pills than in age-matched controls (226). Further, oral contraceptives cause accelerated or malignant hypertension in a small number of patients (227). Genetic characteristics, such as family history of hypertension and black race, as well as environmental characteristics, including preexisting and occult renal disease, obesity, middle age ($>$ 40 years), and duration of oral contraceptive use, increase susceptibility to oral contraceptive-induced hypertension. The diagnosis of oral contraceptive-induced hypertension can be made by documenting the onset of hypertension de novo during contraceptive therapy and the resolution of the hypertension on drug withdrawal. The mechanism of contraceptive-induced hypertension is unclear (194).

Oral contraceptive–induced hypertension can be prevented in part by avoiding the use of these agents in women who are at high risk of developing hypertension. Evidence of thromboembolic disease or chronic hypertension of any cause is a contraindication to use of oral contraceptives. A family history of hypertension and a personal history of preexisting or occult renal disease or of pregnancy complicated by hypertension are relative contraindications to oral contraceptive use. Women over 35 years of age, particularly if obese, should be cautioned about the risk of developing hypertension while ingesting oral contraceptives. Such patients should be followed closely: Blood pressure measurement and a funduscopic examination should be performed, and an interval history obtained on several occasions during the first year of treatment and at yearly intervals thereafter. Although the prevalence of oral contraceptive–induced hypertension is not related to the formulation or dose of estrogen, the incidence of thromboembolic complications is related to estrogen dosage. Therefore, it is preferable to use oral contraceptive preparations of relatively low estrogen content (228).

If hypertension develops in a woman taking oral contraceptives, the pill should be stopped. Blood pressure usually normalizes within a few months. If hypertension persists, antihypertensive treatment should be instituted. When the risks of pregnancy are considered to be greater than the risks of mild hypertension and other contraceptive methods are not suitable, it may be necessary to continue the oral contraceptive. Antihypertensive medications should then be given, and the patient should be carefully monitored.

Hypertension in Pregnancy

The hypertensive disorders of pregnancy can be classified into four diagnostic categories: (1) preeclampsia and eclampsia, (2) chronic hy-

Table 4–4. OMINOUS SIGNS AND SYMPTOMS IN WOMEN WITH PREECLAMPSIA

* Blood pressure ≥ 160 mmHg systolic or ≥ 110 mmHg diastolic
* New onset proteinuria of ≥ 2 g/24 hr (or ≥ 2+ qualitatively)
* Increasing serum creatinine levels (especially > 177 μmol/l [2 mg/dL] unless known to be elevated previously)
* Platelet count < 10 × 10⁹/l or evidence of microangiopathic hemolytic anemia (e.g., schistocytes, and/or increased lactic acid dehydrogenase and direct bilirubin)
* Upper abdominal pain (especially epigastric and upper quadrant)
* Headache, visual disturbances, or other cerebral signs
* Cardiac decompensation (e.g., pulmonary edema, usually associated with underlying heart pathology or chronic hypertension)
* Retinal hemorrhages, exudates, or papilledema—these are extremely rare in the absence of other indicators of severity, and, when present, almost always denote underlying chronic hypertension
* Fetal growth retardation

From Cunningham FG, Lindheim MD. Hypertension in pregnancy. *N Engl J Med* 336:927–932, 1992.

pertension (of whatever cause), (3) preeclampsia superimposed on chronic hypertension, and (4) transient hypertension (229, 230). Since the effects of these disorders on maternal and fetal outcome are very different, correct diagnosis is important. Blood pressure in normal pregnant subjects usually decreases significantly by midpregnancy, so it is inappropriate to use a blood pressure of > 140/90 mmHg as a rigid criterion for diagnosing hypertension in pregnancy. Increases in either systolic or diastolic pressure of ≥ 30 mmHg compared to the average of values prior to 20 weeks of gestation are considered to be pathologic. Further, there is no universal agreement regarding the correct technique for measurement of blood pressure during pregnancy. The World Health Organization and British Hypertension Society recommend use of Korotkoff IV (muffling) to determine diastolic blood pressure in pregnancy (231). However, there is evidence that phase IV may overestimate the intra-arterial diastolic pressure by 7 to 15 mmHg and may be difficult to determine accurately (232). Therefore, the official recommendation of the National High Blood Pressure Education Program (NHBEP) and the Joint National Committee on Detection, Evaluation and Treatment of High Blood Pressure (JNC) is that Korotkoff V (disappearance) be utilized.

Preeclampsia–Eclampsia. Preeclampsia, especially when superimposed on chronic hypertension or renal disease, is the disorder most likely to be associated with severe and even fatal maternal complications and poses the greatest danger to the fetus (230). Preeclampsia occurs primarily in primigravidas after the twentieth week of gestation and is characterized by elevated blood pressure, proteinuria, generalized edema, and, at times, abnormalities of coagulation and liver function. Preeclampsia, even when apparently "mild" in severity may progress rapidly to a convulsive phase, eclampsia, and is thus a potential danger to both mother and fetus. Signs and symptoms that frequently presage progression to eclampsia are summarized in Table 4–4. Some preeclamptic patients develop abnormalities in liver function and reductions in platelet counts even in the presence of minimal hypertension and renal dysfunction and may progress rapidly to the HELLP syndrome (*H*emolysis, *E*levated *L*iver Enzymes, *L*ow *P*latelets), a life-threatening syndrome that requires prompt pregnancy termination (230, 233). Preeclampsia generally resolves spontaneously within 48 hours after delivery, but late postpartum eclampsia, characterized by hypertension, proteinuria, and convulsions, develops occasionally within the first 10 days postpartum (230).

The inciting factor(s) for the development of preeclampsia have not yet been defined, but a number of recent advances in our understanding of the pathophysiology of the disease promise to yield useful preventive and therapeutic strategies. Preeclampsia is characterized by markedly increased peripheral resistance and enhanced sensitivity of the vasculature to endogenous pressor hormones and autocoids, resulting in labile hypertension. Enhanced vascular reactivity in preeclampsia has been attributed to a deficiency of vasodilator prostaglandins, as attested by measurements of reduced renal excretion of prostacyclin metabolites, decreased production of prostacyclin by blood vessels or placenta, and increased thromboxane levels (234). A second popular hypothesis is that preeclampsia is caused by endothelial dysfunction, with enhanced synthesis and release of endothelin and other cytotoxic-mitogenic substances that increase growth factor transcription (235, 236).

The prostacyclin-thromboxane hypothesis has provided the rationale for clinical trials of low-dose aspirin in the prevention of preeclampsia. At low doses (~ 60 mg/day), aspirin has a selective inhibitory effect on thromboxane versus prostacyclin synthesis, thus protecting against vasoconstriction and hypercoagulability. A meta-analysis of 13 small trials of low-dose aspirin therapy begun early in the second trimester showed a significant reduction in "proteinuric preeclampsia" (237). On this basis, some experts recommend the use of low-dose aspirin to prevent preeclampsia; others prefer to await the results of the larger multicenter trials that are now nearing completion (230, 238). Dietary Ca^{2+} supplementation is a second preventive strategy that has reached the clinical trial stage. The rationale behind this approach is that diminished dietary Ca^{2+} intake has been implicated in pregnancy-related hypertension, and hypocalciuria has been demonstrated in preeclamptic patients (239). One recent study from Argentina has shown that Ca^{2+} supplementation reduces the incidence of hypertension (both "gestational hypertension" and preeclampsia) in pregnancy (240). A large multicenter study sponsored by the National Institute of Child Health and Development that has just begun may offer a definitive assessment of the usefulness of Ca^{2+} in preventing preeclampsia in the North American population.

When the diagnosis of preeclampsia is suspected, patients should be hospitalized for further evaluation and careful observation in order to diminish the likelihood of developing eclampsia and life-threatening elevations in blood pressure (224). If the pregnancy is near term, delivery is indicated because removal of the fetus usually cures the syndrome. Delivery is indicated regardless of gestational age in the presence of severe hypertension persisting after 24 to 48 hours of treatment, thrombocytopenia, liver dysfunction (e.g., increasing transaminases), progressive renal dysfunction (including sudden oliguria), premonitory signs of eclampsia (e.g., headache, visual disturbance, hyperreflexia, or epigastric pain), or evidence of fetal distress. If immediate delivery is not contemplated, antihypertensive therapy should be considered. The decision to use antihypertensive drugs should be based on maternal safety because there is no clear-cut fetal benefit to the fetus of lowering blood pressure, and antihypertensive therapy does not cure or reverse preeclampsia. Therapy is generally started when diastolic blood pressure is ≥ 100 mmHg (229). If delivery is not anticipated in 24 hours, an oral agent should be used. Methyldopa is the drug of choice because it has been shown to be both effective and safe for both mother and fetus except in the first trimester of pregnancy (241). Hydralazine, Ca^{2+} antagonists, and beta-blockers are reasonable alternatives. When delivery is imminent, a parenteral antihypertensive agent is preferable. Intravenous hydralazine is effective and safe in pregnancy and is the drug of choice (242). Preliminary data suggest that diazoxide, labetalol, and clonidine are acceptable alternatives. Potent diuretics such as furosemide are not advisable, and sodium nitroprusside should be avoided because of its potential for fetal cyanide poisoning (230). Parenteral magnesium sulfate is the drug of choice in North America for the prevention and treatment of eclampsia (230).

Chronic Hypertension in Pregnancy. The prognosis for pregnancy in women with chronic essential hypertension, unless complicated by superimposed preeclampsia, is generally favorable: > 85% of these women have an uncomplicated pregnancy (230). Most of the excess morbidity in these pregnancies is related to superimposed preeclampsia and correlates with increased age (> 30 yr) of the mother and duration of the hypertension (229, 230, 243). In contrast, women with hypertension secondary to underlying renal parenchymal disease, renal artery stenosis, Cushing's syndrome, pheochromocytoma, and connective tissue disorders, including scleroderma and periarteritis nodosa, frequently do poorly during pregnancy, as do their fetuses (229, 243–245). Accordingly, special care should be taken to detect or rule out these conditions in pregnant women with hypertension. If such a diagnosis is made, the patient should be managed carefully by a specialist in high-risk pregnancy.

Antihypertensive medication should be administered to pregnant women with essential hypertension with diastolic blood pressure of ≥ 100 mmHg, and at lower pressures only if other risk factors such as renal disease or target organ damage are present (229). Aggressive antihypertensive therapy should be avoided because of concern about maintaining adequate uteroplacental blood flow. Alpha-methyldopa is the drug of choice because it has been shown to be safe for mother and fetus

(224). A 7½ year follow-up study of the offspring of mothers treated with alpha-methyldopa during pregnancy has confirmed the absence of fetal toxicity (246). Beta-blockers are effective and safe in the latter part of pregnancy, but their use early in pregnancy may be associated with growth retardation of the fetus (224). Diuretics may be continued if they were taken prior to conception and are particularly useful in women who are NaCl-sensitive (229). ACE inhibitors should be avoided because their use during the second and third trimesters of pregnancy has been associated with serious fetal and neonatal injury, including hypotension, neonatal skull hypoplasia, anuria, reversible or irreversible renal failure, and death. Oligohydramnios has also been reported, presumably resulting from decreased fetal renal function, and has been in turn associated with fetal limb contractures, craniofacial deformation, and hypoplastic lung development. Accordingly, when pregnancy is detected, ACE inhibitors should be discontinued as soon as possible, and infants with histories of in utero exposure to ACE inhibitors should be carefully evaluated for the problems listed above. A boxed warning to this effect appears in the product inserts of all ACE inhibitors (247, 248).

Transient Hypertension of Pregnancy. Transient hypertension of pregnancy is usually characterized by a small elevation in blood pressure that occurs after midpregnancy, generally near term or immediately postpartum (230). The hypertension frequently recurs in subsequent pregnancies but seldom results in an adverse maternal or fetal outcome. Transient hypertension of pregnancy is believed to be a harbinger of essential hypertension later in life (249, 250).

Postmenopausal Estrogen Replacement Therapy

Unlike the synthetic estrogens used in oral contraceptive pills, the conjugated and natural estrogen preparations used for postmenopausal replacement therapy do not appear to cause hypertension or even a tendency toward blood pressure elevation. Prospective studies have shown that conjugated and natural estrogens generally have no effect on blood pressure or tend to reduce it (194, 251). The effects of transdermal estrogen and of progestogen in addition to estrogen replacement on blood pressure in postmenopausal women have not been assessed (194). The presence of hypertension is not a contraindication to postmenopausal estrogen replacement therapy, since postmenopausal estrogens appear to have a beneficial effect on blood pressure as well as on overall cardiovascular risk (150, 252, 253). However, since estrogen replacement may rarely lead to a rise in blood pressure, it is recommended that all women treated with postmenopausal estrogens have their blood pressures monitored (194).

Interaction of Antihypertensive Treatment with Other Cardiovascular Risk Factors

Pharmacologic treatment of hypertension, although of proven efficacy in lowering blood pressure and reducing cardiovascular morbidity and mortality, can be associated with deleterious effects on other cardiovascular risk factors (194). The thiazide diuretics in particular have been shown to increase plasma lipid levels and worsen diabetes control; the beta-adrenergic blockers also increase plasma lipid levels (140). The clinical significance of these adverse effects is uncertain because clinical trials have shown the benefit of these classes of agents in preventing both stroke and coronary artery disease in patients of both genders and all age groups (see earlier section, Clinical Trials of Antihypertensive Therapy).

Quality of Life Issues

Antihypertensive therapy can produce adverse effects on quality of life, including loss of mental acuity, depression, reduced exercise tolerance, and sexual dysfunction, in patients of both genders. Of these, the effects on sexual function, particularly in women, are least well understood (223, 254). The effect of antihypertensive agents on sexual function has been studied almost exclusively in men (255–258). The few reports of female sexual dysfunction due to antihypertensive agents mention only menstrual abnormalities, diminution of vaginal lubrication, and galactorrhea as adverse effects (259–260). When sexual dysfunction has been studied in efficacy trials of specific agents in populations of both genders, it has usually been reported for men only (261–263) or mentioned only briefly for women (264–265). An exception to this generalization is a large study of the efficacy, safety, and quality-of-life effects of captopril in over 30,000 patients, 53% of whom were women, which found similar improvements in sexual function in women and men in whom captopril was substituted for other medications (266). Most recently, methods for detailed study of sexual function in women taking antihypertensive agents have been developed and tested in a small pilot study comparing two antihypertensive agents from different classes (267). Application of these approaches in large clinical trials can give us much needed information about the effects of antihypertensive medication on sexual function in women.

References

1. American Heart Association. *1992 Heart and Stroke Facts.* Dallas, American Heart Association, 1991.
2. Pickering G. Hypertension. Definitions, natural histories and consequences. *Am J Med* 52:570–583, 1972.
3. U.S. Public Health Service, National Institutes of Health. *The 1988 Report of the Joint National Committee on Detection, Evaluation, and Treatment of High Blood Pressure.* NIH Publication No. 88–1088. Washington, D.C., U.S. Department of Health and Human Services, 1988.
4. Rowland M, Roberts J. Blood pressure levels and hypertension in persons ages 6–74 years: United States, 1976–80. Washington, DC, NCHS *Advance Data from Vital and Health Statistics of the National Center for Health Statistics 84,* 1982.
5. Cornoni-Huntley J, LaCroix AZ, Havlik RJ. Race and sex differentials in the impact of hypertension in the United States. The National Health and Nutrition Examination Survey I Epidemiologic Follow-up Study. *Arch Intern Med* 149:780–788, 1989.
6. Vokonas PS, Kannel WB, Cupples LA. Epidemiology and risk of hypertension in the elderly: The Framingham Study. *J Hypertens* 6(Suppl. 1):3–9, 1988.
7. Stamler J, Stamler R, Riedlinger WF, et al. Hypertension screening of 1 million Americans. Community Hypertension Evaluation Clinic (CHEC) program, 1973–1975. *JAMA* 235:2299–2306, 1976.
8. Hypertension Detection and Follow-up Program Cooperative Group. Blood pressure studies in 14 communities: A two-stage screen for hypertension. *JAMA* 237:2385–2391, 1977.
9. Silagy CA, McNeil JJ. Epidemiologic aspects of isolated systolic hypertension and implications for future research. *Am J Cardiol* 69:213–218, 1992.
10. Hjörtland MC, McNamara PM, Kannel WB. Some atherogenic concomitants of menopause: The Framingham Study. *Am J Epidemiol* 103:304–311, 1976.
11. Matthews KA, Meilahn E, Kuller LH. Menopause and risk factors for coronary heart disease. *N Engl J Med* 321:641–646, 1989.
12. Van Berensteyn ECH, Van 'T Hof MA, De Waard H. Contributions of ovarian failure and aging to blood pressure in normotensive perimenopausal women: A mixed longitudinal study. *Am J Epidemiol* 129:947–955, 1989.
13. Staessen J, Bulpitt CJ, Fagard R, et al. The influence of menopause on blood pressure. *J Human Hypertension* 3:427–433, 1989.
14. Weiss NS. Relationship of menopause to serum cholesterol and arterial pressure: The United States Health Examination Survey of Adults. *Am J Epidemiol* 96:237–241, 1972.
15. The WHO Monica Project. Geographical variation in the major risk factors of coronary heart disease in men and women aged 35–64 years. *World Health Statistics Q* 41:115–140, 1988.
16. Nissinen A, Böthig S, Granroth H, et al. Hypertension in developing countries. *World Health Statistics Q* 41:141–154, 1988.
17. Sprafka JM, Burke GL, Folsom AR, et al. Continued decline in cardiovascular disease risk factors: Results of the Minnesota Heart Survey, 1980–1982 and 1985–1987. *Am J Epidemiol* 132:489–500, 1990.
18. Folsom AR, Gomez-Marin O, Sprafka JM, et al. Trends in cardiovascular risk factors in an urban black population, 1973–74 to 1985: The Minnesota Heart Survey. *Am Heart J* 114:1199–1205, 1987.
19. Harlan WR. Economic considerations that influence health policy and research. *Hypertension* 13(Suppl. I):I158–I163, 1989.
20. Littenberg B, Garber AM, Sox HC. Screening for hypertension. *Ann Intern Med* 112:192–202, 1990.
21. Kawachi I, Malcolm LA. The cost-effectiveness of treating mild-to-moderate hypertension: A reappraisal. *J Hypertens* 9:199–208, 1991.
22. Oparil S. Arterial hypertension. In Wyngaarden JB, Smith LH Jr, Bennett JC (Eds.), *Cecil's Textbook of Medicine.* Philadelphia, WB Saunders, 1992, pp. 253–269.
23. Lander ES, Botstein D. Mapping Mendelian factors underlying quantitative traits using RFLP linkage maps. *Genetics* 121:185–199, 1989.
24. Botstein D, White R, Skolnick M, et al. Construction of a genetic linkage map in manusing restriction fragment length polymorphisms. *Am J Hum Genet* 32:314–331, 1980.
25. Riordan JR, Rommens JM, Kerem BS, et al. Identification of the cystic fibrosis gene: Cloning and characterization of complementary DNA. *Science* 245:1066–1073, 1989.
26. Wallace M, Marchuk D, Andersen L, et al. Type 1 neurofibromatosis gene: Identification of large transcript disrupted in three NF1 patients. *Science* 249:181–186, 1990.
27. Cawthon RM, Weiss R, Xu G, et al. A major segment of the neurofibromatosis type 1 gene: cDNA sequence, genomic structure, and point mutations. *Cell* 62:193–201, 1990.
28. Lander ES, Bostein D. Mapping complex genetic traits in humans: New strategies using a complete RFLP linkage map. *Cold Spring Harbor Symp Quant Biol* 51:46–61, 1986.
29. Jacob HJ, Lindpaintner K, Lincoln SE, et al. Genetic mapping of a gene causing hypertension in stroke-prone spontaneously hypertensive rat. *Cell* 67:213–224, 1991.
30. Hilbert P, Lindpaintner K, Beckmann JS, et al. Chromosomal mapping of two genetic loci associated

with blood-pressure regulation in hereditary hypertensive rats. *Nature* 353:521–529, 1991.
31. Nara Y, Nabika T, Ikeda K, et al. Blood pressure cosegregates with a microsatellite of angiotensin I converting enzyme (ACE) in F_2 generation from a cross between original normotensive Wistar-Kyoto rat (WKY) and stroke-prone spontaneously hypertensive rat (SHRSP). *Biochem Biophys Res Commun* 3:941–946, 1991.
32. Mattei MG, Hubert C, Alhenc-Gelas F, et al. Angiotensin converting enzyme maps of chromosome 17. *Cytogenet Cell Genet* 51:1041, 1990.
33. Rapp JP, Wang SM, Dene H. A genetic polymorphism in the renin gene of Dahl rats cosegregates with blood pressure. *Science* 243:542–544, 1989.
34. Kurtz TW, Simonet L, Kabra PM, et al. Cosegregation of the renin allele of the spontaneously hypertensive rat with an increase in blood pressure. *J Clin Invest* 85:1328–1332, 1990.
35. Lindpaintner K, Takahashi S, Ganten D. Structural alterations of the renin gene in stroke-prone spontaneously hypertensive rats: Examination of genotype-phenotype correlations. *J Hypertension* 8:763–773, 1990.
36. Lifton RP, Hunt SC, Williams RR, et al. Exclusion of the Na^+-H^+ antiporter as a candidate gene in human essential hypertension. *Hypertension* 17:8–14, 1991.
37. Lifton RP, Dluhy RG, Powers M, et al. A chimaeric 11 β-hydroxylase/aldosterone synthase gene causes glucocorticoid-remediable aldosteronism and human hypertension. *Nature* 355:262–265, 1992.
38. Guyton AC, Hall JE, Coleman TG, et al. The dominant role of the kidneys in the long-term regulation of arterial pressure in normal and hypertensive states. In Laragh JH, Brenner BM (Eds.), *Hypertension: Pathophysiology, Diagnosis, and Management*. New York, Raven Press, 1990, pp. 1029–1052.
39. Oparil S, Chen YF, Naftilan AJ, et al. Pathogenesis of hypertension. In Fozzard HA, Jennings RB, Katz AM, et al. (Eds.), *The Heart and Cardiovascular System*. New York, Raven Press, 1992, pp. 295–333.
40. Curtis JJ, Luke RG, Dustan HP, et al. Remission of essential hypertension after renal transplantation. *N Engl J Med* 309:1009, 1983.
41. Eich RH, Cuddy RP, Smulyna H, et al. Hemodynamics in labile hypertension. *Circulation* 34:299–307, 1966.
42. Lund-Johansen P. Spontaneous changes in central hemodynamics in essential hypertension—a 10-year follow-up study. In Onesti G, Klimt CR (Eds.), *Hypertension-Determinants, Complications, and Intervention*. New York, Grune & Stratton, 1979, pp. 201–218.
43. Lund-Johansen P, Omvik P. Hemodynamic patterns of untreated hypertensive disease. In Laragh JH, Brenner BM (Eds.), *Hypertension: Pathophysiology, Diagnosis, and Management*. New York, Raven Press, 1990, pp. 305–327.
44. Naftilan AJ, Ryan TJ Jr, Pratt RE, et al. Localization and differential regulation of angiotensinogen mRNA expression in the vessel wall. *J Clin Invest* 87:1300–1311, 1991.
45. Owens GK. Influence of blood pressure on development of aortic medial smooth muscle hypertrophy in spontaneously hypertensive rats. *Hypertension* 9:178–187, 1987.
46. Powell JS, Clozel JP, Muller RKM, et al. Inhibitors of angiotensin-converting enzyme prevent myointimal proliferation after vascular injury. *Science* 245:186–188, 1989.
47. Rosengurt E. Early signals in the mitogenic response. *Science* 234:161–166, 1986.
48. Kannel WB, Doyle JT, Ostfeld AM, et al. Optimal resources for primary prevention of atherosclerotic diseases. Atherosclerosis Study Group. *Circulation* 70:155A–205A, 1984.
49. Gardin JM, Savage DD, Ware JH, et al. Effect of age, sex and body surface area on echocardiographic left ventricular wall mass in normal subjects. *Hypertension* 9:1136–1139, 1987.
50. Devereux RB, Savage DD, Sachs I, et al. Relation of hemodynamic load to left ventricular hypertrophy and performance in hypertension. *Am J Cardiol* 51:171–176, 1983.
51. Devereux RB, Lutas EM, Casale PN, et al. Standardization of M-mode echocardiographic left wall ventricular anatomic measurements. *J Am Coll Cardiol* 4:1222–1230, 1984.
52. Garavaglia GE, Messerli FH, Schmieder RE, et al. Sex differences in cardiac adaptation to essential hypertension. *Eur Heart J* 10:1110–1114, 1989.
53. Koenig H, Goldstone A, Lu CY. Testosterone-mediated sexual dimorphism of the rodent heart. Ventricular lysosomes, mitochondria and cell growth as modulated by androgens. *Circ Res* 50:782–787, 1982.
54. Cabral AM, Vasquez EC, Moyses MR, et al. Sex hormone modulation of ventricular hypertrophy in sinoaortic denervated rats. *Hypertension* 11(Suppl. 1):93–97, 1988.
55. Chen YF, Meng QC. Sexual dimorphism of blood pressure in spontaneously hypertensive rats is androgen dependent. *Life Sci* 48:85–96, 1991.
56. Stumpf WE, Sar M, Aumuller G. The heart: A target organ for estradiol. *Science* 197:319–321, 1977.
57. DeFronzo R. The effect of insulin on renal sodium metabolism. A review with clinical implications. *Diabetologia* 21:165–171, 1981.
58. Stout RW, Bierman EL, Ross R. Effect of insulin on the proliferation of cultured primate arterial smooth muscle cells. *Circ Res* 36:319–327, 1975.
59. Fontbonne A, Tchobroutsky G, Eschwege E, et al. Coronary heart disease mortality risk: Plasma insulin level is a more sensitive marker than hypertension or abnormal glucose tolerance in overweight males. The Paris Prospective Study. *Int J Obes* 12:557–565, 1988.
60. Pyorala K, Savolainen E, Kaukola S, et al. Plasma insulin as coronary heart disease risk factor: Relationship to other risk factors and predictive value during 9½-year follow up of the Helsinki Policeman Study Population. *Acta Med Scand* 701(Suppl.):38–52, 1985.
61. Cullen K, Stenhouse NS, Wearne KL, et al. Multiple regression analysis of risk factors for cardiovascular disease and cancer mortality in Busselton, Western Australia—13-year study. *J Chronic Dis* 36:371–377, 1983.
62. Kannel WB. Hypertension and other risk factors in coronary heart disease. *Am Heart J* 114:918–925, 1987.
63. Modan M, Or J, Karasik A, et al. Hyperinsulinemia, sex, and risk of atherosclerotic cardiovascular disease. *Circulation* 84:1165–1175, 1991.
64. Yamori Y. Physiopathology of the various strains of spontaneously hypertensive rats. In Genest J, Kuchel

O, Hamet P, (Eds.), *Hypertension* (2nd ed.). New York, McGraw-Hill, 1982, pp. 556–581.
65. Bianchi G, Ferrari P, Barber BR. Lessons from experimental genetic hypertension. In Laragh JH, Brenner BM (Eds.), *Hypertension: Pathophysiology, Diagnosis, and Management*. New York, Raven Press, 1990, ch. 78.
66. Cambotti LJ, Cole FE, Gerall AA, et al. Neonatal gonadal hormones and blood pressure in the spontaneously hypertensive rat. *Am J Physiol* 247:E258–E264, 1984.
67. Schlager G, Weibust RS. Genetic control of blood pressure in mice. *Genetics* 55:497–508, 1967.
68. Schlager G. Genetic and physiological studies of blood pressure in mice. *Can J Genet Cytol* 10:833–864, 1968.
69. Dahl LK, Knudsen KD, Ohanian EV, et al. Role of the gonads in hypertension-prone rats. *J Exp Med* 142:748–759, 1975.
70. Iam SG, Wexler BC. Retardation in the development of spontaneous hypertension in SH rats by gonadectomy. *J Lab Clin Med* 90:997–1003, 1977.
71. Iam SG, Wexler BC. Inhibition of the development of spontaneous hypertension in SH rats by gonadectomy or estradiol. *J Lab Clin Med* 94:608–616, 1979.
72. Ouchi Y, Share L, Crofton JT, et al. Sex differences in the development of deoxycorticosterone-salt hypertension in the rat. *Hypertension* 9:172–177, 1987.
73. Ganten U, Schroder G, Witt M, et al. Sexual dimorphism of blood pressure in spontaneously hypertensive rats: Effects of anti-androgen treatment. *J Hypertension* 7:721–726, 1989.
74. Masubuchi Y, Kumai T, Uematsu A, et al. Gonadectomy-induced reduction of blood pressure in adult spontaneously hypertensive rats. *Acta Endocrinologica* 101:154–160, 1982.
75. Crofton JT, Share L, Brooks DP. Gonadectomy abolishes the sexual dimorphism in DOC-salt hypertension in the rat. *Clin Exp Hypertens [A]* 7:1249–1261, 1989.
76. Bachmann J, Feldmer M, Ganten U, et al. Sexual dimorphism of blood pressure: possible role of the renin-angiotensin system. *J Steroid Biochem Mol Biol* 40:511–515, 1991.
77. Chen YF, Naftilan AJ, Oparil S. Androgen dependent angiotensinogen and renin mRNA expression in hypertensive rats. *Hypertension* 19:456–463, 1992.
78. Judy WV, Watanabe AM, Henry DP, et al. Sympathetic nerve activity: Role in regulation of blood pressure in the spontaneously hypertensive rat. *Circ Res* 38:21–29, 1976.
79. Winternitz SR, Katholi RE, Oparil S. Role of the renal sympathetic nerves in the development and maintenance of hypertension in the spontaneously hypertensive rat. *J Clin Invest* 66:971–978, 1980.
80. Dietz R, Schomig A, Rascher W, et al. Contribution of the sympathetic nervous system to the hypertension effects of a high sodium diet in stroke-prone spontaneously hypertensive rats. *Hypertension* 4:773–781, 1982.
81. Lara H, Galleguillos X, Arrau J, et al. Effect of castration and testosterone on norepinephrine storage and on the release of [^{3}H] norepinephrine from rats vas deferens. *Neurochem Int* 7:667–674, 1985.
82. Sar M, Stumpf WE. Distribution of androgen concentrating neurons in rat brain. In Stumpf WE, Grant LD (Eds.), *Anatomical Neuroendocrinology*. Basel, Karger, 1975, pp. 120–133.
83. Heritage AS, Stumpf WE, Sar M, et al. Brainstem catecholamine neurons as target sites for sex steroid hormones. *Science* 207:1377–1379, 1980.
84. Enoch DM, Kerr FWL. Hypothalamic vasopressor and vesicopressor pathways. *Arch Neurol* 16:290–306, 1967.
85. Juskevich JC, Robinson DS, Whitehorn D. Effect of hypothalamic stimulation in spontaneously hypertensive and Wistar-Kyoto rats. *Eur J Pharmacol* 51:429–439, 1978.
86. Takeda K, Bunag RD. Sympathetic hyperactivity during hypothalamic stimulation in spontaneously hypertensive rats. *Clin Invest* 52:642–648, 1978.
87. Bunag RD, Butterfield J, Sasaki S. Hypothalamic pressor responses and salt-induced hypertension in Dahl rats. *Hypertension* 5:460–467, 1983.
88. Winternitz SR, Wyss JM, Oparil S. The role of the posterior hypothalamic area in the pathogenesis of hypertension in the spontaneously hypertensive rat. *Brain Res* 324:51–58, 1984.
89. Barraclough CA, Lookingland KJ, Wise PM. Role of the hypothalamic noradrenergic system in sexual differentiation of the brain. In Serio M, et al (Eds.), *Sexual Differentiation: Basic and Clinical Aspects*. New York, Raven Press, 1983, pp. 99–106.
90. Stumpf WE. Estrogen-neurons and estrogen-neuron systems in the periventricular brain. *Am J Anat* 129:207–218, 1970.
91. Stumpf WE, Sar M, Keefer DA. Atlas of estrogen target cells in rat brain. In Stumpf WE, Grant LD (Eds.), *Anatomical Neuroendocrinology*. Basel, Karger, 1975, pp. 104–119.
92. Wilson CM, Taylor BA. Genetic regulation of thermostability of mouse SMG gene. *J Biol Chem* 257:217–223, 1982.
93. Pratt RE, Dzau VJ, Quellette AJ. Influence of androgen on translatable renin mRNA in the mouse submandibular gland. *Hypertension* 6:605–613, 1984.
94. Catanzaro DF, Mesterovic N, Morris BJ. Studies of the regulation of mouse renin gene by measurement of renin messenger ribonucleic acid. *Endocrinology* 117:872–878, 1985.
95. Ingelfinger JR, Pratt RE, Ellison KE, et al. Multiple sites of regulation of mouse renin expression in ontogeny. *Clin Exp Hypertens* 8:687–694, 1986.
96. Wagner D, Metzger R, Paul M, et al. Androgen dependent and tissue specificity of renin messenger RNA expression in mice. *J Hypertension* 8:45–52, 1990.
97. Ellison KE, Ingelfinger JR, Pivor M, et al. Androgen regulation of rat renal angiotensinogen messenger RNA expression. *J Clin Invest* 83:1941–1945, 1989.
98. Mullins JJ, Peters J, Ganten D. Fulminant hypertension in transgenic rat harbouring the mouse Ren 2 gene. *Nature* 344:541–544, 1990.
99. Kalinyak JE, Perlman AJ. Tissue-specific regulation of angiotensinogen mRNA accumulation by dexamethasone. *J Biol Chem* 262:460–464, 1987.
100. Pratt RE, Zou WM, Naftilan AJ, et al. Altered sodium regulation of renal angiotensinogen mRNA in the spontaneously hypertensive rat. *Am J Physiol* 256:F469–F474, 1989.
101. Nakamura A, Iwao H, Fukui K, et al. Regulation of liver angiotensinogen and kidney renin mRNA levels by angiotensin II. *Am J Physiol* 258:E1–E6, 1990.
102. Naftilan AJ, Zuo WM, Ingelfinger J, et al. Localization of differential regulation of angiotensinogen

mRNA expression in the vessel wall. *J Clin Invest* 87:1300–1311, 1991.
103. Chang E, Perlman AJ. Multiple hormones regulate angiotensinogen messenger ribonucleic acid levels in a rat hepatoma cell line. *Endocrinology* 121:513–519, 1987.
104. Kunapuli SP, Benedict CR, Kumar A. Tissue specific hormonal regulation of the rat angiotensinogen gene expression. *Arch Biochem Biophys* 254:642–646, 1987.
105. Clauser E, Gaillard I, Wei L, et al. Regulation of angiotensinogen gene. *Am J Hypertens* 2:403–410, 1989.
106. Feldmer M, Kaling M, Takahashi S, et al. Glucocorticoid and estrogen responsive elements in the 5′-flanking region of the rat angiotensinogen gene. *J Hypertens* 9:1005–1112, 1991.
107. Carriere PD, De Lean A, Gutkowska J, et al. Chronic estradiol treatment decreases angiotensin II receptor density in the anterior pituitary gland and adrenal cortex but not in the mesenteric artery. *Neuroendocrinology* 43:49–56, 1986.
108. Dzau VJ, Ingelfinger JR, Pratt RE. Regulation of tissue renin and angiotensinogen gene expressions. *J Cardiovasc Pharmacol* 8:S11–S16, 1986.
109. Johannessen A, Nielsen AH, Poulsen K. Sexual dimorphism of inactive renin in rat plasma. *Clin Exp Hypertens* 12:1405–1417, 1990.
110. Nielsen AH, Johannessen A, Poulsen K. Inactive plasma renin exhibits sex difference in mice. *Clin Sci* 76:439–446, 1989.
111. Sealey JE, Atlas SA, Laragh JH. Prorenin and other large molecular weight forms of renin. *Endocrinol Rev* 1:365–391, 1980.
112. Cunard C, Falcon J, Maddox Y, et al. Eicosanoid expression of vascular sexual dimorphism. In Gryglewski RJ, Stock G (Eds.), *Prostacyclin and Its Stable Analogue Iloprost*. Berlin, Springer, 1987, pp. 115–122.
113. Miller VM, Gisclard V, Vanhoutte PM. Modulation of endothelium-dependent and vascular smooth muscle responses by oestrogens. *Phlebology* 224:19–22, 1988.
114. Williams JK, Adams MR, Klopfenstein HS. Estrogen modulates responses of atherosclerotic coronary arteries. *Circulation* 81.1680–1687, 1990.
115. Williams JK, Adams MR, Herrington DM, et al. Effects of short-term estrogen treatment on vascular responses of coronary arteries (abstract). *Circulation* 84(Suppl. II):II272, 1991.
116. Lin AL, McGill HC, Shain SA. Hormone receptors of the baboon cardiovascular system. *Circ Res* 50:610–616, 1982.
117. Lin AL, Gonzalez R Jr, Carey KD, et al. Estradiol-17β affects estrogen receptor distribution and elevates progesterone receptor content in baboon aorta. *Arteriosclerosis* 6:495–504, 1986.
118. Fischer-Dzoga K, Wissler RW, Vesselinovitch D. The effect of estradiol on the proliferation of rabbit aortic medial tissue culture cells induced by hyperlipemic serum. *Exp Mol Pathol* 39:355–363, 1983.
119. Rhee CY, Spaet TH, Gaynor E, et al. Suppression of surgically induced vascular intimal hypertrophy by estrogen (abstract). *Circulation* 49(Suppl. III):III-9, 1974.
120. Rhee CY, Drouet RO, Spaet YH, et al. Growth inhibition of cultured vascular smooth muscle cells by estradiol. *Fed Proc* 37:474, 1978.
121. Weigensberg BI, Lough H, More RH, et al. Effects of estradiol on myointimal thickening from catheter injury and on organizing white mural non-occlusive thrombi. *Atherosclerosis* 52:253–265, 1984.
122. Hough JL, Zilversmit DB. Effect of 17β-estradiol on aortic cholesterol content and metabolism in cholesterol-fed rabbits. *Atherosclerosis* 6:57–63, 1986.
123. Johnson M, Ramey E, Ramwell PW. Androgen-mediated sensitivity in platelet aggregation. *Am J Physiol* 232:H381–H385, 1977.
124. Chang W-C, Nakao J, Orimo H, et al. Stimulation of prostacyclin activity by estradiol in rat aorta smooth muscle cell in culture. *Biochem Biophys Acta* 619:107–118, 1980.
125. Roccella EJ, Bowler AE. Hypertension as a risk factor. *Cardiovasc Clin* 20(3):49–63, 1990.
126. Robinson SC, Brucer M. Range of normal blood pressure: A statistical and clinical study of 11,383 persons. *Arch Intern Med* 64:409–444, 1939.
127. Deubner DC, Tyroler HA, Cassel JC, et al. Attributable risk, population attributable risk, and population attributable fraction of death associated with hypertension in a biracial population. *Circulation* 52:901–908, 1975.
128. Stokes J III, Kannel WB, Wolf PA, et al. Blood pressure as a risk factor for cardiovascular disease. The Framingham Study—30 years of follow-up. *Hypertension* 13(Suppl. I):I13–I18, 1989.
129. Yusuf S, Thom T, Abbott RD. Changes in hypertension treatment and in congestive heart failure mortality in the United States. *Hypertension* 13(Suppl. I):I74–I79, 1989.
130. National High Blood Pressure Education Program. National High Blood Pressure Education Program Working Group report on hypertension and chronic renal failure. *Arch Intern Med* 151:1280–1287, 1991.
131. Whelton PK, Klag MJ. Hypertension as a risk factor for renal disease. Review of clinical and epidemiological evidence. *Hypertension* 13(Suppl. I):I19–I27, 1989.
132. Lindemann RD, Tobin JD, Shock NW. Association between blood pressure and the rate of decline in renal function with age. *Kidney Int* 26:861–868, 1984.
133. Klahr S. The Modification of Diet in Renal Disease Study. *N Engl J Med* 320:864–866, 1989.
134. Shulman NB, Ford CE, Hall WD, et al. On behalf of the Hypertension Detection and Follow-up Program Cooperative Group. Prognostic value of serum creatinine and effect of treatment of hypertension on renal function: Results from the Hypertension Detection and Follow-up Program. *Hypertension* 13(Suppl. I):I80–I93, 1989.
135. Tierney WM, McDonald CJ, Luft FC. Renal disease in hypertensive adults: Effect of race and Type II diabetes mellitus. *Am J Kidney Dis* 13(6):485–493, 1989.
136. Rostand SG, Kirk KA, Rutsky EA, et al. Racial differences in the incidence of treatment for end-stage renal disease. *N Engl J Med* 306:1276–1279, 1982.
137. Whittle JC, Whelton PK, Seidler AJ, et al. Does racial variation in risk factors explain black-white differences in the incidence of hypertensive end-stage renal disease. *Arch Intern Med* 151:1359–1364, 1991.
138. Heistad DD, Lopez JAG, Baumbach GL. Hemodynamic determinants of vascular changes in hypertension and atherosclerosis. *Hypertension* 17(Suppl. III):III7–III11, 1991.

139. O'Kelly BF, Massie BM, Tubau JF, et al. Coronary morbidity and mortality, preexisting silent coronary artery disease, and mild hypertension. *Ann Intern Med* 110:1017–1026, 1989.
140. Working Group on Management of Patients with Hypertension and High Blood Cholesterol. National Education Programs Working Group Report on the Management of Patients with Hypertension and High Blood Cholesterol. *Ann Intern Med* 114:224–237, 1991.
141. Reaven GM. Insulin resistance and compensatory hyperinsulinemia: Role in hypertension, dyslipidemia, and coronary heart disease. *Am Heart J* 121:1283–1288, 1991.
142. Kaplan NM. The deadly quartet. Upper-body obesity, glucose intolerance, hypertriglyceridemia, and hypertension. *Arch Intern Med* 149:1514–1520, 1989.
143. Williams RR, Hunt SC, Hopkins PN, et al. Familial dyslipidemic hypertension: Evidence from 58 Utah families for a syndrome present in approximately 12% of patients with essential hypertension. *JAMA* 259:3579–3586, 1988.
144. Kannel WB, Gordon T, Schwartz MJ. Systolic versus diastolic blood pressure and risk of coronary heart disease. The Framingham Study. *Am J Cardiol* 27:335–346, 1971.
145. Petitti DB, Wingerd J, Pellegrin F, et al. Risk of vascular disease in women. Smoking, oral contraceptives, noncontraceptive estrogens, and other factors. *JAMA* 242:1150–1154, 1979.
146. Beard CM, Kottke TE, Annegers JF, et al. The Rochester Coronary Heart Disease Project: Effect of cigarette smoking, hypertension, diabetes, and steroidal estrogen use on coronary heart disease among 40- to 59-year-old women, 1960 through 1982. *Mayo Clin Proc* 64:1471–1480, 1989.
147. Tyroler HA, Heyden S, Bartel A, et al. Blood pressure and cholesterol as coronary heart disease risk factors. *Arch Intern Med* 128:907–914, 1971.
148. Keil JE, Tyroler HA, Gazes PC. Predictors of coronary heart disease in blacks. *Cardiovasc Clin* 21:227–239, 1991.
149. MacMahon S, Peto R, Cutler J, et al. Blood pressure, stroke and coronary heart disease. Part 1, prolonged differences in blood pressure: Prospective observational studies corrected for the regression dilution bias. *Lancet* 1:765–774, 1990.
150. McFarland KF, Boniface ME, Hornung CA, et al. Risk factors and noncontraceptive estrogen use in women with and without coronary disease. *Am Heart J* 117:1209–1214, 1989.
151. Gruchow HW, Anderson AJ, Barboriak JJ, et al. Postmenopausal use of estrogen and occlusion of coronary arteries. *Am Heart J* 115:954–963, 1988.
152. Dyken ML, Wolf PA, Barnett HJM, et al. Risk factors in stroke. A statement for physicians by the Subcommittee on Risk Factors and Stroke of the Stroke Council. *Stroke* 15:1105–1111, 1984.
153. Kannel WB, Wolf PA, Verter J, et al. Epidemiologic assessment of the role of blood pressure in stroke. The Framingham Study. *JAMA* 214:301–310, 1970.
154. Folsom AR, Prineas RJ, Kaye SA, et al. Incidence of hypertension and stroke in relation to body fat distribution and other risk factors in older women. *Stroke* 21:701–706, 1990.
155. Khaw KT, Barrett-Connor E, Suarez L, et al. Predictors of stroke-associated mortality in the elderly. *Stroke* 15:244–248, 1984.
156. Passero S, Rossi G, Nardini M, et al. Italian Multicenter Study of Reversible Cerebral Ischemic Attacks: Part 5. Risk factors and cerebral atherosclerosis. *Atherosclerosis* 63:211–224, 1987.
157. Inzitari D, Bianchi F, Pracucci G, et al. The Italian Multicenter Study of Reversible Cerebral Ischemic Attacks: IV-Blood pressure components and atherosclerotic lesions. *Stroke* 17:185–191, 1986.
158. Whisnant JP, Homer D, Ingall TJ, et al. Duration of cigarette smoking is the strongest predictor of severe extracranial carotid artery atherosclerosis. *Stroke* 21:707–714, 1991.
159. Homer D, Ingall TJ, Baker HL, et al. Serum lipids and lipoproteins are less powerful predictors of extracranial carotid artery atherosclerosis than are cigarette smoking and hypertension. *Mayo Clin Proc* 66:259–267, 1991.
160. Schneidau A, Harrison MJG, Hurst C, et al. Arterial disease risk factors and angiographic evidence of atheroma of the carotid artery. *Stroke* 20:1466–1471, 1989.
161. Bonithon-Kopp C, Scarabin PY, Taquet A, et al. Risk factors for early carotid atherosclerosis in middle-aged French women. *Arteriosclerosis Thrombosis* 11:966–972, 1991.
162. Crouse JR, Toole JF, McKinney WM, et al. Risk factors for extracranial carotid artery atherosclerosis. *Stroke* 18:990–996, 1987.
163. Rubens J, Espeland MA, Ryu J, et al. Individual variation in susceptibility to extracranial carotid atherosclerosis. *Arteriosclerosis* 8:389–397, 1988.
164. Admani AK, Mangion DM, Naik DR. Extracranial carotid artery stenosis: Prevalence and associated risk factors in elderly stroke patients. *Atherosclerosis* 86:31–37, 1991.
165. Stokes J III, Kannel WB, Wolf PA, et al. The relative importance of selected risk factors for various manifestations of cardiovascular disease among men and women from 35 to 64 years old: 30 years of follow-up in the Framingham Study. *Circulation* 75(Suppl. V):65–73, 1987.
166. Criqui MH, Fronek A, Barret-Conner E, et al. The prevalence of peripheral arterial disease in a defined population. *Circulation* 71:510–515, 1985.
167. Criqui MH, Browner D, Fronek A, et al. Peripheral arterial disease in large vessels is epidemiologically distinct from small vessel disease: An analysis of risk factors. *Am J Epidemiol* 129:1110–1119, 1989.
168. Aronow WS, Sales FF, Etienne F, et al. Prevalence of peripheral arterial disease and its correlation with risk factors for peripheral arterial disease in elderly patients in a long-term health care facility. *Am J Cardiol* 62:644–646, 1988.
169. Boissier C, Carpentier P, Conchonnet P, et al. Influence des facteurs de risque vasculaire dans l'arteriopathie des membres inferieurs de la femme. *J Maladies Vasculaires* 15:296–302, 1990.
170. Effects of treatment on morbidity in hypertension. Results in patients with diastolic blood pressure averaging 115 through 129 mm Hg. *JAMA* 202:1028–1034, 1967.
171. Hamilton M, Thomson EN, Wisniewski TKM. The role of blood-pressure control in preventing complications of hypertension. *Lancet* 1:235–238, 1964.
172. Wolff FW, Lindeman RD. Effects of treatment in hypertension. Results of a controlled study. *J Chron Dis* 19:227–240, 1966.
173. Effects of treatment on morbidity in hypertension.

Results in patients with diastolic blood pressure averaging 90 through 114 mm Hg. *JAMA* 213:1145–1182, 1970.
174. Multiple Risk Factor Intervention Trial. Risk factor changes and mortality results. *JAMA* 248:1465–1477, 1982.
175. Helgeland A. Treatment of mild hypertension: A five year controlled drug trial. The Oslo Study. *Am J Med* 69:725–732, 1982.
176. McFate Smith W. Treatment of mild hypertension. Results of a ten-year intervention trial. U.S. Public Health Service Hospitals Cooperative Study Group. *Circ Res* 40(Suppl. I):98–105, 1977.
177. Hypertension Detection and Follow-up Program Cooperative Group. Five-year findings of the Hypertension Detection and Follow-up Program. Mortality by race, sex, and age. *JAMA* 242:2572–2577, 1979.
178. Hypertension Detection and Follow-up Program Cooperative Group. Five-year findings of the Hypertension Detection and Follow-up Program. Reduction in stroke incidence among persons with high blood pressure. *JAMA* 247:633–638, 1982.
179. Hypertension Detection and Follow-up Program Cooperative Group. The effect of treatment on mortality in mild hypertension. *N Engl J Med* 307:976–980, 1982.
180. Hypertension Detection and Follow-up Program Cooperative Group. Five-year findings of the Hypertension Detection and Follow-up Program. Prevention and reversal of left ventricular hypertrophy with antihypertensive therapy. *Hypertension* 7:105–112, 1985.
181. Schnall PL, Alderman MH, Kern R. An analysis of the HDFP trial. Evidence of adverse effects of antihypertensive treatment on white women with moderate and severe hypertension. *NY State Med J* 84:299–301, 1984.
182. Hypertension Detection and Follow-up Program Cooperative Group. Persistence of reduction in blood pressure and mortality of participants in the Hypertension Detection and Follow-up Program. *JAMA* 259:2113–2122, 1988.
183. Hypertension Detection and Follow-up Program Cooperative Group. Effect of stepped care treatment on the incidence of myocardial infarction and angina pectoris; 5-year findings of the Hypertension Detection and Follow-up Program. *Hypertension* 6(Suppl. I):198–206, 1984.
184. Report by the Management Committee. The Australian Therapeutic Trial in Mild Hypertension. *Lancet* 1:1261–1267, 1980.
185. The Management Committee of the Australian National Blood Pressure Study. Prognostic factors in the treatment of mild hypertension. *Circulation* 69:668–674, 1984.
186. Amery A, Birkenhaeger W, Brixxo P, et al. Mortality and morbidity results from the European Working Party on High Blood Pressure in the Elderly Trial. *Lancet* 1:1349–1354, 1985.
187. Amery A, Birkenhaeger W, Brixxo P, et al. Efficacy of antihypertensive drug treatment according to age, sex, blood pressure, and previous cardiovascular disease in patients over the age of 60. *Lancet* 2:589–592, 1986.
188. Coope J, Warrender TS. Randomised trial of treatment of hypertension in elderly patients in primary care. *Br Med J* 293:1145–1151, 1986.
189. Medical Research Council Working Party. MRC trial of treatment of mild hypertension. Principal results. *Br Med J* 291:97–104, 1985.
190. The Systolic Hypertension in the Elderly Program (SHEP) Cooperative Research Group. Rationale and design of a randomized clinical trial on prevention of stroke in isolated systolic hypertension. *J Clin Epidemiol* 41:1197–1208, 1988.
191. SHEP Cooperative Research Group. Prevention of stroke by antihypertensive drug treatment in older persons with isolated systolic hypertension. Final results of the Systolic Hypertension in the Elderly Program (SHEP). *JAMA* 265:3255–3264, 1991.
192. Dahloef B, Lindholm L, Hansson L, et al. Morbidity and mortality in the Swedish Trial in Old Patients with Hypertension (STOP-Hypertension). *Lancet* 338:1281–1285, 1991.
193. MacMahon SW, Cutler JA, Furberg CD, et al. The effects of drug treatment for hypertension on morbidity and mortality from cardiovascular disease: A review of randomized controlled trials. *Prog Cardiovasc Dis* 29(Suppl. I):99–118, 1986.
194. U.S. Public Health Service, National Institutes of Health. The 1992 Report of the Joint National Committee on Detection, Evaluation, and Treatment of High Blood Pressure. Washington, D.C., U.S. Department of Health and Human Services, (in press, 1992).
195. Frohlich ED, Grim C, Labarthe DR, et al. *Report of a Special Task Force Appointed by the Steering Committee, American Heart Association. Recommendations for Human Blood Pressure Determination by Sphygmomanometers,* (Vol. 5). Dallas, American Heart Association, AHA Publications No. 70–1005 (SA), 1987, pp. i–34.
196. American Society of Hypertension. Recommendations for routine blood pressure measurement by indirect cuff sphygmomanometry. *Am J Hypertens* 5:207–209, 1992.
197. Hypertension Prevention Trial Research Group. The Hypertension Prevention Trial: Three-year effects of dietary changes on blood pressure. *Arch Intern Med* 150:153–162, 1990.
198. Trials of Hypertension Prevention Collaborative Research Group. The effects of nonpharmacologic interventions on blood pressure of persons with high normal levels: Results of the Trials of Hypertension, phase I. *JAMA* 267:1213–1220, 1992.
199. Subcommittee on Nonpharmacologic Therapy of the 1984 Joint National Committee on Detection, Evaluation, and Treatment of High Blood Pressure. Nonpharmacological approaches to the control of high blood pressure: Final Report. *Hypertension* 8(5):444–467, 1986.
200. Treatment of Mild Hypertension Research Group. The Treatment of Mild Hypertension Study. A randomized, placebo-controlled trial of a nutritional-hygienic regimen along with various drug monotherapies. *Arch Intern Med* 151:1413–1423, 1991.
201. Little P, Girling G, Hasler A, et al. A controlled trial of low sodium, low fat, high fiber diet in treated hypertensive patients: Effect on antihypertensive drug requirement in clinical practice. *J Human Hypertens* 5:175–181, 1991.
202. Langford HG, Davis BR, Blaufox MD, et al. Effect of drug and diet treatment of mild hypertension on diastolic blood pressure. *Hypertension* 17:210–217, 1991.
203. Schotte DE, Stunkard AJ. The effects of weight

reduction on blood pressure in 301 obese patients. *Arch Intern Med* 150:1701–1704, 1990.
204. World Hypertension League. Alcohol and hypertension-implications for treatment. *J Human Hypertens* 121:1854–1856, 1991.
205. MacMahon S. Alcohol consumption and hypertension. *Hypertension* 9:111–121, 1987.
206. Maheswaran R, Gill JS, Davies P, et al. High blood pressure due to alcohol: A rapidly reversible effect. *Hypertension* 17:787–792, 1991.
207. World Hypertension League. Physical exercise in the management of hypertension: A consensus statement by the World Hypertension League. *J Hypertens* 9:283–287, 1991.
208. Blair SN, Kohl HW III, Paffenbarger RS Jr, et al. Physical fitness and all-cause mortality: A prospective study of healthy men and women. *JAMA* 262:2395–2401, 1989.
209. American College of Sports Medicine. *Guidelines for Exercise Testing and Prescription* (4th ed.). Philadelphia, Lea & Febiger, 1991.
210. Weinberger MH, Fineberg NS. Sodium and volume sensitivity of blood pressure. Age and pressure change over time. *Hypertension* 18:67–71, 1991.
211. Intersalt Cooperative Research Group: Intersalt: An international study of electrolyte excretion and blood pressure. Results for 24 hour urinary sodium and potassium excretion. *Br Med J* 297:319–328, 1988.
212. Linas SL. The role of potassium in the pathogenesis and treatment of hypertension. *Kidney Int* 39:771–786, 1991.
213. McCarron DA, Morris CD, Henry JH, et al. Blood pressure and nutrient intake in the United States. *Science* 224:1392–1398, 1984.
214. Hamet P, Mongeau E, Lambert J, et al. Interactions among calcium, sodium, and alcohol intake as determinants of blood pressure. *Hypertension* 17(Suppl. I):I-150–I-154, 1991.
215. Joffres MR, Reed DM, Yano K. Relationship of magnesium intake and other dietary factors to blood pressure: The Honolulu Heart Study. *Am J Clin Nutr* 45:469–475, 1987.
216. Expert Panel. Report of the National Cholesterol Education Program Expert Panel on Detection, Evaluation, and Treatment of High Blood Cholesterol in Adults. *Arch Intern Med* 148:36–39, 1988.
217. Sacks FM. Dietary fats and blood pressure: A critical review of the evidence. *Nutr Rev* 47:291–300, 1989.
218. Knapp HR, Fitzgerald GA. The antihypertensive effects of fish oil: A controlled study of polyunsaturated fatty acid supplements in essential hypertension. *N Engl J Med* 320:1037–1043, 1989.
219. van Montfrans GW, Karemaker JM, Wieling W, et al. Relaxation therapy and continuous ambulatory blood pressure in mild hypertension: A controlled study. *Br Med J* 300:1368–1372, 1990.
220. Collins R, Peto R, MacMahon S, et al. Blood pressure, stroke, and coronary heart disease. Part 2. Short-term reductions in blood pressure: Overview of randomized drug trials in their epidemiologic context. *Lancet* 335:827–838, 1990.
221. Cutler JA, MacMahon SW, Furberg CD. Controlled clinical trials of drug treatment for hypertension. A review. *Hypertension* 13(Suppl. I):I-36–I-44, 1989.
222. MacMahon SW, Furberg CS, Cutler JA. Women as participants in trials of the primary and secondary prevention of cardiovascular disease. Part I. Primary prevention: The hypertension trials. In Eaker ED, Packard B, Wenger NK, et al. (Eds.), *Coronary Heart Disease in Women. Proceedings of an NIH Workshop.* New York, Haymarket Doyma, 1987, pp. 233–240.
223. Anastos K, Charney P, Charon RA, et al. Hypertension in women: What is really known? The Women's Caucus, Working Group on Women's Health of the Society of General Internal Medicine. *Ann Intern Med* 115:287–293, 1991.
224. Barron WM, Murphy MB, Lindheimer MD. Management of hypertension during pregnancy. In Laragh JH, Brenner BM (Eds.), *Hypertension: Pathophysiology, Diagnosis, and Management.* New York, Raven Press, 1990, pp. 1809–1827.
225. Woods JW. Oral contraceptives and hypertension. *Hypertension* 11(Suppl. II):II-11–II-15, 1988.
226. Royal College of General Practioners' Oral Contraception Study. *Oral Contraceptives and Health.* New York, Pitman, 1974.
227. Lim KG, Isles CG, Hodsman GP, et al. Malignant hypertension in women of childbearing age and its relation to the contraceptive pill. *Br Med J* 294:1057–1059, 1987.
228. Sondheimer SJ. Update on the metabolic effects of steroidal contraceptives. *Endocrinol Metab Clin North Am* 4:911–923, 1991.
229. National High Blood Pressure Education Program Working Group on High Blood Pressure in Pregnancy. Working Group report on high blood pressure in pregnancy. *Am J Obstet Gynecol* 163:1689–1712, 1990.
230. Cunningham FG, Lindheimer MD. Hypertension in pregnancy. *N Engl J Med* 326:927–932, 1992.
231. WHO Study Group. *The Hypertensive Disorders of Pregnancy,* Technical Report Series 758. Geneva, World Health Organization, 1987, pp. 1–114.
232. Wallenburg HCS. Hemodynamics in hypertensive pregnancy. In Rubin PC (Ed.), *Handbook of Hypertension,* Vol. 10. *(Hypertension in Pregnancy),* Amsterdam, Elsevier, 1988, pp. 66–101.
233. Pritchard JA, Weisman R Jr, Ratnoff OD, et al. Intravascular hemolysis, thrombocytopenia and other hematologic abnormalities associated with severe toxemia of pregnancy. *N Engl J Med* 250:89–98, 1954.
234. Fitzgerald DJ, Fitzgerald GA. Eicosanoids in the pathogenesis of preeclampsia. In Laragh JH, Brenner BM (Eds.), *Hypertension: Pathology, Diagnosis and Management.* New York, Raven Press, 1990, pp. 1789–1807.
235. Roberts JM, Taylor RM, Goldfein A. Clinical and biochemical evidence of endothelial cell dysfunction in the pregnancy syndrome preeclampsia. *Am J Hypertens* 4:700–708, 1991.
236. Taylor RM, Heilbron DC, Roberts JM. Growth factor activity in blood of women destined to develop preeclampsia is elevated from early pregnancy. *Am J Obstet Gynecol* 163:1839–1844, 1990.
237. Collins R. Antiplatelet agents for IUGR and preeclampsia. In Chalmers I (Ed.), *Oxford Data Base for Perinatal Trials. Version 1.2, disk issue 5, 1991; record 4000.* Oxford, Clinical Trials Service Unit, 1991.
238. Cunningham FG, Gant NF. Prevention of preeclampsia—A reality? *N Engl J Med* 321:606–607, 1989.
239. Taufield PA, Ales KL, Resnick LM, et al. Hypocal-

ciuria in preeclampsia. *N Engl J Med* 316:715–718, 1987.
240. Belizan JM, Villar J, Gonzalez L, et al. Calcium supplementation to prevent hypertensive disorders of pregnancy. *N Engl J Med* 325:1399–1405, 1991.
241. Barron WM. Hypertension. In Barron WM, Lindheimer MD (Eds.), *Medical Disorders in Pregnancy*. Chicago, Mosby-Year Book, 1991, pp. 1–42.
242. Pritchard JA, Cunningham FG, Pritchard FA. The Parkland Memorial Hospital protocol for treatment of eclampsia: Evaluation of 245 cases. *Am J Obstet Gynecol* 148:951–963, 1984.
243. Lindheimer MD, Katz AI. Renal physiology and disease in pregnancy. In Seldin DW, Giebisch G (Eds.), *The Kidney: Physiology and Pathophysiology* (2nd ed.). New York, Raven Press, 1992, pp. 3371–3431.
244. Aron DC, Schnall AM, Sheeler LR. Cushing's syndrome and pregnancy. *Am J Obstet Gynecol* 162:244–252, 1990.
245. Greenberg M, Moawad AH, Wieties BM, et al. Extraadrenal pheochromocytoma: Detection during pregnancy using MR imaging. *Radiology* 161:475–476, 1985.
246. Cockburn J, Moar VA, Ounsted M, et al. Final report of study of hypertension during pregnancy: The effects of specific treatment on the growth and development of children. *Lancet* 1:647–649, 1982.
247. Rosa FW, Bosco LA, Graham CF, et al. Neonatal anuria with maternal angiotensin-converting enzyme inhibition. *Obstet Gynecol* 74:371–374, 1989.
248. Hanssens M, Keirse MJNC, Vankelecom D, et al. Fetal and neonatal effects of treatment with angiotensin-converting enzyme inhibitors in pregnancy. *Obstet Gynecol* 78:128–135, 1991.
249. Chesely LC. *Hypertensive Disorders in Pregnancy*. New York, Appleton-Century-Crofts, 1978.
250. Fisher KA, Luger A, Spargo BH, et al. Hypertension in pregnancy: Clinical pathological correlations and late prognosis. *Medicine* 60:267–276, 1981.
251. Wren BG, Rautledge DA. Blood pressure changes: Estrogens in climacteric women. *Med J Aust* 2:528–531, 1981.
252. Colditz GA, Willett WC, Stampfer MJ, et al. Menopause and the risk of coronary heart disease in women. *N Engl J Med* 316:1105–1110, 1987.
253. Stampfer MJ, Colditz GA, Willett WC, et al. Postmenopausal estrogen therapy and cardiovascular disease. Ten-year follow-up from the Nurses' Health Study. *N Engl J Med* 325:756–762, 1991.
254. Drugs that cause sexual dysfunction. *Med Lett Drugs Ther* 29:65–70, 1987.
255. Reichgott MJ. Problems of sexual function in patients with hypertension. *Cardiovasc Med* 4:149–156, 1979.
256. Hogan MJ, Wallin JD, Baer RM. Antihypertensive therapy and male sexual dysfunction. *Psychosomatics* 4:149–156, 1980.
257. Croog SH, Levine S, Sudilovsky A, et al. Sexual symptoms in hypertensive patients: A clinical trial of antihypertensive medications. *Arch Intern Med* 148:788–794, 1988.
258. Hsueh WA. Sexual dysfunction with aging and systemic hypertension. *Am J Cardiol* 61:18H–23H, 1988.
259. Arze RS, Ramos JM, Rashid HU, et al. Amenorrhoea, galactorrhoea, and hyperprolactinaemia induced by methyldopa [clin res]. *Br Med J* 283:194, 1981.
260. Loriaux DL. Spironolactone and endocrine dysfunction. *Ann Intern Med* 85:630–636, 1976.
261. Onesti G, Bock KD, Heimsoth V, et al. Clonidine: A new antihypertensive agent. *Am J Cardiol* 28:74–83, 1971.
262. Michelson EL, Frishman WH, Lewis JE, et al. Multicenter clinical evaluation of long-term efficacy and safety of labetalol in treatment of hypertension. *Am J Med* 75(4A):68–80, 1983.
263. Lipson LG. Treatment of hypertension in diabetic men: Problems with sexual dysfunction. *Am J Cardiol* 53:46A–50A, 1984.
264. Yodfat Y, Fidel J, Bloom DS. Captopril as a replacement for multiple therapy in hypertension: A controlled study. *J Hypertens* 3(Suppl.):S155–S158, 1985.
265. Curb JD, Borhani NO, Blaszkowski TP, et al. Long-term surveillance for adverse effects of antihypertensive drugs. *JAMA* 253:3263–3268, 1985.
266. Schoenberger JA, Testa M, Ross AD, et al. Efficacy, safety, and quality-of-life assessment of captopril antihypertensive therapy in clinical practice. *Arch Intern Med* 150:301–306, 1990.
267. Hodge RH, Harward MP, West MS, et al. Sexual function of women taking antihypertensive agents: A comparative study. *Gen Intern Med* 6:290–294, 1991.

CHAPTER 5

Myocardial Function and Cardiomyopathy

MARC KLAPHOLZ M.D.
PETER BUTTRICK M.D.

The natural history of a number of cardiovascular disorders differs in men and women. Some of these differences, such as survival following a myocardial infarction, may reflect the referral and treatment biases of physicians; others, however, such as the apparent increased incidence of congestive heart failure with normal systolic function in women, may reflect intrinsic or hormonally mediated gender-specific differences in cardiac structure and function. Despite this, very few studies have been performed to study directly sex-related differences in myocardial function and cardiac responses to superimposed hemodynamic loads. The purpose of this chapter is to summarize the existent data on this subject, both in humans and in experimental animals, and then to review the natural history of selected myocardial disorders in light of this discussion. In addition, the clinical presentation and natural history of certain genetic cardiomyopathies that exhibit gender differences will be reviewed.

CARDIAC SIZE

A number of echocardiographic analyses have been done to define left ventricular (LV) dimensions in normal men and women (1, 2, 3). In general, these have shown that LV chamber size and, to a greater degree, LV mass are smaller in women than in men. These differences are detectable even in childhood. The most comprehensive of these studies, the retrospective analysis of the Framingham population, studied 864 healthy adults (out of a total study population of approximately 6000) and defined normal reference values for LV

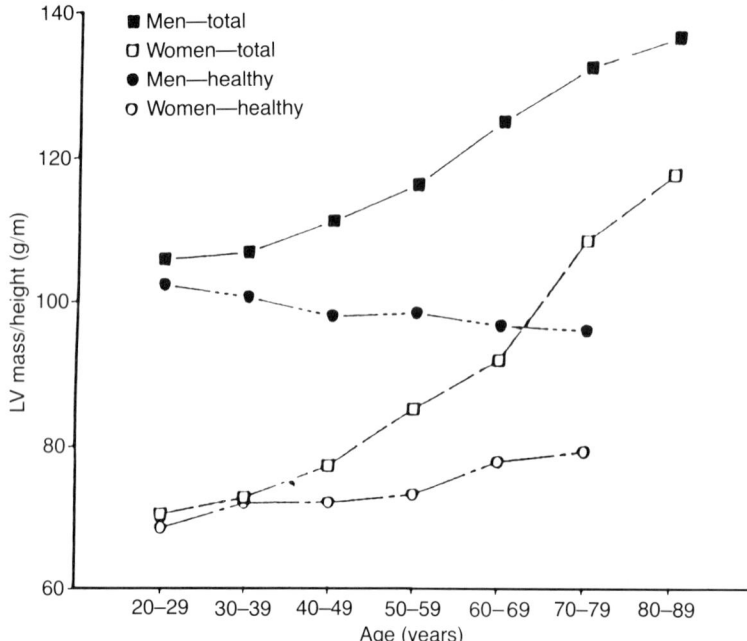

Figure 5-1. Echocardiographic left ventricular (LV) mass by age and sex in the total Framingham study group (2226 men and 2746 women) and in the healthy subgroup (345 men and 517 women). (Adapted from Dannenberg AL, Levy D, Garrison RJ. Impact of age on echocardiographic left ventricular mass in a healthy population (the Framingham Study). *Am J Cardiol* 64:1066–1068, 1989.)

mass and LV mass index (1). Using the Penn convention (4) for the assessment of ventricular dimensions, the authors determined that mean LV mass was 177 g in men and 118 g in women. When the data were normalized to body surface area the mean in males was 92 g/m^2 (53–131; 95% confidence limits), and in females it was 72 g/m^2 (44–100), still a significant difference of more than 20%. Devereux et al. also defined reference values for LV size in a normotensive population and found similar differences between males and females; however, this group also indexed the data to lean body mass, which was significantly reduced in women and showed that this correction eliminated the sex difference (2). Regardless of how the data are presented, the fact remains that males have significantly larger hearts, and, if it is true that the number of myocytes is fixed at birth (and not influenced by gender), then the myocytes from ostensibly normal and nonstressed male hearts must have some degree of hypertrophy relative to females.

The Framingham data also suggest the presence of a significant sexual dimorphism in a normal aging population. There was a slight (~6%) decline in LV mass in males between 20 and 29 and between 70 and 79 years of age, whereas in females there was a small (~15%) increase in LV mass during this time frame. These data are illustrated in Figure 5–1, which shows left ventricular mass estimates in the healthy subset as well as the total cohort of patients. This observation has to be qualified by the fact that the study population represented only a very small percentage of the total patient cohort and was not well controlled or necessarily matched for subtle variables such as activity level, which might have influenced ventricular mass. Nonetheless, since aging is associated with a significant and progressive loss of myocytes and a parallel increase in myocyte volume per nucleus in both males and females (5), it is intriguing to postulate that the remaining myocytes from the large aged male hearts may more closely approach the limits of ventricular hypertrophy than do those in females.

Studies in animals have confirmed the basic observation that heart mass is increased in males. In rats, for example, heart and body weights and growth rates are increased in males (6–9). Koenig et al. (10) have also shown increased heart-body weight ratios in males, although this result has not been consistently observed (8) (probably reflecting the lability in body weight determinations in this species). It appears that the heart weight differences may be, at least in part, hormonally mediated because male rats that are gonadectomized either pre- or postpubertally have smaller hearts than shams, whereas gonadectomized females have increased heart and body weights. Female animals treated with testosterone also show increased heart and body growth rates (8, 11).

BIOCHEMISTRY

Based on studies involving gonadectomy or hormone replacement, it appears that many of the sex-specific differences in structure and function of the heart are mediated by the sex hormones (8, 11–13). Whether these agents affect the heart indirectly, for example, by influencing blood pressure or volume status, or directly is unclear. Both estrogen and androgen receptors have been identified in blood vessels of experimental animals, including the aorta and the epicardial coronary arteries, with androgen receptors predominating in the smooth muscle cells of the media and estrogen receptors localizing primarily to fibroblasts within the adventitia (14). These vascular hormone receptors have been implicated in the discordant vasoreactive responses of men and women and have been postulated to play a role in defining the sex-related differences in both hypertension and coronary artery disease. These topics will be reviewed in other chapters.

Sex hormone receptors have also been found in cardiac tissue: Estrogen receptors have been identified throughout the interstitial tissue of baboon hearts and in atrial but not ventricular rat heart cells (15). In contrast, androgen receptors have been found in both atrial and ventricular myocytes from the rat, monkey, and baboon (14, 16, 17). The presence and specific distribution of these receptors suggest that the sex hormones may play a direct role in modulating cardiac structure and function. A variety of biochemical features that are influenced by sex hormones have been identified in cardiac tissue, and some of them may underlie differences in cardiac performance and susceptibility to various diseases.

Koenig et al. (10) have shown that the ventricles of male mice and rats have a greater specific activity of cytochrome C oxidase, an inner mitochondrial enzyme, than do females. Whether this translates into an augmented respiratory capacity of cardiac mitochondria is conjectural. These same investigators also established that male rodents have greater activities of a number of lysosomal enzymes, including β-glucuronidase, hexosaminidase, β-galactosidase, and arylsulphatase as well as decreased enzyme latency and accelerated lysosomal protein degradation, findings that suggest accelerated protein catabolism. When the mice underwent orchiectomy, ventricular weight, protein content, cytochrome C oxidase, and lysosomal enzyme activity all decreased to female levels and reverted to normal with testosterone administration. Testosterone administration to females increased ventricular weight, protein content, cytochrome C oxidase activity, and total ventricular RNA without affecting total DNA.

Another biochemical axis that appears to be influenced by the sex hormones is cardiac myosin heavy chain gene and protein expression. In cardiac tissue, only the α and β myosin heavy chain genes are expressed, and they in turn form three different isoforms of myosin: V_1 ($\alpha\alpha$), V_2 ($\alpha\beta$), and V_3 ($\beta\beta$), which differ in their ATPase activities, with V_1 being the highest and V_3 the lowest (18). In models of cardiac hypertrophy in the rat, changes in myosin isoform distribution have been observed and correlated with changes in the contractile properties of the intact muscle (19). In general, female rats appear to have higher myosin ATPase activities and a greater percentage of V_1 myosin than males (8, 20), probably reflecting differences in gene transcription (Taylor and Buttrick, personal communication). This result does not predict the mechanical data (outlined below) indicating that male hearts have greater contractile reserve and thus suggests that other components in excitation-contraction coupling are responsible for the gender-specific differences in contraction. However, in response to gonadectomy both male and female rats decrease their cardiac myosin ATPase activity and shift the myosin isoform distribution toward V_3 (males to a greater degree), changes that parallel the depression in contractile indices (8). Also concordant with the mechanical data is the observation that sex-specific hormone replacement prevented or reversed the biochemical changes associated with gonadectomy and that testosterone was able to increase the myosin ATPase activity in female hearts (11).

The role of the sex hormones in modulating other components in excitation-contraction coupling in the heart has not been carefully studied. Testosterone, but not estrogen, has been shown to up-regulate α-adrenergic receptors and rates of gene transcription in a variety of tissue types, including vascular smooth muscle (21) and myometrium (22), but this has never been studied in cardiac myocytes. Similarly, no data exist that might establish a role for the sex hormones in regulating sarcoplasmic reticular function.

Sex hormones influence the deposition of the fibrous proteins, collagen and elastin, in vessel walls. Testosterone has been shown to increase vascular synthesis of these compounds, whereas estradiol administration to male rats resulted in decreased rates of collagen and elastin accumulation (23, 24). Further, in a rat model of hypertension, females had a smaller increase in the volume of connective tissue in the aorta and a more complete return to normal thickness after reversal of hypertension than males (25). No studies have been done directly comparing the volume percentage of collagen or hydroxyproline content in normal or pressure-overloaded male versus female hearts, but it is not unreasonable to presume that cardiac fibroblasts would respond to hormonal signals in a fashion similar to vascular fibroblasts. Since collagen breakdown and subsequent reaccumulation have been shown to play significant roles in the remodeling that occurs following ischemic myocardial injury (26) and also in ventricular rupture (27), it is possible that this dimorphism has major pathophysiologic significance.

VENTRICULAR PERFORMANCE

A paucity of information is available comparing normal ventricular function in males and females. What data do exist are largely derived from isolated perfused rat heart studies. This method allows the quantitation of coronary flow, myocardial oxygen consumption, and pump and muscle function at fixed heart rates under well-controlled loading conditions. In a carefully executed series of experiments, Schaible and Scheuer compared myocardial contractile performance in male and female rats under various loading conditions (9). Representative data from this study are shown in Figure 5–2. In initial studies, they compared hearts from animals of the same age (normalizing cardiac performance to ventricular weight) and established that stroke work was greater in males at all loading conditions, although cardiac output and fractional shortening were greater only at high afterloads. Subsequently, they compared heart function in male and female animals with similar left ventricular size (the females were older) and found that all indices of contractile performance including stroke work, cardiac output, ejection fraction, and fractional shortening were ~25% greater in male hearts at all loading conditions.

These investigators also investigated the role of the sex hormones in determining the differences in cardiac function by comparing the mechanical performance of hearts from both gonadectomized and hormone-repleted animals with that of sham-operated controls (8, 11). As mentioned above, gonadectomized males had smaller heart and body weights, whereas in gonadectomized females body weight and, to a lesser degree, heart weight increased. In both sexes, indices of ventricular performance (adjusted for heart weight) were decreased by gonadectomy, although the differences were more marked in males. Sex-specific hormone replacement (estrogen in females and testosterone in males) prevented and, in the case of testosterone, actually supernormalized these changes in ventricular function. Of further note, testosterone treatment of females also resulted in increased heart and body weights and in augmented ventricular mechanical performance.

In humans, a few studies comparing physiologic responses of normal men and women to acute dynamic exercise have been performed. In general, the physiologic responses and adaptations of women to exercise are similar to those seen in men (28, 29). That is, acute dynamic exercise induces a decrease in peripheral vascular resistance and increases in venous return, stroke volume, and peripheral oxygen extraction. Acute static exercise increases peripheral vascular resistance with relatively modest changes in stroke volume and (A-V) O_2 difference. However, gender-specific differences have been identified. Women, for example, have higher heart rates both at rest and during submaximal exercise (30, 31, 32). This may reflect differences in local adrenergic tone, decreased hemoglobin concentration (on average 15% reduced in adult women), or fundamental differences in Frank-Starling mechanisms. Women also have an approximately 10–15% reduced VO_{2max} relative to age-matched men, even when this measurement is adjusted for lean body mass (28, 30, 33). This difference probably does reflect a true gender-specific difference in oxygen transport and

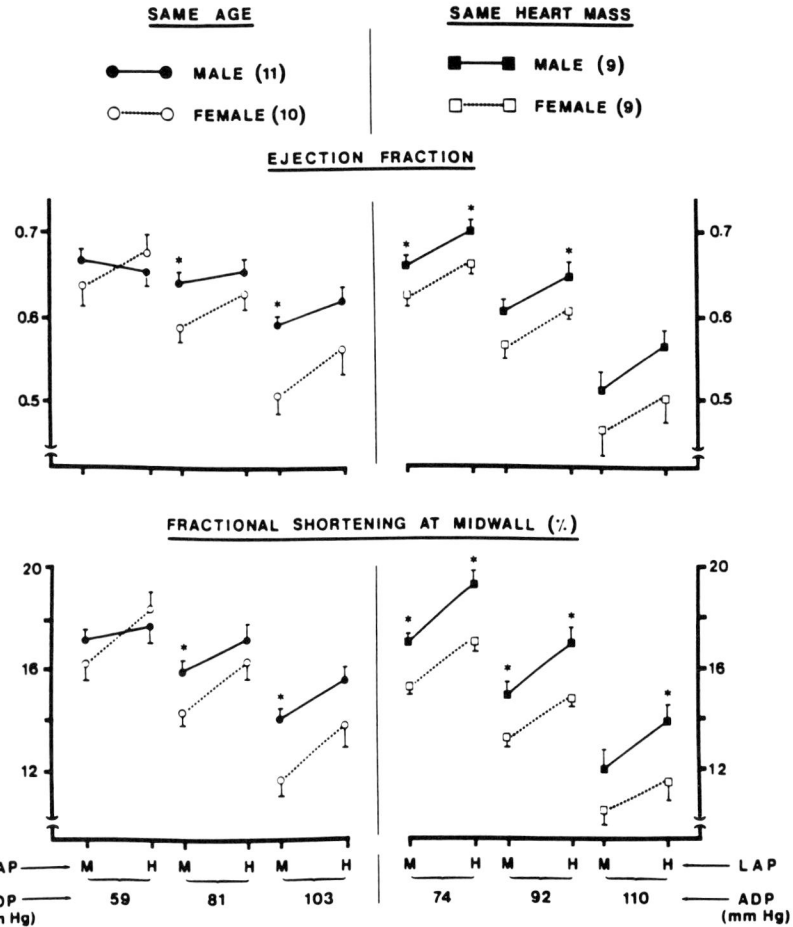

Figure 5-2. Ejection fraction and fractional shortening at midwall in hearts from male and female rats of the same age *(left)* and with the same heart mass *(right)*. Data are at two levels of preload (LAP-left atrial pressure): M, moderate, and H, high; and at three levels of afterload (ADP-aortic diastolic pressure). *p < .05 for male vs. female at any given loading condition. (Adapted from Schaible TF, Scheuer J. Comparison of heart function in male and female rats. *Basic Res Cardiol* 79:402–412, 1984.)

delivery because women have a lower hemoglobin concentration and a smaller blood volume than men. Additional differences in autonomic regulation of the circulation (34, 35), suggested by the female predominance of such diseases as migraine headache and Raynaud's phenomenon, may contribute to the differences in VO_{2max}. Of course, the level of fitness, which might not be comparable between men and women, could contribute to these differences as well.

Differences have been identified in cardiac responses to dynamic exercise in unconditioned men and women using radionucleotide ventriculography. These are highlighted in a paper by Higgenbotham et al. who studied healthy men and women during upright bicycle ergometry (36). Representative data are shown in Figure 5-3. LV function and aerobic capacity were comparable at rest; however, during exercise, men increased their ejection fraction from 0.62 to 0.77, whereas women had a flat ejection fraction response, 0.63 to 0.64. In contrast, end-diastolic volume increased by 30% with exercise in women but was unchanged in men. Stroke volume increased to a similar degree in both sexes reflecting these divergent hemodynamic responses to exercise. Although this study had many limitations that must be acknowledged, including small sample size, it seems to support the animal studies cited above that detail fundamental differences in contractility between male and female hearts. Parenthetically, this study also suggests a clinical caveat—namely, that the lack of a rise in ejection fraction during exercise in

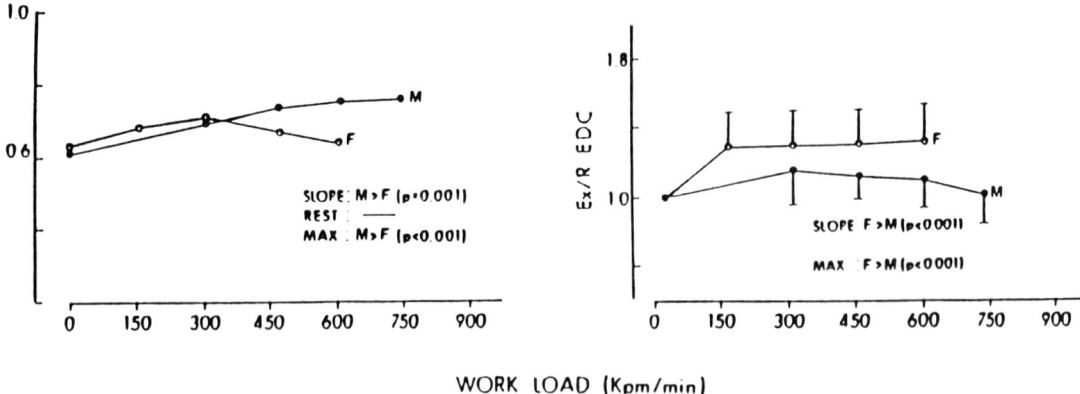

Figure 5-3. Mean ejection fraction responses *(left)* and proportional changes in end-diastolic counts *(right)* in males (M) and females (F) at rest and during submaximal and maximal exercise. (Adapted from Higgenbotham MB, Morris KG, Coleman RE, et al. Sex related differences in the normal cardiac responses to upright exercise. *Circulation* 70(3):357–366, 1984.)

women should not be presumed to reflect cardiac pathology and may in fact be a manifestation of normal physiology.

ADAPTATION TO CHRONIC HEMODYNAMIC LOADS: LEFT VENTRICULAR HYPERTROPHY

The data reviewed thus far details ventricular structure and function in normal male and female animals. Clinical myopathy is a reflection of how normal cardiac muscle adapts to imposed loads such as hypertension or ischemia. Although there are few data in the literature directly comparing these cardiac responses in males and females, information from large epidemiologic data bases as well as a few small clinical and animal studies suggests that there are distinct sex-specific patterns of adaptation and that these are clinically relevant.

The Framingham study is one of the few large epidemiologic studies that assessed sex differences in the incidence of cardiovascular disease. The initial 16-year follow-up analysis of the natural history of congestive heart failure (CHF), published in 1971, noted an increased incidence of CHF in men versus women, 2.3 versus 1.4 per 1000 patients (37). This difference was evident in every age group from age 30 to 62 and was postulated to reflect the increased incidence of coronary disease in men. Interestingly, once the diagnosis of CHF was made, the mean duration of survival was shorter in women. In a more recent 34-year follow-up analysis of this patient cohort, CHF was again noted to predominate in men, but the difference in incidence was slight, especially when contrasted with the marked (46% versus 27%) increase in coronary artery disease seen in men (38). This study suggests that noncoronary factors such as hypertension, which was identified as the most important noncoronary precipitant, may play a more important role in the development of CHF in women than in men. In fact, systolic blood pressure was the strongest predictor of heart failure in women. Pulse pressure was the best predictor in men.

These Framingham studies did not differentiate between congestive heart failure due to systolic and diastolic dysfunction because the criteria used to establish the diagnosis were based solely on clinical observation. An early hint of a sex difference in these patterns of CHF, however, comes from an echocardiographic study of 50 patients (32 men and 18 women) that demonstrated impaired LV systolic function in 72% of the men but only 40% of the women (39). Most of the patients with normal LV systolic function had echocardiographic evidence of left ventricular hypertrophy and impaired diastolic compliance.

Indirect support for the thesis that women are more susceptible to the development of left ventricular hypertrophy associated with diastolic abnormalities comes from other echocardiographic and radionucleotide data (40, 41). As mentioned earlier, analysis of some of the Framingham patients demonstrated a slight

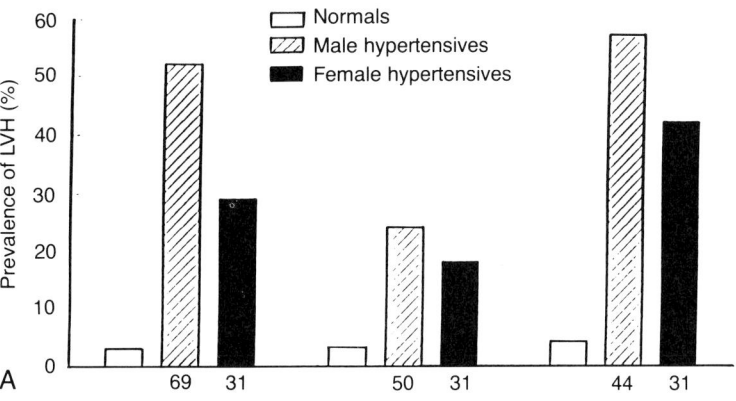

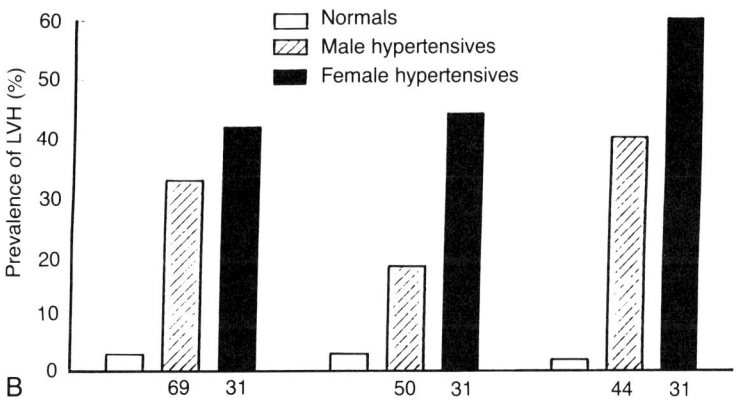

Figure 5–4. Prevalence of left ventricular hypertrophy (LVH) in three independent groups of patients with essential hypertension subdivided by sex. The number of patients in each group is indicated along the abscissa. When the upper limit of normal for both sexes pooled (Panel A) is used, the prevalence of LVH is greater in males, but when sex-specific upper limits are used (panel B), the prevalence of LVH is greater in females. (Adapted from Devereux RB, Pickering TG, Alderman MH, et al. Left ventricular hypertrophy in hypertension: Prevalence and relationship to pathophysiologic variables. *Hypertension* 9 (Suppl. II):II53–II60, 1987.)

age-related increase in LV mass in normal women and a slight decline in men (3). When the total group of subjects was studied (see Fig. 5–1), heart mass increased with age in both men and women, but the percentage increase was greater in women, 54% versus 25%. Lauer et al. (42) correlated long-term blood pressure measurements with LV mass in 299 women and 152 men who were free of intercurrent illness. The 30-year average systolic pressure was shown to correlate with LV mass and wall thickness in both sexes; however, women had higher age-adjusted prevalence rates of left ventricular hypertrophy (LVH) at all levels of blood pressure and a higher odds ratio for the development of LVH when it was indexed to several variables including 30-year average systolic, diastolic, and maximal systolic blood pressure. An increased prevalence of LVH normalized to body mass in women with essential hypertension has also been noted by Devereux et al. (43). Figure 5–4 illustrates data collected from three separate patient groups by Devereux and colleagues, all of which confirm this result.

A recent follow-up analysis of Coronary Artery Surgery Study (CASS) registry patients (44) demonstrated that patients with symptoms of moderate to severe CHF and an LV ejection fraction of >0.45 tended to be older, had a higher incidence of hypertension and diabetes, and were overwhelmingly female compared with a matched cohort of patients with similar ejection fractions without CHF. The 6-year survival rate was significantly reduced in the patients with symptoms of CHF.

The most extreme example of a disproportionate hypertrophic response to chronic overload is the hypertrophic cardiomyopathy of the elderly. This syndrome was first described by Topol et al. (45), who identified a subgroup of elderly patients (mean age 73) who had a history of mild to moderate hypertension and who presented with symptoms of pulmonary congestion. Echocardiography revealed severe concentric LVH that was disproportionate to the severity of the chronic load, a small LV cavity, enhanced systolic function, and markedly impaired diastolic relaxation, particularly during the early filling phase. More than three-quarters of these patients (16/21) were female, and many were black.

Although these clinical data suggest that women have an exaggerated left ventricular hypertrophic response to chronic pressure loads relative to men, none of the studies cited were specifically designed to address this issue. Consequently, this conclusion may be biased by referral patterns, the coincidence of other illnesses (such as ischemic heart disease) that might affect ventricular performance, or other ill-defined factors. However, a few animal studies have been done to assess gender differences in the magnitude of hypertrophy following pressure overload, and these corroborate this clinical suggestion. Malhotra et al. (46), for example, compared the cardiac adaptations in male and female rats subjected to equivalent degrees of renovascular hypertension and found more profound cardiac hypertrophy in females than in males (46% versus 14%). In addition, if hypertensive animals were subjected to the additional load of conditioning by swimming, female animals increased their cardiac mass to 70% as opposed to only 28% in males.

In addition to this apparent discordant myocardial response to pressure overload, animal studies demonstrate that hearts from females respond differently to the physiologic load of chronic exercise conditioning. Chronic conditioning of rats by treadmill exercise, for example, improves contractile performance significantly in males but only marginally in females (13, 47), whereas conditioning by swimming improves contractile performance and increases myosin ATPase activities in both sexes (12, 48). Swimming increased heart weight in females but not in males (48). The presence of an intact sex hormone axis is not necessary for this dimorphism to become manifest because the same patterns of adaptation persisted in both gonadectomized male and female animals (12), suggesting that other neurohumoral factors might mediate the adaptive hypertrophy seen in female animals (49–51).

Finally, females seem to have an increased incidence of LV rupture following myocardial infarction compared to men. This finding has emerged from numerous clinical series, all of which show at least a two- to threefold female predominance, and appears to be independent of the incidence of comorbid diseases (52–54). It is unclear why this should be, especially because the absence of a hypertrophic response to chronic hypertension seems to be a risk factor for ventricular rupture. One possible explanation is suggested by the fact, alluded to above, that sex hormones influence the synthesis and deposition of collagen and elastin in vessel walls, with testosterone leading to an increase and estrogen to a decrease (24). No studies have been done comparing myocardial connective tissue composition in males and females, but it is interesting that rupture commonly occurs in areas of the myocardium that are devoid of connective tissue (27). An alternative explanation might relate to the coronary vasculature. Myocardial capillary-to-fiber ratios are decreased and coronary capacitance (per gram) is reduced in pressure overload hypertrophy (55, 56). It is conceivable, although unexplored, that pressure-overloaded hearts from females, with disproportionately more ventricular hypertrophy, might have more significant reductions in vascularity than hearts from males.

RIGHT VENTRICULAR HYPERTROPHY

In contrast to the data on left ventricular hypertrophy, several studies have suggested that males are more vulnerable to the development of pulmonary hypertension and right ventricular failure than females, especially in the presence of chronic hypoxia (57–60). McMurtry et al. (61), for example, have shown that female swine maintained at high altitudes had less right ventricular hypertrophy (RVH), less pulmonary hypertension, and higher arterial oxygen tension than male animals. The same investigators also studied the effects of the sex hormones on RVH in male gonadectomized rats maintained at altitudes of 1520 and 4000 meters (62). All animals increased their right ventricular weight, but those animals maintained at high altitudes and treated with testosterone had the greatest degree of RVH, an effect that clearly went beyond the anabolic effects of the hormone. Similarly, other investigators have shown that female rats maintained in a hypoxic environment had lower pulmonary and right ventricular pressures than males, an effect that was obviated by ovariectomy (63). Of perhaps more significance is the observation that even under conditions of equivalent hypoxia-induced RVH and pulmonary hypertension, female rats had reduced mortality compared to males, 0% versus 40% (64), and relative resistance to vascular and myocellular injury following an anoxic insult (65, 66). How these animal studies relate to the male predominance of and mortality from such clinical disorders as chronic obstructive pulmonary disease and sleep apnea (67) remains conjectural.

X-LINKED CARDIOMYOPATHIES

In addition to sex-related differences in cardiac performance and biochemistry, genetic factors also affect the presentation of cardiovascular disease. Several cardiomyopathies are X-linked and as such they present differently in males and females. Notable among these are Duchenne's and Becker's muscular dystrophies, both X-linked recessive myopathies. The former, associated with mutations in the gene encoding the dystrophin protein, causes a fulminant peripheral myopathy in affected males, and most patients become wheelchair-bound in their early teens and die in their twenties. Although the cardiomyopathy associated with this disorder is not prominent, largely because of the dramatic peripheral myopathy, characteristic electrocardiographic findings have been described, counterclockwise rotation with tall precordial R waves and deep Q waves in the left lateral leads (68), and abnormal LV systolic function can be demonstrated in most affected individuals (69). Clinical symptoms of myopathy have also been described in heterozygous females as well as elevations in serum creatine phosphokinase levels (70), abnormal electromyograms (71), and focal myopathic changes on muscle biopsy (72). Cardiac findings in heterozygote female carriers include increased R/S ratios in the right precordial leads and occasionally regional wall motion abnormalities, suggesting that occult cardiac involvement may be present (73). An awareness of these manifestations in female carriers is important for genetic counseling, especially because less than 25% of affected males can be linked to an affected individual in a previous generation and because accurate genetic screening is available. Becker's dystrophy is a milder disorder that is also associated with mutations in the dystrophin gene but tends to present later in life; occasional reports have described an associated dilated cardiomyopathy.

A family with a probable X-linked dilated cardiomyopathy was recently described by Berko and Swift (74). Their description of this disease is striking in that both men and women were affected but their clinical course was quite distinct. Affected males presented in their teens and early twenties with a rapidly progressive dilated cardiomyopathy that led to death usually within a year following symptom onset. In contrast, affected women, all of whom were mothers of the affected males, did not develop clinical symptoms until their forties, and their clinical course following disease onset was more protracted, progressing from atypical chest pain to an end-stage dilated cardiomyopathy over a period of more than 10 years. Although the pattern of the disease with a pronounced male predominance and no male-to-male inheritance is most consistent with an X-linked disorder, it is conceivable that the disease is autosomal and that women are in some way protected from its early and aggressive manifestations. Regardless, the distinctly different clinical presentations of this disease in men and women suggest that the environment (male versus female) in which the specific gene responsible is expressed dramatically influences its behavior.

CONCLUSION

In summary, male and female hearts both in humans and in experimental animals have fundamentally different geometric and biochemical features that translate to distinct patterns of pump and muscle performance. The natural history of certain myocardial diseases, such as pressure overload hypertrophy, is distinct in men and women and probably reflects these dimorphisms, and these differences must be acknowledged in clinical management.

References

1. Levy D, Savage DD, Garrison RJ, et al. Echocardiographic criteria for left ventricular hypertrophy: The Framington Heart Study. *Am J Cardiol* 59:956–960, 1987.
2. Devereux RB, Lutas EM, Casale PN, et al. Standardization of M-mode echocardiographic left ventricu-

lar anatomic measurements. *J Am Coll Cardiol* 4(6):1222–1230, 1984.
3. Dannenberg AL, Levy D, Garrison RJ. Impact of age on echocardiographic left ventricular mass in a healthy population (the Framington Study). *Am J Cardiol* 64:1066–1068, 1989.
4. Devereux RB, Reichek N. Echocardiographic determination of left ventricular mass in man: Anatomic validation of a method. Circulation 55:613–618, 1977.
5. Olivetti G, Melissai M, Capasso J, et al. Cardiomyopathy of the aging human heart: Myocyte loss and reactive cellular hyperplasia. *Circ Res* 68:1560–1568, 1991.
6. Grunt JA. Effect of adrenalectomy and gonadectomy on growth and development in the rat. *Endocrinology* 75:446–451, 1964.
7. KoosSlob A, Van DerWeff T, Bosch JJ. Sex differences in body growth in the rat. *Physiol Behavior* 14:353–361, 1975.
8. Schaible TF, Malhotra A, Ciambrone G, et al. The effect of gonadectomy on left ventricular function and cardiac contractile proteins in male and female rats. *Circ Res* 54:38–49, 1984.
9. Schaible TF, Scheuer J. Comparison of heart function in male and female rats. *Basic Res Cardiol* 79:402–412, 1984.
10. Koenig H, Goldstone A, Lu Cy. Testosterone-mediated sexual dimorphism of the rodent heart. *Circ Res* 50:782–787, 1982.
11. Scheuer J, Malhotra A, Schaible TF, et al. Effects of gonadectomy and hormonal replacement on rat hearts. *Circ Res* 61:12–19, 1987.
12. Malhotra A, Buttrick P, Scheuer J. Effects of sex hormones on development of physiological and pathological cardiac hypertrophy in male and female rats. *Am J Physiol* 259 (*Heart Circ Physiol* 28):H866–H871, 1990.
13. Schaible TF, Penpargkul S, Scheuer J. Differences in male and female rats in cardiac conditioning. *J Appl Physiol* 50:112–117, 1981.
14. McGill HC, Sheridan PJ. Nuclear uptake of sex steroid hormones in the cardiovascular system of the baboon. *Circ Res* 48:238–246, 1981.
15. Stumpf WE, Sar M, Anmuller G. The heart: A target organ for estradiol. *Science* 196:319–321, 1977.
16. Krieg M, Smith K, Bartsch W. Demonstration of specific androgen receptors in rat heart muscle: Relationship between binding, metabolism and tissue levels of androgens. *Endocrinology* 103:1686–1694, 1978.
17. McGill HC, Anselmo VC, Buchanan JM, et al. The heart is a target organ for androgen. *Science* 207:775–777, 1980.
18. Hoh JFY, McGrath PA, Hoh H. Electrophoretic analysis of multiple forms of rat cardiac myosin: Effects of hypophysectomy and thyroxine replacement. *J Mol Cell Cardiol* 10:1053–1076, 1978.
19. Lompre AM, Schwartz K, D'Albris A, et al. Myosin isoenzyme distribution in chronic heart overload. *Nature* 282:105–107, 1979.
20. Schaible TF, Scheuer J. Cardiac adaptations to chronic exercise. *Prog Cardiovasc Dis* 27:297–324, 1985.
21. Sakaue M, Hoffman BB. Glucocorticoids induce transcription and expression of the α_1 β-adrenergic receptor. *J Clin Invest* 88:385–389, 1991.
22. Bottari SP, Vokaer A, Kaivez E, et al. Regulation of α and β adrenergic subclasses of gonadal steroids in human myometrium. *Acto Physiol Hung* 65:335–346, 1985.
23. Wolinsky H. Effects of androgen treatment on the male rat aorta. *J Clin Invest* 51:2552, 1972.
24. Fischer GM, Swain ML. Effects of sex hormones on blood pressure and vascular connective tissue in castrated and noncastrated male rats. *Am J Physiol* 232:H617–621, 1977.
25. Wolinsky H. Effects of hypertension and its reversal on the thoracic aorta of male and female rats. *Circ Res* 28:622–637, 1971.
26. Zhao MJ, Zhang H, Robinson TF, et al. Profound structural alterations in the extracellular matrix in post ischemic dysfunctional but viable myocardium. *J Am Coll Cardiol* 10:1322–1334, 1987.
27. Factor SM, Robinson TF, Dominitz R, et al. Alterations of the myocardial skeletal framework in acute myocardial infarction with and without ventricular rupture. A preliminary report. *Am J Cardiovasc Pathol* 1:91–97, 1987.
28. Drinkwater BL. Women and exercise: Physiological aspects. *Exerc Sport Sci Rev* 12:21–51, 1984.
29. Martin D, Ranwell GPH. Continuous assistive-passive exercise and cycle ergometry training in sedentary women. *Med Sci Sports Exerc* 22:523–527, 1990.
30. Astrand PO, Rodahl K. *Textbook of Work Physiology, Physiologic Basics of Exercise.* New York, McGraw-Hill, 1986, pp. 343–344.
31. Becklake MR, Frank H, Dagenais GR, et al. Influence of age and sex on exercise cardiac output. *J Appl Physiol* 20(5):938–947, 1965.
32. Hossack KF, Bruce RA. Maximal cardiac function in normal sedentary men and women: Comparison of age-related changes. *J Appl Physiol* 53:799–804, 1982.
33. Drinkwater BL. Physiological responses of women to exercise. *Exerc Sport Sci Rev* 1:126–154, 1973.
34. Rowell LB. *Human Circulation: Regulation During Physical Stress.* Vol. 1. New York, Oxford University Press, 1986, pp. 4–16.
35. Mitchell JH. Neural control of the circulation during exercise. *Med Sci Sports Exerc* 22:141–158, 1990.
36. Higginbotham MB, Morris KG, Coleman RE, et al. Sex related differences in the normal cardiac responses to upright exercise. *Circulation* 70:(3)357–366, 1984.
37. McKee PA, Castelli WP, McNamara PM, et al. The natural history of congestive heart failure: The Framington study. *N Engl J Med* 285:(26)1441–1446, 1971.
38. Kannel WB, Belanger AJ. Epidemiology of heart failure. *Am Heart J* 121:951, 1991.
39. Echeverria HH, Bilsker MS, Myerburg RJ, et al. Congestive heart failure: Echocardiographic insights. *Am J Med* 75:750–755, 1983.
40. Soufer R, Wohlgelernter D, Vita NA, et al. Intact systolic left ventricular function in clinical congestive heart failure. *Am J Cardiol* 55:1032–1036, 1985.
41. Dougherty AH, Naccarelli GV, Gray EL, et al. Congestive heart failure with normal systolic function. *Am J Cardiol* 54:778–782, 1984.
42. Lauer MS, Anderson KM, Levy D. Influences of contemporary versus 30-year blood pressure levels on left ventricular mass and geometry: The Framingham Heart study. *J Am Coll Cardiol* 18:1287–1294, 1991.
43. Devereux RB, Pickering TG, Alderman MH, et al. Left ventricular hypertrophy in hypertension: Prevalence and relationship to pathophysiologic variables. *Hypertension* 9(Suppl. II):II53–II60, 1987.
44. Judge KW, Pawitan Y, Caldwell J, et al. Congestive

heart failure symptoms in patients with preserved left ventricular function: Analysis of the CASS Registry. *J Am Coll Cardiol* 18:377–382, 1991.
45. Topol EJ, Traill TA, Fortuin NJ. Hypertensive hypertrophic cardiomyopathy of the elderly. *N Engl J Med* 312:277–283, 1985.
46. Malhotra A, Schaible TF, Capasso J, et al. Correlation of myosin isoenzyme alterations with myocardial function in physiologic and pathophysiologic hypertrophy. *Eur Heart J* 5 Suppl(F):61–67, 1984.
47. Schaible TF, Scheuer J. Cardiac function in hypertrophied hearts from chronically exercised female rats. *J Appl Physiol* 50(6):1140–1145, 1981.
48. Scheuer J, Malhotra A, Hirsch C, et al. Physiologic cardiac hypertrophy corrects contractile protein abnormalities associated with pathologic hypertrophy in rats. *J Clin Invest* 70:1300–1305, 1982.
49. Whitehorn WV. Effects of hypophyseal hormones on cardiac growth and function. In Albert NR (Ed.), *Cardiac Hypertrophy*. New York, Academic, 1971, pp. 27–37.
50. Baker PJ, Ramey ER, Ramwell PW. Androgen mediated sex differences of cardiovascular responses in rats. *Am J Physiol* 235 (*Heart Circ. Physiol* 4):H242–H246, 1978.
51. Colucci WS, Giambrone MA, McLaughlin MK, et al. Increased vascular catecholamine sensitivity and α adrenergic receptor affinity in female and estrogen treated male rats. *Circ Res* 50:805–811, 1982.
52. Dellborg M, Held P, Swedberg K, et al. Rupture of the myocardium: Occurrence and risk factors. *Br Heart J* 54:11–16, 1985.
53. Shapira I, Isakov A, Burke M, et al. Cardiac rupture in patients with acute myocardial infarction. *Chest* 92(2):219–223, 1987.
54. Batts KB, Ackerman DM, Edwards WD. Postinfarction rupture of the left ventricular free wall: Clinicopathologic correlates in 100 consecutive autopsy cases. *Hum Pathol* 21:530–535, 1990.
55. Mueller TM, Marcus ML, Herber RE, et al. Effect of renal hypertension and left ventricular hypertrophy on the coronary circulation in dogs. *Circ Res* 42:543–549, 1978.
56. Buttrick PM, Schaible TF, Scheuer J. Combined effects of hypertension and conditioning in coronary vascular reserve in rats. *J Appl Physiol* 60(1):275–279, 1985.
57. Arias-Stella J. Chronic mountain sickness; Pathology and definition. In Porter R, Knight J (Eds.), *High Altitude Physiology: Cardiac and Respiratory Aspects*. Ciba Foundation Symposium. Edinburgh, Churchill Livingtone, 1971, pp. 31–40.
58. Penaloza D, Sime F, Ruiz L. Cor pulmonale in chronic mountain sickness: Present concept of Monge's disease. In Porter R, Knight J (Eds.), *High Altitude Physiology: Cardiac and Respiratory Aspects*. Ciba Foundation Symposium. Edinburgh, Churchill Livingtone, 1971, pp. 41–52.
59. Silau AH, Cueva S, Morales P. Pulmonary arterial hypertension in male and female chickens at 3300 m. *Eur J Physiol* 386:269–275, 1980.
60. Cudkowicz L, Spielvogel H, Zubieta G. Respiratory studies in women at high altitude: 3,600 m and 5,200 m. *Respiration* 29:393–426, 1972.
61. McMurtry IF, Frith CH, Will DH. Cardiopulmonary responses of male and female swine to simulated high altitude. *J Appl Physiol* 35:459–462, 1973.
62. Moore LG, McMurtry IF, Reeves JT. Effects of sex hormones on cardiovascular and hematologic responses to chronic hypoxia in rats. *Proc Soc Exp Bio Med* 158:658–662, 1978.
63. Kentera D, Susic D, Zdravkovic M. A sex difference in the hemodynamic effects of chronic normobaric hypoxia in rats. *Respiration* 44:38–43, 1983.
64. Ou LC, Smith RP. Strain and sex differences in the cardiopulmonary adaptation of rats to high altitude. *Proc Soc Exp Biol Med* 177:308–311, 1981.
65. Ostadal B, Prochazka J, Pelouch V, et al. Comparison of cardiopulmonary responses of male and female rats to intermittent high altitude hypoxia. *Physiol Bohemslovaca* 33(2):129–138, 1984.
66. Rabinovitch M, Gamble WJ, Meittinen OS, et al. Age and sex influence on pulmonary hypertension of chronic hypoxia and on recovery. *Am J Physiol* 240:H62–H72, 1981.
67. Webster JR, Kettel LJ, Moran F, et al. Chronic obstructive pulmonary disease: A comparison between men and women. *Am Rev Resp Dis* 98:1021–1026, 1968.
68. Perloff JK, Roberts WC, Deleon AC, et al: The distinctive electocardiogram of Duchenne's progressive muscular dystrophy: An electrocardiographic-pathologic correlative study. *Am J Med* 42:179–188, 1967.
69. Perloff JK, Deleon AC, O'Doherty D. The cardiomyopathy of progressive muscular dystrophy. *Circulation* 33:625, 1966.
70. Wilson KM, Evans KA, Carter CO. Creatine kinase levels in women who carry genes for three types of muscular dystrophy. *Br Med J* 1:750–753, 1966.
71. Gersten JW, Stillwell DM, Rose NA. Harmonic analysis in carriers of Duchenne muscular dystrophy. *Arch Phys Med Rehabil* 48:164–169, 1967.
72. Pearson CM. Muscular dystrophy: Review and recent observations. *Am J Med* 35:632–645, 1966.
73. Lane RJM, Gardner-Medwin D, Roses AD. Electrocardiographic abnormalities in carriers of Duchenne muscular dystrophy. *Neurology* 30:497–501, 1980.
74. Berko BA, Swift M. X-linked dilated cardiomyopathy. *N Engl J Med* 316:1186–1191, 1987.

CHAPTER 6

Valvular Heart Disease

RICHARD B. DEVEREUX, M.D.

From the time cardiac auscultation was introduced by Laennec until the late nineteenth century, most attention in cardiology was focused on diseases of the heart valves. Due both to advances in diagnostic nosology and to changes in the epidemiologic prevalences of diseases, this situation was radically altered in the twentieth century by the recognition that coronary artery disease is the leading cause of morbidity and mortality in the general population (1). The focus on the primary importance of coronary and other forms of atherosclerotic cardiovascular disease has been reinforced by the long decline in the frequency of rheumatic fever, traditionally considered the predominant cause of valvular heart disease. However, these changes have resulted in underappreciation of the substantial number of individuals affected by diseases of the heart valves. This situation may also have led to overstatement of the greater comparative burden of cardiovascular disease in men because several forms of valvular heart disease affect women predominantly as opposed to the greater prevalence of atherosclerotic cardiovascular diseases in men.

MAGNITUDE OF THE PROBLEM

Although less information is available on the epidemiology of valvular heart diseases than on that of the atherosclerotic diseases, several lines of evidence indicate that they are both common and are associated with appreciable morbidity and mortality. For instance, data from the National Hospital Discharge Survey reveal that in 1987 an estimated 123,000 patients were discharged from United States hospitals with diagnoses of aortic or mitral valve disease (2). Of note, 87,000 (71%) of those with valvular heart disease were women, as opposed to 334,000 (39%) of the 872,000 who were discharged with diagnoses of acute myocardial infarction. Put another way, the ratio of myocardial infarction to valvular heart disease diagnoses among patients hospitalized in the United States was 3.8:1 among women and 14.9:1 among men (2). Similarly, mitral valve prolapse, the commonest heart valve abnormality in industrialized nations, affects approximately 5% of adult women but only about 3% of adult men (3–4). Rheumatic heart disease, which remains a common form of chronic valvular disease in industrialized nations and is endemic in some less developed countries, also affects women about one and a half times as frequently as men (5–6). The relation between gender and various forms of valvular heart disease has received relatively little attention in standard textbooks (e.g., [7]), but this situation has begun to change recently (8).

To judge the population burden imposed by different medical conditions it is desirable to assess the rates of death or of major morbidity caused by these conditions. Although sound estimates of mortality rates due to valvular heart disease in industrialized countries are not currently available, most decisions to replace or repair a cardiac valve are closely enough related to a need to relieve limiting symptoms or to prolong life to provide a reasonable "surrogate end point." Data collected by the National Center for Health Statistics estimated that in 1987 about 46,000 heart valve replacements or repairs were performed in the United States (2). Of these, about 60% were in women compared with 29% of 518,000 coronary artery bypass graft procedures or angioplasties that year that were performed in women (2).

These data suggest that the current level of attention paid to valvular heart disease is relatively low compared with its population prevalence and underemphasizes forms of heart disease that are proportionately more common in women than in men.

It is the purpose of this chapter to consider the relation of gender to the prevalence, manifestations, and prognosis of valvular heart disease. Primary emphasis is given to those forms of valvular heart disease that are encountered in industrialized countries. Aspects of normal valvular anatomy are reviewed as needed to understand the impact of body and heart size on specific valvular diseases. Topics that will be considered in turn are (1) mitral valve prolapse, (2) rheumatic heart disease, (3) other diseases of the mitral valve, (4) nonrheumatic aortic valve disease, and (5) the Marfan syndrome. Diseases of the tricuspid and pulmonic valves are not reviewed because of their low population prevalences and because of the lack of data on gender influences on them.

MITRAL VALVE PROLAPSE

Inheritance and Expression of Mitral Valve Prolapse

The phenomenon of mitral valve prolapse—systolic displacement of the mitral leaflets in a posterior and superior direction from their usual position—may occur as a secondary feature of a number of cardiovascular connective tissue conditions (e.g., the Marfan syndrome, discussed below) or in situations in which the left ventricle is disproportionately small in relation to the size of the mitral valve (e.g., atrial septal defect [9] or anorexia nervosa [10]). However, most instances of mitral valve prolapse (MVP) occur independently of any other recognized cardiovascular condition and may be considered "primary" MVP (11).

Most evidence now favors a genetic etiology (or etiologies) of primary MVP. This was first documented by Weiss and coworkers (12), who used echocardiography to show that in families of 17 probands selected from a cardiologic population, about 50% of first-degree relatives were affected. A similar 50% prevalence was reported by Strahan and associates (13) in a study of 12 families. However, a lower prevalence (18 of 59, or 31%) was reported by Scheele and colleagues (14). In our own studies of two sequential groups of families (11, 15), 30% (54 of 179 and 51 of 171) of first-degree relatives had echocardiographic MVP. Lower prevalences of MVP (11–21%) have been found by other investigators (16–18), but even the lowest prevalence of MVP in family studies exceeds by at least a factor of 5 the prevalence of MVP among unselected subjects studied by the same laboratories. Differences in criteria for diagnosis of MVP and for selection of probands and studied relatives are the most likely explanations for these differences in findings. For instance, relatives with known heart murmurs or other evidence of MVP were excluded in a study by Hickey and Wilcken (18), resulting in a negative selection bias that most likely caused significant understatement of the prevalence of MVP among first-degree relatives.

Relation of Gender and Age to Prevalence of Mitral Valve Prolapse

Expression of the MVP gene is affected by gender. In the initial family study by Weiss and associates (12), only 27% (6 of 22) of male first-degree relatives but 60% (21 of 35) of female first-degree relatives were affected. Our own findings confirm these reports in that 70% (123 of 175) of clinically recognized probands were female (19), whereas among first-degree relatives in 93 families, 37% (69 of 188) of female relatives but only 22% (36 of 162) of male relatives were affected (11).

Available evidence also indicates that the expression of MVP is age dependent. About 6% of neonates had M-mode echocardiographic MVP in one study (20) at a time when the left ventricle is relatively underdeveloped owing to the predominant role of the right ventricle in the fetal circulation. As the left ventricle enlarges in early childhood, the prevalence of MVP decreases to approximately 1% (21–22). With adolescence and adulthood, the frequency returns to about 3–4%. This is reflected in family studies; e.g., Scheele and coworkers (14) found echocardiographic MVP in 46% (13 of 28) of first-degree relatives over the age of 20 but in only 16% (5 of 31) below this age. Strahan and colleagues (13) also assessed the age-dependent expression of MVP in a study of 12 probands and 70 of their first-degree relatives. A mathematical analysis of the data revealed a latency stage followed by a manifestation stage; the mean age of expression of the condition was calculated to be approximately 9 years (13). Similarly, among first-degree relatives in 93 families studied at Cornell, 4% (1 of 24) of subjects under 10, 28% (18 of 64) of subjects aged 19 to 20, and 33% (86 of 262) of older subjects manifested mitral valve prolapse (p < .01).

In older subjects there may also be a decline in gene expression, which is more apparent in women. Our family studies revealed a lower prevalence of mitral valve prolapse among female first-degree relatives 50 years of age and older (14 of 52, or 27%) than among those aged 20 to 49 years of age (44 of 90, or 49%, p < .01), without a significant decrease in prevalence among older male first-degree relatives (11). The study by Strahan and colleagues (13) also provided evidence of a reduced prevalence of MVP among first-degree relatives older than 50 years of age (3 of 12, or 25%) compared with those 21 to 50 (14 of 17, or 51%), although they noted no sex difference. The explanation for the reduced prevalence of MVP in older women is not yet clear. Excess mortality among subjects with MVP may play a role; however, clinical and autopsy studies suggest that severe complications of MVP occur disproportionately in men, reach their peak incidence after the sixth decade, and do not shorten the average life span among individuals with MVP (23–32). A more attractive explanation may be that expression of MVP is reduced because of age-related secondary valvular thickening, a phenomenon that we have documented in adults with MVP using quantitative echocardiography (33). This could result in stiffened, poorly mobile leaflets that cannot prolapse, especially in individuals who develop calcification of the posterior mitral leaflet apparatus (see section, Mitral Anular Calcification, below).

In addition to information from family studies, important data concerning the relation of gender and age to the expression of MVP have been derived from population surveys. Among 4697 members of the Framingham population sample who ranged in age from 20 to 91 years, 206 of 2743, or 7.6%, of women and 56 of 2224, or 2.5%, of men exhibited M-mode echocardiographic findings of MVP (34). Among women, the prevalence of MVP declined with increasing age, a phenomenon that may have been overstated due to the limitations of the M-mode echocardiographic methods and criteria that were used. In a smaller group of unselected adults studied at Cornell, we also found a difference in the prevalence of MVP between women (6 of 111, or 5.4%) and men (5 of 167, or 3.0%) (3).

The Phenotype of Hereditary Mitral Valve Prolapse

During the past two decades numerous investigators have reported that MVP is associated with a variety of symptoms and clinical signs that have been considered to represent a "mitral prolapse syndrome" (35–37). These features have included chest pain, dyspnea, palpitations, syncope, anxiety, panic attacks, skeletal abnormalities and altered body habitus, and electrocardiographic abnormalities. However, because these symptoms prompt medical attention and recognition of MVP, the high prevalence of these features in clinical series of patients with MVP may reflect ascertainment bias (38). Several studies have examined the strength of association between components of the "mitral prolapse syndrome" by comparing comparably selected or unselected patients with echocardiographically documented MVP and control subjects (39–47).

Two studies found equally high prevalences of cardiac and psychiatric symptoms in patients with MVP and control groups of cardiovascularly normal individuals evaluated in the same clinical setting (42, 44). Similarly, no difference in the prevalence of chest pain, dyspnea, or electrocardiographic (ECG) repolarization abnormalities was found between individuals with and without echocardiographic MVP in the Framingham population sample (40).

We have compared the prevalence of the full range of features of the mitral prolapse syndrome in affected first-degree relatives of referred MVP patients and in the control groups of genetically related and unrelated adults without MVP, composed of the first-degree relatives and spouses without MVP whom we evaluated in our family studies (46). The data in Table 6–1 demonstrate associations between echocardiographic MVP and midsystolic clicks and mitral systolic murmurs as well as the statistically significant but less close associations between MVP and thoracic bony abnormalities, low body weight and systolic blood pressure, and palpitations. In contrast, no association at all was found between MVP and chest pain, dyspnea, anxiety, panic attacks, or inferior lead repolarization abnormalities. In a separate study (47), we found that subjects with MVP and nonspecific cardiovascular and psychologic symptoms were significantly more likely to experience orthostatic hypotension and syncope than similarly symptomatic subjects without MVP. Thus, the results of controlled studies indicate that the spectrum of clinical features associated with MVP is narrower than initially thought. Even those clinical features truly associated with heritable primary MVP (e.g., palpitations, asthenic body habitus, or thoracic bony abnormalities) are not sufficiently specific in individuals with MVP to be useful as diagnostic features.

The results of these controlled studies suggest that the acceptance by many clinicians that MVP is the cause of a distinctive syndrome of chest pain, dyspnea, and anxiety may lead to the erroneous diagnosis of MVP in patients who experience these symptoms. An additional problem that led to many erroneous diagnoses of MVP in the 1970s and 1980s was the acceptance of echocardiographic criteria with low specificity for the diagnosis of MVP, especially holosystolic prolapse on M-mode recordings without two-dimensional echocardiographic confirmation or protrusion of the mitral valve leaflets across the mitral annular plane in the apical four-chamber two-dimensional view. In one study (48), the four-chamber echocardiogram yielded apparently false-positive diagnoses of MVP in about one-fifth of clinically normal young adults. This unfortunate situation developed because the initial study proposing this approach to diagnosis had not included any validation by an independent reference standard (49), and also because it had not been recognized that the mitral anulus

Table 6–1. ASSOCIATION BETWEEN CLINICAL FEATURES OF THE MITRAL PROLAPSE SYNDROME AND ECHOCARDIOGRAPHICALLY DOCUMENTED MITRAL VALVE PROLAPSE

	Adult First-Degree Relatives With MVP	p Value	Adult First-Degree Relatives and Spouses Without MVP
Systolic clicks and/or mitral murmurs	55/81 = 68%	<.0001	17/232 = 7%
Thoracic bony abnormalities	33/81 = 41%	<.001	34/232 = 15%
Palpitations	32/81 = 40%	<.01	53/232 = 23%
Atypical chest pain	14/81 = 17%	NS	37/232 = 16%
Dyspnea	5/81 = 6%	NS	21/232 = 9%
Panic attacks	6/81 = 7%	NS	11/232 = 5%
Trait anxiety score >50	5/81 = 6%	NS	14/232 = 6%
Inferior lead ECG repolarization abnormalities	9/81 = 11%	NS	23/232 = 10%

ECG = electrocardiographic; MVP = mitral valve prolapse; NS = not significant.
Adapted from Devereux RB, Kramer-Fox R. Gender differences in mitral valve prolapse. *Cardiovasc Clin* 19:243–258, 1988.

had a "saddle" shape as opposed to being a flat plane (50). Criteria that allow accurate echocardiographic diagnosis of MVP include (1) late systolic posterior motion of continuous mitral leaflet interfaces at least 2 mm behind the valve's systolic closure line on M-mode echocardiography or (2) clear-cut systolic protrusion of one or both mitral leaflets across the mitral anular plane in parasternal or apical two-dimensional long-axis views (11, 50–51).

Clinical Features of Mitral Valve Prolapse in Women and Men

Because women and men differ in the prevalence of MVP in families in which the condition is due to the same underlying MVP gene(s), it is reasonable to inquire whether gender effects also contribute to either the true associations between MVP and certain clinical features or to the erroneous associations between MVP and other cardiologic and psychologic features of the mitral prolapse syndrome reported in uncontrolled studies. These questions can be best answered by comparing findings in relatively unselected men and women with and without MVP such as the groups we have identified in the course of our family studies.

The most important extracardiac feature of inherited MVP is the occurrence of slightly low body weight and blood pressure in many subjects with MVP. This association may explain the otherwise counterintuitive situation of a mendelian inherited condition with a clinically perceptible risk of severe complications being common in the general population. Our discovery (41) that adults with MVP in our families weighed less than blood relatives and spouses without MVP in the same families by approximately 8% among women and 11% among men has been confirmed by other investigators (34, 39, 52) and by findings in our enlarged family series (see Table 6–1). In our initial report, we also found a difference between subjects with MVP and normal subjects of 9 mmHg for systolic blood pressure and 4 mmHg for diastolic pressure (41). Evaluation of a general population sample aged 20 to 72 years in Framingham revealed that systolic blood pressure was 14 mmHg lower among women with MVP compared with normal women and 7 mmHg lower among men with MVP, whereas differences in diastolic blood pressure were considerably smaller (40). Differences in blood pressure of this magnitude among young women might confer a significant reproductive advantage because it has been calculated that a 5-mmHg difference in mean arterial pressure would be associated with a difference of 0.5% in the combined rate of third trimester stillbirths and perinatal mortality (53).

Other biologic features appear to be equally strongly associated with MVP among women and men, including the occurrence of minor abnormalities of the thoracic skeleton and of palpitations. Thus, pectus excavatum, scoliosis, and an abnormally straight thoracic spine occurred in 45% of women and 40% of men with MVP in our family study as opposed to 20% and 14% of control women and men (both p < .01) (4). Similarly, palpitations were reported by 48% and 44% of women and men with MVP as opposed to 29% and 18% of control subjects of the same gender (both p < .05) (4).

Gender Differences in Prevalence of Nonspecific Cardiac and Psychologic Symptoms

As discussed earlier, studies at Cornell and other centers in which comparably selected subjects with MVP and control subjects have been compared have disproved previously reported associations between a variety of symptoms (including nonanginal chest pain, dyspnea occurring at rest or with mild exertion, high levels of anxiety and panic attacks) and MVP. Although part of the reason for these apparent misattributions was undoubtedly selection of highly symptomatic patient groups with multiple conditions for study, an additional factor appears to have been true gender differences in the frequency of these symptoms. Thus, when the women and men in our families were compared (Table 6–2), women were more likely, regardless of the presence or absence of MVP, to experience each of these symptoms, the discrepancy being even greater for panic attacks and high trait anxiety than for nonanginal chest pain and dyspnea. This gender difference has undoubtedly contributed importantly to the impression of researchers and clinicians alike that patients with MVP, a majority of whom are women, are disproportionately likely to complain of a variety of symptoms than are patients with coronary artery disease, most of whom are men.

Table 6–2. FINDINGS FROM THE CORNELL FAMILY STUDY ON THE PREDOMINANCE IN WOMEN OF FEATURES OF THE MITRAL PROLAPSE SYNDROME

	Women—n = 216 n (%)	Men—n = 185 n (%)	p Value
Nonanginal chest pain	63 (29)	24 (13)	<.001
Dyspnea	50 (23)	15 (8)	<.001
Panic attacks	29 (13)	4 (2)	<.001
High trait anxiety	23 (11)	6 (3)	<.01
Inferior lead ST-T abnormalities	44 (20)	12 (6)	<.001

From Devereux RB, Kramer-Fox R, Kligfield P. Mitral valve prolapse: Etiology, clinical manifestations and management. *Ann Intern Med* 111:305–317, 1989. Reproduced with permission of the American College of Physicians.

Gender as a Risk Factor for Complications of Mitral Valve Prolapse

Although most individuals with MVP have an entirely benign prognosis, serious complications occur in a minority of patients with this condition. The most persuasive evidence in favor of the association between MVP and major complications is the fact that whereas individuals with MVP comprise 3–4% of unselected adult populations, they account for as many as 25% of patients currently needing mitral valve replacement or repair (54) and about 13% of patients with infective endocarditis (26).

Combining these estimates with other information concerning the frequency of these complications suggests that in the United States as many as 4000 adults with MVP require mitral valve surgery, and more than 1000 develop infective endocarditis annually (4). Kligfield and associates (55) have calculated that as many as 4000 sudden deaths in MVP subjects may occur annually, mostly in patients with severe mitral regurgitation due to MVP. Some progress has been made in identifying features of mitral valve anatomy that are associated with serious complications. Several studies have suggested that subjects with MVP with thickened mitral leaflets are at high risk of complications (56–58), but this association appeared weaker in a less selected group of MVP patients studied at Cornell (33). A controlled study at Cornell (59) indicates that MVP patients with severe mitral regurgitation have substantially larger mitral leaflets and anuli than subjects with uncomplicated MVP.

Available data suggest that gender is an especially important risk factor for complications of MVP. In contrast to the situation with gene expression, in which women are more likely than men to exhibit typical cardiac findings of MVP, the major complications of MVP are more likely to occur in affected men. This is true of both infective endocarditis and severe mitral regurgitation. Although hemodynamically important mitral regurgitation is a major factor predisposing to sudden death, a similar sex difference has not yet been established with regard to the risk of sudden death in MVP patients (60–62).

The surprising fact that most MVP patients with hemodynamically important mitral regurgitation were men was first noted by Higgins and colleagues (63). Subsequent reports have consistently confirmed this male predominance, showing that 53–91% of patients with severe mitral regurgitation are men (24–25, 54, 64–69) (Table 6–3). The reasons for the increased risk of severe mitral regurgitation in men with MVP are unclear, but our observation that prolapse patients with mitral regurgitation had higher blood pressures than subjects with uncomplicated MVP (69), coupled with the fact that in the general population arterial pressure is slightly higher in men than in women (70), provides one possible reason why damage of potentially vulnerable prolapsed mitral valves due to hemodynamic stress occurs disproportionately in men with MVP.

MVP is also increasingly recognized as one of the most frequent predisposing conditions among patients who develop infective endocarditis (25–26, 71–77). Like the situation with mitral regurgitation, male predominance also exists among MVP patients who develop infective endocarditis. This fact was first noted by Corigal and coworkers (71) and has been subsequently confirmed by studies in the United States (25–26, 74), Australia (72–73), France (75), and Israel (77) (Table 6–4). Analysis of our experience at Cornell suggests that male gender increases risk for infective endocarditis

Table 6–3. GENDER OF MITRAL VALVE PROLAPSE PATIENTS WITH SEVERE MITRAL REGURGITATION

Author	Reference	N	Number Male (%)
Tresch et al.	24	30	20 (57%)
Kolibash et al.	65	86	53 (62%)
Devereux et al.	27	17	9 (53%)
Caidahl et al.	66	11	10 (91%)
Roberts et al.	67	83	57 (69%)
Olson et al.	54	100	76 (76%)
Danielsen et al.	68	21	15 (71%)
Jerasaty et al.	64	25	16 (64%)
Cornell	Unpublished	88	44 (50%)
Total[a]		451	300 (67%)

[a] Adjusted for overlap between studies from the same institution.
Adapted from Devereux RB, Kramer-Fox R. Gender differences in mitral valve prolapse. *Cardiovasc Clin* 19:243–258, 1988.

independent of the effects of preexisting mitral regurgitation or older age among patients with MVP (26). At present, this situation is unexplained.

Risk Level and Management

The best care of the patient with MVP should combine a high level of diagnostic accuracy and therapeutic efficacy with an efficient approach that minimizes both costs and demands on the patient's time (78) (Table 6–5). The diagnosis of MVP can be made accurately when a clear-cut midsystolic click and a late systolic murmur can be made to respond appropriately to maneuvers (moving earlier with sitting and standing, becoming louder when blood pressure rises in response to isometric handgrip exercise) (79). Hemodynamically important mitral regurgitation is unlikely to be present if the late systolic murmur is confined to the second half of systole and the left ventricular impulse is clearly normal in size (less than the diameter of a U.S. quarter) and location (at or to the right of the midclavicular line) on physical examination (80).

Echocardiography is indicated when the auscultatory features are less clear, when symptoms or physical signs suggest more than very mild mitral regurgitation, or when a previous diagnosis of MVP appears to have been erroneous and needs to be disproved. Another efficient use of echocardiography is to screen first-degree relatives (parents, siblings, and children) of patients with MVP because of the 30% yield of affected individuals. When echocardiography is performed, it is important to use strict criteria for the diagnosis of MVP and to pay particular attention to the features—such as leaflet and anular enlargement, prominent or asymmetric prolapse of the leaflets,

Table 6–4. GENDER OF MITRAL VALVE PROLAPSE PATIENTS WITH INFECTIVE ENDOCARDITIS

Author	Reference	N	Number Male (%)
Corigal et al.	71	21[a]	13 (62%)
MacMahon et al.	73	19	13 (68%)
Devereux et al.	27	11	8 (73%)
MacMahon et al.	26	21	13 (62%)
McKinsey et al.	74	18	7 (39%)
Danchin et al.	75	9	7 (78%)
Awadallah et al.	76	7	1 (14%)
Weinberger et al.	77	19	12 (63%)
Total[b]		114	66 (58%)

MVP = mitral valve prolapse.
[a] Excluded patients from a Veterans Administration Hospital.
[b] Adjusted for overlap between studies.
Adapted from Devereux RB, Kramer-Fox R. Gender differences in mitral valve prolapse. *Cardiovasc Clin* 19:243–258, 1988.

Table 6–5. MATCHING RISK AND MANAGEMENT IN MITRAL VALVE PROLAPSE

Lowest risk:	Subjects without mitral regurgitant murmurs or Doppler regurgitation, especially women < 45 years. Management: Reassurance; no clear need for antibiotics; reevaluation and echocardiogram at moderate intervals (5 years).
Moderate risk:	Subjects with intermittent or persistent mitral murmurs and mild Doppler regurgitation. Management: Antibiotic proplylaxis with amoxicillin or erythromycin; treat even mild established hypertension; reevaluation and echocardiography more frequently (2–3 years).
High risk:	Patients with moderate or severe mitral regurgitation. Management: Antibiotic prophylaxis with amoxicillin (unless allergic); optimize afterload (arterial pressure); reevaluate with Doppler echocardiogram and other tests if needed annually. Consider valve repair or replacement for exertional dyspnea or decline of left ventricular function into low-normal range.

Adapted from Devereux RB, Kligfield P. Mitral valve prolapse. In Rakel RE (Ed.), *Current Therapy, 1992.* Philadelphia, WB Saunders, pp. 237–241.

and severe leaflet thickening (33, 51, 58, 81)—that may be useful markers of more severe valve involvement.

The need for follow-up and treatment of the patient with MVP is primarily determined by the presence and severity of mitral regurgitation. An approach to matching the extent of evaluation and treatment to the level of risk in MVP patients that we have developed from our experience at Cornell is given in Table 6–4 (78). Analyses performed for cost-effectiveness (82) suggest that erythromycin ethyl succinate may be preferable to ampicillin or other penicillins for prevention of bacterial endocarditis in MVP patients with mild mitral regurgitation because of the lack of risk of anaphylaxis with this agent. Additional aspects of the management of the patient with MVP have recently been reviewed in more detail (78).

RHEUMATIC HEART DISEASE

For many years acute rheumatic fever appeared to be on its way to extinction in industrialized countries, but this trend has been reversed in recent years, and at least a small increase in the incidence of acute rheumatic fever has been noted in the United States (83). This may pose a problem for contemporary physicians who are unaccustomed to the clinical syndrome of rheumatic fever. A high index of suspicion of this diagnosis is needed when one encounters, singly or in combination, the clinical features of migratory polyarthritis, new heart murmurs, pericardial rubs or electrocardiographic abnormalities, skin lesions, and chorea in association with evidence of a streptococcal infection (84). Although males have predominated in some studies of acute rheumatic fever (85), girls have predominated among patients who manifest the unusual neurologic feature of chorea (86). Reasons for gender differences in the prevalence of different manifestations of rheumatic fever are unclear but may reflect an interaction between gender-specific factors and genetic predispositions that have been identified by genetic studies performed in the pre-antibiotic era (87) and by more recent research on genes that influence immune responsiveness (88).

Chronic Rheumatic Valvular Disease

The prevalence of chronic rheumatic heart disease has declined to a lesser extent than that of acute rheumatic fever. This discordance is due in part to the long lag phase before the chronic condition becomes manifest in some individuals and to the immigration to industrialized countries of people from areas where rheumatic fever is endemic. Twenty percent or more of individuals with rheumatic-type heart disease have no history of acute rheumatic fever (89), and it has been shown that some viruses can produce experimental valvulitis that resembles the acute phase of rheumatic heart disease (90). Both this long-term decline and the continued importance of rheumatic heart disease as a cause of morbidity are exemplified by the findings of Olson et al (54) that the proportion of mitral valve operations at the Mayo Clinic performed for mitral stenosis—the valvular lesion most characteristic of rheumatic disease—were 69% and 33%, respectively, in 1975, 40% and 28% in 1980, and 35% and 26% in 1985. The clinical and echocardiographic features that are most useful for the diagnosis of chronic rheumatic valvular lesions do not differ between women and men and have been well described elsewhere (91–92).

Mitral Stenosis

Although inflammation of the cardiac valves, pericardium, and on occasion the myocardium may cause valvular regurgitation, pericarditis, and, rarely, severe myocarditis during the acute phase of rheumatic fever, the mitral valve obstruction that is the most characteristic lesion of rheumatic valvular disease (5, 93) develops only gradually as acute inflammation of the mitral leaflets' zones of apposition gives way to gradual fusion of the commissures between the anterior and posterior mitral leaflets (94). In response to repeated attacks of rheumatic fever or to indolent inflammation that may occur without clinical evidence of rheumatic fever in individuals not receiving antibiotic prophylaxis (95), progressive fusion of the mitral commissures and fibrosis and contraction of the mitral leaflets and subvalvular apparatus may develop (94). The latter distortion of the mitral subvalvular apparatus may on occasion impair left ventricular filling in patients whose rheumatic disease has not significantly narrowed the mitral valve orifice (96).

In all large clinical series of patients with mitral stenosis there is a strong female predominance, with an overall female-male ratio of about 3:1 (5, 97–99) (Table 6–6). It is thought that the development of mitral stenosis in patients who did not have clinically evident carditis during the initial acute rheumatic fever and the likelihood of progressive stenosis in the absence of recurrent acute episodes are both more likely in women than men (8). In the period before effective antibiotic prophylaxis was widely used, the average interval from the occurrence of the first episode of rheumatic fever until the development of symptoms due to mitral stenosis averaged about 19 years (5), with a subsequent period of about 7 years before congestive heart failure supervened. In women with mitral stenosis, congestive heart failure is often precipitated first during pregnancy, when the narrowed mitral valve orifice cannot accommodate the demand for increased cardiac output without an excessive increase in the transmitral valve gradient and hence in the left atrial and pulmonary venous pressure (see Chap. 17). One unusual clinical manifestation of moderately severe rheumatic mitral stenosis that appears more commonly in women than men is the occurrence of hemoptysis when tachycardia due to exercise or arrhythmia shortens the proportion of each minute occupied by diastole and, as a consequence, raises left atrial and pulmonary venous pressure above the level that can be withstood by the vessels. In Wood's series (5), this occurred during 12 of 140 pregnancies in women with mitral stenosis.

Once mitral stenosis is clinically evident, the prognosis appears to be generally similar in women and men. However, the tendency of stenotic mitral valves to become heavily calcified at an older age in women may afford them an advantage with regard to treatment options. In keeping with the theory that "wear-and-

Table 6–6. GENDER PREDOMINANCES IN RHEUMATIC AND OTHER DISEASES OF THE MITRAL AND AORTIC VALVES

	Gender Predominance	Approximate Female-Male Ratio
Rheumatic heart disease		
Mitral stenosis	Female	3:1
Mitral regurgitation	Male	1:1.5
Aortic regurgitation	Male	3:1
Aortic stenosis		
Bicuspid aortic valve	Male	3–4:1
Degenerative aortic calcification	Female	1:1.5
Aortic regurgitation		
Bicuspid aortic valve	Male	3:1
Anuloaortic ectasia	Male	?
Other mitral valvular diseases		
Mitral anular calcification	Female	1.5–2.0:1
Rheumatic inflammatory disease	Female	?

See text for sources.

tear" due to turbulent blood flow across a partially stenotic mitral valve may accelerate the progression of stenosis, there is some evidence (100) that performance of mitral commissurotomy at a stage when the mitral valve is susceptible to conservative repair may delay the time at which valve replacement is needed. Because of gender differences in the dynamics of valve calcification, this option may benefit a higher proportion of women than men with mitral stenosis. In the large series of patients undergoing the catheterization laboratory procedure of percutaneous balloon mitral valvotomy that was reported by Absacal et al (101) and Reid et al (102), 107 of 130 (82%) and 456 of 555 (82%) were women. Conversely, some women with mitral stenosis who desire to become pregnant but require valve replacement may need to receive a bioprosthetic valve despite the known likelihood that these valves may require replacement after an average interval of 10 years or less. The rare instances of nonrheumatic mitral stenosis due to entrapment of the mitral leaflets in heavy degenerative calcification occur at least as often in women as in men (103).

Mitral Regurgitation

Although rheumatic heart disease was traditionally considered the predominant cause of mitral regurgitation, this is no longer the case due both to a true decrease in the prevalence of rheumatic heart disease and to the recognition that many instances of pure mitral regurgitation that would have been classified as "rheumatic" prior to 1965 are in fact due to mitral valve prolapse (94). However, instances of pure or predominant mitral regurgitation do occur in which rheumatic fever is the apparent cause. For example, among 101 patients with valvular causes of severe mitral regurgitation in an ongoing natural history study at Cornell that has been previously reported in part (104–105), the cause appeared to be rheumatic fever in 15%, whereas 54% of cases were due to primary mitral prolapse. However, in a pathologic study that did not consider a history of rheumatic fever in making an etiologic diagnosis and that excluded patients with even slight anatomic mitral stenosis, Waller and coworkers (106) identified rheumatic heart disease and mitral prolapse as the cause of 3% and 62%, respectively, in 97 patients requiring valve replacement for isolated severe regurgitation. In these series, there was a slight male predominance among patients with rheumatic mitral regurgitation. However, even among men who have suffered rheumatic fever, mitral stenosis is more frequent than pure mitral regurgitation.

On anatomic inspection, valves affected by rheumatic mitral regurgitation are distinguished from those with stenosis by the presence of relatively little commissural fusion, but they share the features of thickening and variable retraction of the leaflets and chordae tendineae (94). We identified mitral anular dilatation as an additional feature of severe chronic rheumatic mitral regurgitation in a study using quantitative echocardiography (59), paralleling the pathologic finding that anular dilatation contributed to mitral regurgitation in patients with MVP or the Marfan syndrome (107).

Aortic Regurgitation

The rheumatic processes of commissural fusion and leaflet retraction that result in mitral stenosis also affect the aortic valve, but in this case they result in aortic regurgitation because few if any instances of pure aortic stenosis occur as late consequences of rheumatic fever (93, 108). The relative importance of rheumatic fever as a cause of aortic regurgitation can be appreciated by its occurrence in 26 of 100 or 26% of cases in Davies' pathologic series (10 of 84 or 12%, if immigrants to England were excluded [94]), and in 15 of 102 or 15% of cases in the series of Roman and colleagues of patients studied at Cornell by echocardiography (109). In our experience, as well as that of other investigators (5, 110), there is an approximately 3:1 ratio of men to women among patients with rheumatic aortic regurgitation.

One interesting and superficially counterintuitive aspect of the natural history of aortic regurgitation is the fact that the markers of extreme left ventricular enlargement that have been found to be useful indicators of a poor prognosis do not differ between women and men despite the clear gender difference in normal body size and left ventricular size (111–112). Thus, an end-systolic left ventricular internal dimension that exceeds 55 mm on echocardiography has been found to be as strong a predictor of poor postoperative outcome in women as in men with aortic regurgitation (113–115). This result parallels the finding in other studies (116–117) that the same partition values for indexed left ventricular mass predict an adverse prognosis in female and male hypertensive patients or members of the general population despite the well known difference in ventricular mass between normal women and men (111–112). These findings suggest the hypothesis that one reason why more men suffer severe morbid consequences of several forms of cardiovascular disease may be that normal men have mild degrees of "physiologic" left ventricular dilatation and hypertrophy that encroach on the "reserves" that they would use to adapt to several forms of hemodynamic overload. In any case, both women and men with aortic regurgitation appear to do well if valve replacement is performed when symptoms of exertional dyspnea or objective evidence of left ventricular dysfunction develop (115).

OTHER DISEASES OF THE MITRAL VALVE

Mitral Anular Calcification

This condition is actually partially misnamed because the degenerative calcification it describes commonly involves the posterior (and occasionally the anterior) mitral leaflet in addition to the mitral anulus (94). Women tend to develop mitral anular calcification at an earlier age and, in most studies, to a more severe degree than men (118–119). In necropsy and echocardiographic studies the female-male ratio has ranged from 1.6 to 2.2:1 (120–121). Although many instances of mitral anular calcification are clinically silent and are only discovered as an incidental finding on echocardiograms performed for other purposes, this condition is also a common cause of late systolic murmurs that mimic those due to mitral valve prolapse. The mild mitral regurgitation that underlies these late systolic murmurs is generally benign regardless of the etiology (122). However, 1% or 2% of cases of severe mitral regurgitation are presently due to severe degenerative calcification of the mitral valve in older individuals. This lesion has also been reported to be a potential site of infective endocarditis (123), although the risk appears to be low. The decision to use endocarditis prophylaxis depends on the presence of a mitral regurgitant murmur, as it does for other conditions (82, 124).

Infective Endocarditis

Infections with a wide variety of organisms may occur on previously normal mitral valves, but in most instances there is an underlying valvular abnormality due to rheumatic disease, mitral prolapse, or other conditions. As with endocarditis on other heart valves, there is a male predominance in cases of mitral valve endocarditis, the cause of which is unknown.

Nonrheumatic Inflammatory and Immunologic Conditions

Systemic lupus erythematosus, a condition with a female predominance that approaches 90%, may be associated with both acute (Libman-Sacks) noninfectious endocarditis, and with chronic stenosis or insufficiency of the mitral valve. In the pathologic series of Bulkley and Roberts (125), among 36 patients with lupus (33 [92%] of whom were women), 18 (50%) had noninfectious vegetations and two (6%) had severe mitral regurgitation causing heart failure. Patients with systemic lupus erythematosus and individuals with no evidence of a known collagen vascular disease may develop high titers of circulating anticardiolipin antibodies, a condition associated with the presence of valvular thickening and with strokes or other peripheral emboli (126).

NONRHEUMATIC AORTIC VALVE DISEASES

Bicuspid Aortic Valve

The bicuspid aortic valve is the commonest form of congenital heart disease and has a prevalence that is estimated to be between 0.5% and 1.5% (94, 127). Like other diseases of the aortic valve and aorta, there is a nearly 3:1 male-female predominance among patients with bicuspid aortic valves in clinical and autopsy studies (127–129). The proportion of men among individuals with severe aortic stenosis or regurgitation due to bicuspid valves may exceed 80%, whereas the sex ratio was more nearly even among those with functionally normal bicuspid aortic valves in a study at Cornell (129). Dilatation of the aortic root and ascending aorta is common in patients with bicuspid aortic valves and may contribute to the development of aortic regurgitation (129–131). Whether this feature of the bicuspid valve complex or the association between bicuspid valves and coarctation of the aorta differs between the genders has not been fully evaluated.

Aortic Stenosis

Well over 90% of cases of aortic stenosis in adults occur at the valvular level, the remainder being largely split among instances of fixed subvalvular obstruction or dynamic obstruction due to hypertrophic cardiomyopathy. Valvular aortic stenosis resembles other aortic conditions in that it has a striking male predominance. In the pathologic series of Davies (94), 56% of cases were men, as were 1881 of 2763 (68%) of patients in 26 clinic studies of aortic stenosis reviewed by Mautner and Roberts (132). The mix of both etiologies and genders varies among patient groups of different ages and between patients with isolated aortic stenosis or with mixed aortic and mitral valvular disease. Thus, most middle-aged patients with pure aortic stenosis are men with bicuspid aortic valves, whereas patients over the age of 65 are more likely to be women with degenerative calcification of tricuspid aortic valves (94, 133). Aortic stenosis in patients with rheumatic heart disease is usually associated with rheumatic-type mitral valve disease (94, 99), which may be detected by echocardiography even when it is too mild to produce typical physical signs. Coronary atherosclerosis is commonly associated with aortic stenosis, at least in part due to common associations with advancing age and male gender and may contribute to impairment of left ventricular function in some patients with this valvular lesion (132, 134).

Anuloaortic Ectasia (Idiopathic Aortic Root Dilatation)

With the more accurate classification of the causes of aortic regurgitation that has been made possible by echocardiography, it has become clear that as many as 30% of instances of aortic regurgitation in adults may be due to idiopathic aortic root dilatation in the absence of a specific valvular cause (94, 109, 131). This condition may run in families (135–136) but tends to become manifest in middle or older age when aortic regurgitation of a clinically detectable degree develops. Pathologic examination of severe cases reveals cystic medial necrosis and degeneration of elastin fibers that may be indistinguishable from the changes found in the aorta of patients with the Marfan syndrome (137), but extracardiac features of the latter condition are not found in individuals with anuloaortic ectasia. Identification of aortic root dilatation as the cause of aortic regurgitation is aided by clinical and echocardiographic exclusion of specific valvular etiologies (history of rheumatic fever or other inflammatory condition or visualization of commissural fusion, bicuspid valve, or a vegetation) in combination with the demonstration by two-dimensional echocardiography that the aortic root diameter at the level of the sinus of Valsalva exceeds established normal limits (138) (Fig. 6–1).

THE MARFAN SYNDROME

The Marfan syndrome is an autosomal disorder affecting the connective tissue with multiple progressive changes involving the cardiovascular and musculoskeletal system, eyes, and lungs. The cause of the connective tissue abnormalities in the Marfan syndrome has recently been related to the microfibrillar protein fibrillin (139) by both genetic linkage studies (140–142) and detection of causative mutations (143). Cardiovascular complications cause most deaths of untreated patients with the Marfan syndrome, whose average life span prior to the availability of preventive treatment was about 40 years in men and 50 years in women (144). Diagnostic criteria and other manifestations of the Marfan syndrome have been discussed in recent reviews (145–147).

Cardiovascular Manifestations of The Marfan Syndrome

Structural cardiovascular abnormalities occur in the majority of patients with the Marfan syndrome, with from 82–100% of patients in several series manifesting one or more defects,

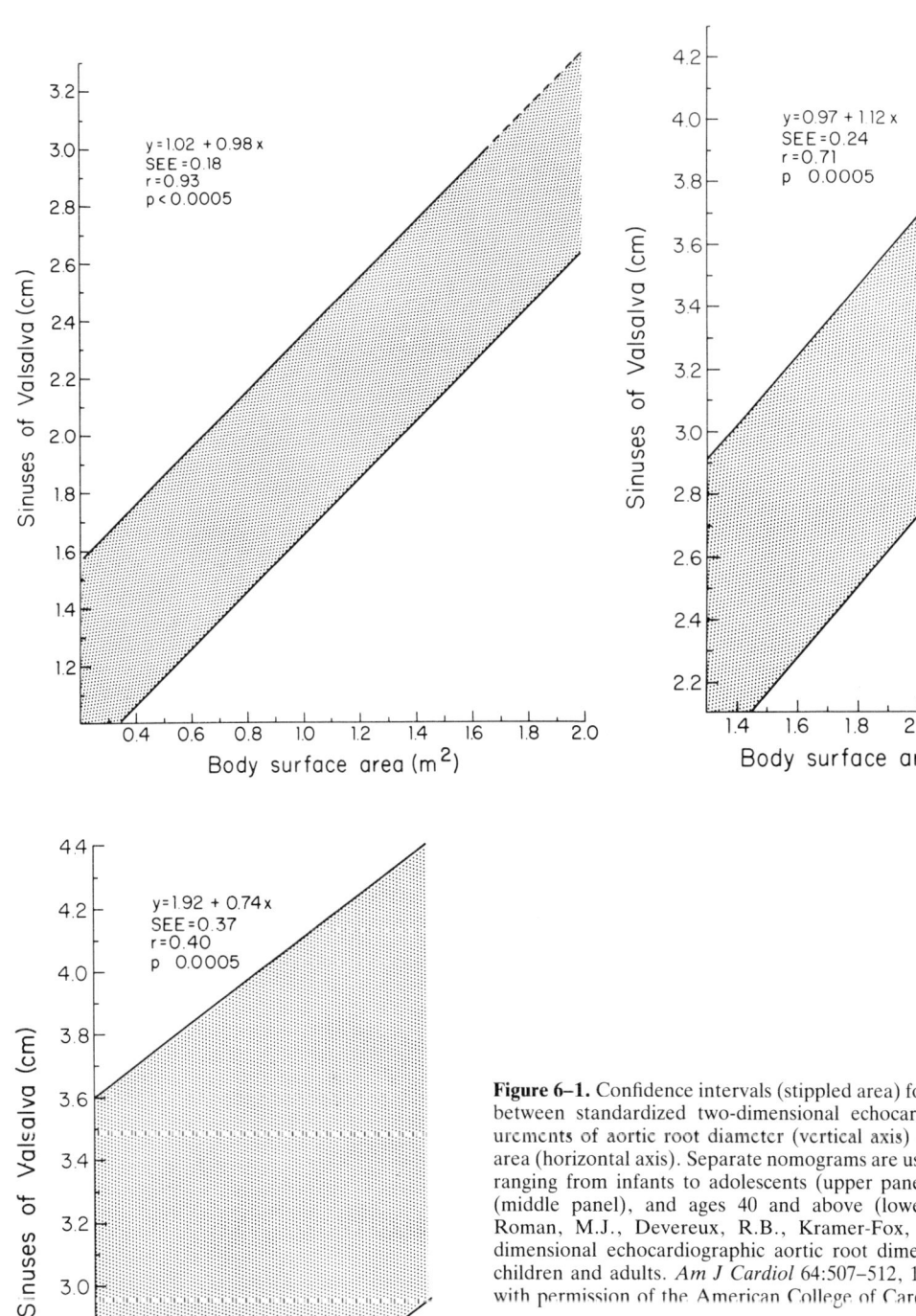

Figure 6–1. Confidence intervals (stippled area) for the relationship between standardized two-dimensional echocardiographic measurements of aortic root diameter (vertical axis) and body surface area (horizontal axis). Separate nomograms are used for individuals ranging from infants to adolescents (upper panel), ages 20 to 39 (middle panel), and ages 40 and above (lower panel). (From Roman, M.J., Devereux, R.B., Kramer-Fox, R., et al. Two-dimensional echocardiographic aortic root dimensions in normal children and adults. *Am J Cardiol* 64:507–512, 1989. Reproduced with permission of the American College of Cardiology.)

the most common of which are mitral valve prolapse, aortic root dilatation, and aortic regurgitation (147–159). Echocardiography has proved to be a far more sensitive technique for detecting cardiac manifestations of the Marfan syndrome than either physical examination or chest roentgenography (153, 156, 160).

The prevalence of different cardiac manifestations of the Marfan syndrome shows moderate variability among reported series. One factor contributing to this situation is the different proportions of patients referred to specific institutions because they had already developed complications of this syndrome. Another factor seems to be a difference in the age at which specific cardiac complications of the Marfan syndrome tend to occur. Thus, Sisk et al (150) reported that most cardiac morbidity in patients with the Marfan syndrome under the age of 4 is due to complications of mitral valve prolapse, whereas in series composed of older patients aortic root dilatation, aortic regurgitation, and aortic dissection occur more commonly (151, 153–154, 157). Of note, the valvular abnormalities underlying mitral valve prolapse in the Marfan patients (159) differ partially from the abnormalities found in patients with primary mitral valve prolapse (161). All chordae supporting the posterior mitral leaflet that could be seen in long-axis two-dimensional echocardiographic views arose from the posterior left ventricular wall in almost half the Marfan syndrome patients with mitral valve prolapse, a pattern we have not encountered in primary MVP. Mitral regurgitation (162) and mitral valve prolapse (159) occur in a higher proportion of women than men with the Marfan syndrome, whereas aortic dilatation and aortic regurgitation are more common in men with the Marfan syndrome than women.

Natural History and Management

The natural history of patients with cardiovascular abnormalities due to the Marfan syndrome is not precisely known because improving methods of diagnosis have allowed the condition to be detected in increasing numbers of patients whose disease is mild or at an early stage, and improvements in medical and surgical treatment are prolonging survival. Unfortunately, the only available study in which life-table analyses of survival were performed, that by Murdoch et al (144), was completed more than 20 years ago. This study, based on 257 patients, suggested a median age of death of approximately 40 years in males and 50 years in females (144). In this series, cardiac complications of the Marfan syndrome were responsible for 93% of deaths of known cause. It appears from these data and from clinical experience that as many as two-thirds to three-quarters of untreated patients with the Marfan syndrome would ultimately develop severe aortic or mitral regurgitation or dissection of the aortic root or distal aortic segments. Despite the survival advantage among women with the Marfan syndrome, severe valvular or aortic complications, including aortic dissection, still account for most premature deaths among affected women.

Management of Marfan syndrome patients revolves around prevention of complications and correction of them when they do occur. To prevent progressive aortic root dilatation and aortic regurgitation, or aortic dissection, which may result in aortic rupture or may prove fatal by causing overwhelming aortic regurgitation or myocardial infarction due to dissection of a coronary artery, preventive measures to reduce stress on the aorta are generally required. Based on a study reported in preliminary form by Pyeritz (163), beta-blockers or other hypotensive agents are recommended to most patients with the Marfan syndrome. In their study of 70 patients, including both children and adults, randomized to treatment or to receive beta-blockers in a dose sufficient to depress left ventricular contractility, the rate of aortic root enlargement was reduced in the beta-blocker group among both skeletally mature and skeletally immature patients. As an extension of this logic, it is also recommended that Marfan patients avoid athletics or other strenuous activity.

A major issue for women with the Marfan syndrome concerns the potential risk of pregnancy. It is well known that a disproportionate share of aortic dissections in individuals under 40 years of age occur in women who are pregnant or have just delivered (164–165). A large number of case reports of women with the Marfan syndrome who suffered aortic dissection during pregnancy suggests that pregnancy may also carry this risk in patients with the Marfan syndrome (reviewed by Godfrey [146]). No aortic dissections or other serious complications were reported in the one published, relatively small series (n = 26) of women with the Marfan syndrome who were prospectively studied before and after pregnancy (166). Instances of aortic dissection prior to or just after delivery have occurred in women whose aortic root diameters were only mildly enlarged (4.2 and 3.8 cm) prior to pregnancy (R.E. Pyeritz and R. Boxer, personal communication). Accordingly, we advise women with the Marfan syndrome whose aortic root diameter on two-dimensional echocardiography is within normal limits (138) that the risk of acute complications is too low to be calculated at present, whereas if there is even slight aortic enlargement there is a risk that begins at perhaps 1% and rises with increasing aortic dilatation (Table 6–7). There is also a chance that enlargement of the aorta will accelerate during pregnancy, but the probability of this and of dissection at different aortic sizes requires a future multicenter study for resolution. Whether the mother or father is affected by the Marfan syndrome, the chance that a child will inherit the condition—which may be more or less severe than that in the parent—is 50%. With advances in knowledge, it will gradually become possible to perform antenatal testing to determine whether a fetus is affected by detecting either the responsible mutation or by establishing linkage to the fibrillin allele that is responsible for the Marfan syndrome in the parent (167).

A therapeutic advance of great importance to patients with Marfan syndrome is the development and refinement of surgical techniques for repair of the dilated or dissected aortic root, with simultaneous replacement of the aortic valve when needed. As surgical expertise with the use of aortic root and valve composite grafts has improved (168–171), operative mortality has fallen to 2–3% or possibly less in Marfan syndrome patients undergoing elective composite graft repair. Our practice is to recommend performance of aortic root repair on a prophylactic basis in Marfan syndrome patients whose aortic root dimension exceeds 6.0 cm regardless of the degree of aortic regurgitation, and in those with severe aortic regurgitation whose aortic root diameter exceeds 5.5 cm. Interestingly, these criteria do not appear to need adjustment for the known differences in body size and aortic root diameter between normal women and men (138), paralleling the situation with regard to left ventricular size in patients with aortic regurgitation (see earlier discussion).

Continuation of hypotensive medication and restriction of exercise is still needed postoperatively because Marfan syndrome patients remain vulnerable to dissection of more distal segments of the aorta as well as to rare complications of the repair itself, such as development of paragraft false aneurysms (172) or partial dehiscence of a coronary artery from the graft (173). In our experience at Cornell (174), arterial complications requiring additional surgery have occurred at a rate of 1–2%/year in patients who underwent elective composite graft repair but at a rate of nearly 10%/year in those who had suffered an initial aortic dissection. This difference emphasizes the need to combine careful medical management with surveillance in order to time elective surgery before dissection supervenes. An additional recommendation for the protection of patients with composite grafts is to use parenteral antibiotics for endocarditis prophylaxis (175) because of the increased difficulty associated with replacement of an infected composite graft.

Table 6–7. PREGNANCY AND THE WOMAN WITH THE MARFAN SYNDROME

Maternal Risks
Normal aortic size[a]: Minimal risk of aortic dissection or severe regurgitation; possible progression of aortic enlargement.
Mild aortic dilatation: Low (perhaps 1%) risk of major complications during pregnancy; possible progression of aortic enlargement.
Moderate-severe aortic dilatation: Higher, but not yet quantitated, risk of dissection or progression to severe aortic regurgitation; greater likelihood of progressive aortic enlargement.

Recurrence Risk in Offspring
Fifty percent whether mother or father is affected. The condition may be milder or more severe in an affected child.

[a]Compared to two-dimensional echocardiographic normal limits for age and body size (138).

Acknowledgment

I would like to thank Virginia Burns for her assistance in preparation of this chapter.

References

1. Kannel WB, Thom TJ. Incidence, prevalence, and mortality of cardiovascular diseases. In Hurst JW, Schlant RC, Rackley CE, et al, (Eds.), *The Heart, Arteries and Veins* (7th ed.). New York, McGraw-Hill, 1990, pp. 627–638.

2. Graves E. Detailed diagnoses and procedures. National Hospital Discharge Survey, 1987. Data from the National Health Survey, No. 100. *Vital and Health Statistics*, Series 13. DHHS Publication No. (PHS) 89-1761. Washington, D.C., U.S. Government Printing Office, 1987.
3. Devereux RB, Kramer-Fox R. Gender differences in mitral valve prolapse. *Cardiovasc Clin* 19:243–258, 1988.
4. Devereux RB, Kramer-Fox R, Kligfield P. Mitral valve prolapse: Etiology, clinical manifestations and management. *Ann Intern Med* 111:305–317, 1989.
5. Wood P. An appreciation of mitral stenosis. Part I. Clinical features. *Br Med J* 1:1051–1063, 1954.
6. National Center for Health Statistics. *Vital Statistics of the United States, 1984*. Vol. II. *Mortality*: Part B. DHHS Pub. No. (PHS) 87-1114. Washington, D.C., U.S. Public Health Service, 1987.
7. Dalen JE, Alpert JS (Eds.). *Valvular Heart Disease*. Boston, Little, Brown, 1981.
8. Douglas PS. Rheumatic heart disease and other valvular disorders in women. *Cardiovasc Clin* 19:259–265, 1988.
9. Schreiber TL, Feigenbaum H, Weyman AE. Effect of atrial septal defect repair on left ventricular geometry and degree of mitral valve prolapse. *Circulation* 61:888–896, 1980.
10. Meyers DG, Starke H, Pearson PH, et al. Mitral valve prolapse in anorexia nervosa. *Ann Intern Med* 105:384–386, 1986.
11. Devereux RB, Kramer-Fox R, Shear MK, et al. Diagnosis and classification of severity of mitral valve prolapse: Methodologic, biologic and prognostic considerations. *Am Heart J* 113:1265–1280, 1987.
12. Weiss AN, Mimbs JW, Ludbrook PA, et al. Echocardiographic detection of mitral valve prolapse. Exclusion of false positive diagnosis and determination of inheritance. *Circulation* 52:1091–1096, 1975.
13. Strahan NV, Murphy EA, Fortuin NJ, et al. Inheritance of the mitral valve prolapse syndrome. Discussion of a three-dimensional penetrance model. *Am J Med* 74:967–972, 1983.
14. Scheele W, Allen NH, Kraus R, et al. Familial prevalence and genetic transmission of mitral valve prolapse. *Circulation* 56 (Suppl. 3):III-111, 1987.
15. Devereux RB, Brown WT, Kramer-Fox R, et al. Inheritance of mitral valve prolapse: Effect of age and sex on gene expression. *Ann Intern Med* 97:826–832, 1982.
16. Chen WWC, Chan FL, Wong PHC, et al. Familial occurrence of mitral valve prolapse: Is this related to the straight back syndrome? *Br Heart J* 50:97–100, 1983.
17. Wilcken DEL, Hickey AJ, Cole WG, et al. The pathogenesis of the floppy mitral valve. *Circulation* 70 (Suppl. 2):102, 1984.
18. Hickey AJ, Wilcken DEL. Age and the clinical profile of idiopathic mitral valve prolapse. *Br Heart J* 55:582–586, 1986.
19. Kramer-Fox R, Devereux RB, Brown WT, et al. Lack of association between dermal arches and mitral valve prolapse: Relation to anxiety. *Am J Cardiol* 53:148–152, 1984.
20. Chandraratna PAN, Vlahovich G, Kong Y, et al. Incidence of mitral valve prolapse in one hundred clinically stable newborn baby girls: An echocardiographic study. *Am Heart J* 98:312–314, 1979.
21. Rizzon P, Biasco G, Brindicci G, et al. Familial syndrome of midsystolic click and late systolic murmur. *Br Heart J* 35:245–259, 1973.
22. McLaren MJ, Hawkins DM, Lachman AS, et al. Non-ejection systolic clicks and mitral systolic murmurs in Black schoolchildren of Soweto, Johannesburg. *Br Heart J* 38:718–724, 1976.
23. Davies MJ, Moore BP, Braimbridge MV. The floppy mitral valve: Study of incidence, pathology, and complications in surgical, necropsy, and forensic material. *Br Heart J* 40:468–481, 1978.
24. Tresch DD, Doyle TP, Boncheck LI. Mitral valve prolapse requiring surgery. Clinical and pathologic study. *Am J Med* 78:245–250, 1985.
25. Kolibash AJ, Bush CA, Fontana MB, et al.: Mitral valve prolapse syndrome: Analysis of 62 patients aged 60 years and older. *Am J Cardiol* 52:534–539, 1983.
26. MacMahon SW, Roberts JK, Kramer-Fox R, et al. Mitral valve prolapse and infective endocarditis. *Am Heart J* 113:1291–1298, 1987.
27. Devereux RB, Hawkins I, Kramer-Fox R, et al. Complications of mitral valve prolapse. Disproportionate occurrence in men and older patients. *Am J Med* 81:751–758, 1986.
28. Guy FC, MacDonald RP, Fraser DB, et al. Mitral valve prolapse as a cause of hemodynamically important mitral regurgitation. *Can J Surg* 23:166–170, 1980.
29. Naggar CA, Pearson WN, Seljan MP. Frequency of complications of mitral valve prolapse in subjects aged 60 years and older. *Am J Cardiol* 58:1209–1212, 1986.
30. King BD, Clark MA, Baba N, et al. "Myxomatous" mitral valves: Collagen dissolution as the primary defect. *Circulation* 66:288–296, 1982.
31. Wilcken DE, Hickey AJ. Lifetime risk for patients with mitral prolapse of developing severe valve regurgitation requiring surgery. *Circulation* 78:10–14, 1988.
32. Lucas RV Jr, Edwards JE. The floppy mitral valve. *Curr Probl Cardiol* 7:1–48, 1982.
33. Weissman N, Pini R, Roman MJ, et al. In vivo mitral valve morphology and motion in mitral valve prolapse. *Clin Res* 40:364A, 1992.
34. Savage DD, Garrison RJ, Devereux RB, et al. Mitral valve prolapse in the general population. I. Epidemiologic features: The Framingham Study. *Am Heart J* 106:571–576, 1983.
35. Popp RL, Winkel RA. Mitral valve prolapse syndrome. *JAMA* 236:867–870, 1976.
36. Beton DC, Brear SG, Edwards JD, et al. Mitral valve prolapse: An assessment of clinical features, associated conditions and prognosis. *Q J Med* 52:150–164, 1983.
37. Boudoulas H, Wooley CF. Mitral valve prolapse and the mitral valve prolapse syndrome. *Progr Cardiovasc Dis* 14:275–309, 1986.
38. Motulsky AG. Biased ascertainment and the natural history of diseases. *N Engl J Med* 298:1196–1197, 1978.
39. Hickey AJ, Narunsky L, Wilcken DEL. Bodily habitus and mitral valve prolapse. *Aust NZ J Med* 15:326–330, 1985.
40. Savage DD, Devereux RB, Garrison RJ, et al. Mitral valve prolapse in the general population. 2. Clinical features: The Framingham Study. *Am Heart J* 106:577–581, 1983.
41. Devereux RB, Brown WT, Lutas EM, et al. Asso-

ciation of mitral valve prolapse with low body weight and low blood pressure. *Lancet* 2:792–795, 1982.
42. Uretsky BF. Does mitral valve prolapse cause nonspecific symptoms? *Int J Cardiol* 1:435–442, 1982.
43. Hartman N, Kramer R, Brown WT, et al. Panic disorder in patients with mitral valve prolapse. *Am J Psychiatry* 139:669–670, 1982.
44. Retchin SM, Fletcher RHJ, Earp J, et al. Mitral valve prolapse. Disease or illness? *Arch Intern Med* 146:1081–1084, 1986.
45. Hickey AJ, Andrews G, Wilcken DEL. Independence of mitral valve prolapse and neurosis. *Br Heart J* 50:333–336, 1983.
46. Devereux R, Kramer-Fox R, Brown WT, et al. Relation between clinical features of the mitral prolapse syndrome and echocardiographically documented mitral valve prolapse. *J Am Coll Cardiol* 8:763–772, 1986.
47. Weissman N, Shear MK, Kramer-Fox R, et al. Contrasting patterns of autonomic dysfunction in patients with mitral valve prolapse and panic attacks. *Am J Med* 82:880–888, 1987.
48. Warth DC, King ME, Cohen J, et al. Prevalence of mitral valve prolapse in normal children. *J Am Coll Cardiol* 5:1173–1177, 1985.
49. Morganroth J, Jones RH, Chen CC, et al. Two dimensional echocardiography in mitral, aortic and tricuspid valve prolapse. The clinical problem, cardiac nuclear imaging considerations, and a proposed standard for diagnosis. *Am J Cardiol* 46:1164–1177, 1980.
50. Levine RA, Triulzi MO, Harrigan P, et al. The relationship of mitral annular shape to the diagnosis of mitral valve prolapse. *Circulation* 75:756–767, 1987.
51. Levine RA, Stathogiannis E, Newell JB, et al. Reconsideration of echocardiographic standards for mitral valve prolapse: Lack of association between leaflet displacement isolated to the apical four chamber view and independent echocardiographic evidence of abnormality. *J Am Coll Cardiol* 11:1010–1019, 1988.
52. Zema MJ, Chiaramida S, DeFilipp GJ, et al. Somatype and idiopathic mitral valve prolapse. *Cathet Cardiovasc Diagnosis* 8:105–111, 1982.
53. Page EW, Christianson R. The impact of mean arterial pressure in the middle trimester upon the outcome of pregnancy. *Am J Obstet Gynecol* 125:740–746, 1976.
54. Olson LJ, Subramanian R, Ackermann DM, et al. Surgical pathology of the mitral valve: A study of 712 cases spanning 21 years. *Mayo Clin Proc* 62:22–34, 1987.
55. Kligfield P, Levy D, Devereux RB, et al. Arrhythmias and sudden death in mitral valve prolapse. *Am Heart J* 113:1298–1307, 1987.
56. Chandraratna PAN, Nimalasuriya A, Kawanishi D, et al. Identification of the increased frequency of cardiovascular abnormalities associated with mitral valve prolapse by two-dimensional echocardiography. *Am J Cardiol* 54:1283–1285, 1984.
57. Nishimura RA, McGoon MD, Shub C, et al. Echocardiographically documented mitral-valve prolapse: Long-term follow-up of 237 patients. *N Engl J Med* 313:1305–1309, 1985.
58. Marks AR, Choong CY, Sanfilippo AJ, et al. Identification of high-risk and low-risk subgroups of patients with mitral-valve prolapse. *N Engl J Med* 320:1031–1036, 1989.
59. Pini R, Devereux RB, Greppi B, et al. Comparison of mitral valve prolapse with severe mitral regurgitation to uncomplicated mitral valve prolapse and to mitral regurgitation without mitral valve prolapse. *Am J Cardiol* 62:257–263, 1988.
60. Boudoulas H, Schaal SF, Stang JM, et al. Mitral valve prolapse: Cardiac arrest with long-term survival. *Int J Cardiol* 26:37–44, 1990.
61. Dollar AL, Roberts WC. Morphologic comparison of patients with mitral valve prolapse who died suddenly with patients who died from severe valvular dysfunction or other conditions. *J Am Coll Cardiol* 17:921–931, 1991.
62. Farb A, Tang AL, Atkinson JB, et al. Comparison of cardiac findings in patients with mitral valve prolapse who die suddenly to those who have congestive heart failure from mitral regurgitation and to those with fatal noncardiac conditions. *Am J Cardiol* 70:234–239, 1992.
63. Higgins CB, Reinke RT, Gosink BB, et al. The significance of mitral valve prolapse in middle-aged and elderly men. *Am Heart J* 91:292–296, 1976.
64. Jerasaty RM, Edwards JE, Chawla SK. Mitral valve prolapse and ruptured chordae tendineae. *Am J Cardiol* 55:138–142, 1985.
65. Kolibash AJ Jr, Kilman JW, Bush CA, et al. Evidence for progression from mild to severe mitral regurgitation in mitral valve prolapse. *Am J Cardiol* 58:762–767, 1986.
66. Caidahl K, Larsson S, Sudow G, et al. Conservative surgery for mitral valve prolapse with regurgitation: Clinical follow-up and noninvasive assessment. *Eur Heart J* 8:384–894, 1987.
67. Roberts WC, McIntosh CL, Wallace RB. Mechanisms of severe mitral regurgitation in mitral valve prolapse determined from analysis of operatively excised valves. *Am Heart J* 113:1316–1323, 1987.
68. Danielsen R, Nordrehaug JE, Vik-Mo H. High occurrence of mitral valve prolapse in cardiac catheterization patients with pure isolated mitral regurgitation. *Acta Med Scand* 221:33–38, 1987.
69. Capucci R, Devereux RB, Hochreiter C, et al. Risk factors for severe mitral regurgitation in patients with mitral valve prolapse. *Clin Res* 35:785a, 1987.
70. MacMahon SW, Blocket RB, Macdonald GJ, et al. Obesity, alcohol consumption and blood pressure in Australian men and women. The National Heart Foundation of Australia Risk Factor Prevalence Study. *J Hypertens* 2:85–91, 1984.
71. Corigal D, Bolen J, Hancock EW, et al. Mitral valve prolapse and infective endocarditis. *Am J Med* 63:215–222, 1977.
72. Hickey AJ, MacMahon SW, Wilcken DE. Mitral valve prolapse and bacterial endocarditis: When is antibiotic prophylaxis necessary? *Am Heart J* 109:431–435, 1985.
73. MacMahon SW, Hickey AJ, Wilcken DEL, et al. Risk of infective endocarditis in mitral valve prolapse with and without precordial systolic murmurs. *Am J Cardiol* 59:105–108, 1987.
74. McKinsey DS, Ratts TE, Bisno AL. Underlying cardiac lesions in adults with infective endocarditis. The changing spectrum. *Am J Med* 82:681–688, 1987.
75. Danchin A, Voiriot P, Briancon S, et al. Mitral valve prolapse as a risk factor for infective endocarditis. *Lancet* 1:743–745, 1989.

76. Awadallah SM, Kavey R-EW, Byrum CJ, et al. The changing pattern of infective endocarditis in childhood. *Am J Cardiol* 68:90–94, 1991.
77. Weinberger I, Rotenberg Z, Zacharovitch D, et al. Native valve endocarditis in the 1970s versus the 1980s: Underlying cardiac lesions and infecting organisms. *Clin Cardiol* 13:94–98, 1990.
78. Devereux RB, Kligfield P. Mitral valve prolapse. In Rakel RE (Ed.), *Current Therapy 1992*. Philadelphia, W.B. Saunders, 1992, pp. 237–241.
79. Perloff JK. *Physical Examination of the Heart and Circulation*. Philadelphia, W.B. Saunders, 1982, pp. 171–237.
80. Conn RD, Cole JS. The cardiac apex impulse. Clinical and angiographic correlations. *Ann Intern Med* 75:185–188, 1971.
81. Nidorf SM, Weyman AE, Levine RA. A new two-dimensional echocardiographic classification of mitral valve prolapse which relates mitral valve morphology to mitral valve function. *J Am Coll Cardiol* 19:157A, 1992.
82. Frary C, Devereux RB, Kramer-Fox R. Infective endocarditis and mitral valve prolapse: Clinical consequences and cost-effectiveness of prevention. *Circulation* 84 (Suppl. II):II-148, 1991.
83. Congeni B, Rizzo C, Congeni J, et al. Outbreak of acute rheumatic fever in northeast Ohio. *J Pediatr* 111:176–179, 1987.
84. Stollerman GH, Markowitz M, Taranta A, et al. Jones criteria (revised) for guidance in the diagnosis of rheumatic fever. *Circulation* 32:664–668, 1965.
85. Gordis L, Lillienfeld A, Rodriguez R. Studies in the epidemiology and preventability of rheumatic fever. I. Demographic factors and the incidence of acute attacks. *J Chron Dis* 21:645–654, 1969.
86. Aron AM, Freeman JM, Carter S. The natural history of Sydenham's chorea. Review of the literature and long-term evaluation with emphasis on cardiac sequelae. *Am J Med* 38:83–95, 1965.
87. Wilson MG, Schweitzer MD, Lubschez R. The familial epidemiology of rheumatic fever: Genetic and epidemiologic studies. *J Pediatr* 22:468–492 and 581–611, 1943.
88. Zabriskie JB. Rheumatic fever: The interplay between host, genetics and microbe. *Circulation* 71:1077–1086, 1985.
89. Pomerance A. Pathology and valvular heart disease. *Br Heart J* 34:437–443, 1972.
90. Burch GE, Giles TD. The role of viruses in the production of heart disease. *Am J Cardiol* 29:231–240, 1972.
91. Reichek N, Shelbourne JC, Perloff JK. Clinical aspects of rheumatic valvular disease. *Progr Cardiovasc Dis* 15:491–537, 1973.
92. Feigenbaum H. *Echocardiography* (4th ed.). Philadelphia, Lea & Febiger, 1986, pp 249–312.
93. Bland EF, Jones TD. Rheumatic fever and rheumatic heart disease. A twenty year report on 1000 patients followed since childhood. *Circulation* 4:836–843, 1951.
94. Davies MJ. *Pathology of Cardiac Valves*. London, Butterworth, 1980.
95. Edwards WD, Peterson K, Edwards JE. Active valvulitis associated with chronic rheumatic valvular disease and active myocarditis. *Circulation* 57:181–185, 1978.
96. Traill TA, St John Sutton MG, Gibson DG. Mitral stenosis with high left ventricular diastolic pressure. *Br Heart J* 41:405–411, 1979.
97. Clawson BJ. Rheumatic heart disease. An analysis of 796 cases. *Am Heart J* 20:454–474, 1940.
98. Rowe JC, Bland EF, Sprague HB, et al. The course of mitral stenosis without surgery: ten and twenty-year perspectives. *Ann Intern Med* 52:741–749, 1960.
99. Olesen KH. The natural history of 271 patients with mitral stenosis under medical treatment. *Br Heart J* 24:349–357, 1962.
100. Mullin MJ, Engleman RM, Isom OW, et al. Experience with open mitral commissurotomy in 100 consecutive patients. *Surgery* 76:974–982, 1974.
101. Absacal VM, Wilkins GT, O'Shea JP, et al. Prediction of successful outcome in 130 patients undergoing percutaneous balloon mitral valvotomy. *Circulation* 82:448–456, 1990.
102. Reid CL, Otto CM, Cavis KB, et al. Influence of mitral valve morphology on mitral balloon commissurotomy: Immediate and six-month results from the NHLBI Balloon valvuloplasty registry. *Am Heart J* 124:657–665, 1992.
103. Osterberger LE, Goldstein S, Khaja F, et al. Functional mitral stenosis in patients with massive mitral anular calcification. *Circulation* 64:472–476, 1981.
104. Hochreiter C, Niles N, Devereux RB, et al. Mitral regurgitation: Relationship of noninvasive descriptors of right and left ventricular performance to clinical and hemodynamic findings and to prognosis in medically and surgically treated patients. *Circulation* 73:900–912, 1986.
105. Rosen S, Borer JS, Hochreiter C, et al. Natural history of asymptomatic severe mitral regurgitation: dissociation of symptom development and ventricular performance. *J Am Coll Cardiol* 15:236A, 1990.
106. Waller BF, Morrow AG, Maron BJ, et al. Etiology of clinically isolated, severe, chronic, pure mitral regurgitation: Analysis of 97 patients over 30 years of age having valve replacement. *Am Heart J* 104:276–288, 1982.
107. Bulkley BH, Roberts WC. Dilatation of the mitral anulus: A rare cause of mitral regurgitation. *Am J Med* 59:457–463, 1975.
108. Roberts WC. Anatomically isolated aortic valvular disease. The case against its being of rheumatic etiology. *Am J Med* 49:151–159, 1970.
109. Roman MJ, Devereux RB, Niles NW, et al. Aortic root dilatation as a cause of isolated, severe aortic regurgitation. Prevalence, clinical and echocardiographic features, and relation to left ventricular hypertrophy and function. *Ann Intern Med* 106:800–807, 1987.
110. Goldschlager N, Pfeifer J, Cohn K, et al. The natural history of aortic regurgitation. A clinical and hemodynamic study. *Am J Med* 54:577–588, 1973.
111. Devereux RB, Lutas EM, Casale PN, et al. Standardization of M-mode echocardiographic left ventricular anatomic measurements. *J Am Coll Cardiol* 4:1222–1230, 1984.
112. de Simone G, Daniels SR, Devereux RB, et al. Left ventricular mass and body size in normotensive children and adults: Assessment of allometric relations and of the impact of overweight. *J Am Coll Cardiol* 20:1251–1260, 1992.
113. Henry WL, Bonow RO, Borer JS, et al. Observations on the optimum time for operative intervention for aortic regurgitation. I. Evaluation of the results

of aortic valve replacement in symptomatic patients. *Circulation* 61:471–483, 1980.
114. Roman MJ, Klein L, Devereux RB, et al. Reversal of left ventricular dilatation, hypertrophy and dysfunction by valve replacement in aortic regurgitation. *Am Heart J* 118:553–563, 1989.
115. Bonow RO, Dodd JT, Maron BJ, et al. Long-term serial changes in left ventricular function and reversal of left ventricular dilatation after valve replacement for chronic aortic regurgitation. *Circulation* 78:1108–1120, 1988.
116. Levy D, Garrison RJ, Savage DD, et al. Prognostic implications of echocardiographically determined left ventricular mass in the Framingham Heart Study. *N Engl J Med* 322:1561–1566, 1990.
117. Koren MJ, Devereux RB, Casale PN, et al. Relation of left ventricular mass and geometry to morbidity and mortality in men and women with essential hypertension. *Ann Intern Med* 114:345–352, 1991.
118. Sell S, Scully RE. Aging changes in the aortic and mitral valves. Histologic and histochemical studies, with observations on the pathogenesis of calcific aortic stenosis and calcification of the mitral annulus. *Am J Pathol* 46:345–365, 1965.
119. Roberts WC, Perloff JK. Mitral valvular disease: A clinicopathologic survey of the conditions causing the mitral valve to function abnormally. *Ann Intern Med* 77:939–975, 1972.
120. Simon MA, Liu SF. Calcification of the mitral valve annulus and its relation to functional valvular disturbance. *Am Heart J* 48:497–505, 1954.
121. Mellino M, Salcedo EE, Lever HM, et al. Echographic quantified severity of mitral anulus calcification: Prognostic correlation to related hemodynamic, valvular, rhythm, and conduction abnormalities. *Am Heart J* 103:222–225, 1982.
122. Leatham A, Brigden W. Mild mitral regurgitation and the mitral valve prolapse fiasco. *Am Heart J* 99:659–664, 1980.
123. DeSanctis RW. Calcification in the region of the aortic and mitral valves. In Castleman B, DeSanctis RW (Eds.), *Cardiac Clinicopathologic Conferences of the Massachusetts General Hospital.* Boston, Little-Brown, 1972, pp. 183–193.
124. Dajani AS, Bisno AL, Chung DJ, et al. Prevention of bacterial endocarditis. Recommendations by the American Heart Association. *JAMA* 264:2919–2922, 1990.
125. Bulkley BH, Roberts WC. The heart in systemic lupus erythematosus and the changes induced in it by corticosteroid therapy. A study of 36 necropsy patients. *Am J Med* 58:243–264, 1975.
126. Barbut D, Borer JS, Gharavi A, et al. Prevalence of anticardiolipin antibody in isolated mitral regurgitation and/or aortic regurgitation and possible relation to cerebral ischemic events. *Am J Cardiol* 70:901–905, 1992.
127. Roberts WC. Congenitally bicuspid aortic valve: A study of 85 autopsy cases. *Am J Cardiol* 26:72–83, 1970.
128. Campbell M. Calcific aortic stenosis and bicuspid aortic valve. *Br Heart J* 30:606–616, 1968.
129. Hahn R, Roman MJ, Mogtader AH, et al. Association of aortic dilatation with regurgitant, stenotic and functionally normal bicuspid aortic valves. *J Am Coll Cardiol* 19:283–288, 1992.
130. Olson LJ, Subramanian R, Edwards WD. Surgical pathology of pure aortic insufficiency: A study of 225 cases. *Mayo Clin Proc* 59:835–841, 1984.
131. Guiney TE, Davies MJ, Parker DJ, et al. The aetiology and course of isolated severe aortic regurgitation: A clinical, pathological, and echocardiographic study. *Br Heart J* 58:358–368, 1987.
132. Mautner GC, Roberts WC. Reported frequency of coronary arterial narrowing by angiogram in patients with valvular aortic stenosis. *Am J Cardiol* 70:539–540, 1992.
133. Roberts WC, Perloff JK, Constantino T. Severe valvular aortic stenosis in patients over 65 years of age. *Am J Cardiol* 27:497, 1971.
134. Vekshtein VI, Alexander RW, Yeung AC, et al. Coronary atherosclerosis is associated with left ventricular dysfunction and dilatation in aortic stenosis. *Circulation* 82:2068–2074, 1990.
135. Nicod P, Bloor C, Godfrey M, et al. Familial aortic dissecting aneurysms. *J Am Coll Cardiol* 13:811–819, 1989.
136. Roman MJ, Devereux RB. Heritable aortic disease. In Lindsay J (Ed.), *Diseases of the Aorta.* Andover Press (in press, 1992).
137. Lemon DK, White CW. Anuloaortic ectasia: Angiographic, hemodynamic and clinical comparison with aortic valve insufficiency. *Am J Cardiol* 41:482–486, 1978.
138. Roman MJ, Devereux RB, Kramer-Fox R, et al. Two-dimensional echocardiographic aortic root dimensions in normal children and adults. *Am J Cardiol* 64:507–512, 1989.
139. Hollister DW, Godfrey MP, Sakai LY, et al. Immunohistologic abnormalities of the microfibrillar-fiber system in the Marfan syndrome. *N Engl J Med* 323:152, 1990.
140. Lee B, Godfrey M, Vitale E, et al. Linkage of Marfan syndrome and a phenotypically related disorder to two different fibrillin genes. *Nature* 352:330–334, 1991.
141. Maslen CL, Corson GM, Maddox BK, et al. Partial sequence of a candidate gene for the Marfan syndrome. *Nature* 352:334–337, 1991.
142. Tsipouras P, Del Maestro R, Sarfarasi M, et al. Linkage of Marfan Syndrome, dominant ectopia lentis and congenital contractural arachnodactyly to the fibrillin genes on chromosomes 15 and 5. *N Engl J Med* 326:905–910, 1992.
143. Dietz HC, Cutting GR, Pyeritz RE, et al. Marfan syndrome caused by a recurrent de novo missense mutation in the fibrillin gene. *Nature* 352:337–339, 1991.
144. Murdoch JL, Waler BA, Halpern BL, et al. Life expectancy and causes of death in the Marfan syndrome. *N Engl J Med* 286:804–808, 1972.
145. Beighton P, de Paepe A, Danks D, et al. International nosology of heritable disorders of connective tissue, Berlin, 1986. *Am J Med Genet* 29:581–594, 1988.
146. Godfrey M. The Marfan syndrome. In Beighton P (Ed.), *McKusick's Heritable Disorders of Connective Tissue.* St. Louis, Mosby-Year Book, (in press, 1993).
147. Devereux RB, Brown WT. Structural heart disease. In King RA, Motulsky AG, Rotter JI (Eds.), *The Genetic Basis of Common Disease.* New York, Oxford University Press, (in press, 1993).
148. Roman MJ, Devereux RB, Kramer-Fox R, et al. Comparison of cardiovascular and skeletal features

of primary mitral valve prolapse and Marfan syndrome. *Am J Cardiol* 63:317–321, 1989.
149. Payvandi MN, Kerber RE, Phelps CD, et al. Cardiac, skeletal and ophthalmologic abnormalities in relatives of patients with the Marfan syndrome. *Circulation* 55:797–802, 1977.
150. Sisk HE, Zahka KG, Pyeritz RE. The Marfan syndrome in early childhood: Analysis of 15 patients diagnosed at less than 4 years of age. *Am J Cardiol* 52:353–358, 1983.
151. Roberts WC, Honig HS. The spectrum of cardiovascular disease in the Marfan syndrome: A clinicomorphologic study of 18 necropsy patients and comparison to 151 previously reported necropsy patients. *Am Heart J* 104:115–135, 1982.
152. Freed C, Schiller NB. Echocardiographic findings in Marfan's syndrome. *West J Med* 126:87–90, 1977.
153. Brown OR, DeMots H, Kloster FE, et al. Aortic root dilatation and mitral valve prolapse in Marfan's syndrome. An echocardiographic study. *Circulation* 52:651–657, 1975.
154. Spangler RD, Nora JJ, Lortsher RH, et al. Echocardiography in Marfan's syndrome. *Chest* 69:72–78, 1976.
155. Pyeritz RE, Wappel MA. Mitral valve dysfunction in the Marfan syndrome. Clinical and echocardiographic study of prevalence and natural history. *Am J Med* 74:797–807, 1983.
156. Come PC, Fortuin NJ, White RI Jr, et al. Echocardiographic assessment of cardiovascular abnormalities in the Marfan syndrome. Comparison with clinical findings and roentgenographic estimation of aortic root size. *Am J Med* 74:465–474, 1983.
157. Chan K-L, Callahan JA, Seward JB, et al. Marfan syndrome diagnosed in patients 32 years of age or older. *Mayo Clin Proc* 62:589–594, 1987.
158. Marsalese DL, Moodie DS, Vacange M, et al. Marfan's syndrome: Natural history and long-term follow-up of cardiovascular involvement. *J Am Coll Cardiol* 14:422–428, 1989.
159. Pini R, Roman MJ, Kramer-Fox R, et al. Mitral valve dimensions and motion in Marfan patients with and without mitral valve prolapse. *Circulation* 80:915–924, 1989.
160. Pyeritz RE, McKusick VA. The Marfan syndrome: Diagnosis and management. *N Engl J Med* 300:772–777, 1979.
161. Pini R, Greppi B, Kramer-Fox R, et al. Mitral valve dimensions and motion and familial transmission of mitral valve prolapse with and without leaflet billowing. *J Am Coll Cardiol* 12:1423–1431, 1988.
162. Phornphutkul C, Rosenthal A, Nadas AS. Cardiac manifestations of Marfan syndrome in infancy and childhood. *Circulation* 57:587–596, 1973.
163. Pyeritz RE. Effectiveness of beta-adrenergic blockade in the Marfan syndrome: Experience over 10 years (abstract). *Am J Med Genet* 32:245, 1988.
164. Schnitker MA, Bayer CA. Dissecting aneurysms of the aorta in young individuals, particularly in association with pregnancy. *Ann Intern Med* 20:486–511, 1944.
165. Pedowitz P, Perell A. Aneurysms complicated by pregnancy. I. Aneurysms of the aorta and its major branches. *Am J Obstet Gynecol* 73:720–735, 1957.
166. Pyeritz RE. Maternal and fetal complications of pregnancy in the Marfan syndrome. *Am J Med* 71:784–790, 1981.
167. Biesecker BB. Special report: Discovery of the Marfan syndrome gene—update on the implications for families. *Connective Issues*. Port Jefferson NY, National Marfan Foundation (in press, 1992).
168. Gallotti R, Ross DN. The Marfan syndrome: Surgical technique and follow-up in 50 patients. *Ann Thoracic Surg* 29:428–433, 1980.
169. McDonald GR, Schaff HV, Pyeritz RE, et al. Surgical management of patients with the Marfan syndrome and dilatation of the ascending aorta. *J Thorac Cardiovasc Surg* 81:180–186, 1981.
170. Gott VL, Pyeritz RE, Magovern GJ Jr, et al. Surgical treatment of aneurysms of the ascending aorta in the Marfan syndrome. *N Engl J Med* 314:1070–1074, 1986.
171. Crawford ES, Crawford JL. Marfan's syndrome. In Crawford ES, Crawford JL (Eds.), *Disorders of the Aorta*. Baltimore, Williams & Wilkins, 1984.
172. Josephson RA, Singer I, Levine JH, et al. Systolic expansion of the aortic root: An echocardiographic and angiographic sign of aortic composite graft dehiscence. *Cathet Cardiovasc Diagn* 14:105–107, 1988.
173. Barbetseas J, Crawford ES, Safi HJ, et al. Doppler echocardiographic evaluation of pseudoaneurysms complicating composite grafts of the ascending aorta. *Circulation* 85:212–222, 1992.
174. Aldrich HR, Labarre RL, Roman MJ, et al. Color flow and conventional echocardiography of the Marfan syndrome. *Echocardiography: A Review of Cardiovascular Ultrasound.* 9:627–636, 1992.
175. Devereux RB, Gott VL, Pyeritz RE. Endocarditis prophylaxis for people with Marfan syndrome who have had cardiac surgery. *Connective Issues* 10(4):3–4, 1991.

CHAPTER 7

Stroke and Peripheral Vascular Diseases

ROBERT D. LANGER, M.D., M.P.H.
MICHAEL H. CRIQUI, M.D., M.P.H.

STROKE

Perhaps because rates of stroke have declined rapidly in the United States during the current century, with this trend apparently starting before major programs to reduce cardiovascular disease were begun, it has received considerably less attention than coronary disease (1,2). After a greater than 50% decrease in the annual rate of stroke in whites from 1920 to 1980 (2), in 1985 the United States had the seventh lowest age-standardized rate of stroke mortality in women among 27 developed countries and the third lowest rate in men (3) (Fig. 7–1).

Epidemiology and Trends

There are marked ethnic differences in stroke rates in the United States. Stroke mortality among black women is almost twice that of white women (2,4,5). The overall age-adjusted stroke mortality in the United States in 1988 was 30/100,000/year but ranged from 26/100,000 in white women to 58/100,000 in black men. Geographic differences also exist: An area of the coastal plains in the southeastern United States known as the "stroke belt" has stroke rates about two times higher than the U.S. average (6), although that clustering has become more diffuse in recent decades.

Although men have about a 30% greater

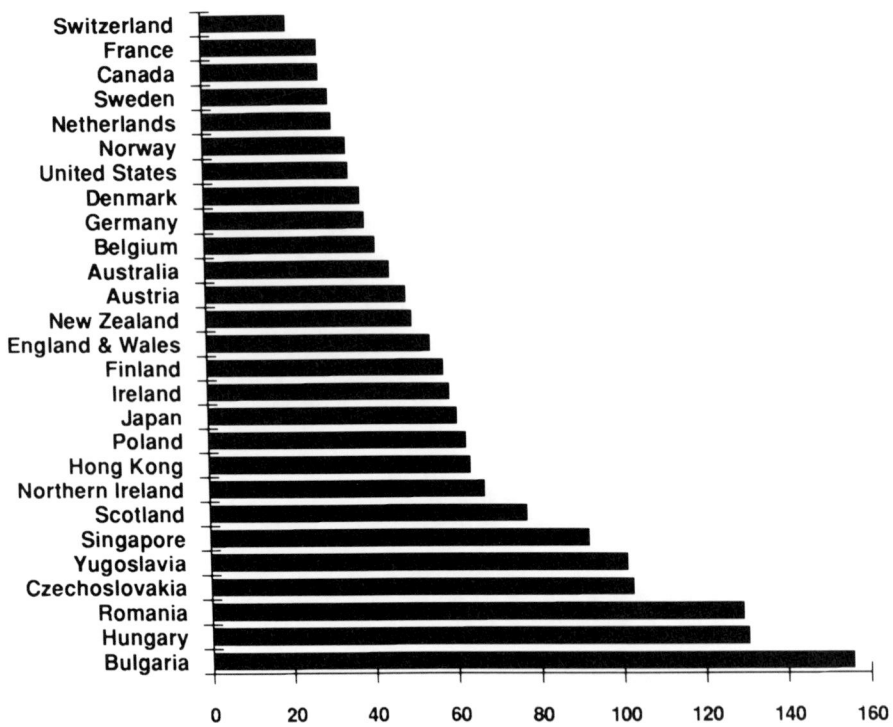

Figure 7-1. International age-adjusted rates per 100,000 population of stroke in women. (From Bonita R, Stewart A, Beaglehole R. International trends in stroke mortality: 1970–1985. *Stroke* 21:989–992, 1990.)

death rate from stroke than women (7) (Fig. 7–2), this statistic is biased by earlier mortality in men and obscures the fact that stroke may be a more important entity within the scope of women's health. Stroke in the United States accounts for a higher percentage of deaths in women than men in all stages of life (5). Since stroke mortality rates increase with age (Fig. 7–3), the biggest discrepancy is seen in the oldest old, those aged 85 years or more, in whom stroke accounts for 12% of mortality in women compared with 9% in men. Also, as shown in Figure 7–3, among survivors after age 85 years, the race and sex trends for stroke are reversed, with white women having the highest mortality.

Estimates of morbidity are much harder to obtain. One source is hospital discharge rates from the National Hospital Discharge Survey (5). According to those data, women had about 15% fewer hospital discharges for first listed diagnosis of stroke than men in 1980 but a 5% higher rate in 1989.

Some data suggest that the long decline in stroke morbidity and mortality may be at an end. An ongoing community-based study in Rochester, Minnesota (8) documented a 46% decline in combined morbidity and mortality for stroke between 1950 and 1979, a decline that appeared earlier in women than in men; a reversal of this trend followed, with a 15% increase in stroke morbidity and mortality in women (and a 19% increase in men) between 1979 and 1984. The trend toward an increase also began earlier in women. Stroke incidence rates continued to increase beyond age 75 years in women, whereas they did not in men. Overall age-adjusted stroke rates for the period 1980 to 1984 were 110/100,000/year in women and 168/100,000/year in men. Cerebral infarction accounted for 102 events/100,000/year, cerebral hemorrhage accounted for 14/100,000, and subarachnoid hemorrhage for 10/100,000. The increase in rates between 1975 and 1979 and between 1980 and 1984 was apparent for cerebral infarction and cerebral hemorrhage, whereas subarachnoid hemorrhage rates have not changed since 1950.

A community-based study in an older population in Sweden (9) (where stroke rates are very close to those in the United States) also found an increase in stroke morbidity and mortality in women when rates for the years 1975 to 1978 were compared with those for 1983 to 1986. The largest increase (232%) was seen in women aged 45 to 64, although increased rates were seen in all age groups for women; smaller and less consistent trends were found in men. The authors noted a parallel finding in women of North Karelia (Finland). Other recent population-based reports from the United States (2,3,7) have shown a slowing in the rate of decline in stroke mortality but not a reversal of the trend. This could be because morbidity data were not included. The suggestion of a reversal in the decline of stroke is controversial and awaits confirmation. If true, it could be the result of increased diagnosis of less significant events since the advent of computed tomographic (CT) and magnetic resonance imaging (MRI) scanners (8). However, it could also be an accurate reflection of higher rates in older women—a very rapidly growing demographic segment.

Diagnosis and Classification

Evaluation of trends in stroke is complicated by problems of diagnosis and classification. Cogent arguments have been made that the decline in stroke that preceded intervention earlier in this century was more a change in diagnostic style than in disease (10). Ischemic stroke is classified by using several overlapping systems, which complicate comparisons across studies. Some of these lump all ischemic events together, whereas others attempt to separate stenotic or thrombotic from embolic causes. Even the more basic distinction between ischemic and hemorrhagic stroke was prone to error in the absence of autopsy before CT and MRI imaging became available. The advent of these imaging techniques has not only vastly improved case-finding, they have also provided invaluable information on the extent and location of the lesion. Despite these earlier problems of classification, data have consistently indicated that young women have about a 50% increased incidence of the least common form of stroke, subarachnoid hemorrhage (1,7,11), although the reason for this excess is unknown.

Carotid Disease and Stroke

The relation between asymptomatic carotid bruit and stroke remains controversial. Inves-

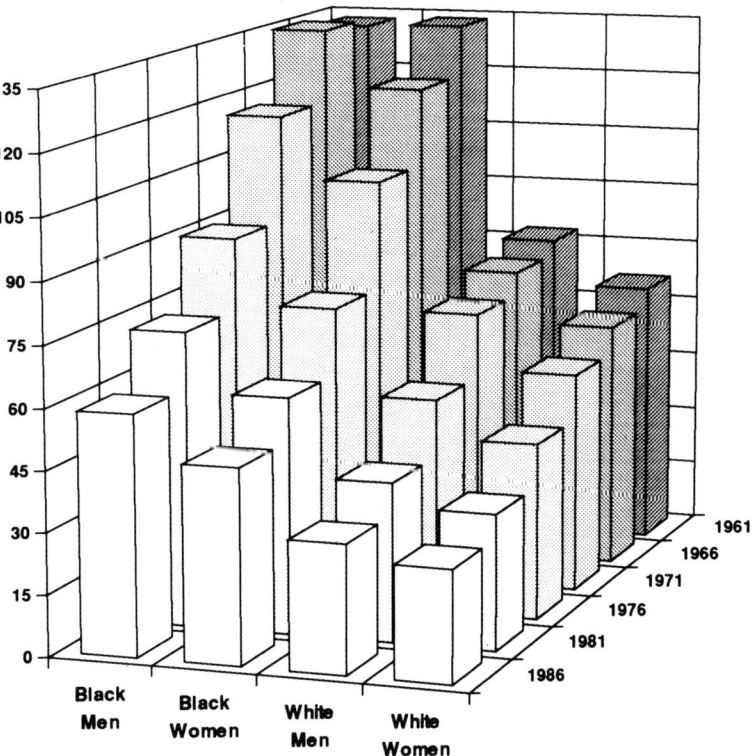

Figure 7-2. United States stroke rates per 100,000 population by sex and race, 1961–1986. (From United States Public Health Service, Centers for Disease Control. *Health United States 1990*, Washington, D.C., U.S. Government Printing Office 1991, pp. 85–148.)

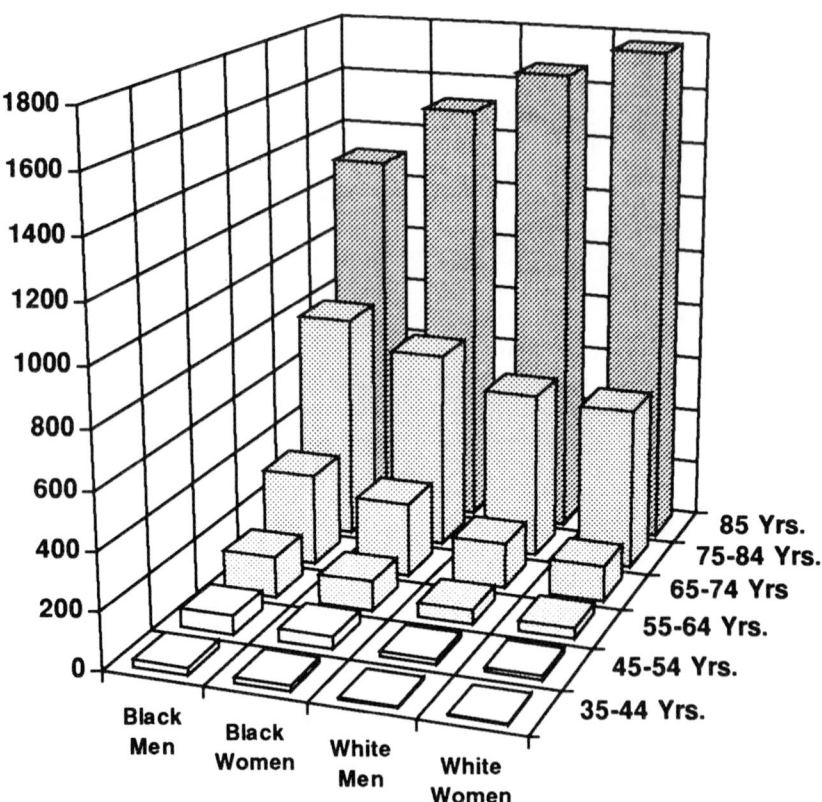

Figure 7–3. United States stroke rates per 100,000 population by sex, race, and age, 1988. (From United States Public Health Service, Centers for Disease Control, *Health United States 1990*. Washington, D.C., U.S. Government Printing Office, 1991, pp. 85–148.)

tigators from the Framingham study reported that the presence of a carotid bruit increased the risk of both stroke and myocardial infarction, but those incident strokes often occurred in an anatomic location unrelated to the bruit. They concluded that an asymptomatic bruit is a marker for atherosclerotic disease but not necessarily a direct cause of stroke (12). A large population study in Evans County, Georgia, found a higher prevalence of carotid bruit in women than in men (5.9% versus 2.6%), but the presence of a bruit was not associated with incident stroke after 6 years in women, whereas it was in men (13).

Doppler ultrasound examination allows better noninvasive characterization of carotid disease. In a study of 659 consecutive patients referred to a vascular laboratory for Doppler evaluation of asymptomatic bruits, women with disease had less stenosis than men (84% of women and 68% of men had less than 75% stenosis), and male sex, existing heart disease, and greater stenosis were the best predictors of stroke (14). Available data suggest that the risk of stroke from asymptomatic carotid disease associated with less than 75% stenosis is low. The use of carotid endarterectomy to correct these asymptomatic lesions with marginal decrements in flow is highly controversial.

Risk Factors

Ischemic Stroke. Elevated blood pressure is the strongest and most consistent risk factor for stroke. Although most studies have found no sex difference in the association of blood pressure with stroke, a community-based study of the elderly in England suggested that there may not be a relationship between blood pressure and stroke in older women (15). Cigarette smoking is a powerful risk factor for ischemic stroke just as for coronary disease. Diabetes, elevated blood cholesterol, and a history of myocardial infarction or past stroke are also strongly associated with incident stroke. Besides these well-known atherosclerotic risk factors (7), ischemic stroke risk factors associated with female gender or that are more prevalent in women include pregnancy (toxemia, postpartum cerebral thrombosis, and hypercoagulable state), autoimmune diseases, mitral valve prolapse, oral contraceptive use, and migraine (1,7). In the very old, chronic atrial fibrillation may be the most important predictor of ischemic stroke (16), whereas traditional risk factors may be less important, and other still uncharacterized risk factors may also play a role. Observational studies have suggested that postmenopausal hormone replacement with unopposed conjugated equine estrogen reduces the incidence of stroke by about 50% (1,17), but this effect has not been tested in a randomized clinical trial. Diabetes and smoking are associated with greater relative risks for stroke in women than in men, a pattern similar to that seen for coronary disease (18,19).

Hemorrhagic Stroke. Elevated blood pressure and heavy alcohol use are the only consistently documented risk factors for hemorrhagic stroke (1,7). Cross-cultural observations of a much higher incidence of hemorrhagic stroke in countries with low serum cholesterol levels have given rise to a controversial hypothesis that low cholesterol may be a risk factor for hemorrhagic stroke. Recent changes in the rates of stroke in Japan have led to speculation that dietary fat and serum cholesterol may be inversely related to hemorrhagic stroke (20), such that the higher levels of serum cholesterol seen in the United States may be associated with a lower risk of cerebral hemorrhage than the traditionally lower levels of serum cholesterol found in Japan. Although early studies of this effect included only Hawaiian and Japanese men (21,22), some have included women (23), and one has demonstrated this relation in U.S. men (24). These data are confounded by additional risk factors including hypertension, alcohol consumption, and smoking that could at least partially account for the observation. Nevertheless, this association cannot be excluded based on currently available data.

Disability, Sequelae, and Economic Impact

In addition to its substantial impact on mortality, nonfatal stroke is often associated with considerable disability. About 70% of stroke victims survive the event, and women are more likely to survive than men. In the United States in 1986, there were about 500,000 incident strokes and about 2,000,000 stroke survivors (prevalent cases) (25). Data from some community-based studies suggest that stroke may account for less severe disability in elderly women than men (26,27). Stroke-related disability that affects the patient's usual activities resolves within the first year in the majority of stroke victims who survive the event. Estimates of residual disability affecting independence in daily activities range from about 25% to 50%, with greater residual disability in survivors of recurrent strokes.

Since women tend to suffer strokes later in life than men, female stroke survivors often become nursing home residents due to the absence of a suitable caretaker at home. Cerebrovascular disorders account for the highest percentage of nursing home admissions in patients aged 65 years or older admitted from short-stay hospitals (28). Women make up 76.0% of this group. Marital status and age at the time of the stroke also predict nursing home admission; 75.1% of the elderly entering nursing homes for stroke have no spouse, 33.6% are 85 or more years old, 42.3% are 75 to 84 years old, and just 24.1% are aged 65 to 74 years (29). Stroke-related costs in the United States were estimated to be $13.5 billion in 1989, of which $9.8 billion (73%) were attributed to hospital and nursing home services (25). Gender differences in use of rehabilitation have not been examined.

Prevention and Intervention

Interventions to reduce atherosclerotic risk including blood pressure control, achieving a moderate serum cholesterol level, quitting smoking, and avoiding diabetes will also reduce stroke risk in both sexes. Also, as noted above, observational data suggest that postmenopausal estrogen replacement may reduce stroke risk, but clinical trial data are lacking. Recent observational reports have suggested that aspirin may prevent stroke in women (30), although clinical trials have failed to show this benefit (1), perhaps because they have generally enrolled fewer women than men while event rates require more women than men for the same statistical power. Case series of carotid endarterectomy also suggest that women are less likely to receive this intervention; studies of 206 and 221 consecutive cases had only 26% and 27% women, respectively (31,32). As noted above, endarterectomy appears to be beneficial for those with symptomatic carotid stenosis of at least 75%, but sex-specific data on benefit are lacking. Clinical trials of stroke prevention in persons with atrial fibrillation have demonstrated a reduction in stroke with anticoagulant therapy including warfarin (33,34,35) and aspirin (33). Most participants in these studies were male, and results were not reported by sex.

PERIPHERAL VASCULAR DISEASE

Peripheral vascular disease, like stroke, is complicated by a lack of generally accepted standards for diagnosis and nomenclature. However, a preliminary stratification between venous and arterial disease is easily accomplished. Relatively few studies have addressed the epidemiology of these diseases in either sex.

Venous Disease

Venous disease can be further divided into superficial and deep anatomic locations. *Varicose veins* are by far the most prevalent of these conditions (36,37,38). As shown in Table 7–1, which is based on interview, not examination data, this form of superficial venous disease increases with age and is reported more than twice as often in women as in men at any age. Population studies using clinical examination data indicate a prevalence of about 80% in women over age 60 (36,38). Additional risk factors for varicose veins include pregnancy, sedentary life style, family history, and obesity (36,37). Although rarely associated with medical complications, this condition accounts for substantial health care costs related to both conservative and surgical treatment (37).

Deep venous thromboses (DVT) have more serious medical implications. Often ignored as a condition of importance, DVT is both quite common and associated with a poor prognosis. Since invasive diagnostic procedures are rarely warranted, prior to the advent of Duplex ultrasonography study of DVT was quite limited, and diagnosis was problematic. In a 6-year series of consecutive scans obtained between 1982 and 1988 from 485 women and 468 men referred to a vascular laboratory for evaluation (40), there were no sex differences in the incidence rates for this condition. However, women were significantly older (62.9 versus 58.8 years) and had a higher rate of unilateral single thrombi (34% versus 25%). There were no significant differences between women and men in the anatomic locations of disease.

Based on projections from a study of short-stay hospitalizations in the Worcester Standard Metropolitan Statistical Area (SMSA) conducted in 1985 and 1986, the annual attack rate is 107/100,000 population, and age-adjusted DVT incidence rates are 48/100,000/year in each sex (41). Extrapolation of these rates to the U.S. population predicts 116,000 new cases of DVT per year. The hospital case-fatality rate for the Worcester SMSA was 5%, and the 3-year case-fatality rate in patients surviving to be discharged was 30%. The incidence rate and case-fatality rate both increased dramatically with age. Figure 7–4 plots the trends in incidence rates by age and sex.

Risk factors for DVT include cancer, congestive heart failure, fracture, myocardial infarction, obesity, stroke, surgery, and trauma (41). The considerable mortality associated with DVT may be explained in part by the frequency of comorbidity with other serious diseases. In the Worcester study, 80% of patients aged 40 years or older had three or more of the risk factors listed above. Although the incidence of DVT in women of childbearing age is low, retrospective studies suggest that oral contraceptives are associated with an elevated risk of these events (42,43). A case-control study found that this risk was associated with current or recent use and was no different for high- compared with low-dose estrogen preparations (42).

Table 7–1. PREVALENCE OF VARICOSE VEINS PER 1000 PERSONS BY AGE AND SEX, FROM THE NATIONAL HEALTH INTERVIEW SURVEY, U.S., 1984

	Under 45 Years	45–64 Years	65–74 Years	Over 74 Years
Women	24.8	97.3	87.5	112.5
Men	4.0	29.5	39.7	44.2
Ratio: women/men	6.2	3.3	2.2	2.6

From National Center for Health Statistics. Current estimates from the National Health Interview Survey: United States, 1984. *Vital and Health Statistics*, Series 10, No. 156, p. 84 (39).

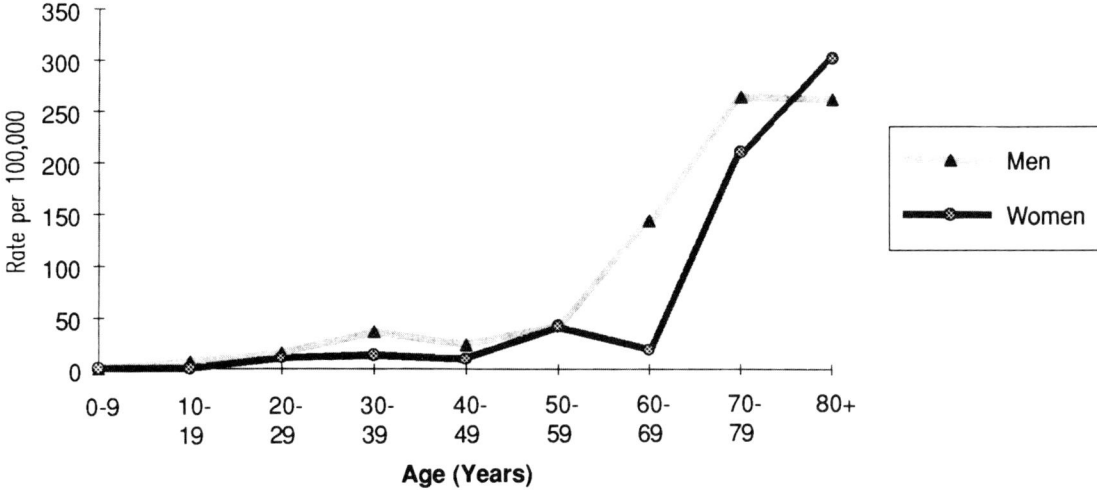

Figure 7-4. Annual incidence of deep vein thrombosis per 100,000 population by age and sex in patients treated in short-stay hospitals, Worcester SMSA. (From Anderson FA, Wheeler B, Goldberg RJ, et al. A population-based perspective of the hospital incidence and case fatality rates of deep vein thrombosis and pulmonary embolism. *Arch Intern Med* 151:933–938, 1991.)

Peripheral Arterial Disease

Peripheral arterial disease (PAD) usually results from atherosclerotic narrowing of the arterial lumen. Although rarely the proximal cause of death, PAD is associated with significant cardiovascular mortality from other causes (44). Diagnostic standards vary for this condition, which complicates interpretation of the literature.

Definition, Prevalence, and Incidence

Traditional epidemiologic assessment of PAD has employed the Rose questionnaire for intermittent claudication, which by definition detects only persons with classic symptoms of PAD (45). Using this instrument, it has been demonstrated that classic claudication is uncommon in persons less than 50 years of age but increases sharply with age. At approximately 60 years of age, rates in various studies have ranged between 1% and 6% (46–53). Rates in women are generally 25% to 50% lower than those in men. This contrasts with the known excess of angina pectoris in women (54,55). However, in young women angina may be a poor marker for coronary disease (54).

Not all patients with symptomatic PAD have classic intermittent claudication. "Possible" claudication, defined as any exercise calf pain not present at rest, has considerable validity as a marker for PAD (56). In a population-based study in an older southern California cohort with an average age of 66 years, possible claudication was present in 4.9% of women and 7.2% of men (57). Age-specific rates for both sexes combined were 3.1% at less than 60 years of age, 5.4% at 60 to 69 years of age, and 7.7% in the group aged 70 to 82 years. Interestingly, the rates for reduced or absent pulses in the lower extremity, another traditional clinical marker for PAD, were quite similar in women and men, 22.1% and 20.3%, respectively.

The sensitivity, specificity, and predictive value of traditional PAD clinical assessments are perhaps lower than one might expect compared with the results of accurate and reliable noninvasive testing (58). For example, among patients with definitive PAD by noninvasive testing, only 27% have exercise calf pain, and only 14% have classic claudication. Among patients with exercise calf pain, only 40% have PAD, and even among patients with classic intermittent claudication, only about half have PAD. Prevalence rates of PAD by noninvasive testing are more accurate and considerably higher because they include flow limiting but asymptomatic PAD, and all but eliminate false-positive symptoms. Figure 7–5 shows

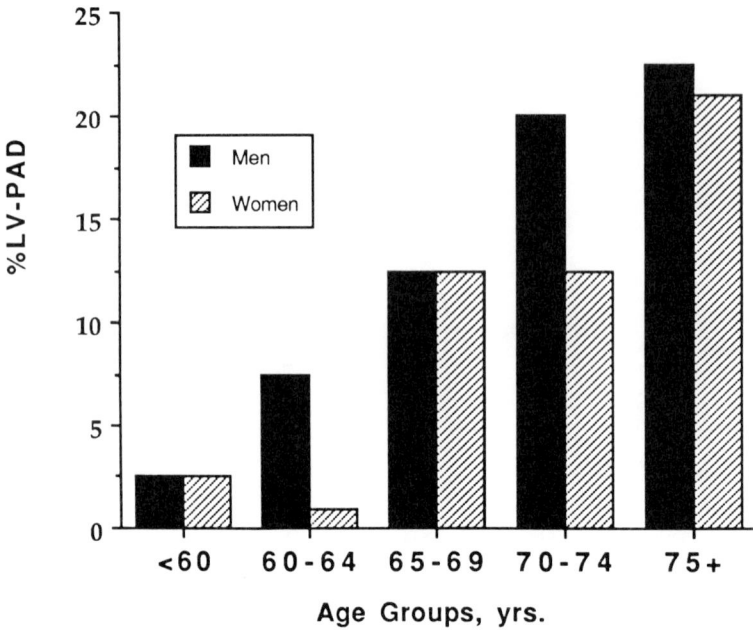

Figure 7–5. Prevalence of large-vessel peripheral arterial disease by age and sex, Rancho Bernardo, California, 1978–1980. (From Criqui MH, Fronek A, Barrett-Connor E, et al. The prevalence of peripheral arterial disease in a defined population. *Circulation* 71: 510–515, 1985.)

age- and sex-specific rates of PAD for men and women as determined by noninvasive testing in 565 community-dwelling older men and women. The results shown in Figure 7–5 indicate a somewhat higher prevalence of PAD in men than in women. Overall, adjusted for age and hyperlipidemia, the excess in men was 27% (57). Incidence data for PAD require repeated assessments in a stable population over time. Such data for intermittent claudication are available from the Framingham study, and age- and sex-specific data are shown in Table 7–2. These Framingham data are based on typical claudication and have the limitations noted above. Nonetheless, like the noninvasive prevalence data, they show a strikingly higher incidence in men up to age 65, but, in a pattern reminiscent of coronary disease and stroke rates, this gap narrows substantially at older ages.

Natural History

Dormandy and colleagues noted that if patients survive for several years after diagnosis, two-thirds to three-quarters will have no worse than stable symptoms, whereas the remaining one-third to one-quarter will show progression of PAD (60). Up to 5% will deteriorate to the point where amputation is required. These percentages by definition reflect the natural history in survivors. However, PAD is strongly associated with early mortality. More dramatic progression of PAD probably occurs in patients at greater risk for early mortality.

Although in population studies of PAD the sex ratio (men-women) is generally less than 2, Dormandy has noted that in clinical studies of more advanced disease the sex ratio is often higher, varying from 3 to 13 (60). He believes that this observation suggests that the prognosis of local disease in women is much better than that in men. However, the degree to which selective factors, such as employment, physician attention, or group studied might create a bias toward a large excess of diagnosed cases in men is unclear.

Table 7–2. ANNUAL INCIDENCE RATES OF CLAUDICATION PER 1000 PERSONS BY AGE AND SEX, FRAMINGHAM

Age at Biennial Examination (Yr)	Women	Men
30–44	0.3	0.6
45–54	0.7	1.9
55–64	1.8	5.3
65–74	5.4	6.1
Total	1.2	2.6

Adapted from Kannel WB, Skinner JJ, Schwartz MJ, et al. Intermittent claudication: Incidence in the Framingham study. *Circulation* 41:875, 1970 (59).

Table 7–3. PERCENT MORTALITY AND AGE-ADJUSTED RELATIVE RISK FOR SPECIFIC CAUSES OF DEATH BY PAD STATUS AND SEX, RANCHO BERNARDO, CALIFORNIA

	Men			Women		
	Normal	*PAD*	*RR*	*Normal*	*PAD*	*RR*
N	183	34	—	225	33	—
All-cause	16.9	61.8	3.3	11.6	33.3	2.5
CVD	7.7	41.7	5.1	3.6	18.2	4.8
CHD	5.5	35.3	5.8	2.2	9.1	4.8
Other	9.3	14.7	1.6	8.0	15.2	1.6

CVD = cardiovascular disease; CHD = coronary heart disease (a subset of cardiovascular disease mortality); PAD = peripheral arterial disease; RR = relative risk.
Adapted from Criqui MH, Langer RD, Fronek A, et al. Mortality over 10 years in patients with peripheral arterial disease. *N Engl J Med* 326:381–386, 1992.

Data from the U.S. National Hospital Discharge Survey indicate that the sex ratio in clinically recognizable disease may be less than 2 (61). The sex ratio for chronic PAD was 1.3 to 1.8, although women tended to be older at the time of diagnosis. The sex ratio for arteriography of femoral and other lower extremity arteries was 1.5, and the sex ratio for acute PAD hospitalization at age 65 and above was 1.5. Men had a 2.1 times greater rate of aortoiliac-femoral bypass at ages 65 and older and were 2.0 times more likely than women to have other peripheral shunt or bypass procedures. However, the sex ratio for amputation at age 65 and above was only 1.6.

Prognostic Significance of PAD for Mortality

PAD is a relatively uncommon primary cause of death (61). However, coronary disease prevalence may be as high as 50% in patients with PAD, and PAD patients have an excess of cerebrovascular occlusive disease as well (60). Such comorbidity is to some degree predictable, given the overlap of risk factors for atherosclerosis in these three anatomic locations (62). Intermittent claudication has been known for some time to be associated with about a twofold excess of all-cause mortality (52,63,64). Whether this increase in risk represents an independent effect or can be attributed to the known excess of cardiovascular comorbidity or the high levels of cardiovascular risk factors in PAD patients remains controversial. One study suggested a sex difference in the risk associated with symptomatic claudication, with women experiencing about a 50% greater mortality after 10 years than men (65). Those results are not validated by other studies and probably are an artifact of the older age of onset for PAD in women since no adjustment was made for age or the poor specificity of claudication as a means of diagnosing PAD.

Ten years of follow-up in older community-dwelling men and women in whom PAD was accurately diagnosed using noninvasive tests has revealed sharply elevated relative risks of coronary heart disease mortality, cardiovascular disease mortality, and all-cause mortality in both men and women with PAD. Table 7–3 shows sex-specific crude percent mortality rates and age-adjusted relative risks for coronary heart disease mortality, cardiovascular disease mortality, and all-cause mortality. Absolute mortality rates in women were lower than those in men, both in normal subjects and in subjects with PAD. However, the relative risk, or ratio of incidence rates, was nearly identical in men and women. The increase in all-cause mortality was due almost exclusively to the increase in cardiovascular disease mortality, since other causes of mortality were not significantly increased.

Additional analyses excluding subjects with known cardiovascular disease at baseline and controlling for other cardiovascular disease risk factors gave similar results. Further analyses revealed that the mortality risk was particularly high in persons with severe and symptomatic PAD. Thus, PAD appears to be an independent marker for a sharply elevated risk of mortality in both men and women, even after known clinical coronary heart disease and cardiovascular disease risk factors are taken into account.

Treatment

Initial treatment for mild to moderate claudication should address risk factors including cigarette smoking, dyslipidemia, hypertension, obesity, diabetes, and sedentary life style. Daily walking may double or triple the average walking distance possible (66). Pentoxifylline has rheologic effects, and ketanserin blocks peripheral S2 serotonin receptors, but benefits of these drugs are modest at best (67). Intra-arterial and intravenous prostacyclin may be of benefit in selected patients, presumably due to their platelet anti-aggregatory and vasodilatory effects (68). Vasodialator drugs are not useful (67,69).

For patients with debilitating or disabling claudication, surgery may be considered. The development of lower-risk procedures has lowered operative mortality and reduced the degree of reconstruction necessary. Clinical reports suggest a nearly 90% early success rate with femoropopliteal percutaneous transluminal angioplasty. The largest decline in patency occurs in the first 6 to 12 months after the procedure, with little further decline occurring after 2 years [70]. This technique is most effective in short iliac artery stenoses.

Thrombolytic therapy is currently being evaluated for chronic use. For acute ischemia, thrombolysis should be considered. Treatment hinges on the viability of the limb (71,72).

Economic Implications of PAD

Women live longer than men, and PAD rates in elderly women approach those in men. Thus, a significant PAD burden exists and is projected to grow in older women as the population ages. Data from Maryland show that between 1979 and 1989 the annual age- and sex-adjusted rate for performance of percutaneous transluminal angioplasty for PAD rose from 1 to 24/100,000 residents (73). Despite the presumed benefit from restored flow, the annual rate of peripheral bypass surgery also increased from 32 to 65/100,000, and despite the increase in both these interventions, the annual rate of amputation was stable at 30/100,000. Although focused, selected efforts by an expert vascular surgery team can produce a reduction in amputations (74), current overall medical community treatment of PAD apparently does not, perhaps because of some inappropriate treatment and some treatment in hospitals with limited expertise (75).

In the Maryland study, 41% of the patients receiving both angioplasty and bypass surgery were women, and 49% of the amputations were performed in women. Fifteen percent of the angioplasty procedures were performed in blacks, whereas 24% of the bypass surgeries and 40% of the amputations were performed in blacks. These data suggest the possibilities of both gender and racial bias in access to early PAD interventions.

In constant dollars and adjusted for the aging of the population, total hospital charges for PAD procedures in Maryland rose from $14.7 million in 1979 to $30.5 million in 1989, and the number of hospital days increased from 20,695 to 33,830 (73). Such figures are daunting, given the economic burden of current medical care costs. As with so many other diseases, risk factor modification, particularly cigarette smoking cessation, may offer the best hope of reducing disease incidence and medical expenditures.

Isolated Small-Vessel PAD

Isolated small-vessel PAD, defined as disease of the arterioles of <2 mm in diameter without disease higher in the vascular tree, was more prevalent than large-vessel PAD in a community-based study, affecting 16% of older women and 15% of men (57). This condition was not associated with any of the usual cardiovascular risk factors but doubled the risk of cardiovascular mortality in both women and men compared with normal participants after 10 years (58). It may represent a reactive vasospastic phenomenon not unlike microvascular angina. Diagnosis of isolated small-vessel PAD requires noninvasive testing, both to identify this disorder and to exclude large-vessel disease. Accordingly, it has been characterized in only one population study to date, and additional research is necessary.

SUMMARY

With two exceptions, subarachnoid hemorrhage and varicose veins, stroke and peripheral vascular diseases, like coronary artery disease, occur at later ages in women than in men. The factors underlying the delayed onset of atherosclerotic diseases in women are not fully understood, but hormonal influences, particularly the effects of estrogen, are believed to be important. Nevertheless, since women live longer than men, these diseases account for significant morbidity, mortality, disability, and social and economic hardship in women, particularly at older ages. For many very old women, limited social support complicates the disability associated with non-fatal stroke or significant PVD and imposes the need for custodial or institutional care.

Data are sparse on the natural history of peripheral arterial disease in both sexes. Available studies suggest that the population-wide excess mortality associated with PAD may be somewhat lower in women than in men. However, this may be an artifact of the delayed development of atherosclerotic disease in women and the limitations of currently available follow-up data in which men and women have been followed for the same amount of time. It remains to be seen whether women will approach the same excess risk associated with PAD as men when they reach the oldest ages. At both younger and older ages, once PAD has developed, the relative risk of mortality is similar in men and women.

References

1. Barnett HJM. Stroke in women. *Can J Cardiol* 6(Suppl. B):11B–17B, 1990.
2. Cooper R, Sempos C, Hsieh SC, et al. Slowdown in the decline of stroke mortality in the United States, 1978–1986. *Stroke* 21:1274–1279, 1990.
3. Bonita R, Stewart A, Beaglehole R. International trends in stroke mortality: 1970–1985. *Stroke* 21:989–992, 1990.
4. Kittner SJ, White LR, Losonczy KG, et al. Black-white differences in stroke incidence in a national sample. *JAMA* 264:1267–1270, 1990.
5. Public Health Service, Centers for Disease Control. *Health United States 1990*. Washington, D.C., Public Health Service, 1991, pp. 85–148.
6. Wing S, Casper M, Davis WB, et al. Stroke mortality maps: United States whites aged 35–74 years, 1962–1982. *Stroke* 19;1507–1513, 1988.
7. Wong MCW, Giuliani MJ, Haley C. Cerebrovascular disease and stroke in women. *Cardiology* 77(Suppl 2):80–90, 1990.
8. Broderick JP, Phillips SJ, Whisnant JP, et al. Incidence rates of stroke in the eighties: The end of the decline in stroke? *Stroke* 20:577–582, 1989.
9. Terent A. Increasing incidence of stroke among Swedish women. *Stroke* 19:598–603, 1988.
10. Homer D, Whisnant JP, Schoenberg BS. Trends in the incidence rates of stroke in Rochester, Minnesota, since 1935. *Ann Neurol* 22:245–251, 1987.
11. Suzuki K, Kutsuzawa T, Takita K, et al. Clinico-epidemiologic study of stroke in Akita, Japan. *Stroke* 18:402–406, 1987.
12. Wolf PA, Kannel WB, Sorlie P, et al. Asymptomatic carotid bruit and risk of stroke. *JAMA* 245:1442–1445, 1981.
13. Heyman A, Wilkinson WE, Heyden S, et al. Risk of stroke in asymptomatic persons with cervical arterial bruits: A population study in Evans County, Georgia. *N Engl J Med* 302:838–841, 1980.
14. Chambers BR, Norris JW. Outcome in patients with asymptomatic neck bruits. *N Engl J Med* 315:860–865, 1986.
15. Evans JG. Blood pressure and stroke in an elderly English population. *J Epidemiol Commun Hlth* 41:275–282, 1987.
16. Wolf PA, Abbott RD, Kannel WB. Atrial fibrillation: A major contributor to stroke in the elderly. *Arch Intern Med* 147:1561–1564, 1987.
17. Paganini-Hill A, Ross RK, Henderson BE. Postmenopausal oestrogen treatment and stroke: A prospective study. *Br Med J* 297(6647):519–522, 1988.
18. Thompson SG, Greenberg G, Meade TW. Risk factors for stroke and myocardial infarction in women in the United Kingdom as assessed in general practice: A case-control study. *Br Heart J* 61:403–409, 1989.
19. Shimamoto T, Komachi Y, Inada H, et al. Trends for coronary heart disease and stroke and their risk factors in Japan. *Circulation* 79:503–515, 1989.
20. Colditz GA, Bonita R, Stampfer MJ, et al. Cigarette smoking and risk of stroke in middle-aged women. *N Engl J Med* 318:937–941, 1988.
21. Kagan A, Popper JS, Rhoads GG. Factors related to stroke incidence in Hawaiian Japanese men. *Stroke* 11(1):14–21, 1980.
22. Kagan A, Popper JS, Rhoads GG, et al. Dietary and other risk factors for stroke in Hawaiian Japanese men. *Stroke* 16(3):390–396, 1985.
23. Tanaka H, Ueda Y, Hayashi M, et al. Risk factors for cerebral hemorrhage and cerebral infarction in a Japanese rural community. *Stroke* 13(1):62–73, 1982.
24. Iso H, Jacobs DR Jr, Wentworth D, et al. Serum cholesterol levels and six-year mortality from stroke in 350,977 men screened in the multiple risk factor intervention trial. *N Engl J Med* 320(14):904–910, 1989.
25. American Heart Association. *1989 Stroke Facts*. American Heart Association, Dallas, TX, 1988.
26. Jette AM, Pinsky JL, Branch LG, et al. The Framingham disability study: Physical disability among community-dwelling survivors of stroke. *J Clin Epidemiol* 41:719–726, 1988.
27. Ueda K, Fujii I, Kawano H, et al. Severe disability related to cerebral stroke: Incidence and risk factors observed in a Japanese community, Hisayama. *J Am Geriatr Soc* 35:616–622, 1987.
28. National Center for Health Statistics. The National Nursing Home Survey: 1985. *Vital & Health Statistics*, Series 13, No. 97, p. 43, 1989.
29. National Center for Health Statistics. The National Nursing Home Survey: 1985. *Vital & Health Statistics*, Series 13; No. 97, p. 44, 1989.
30. Manson JE, Stampfer MJ, Colditz GA, et al. A prospective study of aspirin use and primary prevention of cardiovascular disease in women [see comments]. *JAMA* 266(4):521–527, 1991.
31. Healy DA, Zierler RE, Nicholls SC, et al. Long-term follow-up and clinical outcome of carotid restenosis. *J Vasc Surg* 10:662–669, 1989.
32. Loftus CM, Biller J, Godersky JC, et al. Carotid endarterectomy in symptomatic elderly patients. *Neurosurgery* 22:676–680, 1980.
33. SPAF Investigators. Special Report: Preliminary report of the Stroke Prevention in Atrial Fibrillation Study. *N Engl J Med* 322:863–868, 1990.

34. Petersen P, Boysen G, Godtfredsen J, et al. Placebo-controlled, randomized trial of warfarin and aspirin for prevention of thromboembolic complications in chronic atrial fibrillation the Copenhagen AFASAK Study. *Lancet,* 1:175–179, 1989.
35. The Boston Area Anticoagulation Trial for Atrial Fibrillation Investigators. The effect of low dose warfarin on the risk of stroke in patients with atrial fibrillation. *N Engl J Med,* 323:1505–1511, 1990.
36. Widmer LK, Stahelin HB, Nissen C, et al. *Venen Arperien, Klankheiten koronare Herzkrankheit bei Berufstatigen.* Bern, Switzerland, Hubert Bernt, 1989.
37. Brand FN, Dannenberg AL, Abbott RD, et al. The epidemiology of varicose veins: The Framingham study. *Am J Prev Med* 4:96–101, 1988.
38. Hirai M, Naiki K, Nakayama R. Prevalence and risk factors of varicose veins in Japanese women. *Angiology J Vasc Dis* 41:228–232, 1991.
39. National Center for Health Statistics. Current estimates from the National Health Interview Survey: United States, 1984. *Vital & Health Statistics,* Series 10, No. 156, 1986, p. 84.
40. Kerr TM, Cranley JJ, Johnson JR, et al. Analysis of 1084 consecutive lower extremities involved with acute venous thrombosis diagnosed by Duplex scanning. *Surgery* 108:520–527, 1990.
41. Anderson FA, Wheeler B, Goldberg RJ, et al. A population-based perspective of the hospital incidence and case-fatality rates of deep vein thrombosis and pulmonary embolism. *Arch Intern Med* 151:933–938, 1991.
42. Helmrich SP, Rosenberg L, Kaufman DW, et al. Venous thromboembolism in relation to oral contraceptive use. *Obstet Gynecol* 69:91–95, 1987.
43. Gerstman BB, Piper JM, Freiman JP, et al. Oral contraceptive oestrogen and progestin potencies and the incidence of deep venous thromboembolism. *Int J Epidemiol* 19(4):931–936, 1990.
44. Criqui MH, Langer RD, Fronek A, et al. Mortality over 10 years in patients with peripheral arterial disease. *N Engl J Med* 326:381–386, 1992.
45. Rose GA. The diagnosis of ischaemic heart pain and intermittent claudication in field surveys. *Bull WHO* 27:645–658, 1962.
46. Isaacson S. Venous occlusion plethysmography in 55-year-old men: A population study in Malmo, Sweden. *Acta Med Scand* 537(Supp.):1, 1972.
47. Gyntelberg F. Physical fitness and coronary heart disease: Male residents in Copenhagen aged 40–59. *Dan Med Bull* 20:1, 1973.
48. Reid DD, Brett GZ, Hamilton PJS, et al. Cardiorespiratory disease and diabetes among middle-aged male civil servants: A study of screening and intervention. *Lancet* 1:469, 1974.
49. Hughson WG, Mann JI, Garrod A. Intermittent claudication: Prevalence and risk factors. *Br Med J* 1:1379, 1978.
50. DeBacker IG, Kornitzer M, Sobolski J, et al. Intermittent claudication—epidemiology and natural history. *Acta Cardiol* 34:115, 1979.
51. Schroll M, Munck O. Estimation of peripheral arteriosclerotic disease by ankle blood pressure: Measurements in a population study of 60-year-old men and women. *J Chron Dis* 34:261, 1981.
52. Reunanen A, Takkunen H, Aromaa A. Prevalence of intermittent claudication and its effect on mortality. *Acta Med Scand* 211:249, 1982.
53. Fowkes FGR, Housley E, Cawood EHH, et al. Edinburgh artery study: Prevalence of asymptomatic and symptomatic peripheral arterial disease in the general population. *Int J Epidemiol* 20:384–392, 1991.
54. Wilcosky T, Harris R, Weissfeld L. The prevalence and correlates of Rose questionnaire angina among women and men in the Lipid Research Clinics Program Prevalence Study Population. *Am J Epidemiol* 125:400–409, 1987.
55. La Croix AZ, Guralnik JM, Curb JD, et al. Chest pain and coronary heart disease mortality among older men and women in three communities. *Circulation* 81:437–446, 1990.
56. Criqui MH. Peripheral arterial disease and subsequent cardiovascular mortality: A strong and consistent association. *Circulation* 82:2246–2247, 1990.
57. Criqui MH, Fronek A, Barrett-Connor E, et al. The prevalence of peripheral arterial disease in a defined population. *Circulation* 71:510–515, 1985.
58. Criqui MH, Fronek A, Klauber MR, et al. The sensitivity, specificity, and predictive value of traditional clinical evaluation of peripheral arterial disease: Results from a non-invasive testing in a defined population. *Circulation* 71:516–521, 1985.
59. Kannel WB, Skinner JJ, Schwartz MJ, et al. Intermittent claudication: Incidence in the Framingham study. *Circulation* 41:875, 1970.
60. Dormandy J, Mahir M, Ascady G, et al. Fate of the patient with chronic leg ischaemia. *J Cardiovasc Surg* 30:50–57, 1989.
61. Gillum RF. Peripheral arterial occlusive disease of the extremities in the United States: Hospitalization and mortality. *Am Heart J* 120:1414–1418, 1990.
62. Criqui MH, Browner D, Fronek A, et al. Peripheral arterial disease in large vessels is epidemiologically distinct from small vessel disease: An analysis of risk factors. *Am J Epidemiol* 129:1110–1119, 1989.
63. Peabody CN, Kannel WB, McNamara PM. Intermittent claudication: Surgical significance. *Arch Surg* 109:693, 1974.
64. Hughson WG, Mann JI, Tibbs DJ, et al. Intermittent claudication: Factors determining outcome. *Br Med J* 1:1377, 1978.
65. Peabody CN, Kannel WB, McNamara PM. Intermittent claudication. *Arch Surg* 109:693–697, 1974.
66. Clifford PC, Davies PW, Hayne JA, et al. Intermittent claudication: Is a supervised exercise class worth while? *Br Med J* 280:1503, 1980.
67. Taylor LM, Porter JM. Drug treatment of claudication: Vasodilators, hemorrheologic agents, and anti-serotonin drugs. *J Vasc Surg* 3:374–381, 1986.
68. Belch JJF, McKay A, McArdle B, et al. Epoprostenol (prostacyclin) and severe arterial disease. *Lancet* 1:315–317, 1983.
69. Coffman JD. Vasodilator drugs in peripheral vascular disease. *N Engl J Med* 300:713–717, 1979.
70. Morin JF, Johnston KW, Wasserman L, et al. Factors that determine the long term results of percutaneous transluminal dilatation for peripheral arterial occlusive disease. *J Vasc Surg* 4:68–72, 1986.
71. Koltun WA, Gardiner A Jr, Harrington DP, et al. Thrombolysis in the treatment of peripheral arterial vascular occlusions. *Arch Surg* 122:901–905, 1987.
72. Van Breda A, Katzan BT, Deutsch AF. Urokinase vs. streptokinase in local thrombolysis. *Radiology* 65:109, 1987.
73. Tunis SR, Bass EB, Steinberg EP. The use of angioplasty, bypass surgery, and amputation in the man-

agement of peripheral vascular disease. *N Engl J Med* 325:556–562, 1991.
74. Veith FJ, Gupta SK, Wengerter KR, et al. Changing arteriosclerotic disease patterns and management strategies in lower-limb-threatening ischemia. *Ann Surg* 402–414, 1990.
75. Coffman JD. Intermittent claudication—Be conservative. *N Engl J Med* 325:577–578, 1991.

SECTION 3

Coronary Heart Disease: Risk Factors and Their Clinical Modification

CHAPTER 8

Hormones, Hormone Replacement Therapy, and Heart Disease

ROGERIO A. LOBO, M.D.

Reproductive hormones have extremely potent effects on many organ systems, including the cardiovascular (CV) system. Since heart disease is the leading cause of death in women, an in-depth understanding of the impact of reproductive hormones on the CV system is extremely important and will be the focus of this chapter.

The chapter is divided into four sections. First is a brief review of reproductive hormonal changes in premenopausal women as well as in the peri- and postmenopausal periods. The second section reviews the impact of estrogen deprivation on the CV system. Third, the effects of contraceptive steroids on the CV system are discussed, including an overview of the pharmacology of these agents. Finally, section four focuses on the treatment of postmenopausal (PM) women. The impact of estrogens and progestins on the CV system of PM women is discussed, and a discussion of the types of hormones available for "replacement" therapy and various prescribing regimens is also included.

REPRODUCTIVE ENDOCRINOLOGY

The ovary combines two important functions: gametogenesis and sex hormone production. The integration of ovarian steroid hormone biosynthesis and secretion with follicle maturation, ovulation, and corpus luteum function is essential for (1) the intraovarian control of morphologic and hormone activity, (2) hypothalamic-pituitary feedback control of gonadotropin release, which in turn regulates morphologic changes and steroid hormone production in the ovary, and (3) timing and support of events associated with fertilization and nidation through the effects of estradiol (E_2) or progesterone on tubal motility and secretion, endometrial proliferation, and the properties of cervical mucus. The functional interdependence of germ cells and hormone-producing cells, arranged in close anatomic proximity, allows the ovary to regulate the proper sequence of follicle maturation, ovulation, corpus luteum formation, and the ovary's function and regression through its own hormonal signals.

The hypothalamus and anterior pituitary regulate the sequence and extent of these morphologic and endocrine events in the ovary through the secretion of gonadotropin-releasing hormone and gonadotropins, respectively. Although both gonadotropins act synergistically, follicle-stimulating hormone (FSH) primarily stimulates follicle growth and luteinizing hormone (LH) mainly affects gonadal steroid biosynthesis. As shown in Figure 8–1, the granulosa cells of the developing follicle also secrete peptides that control the release of FSH. Inhibin inhibits, whereas activin stimulates FSH secretion. Another peptide not structurally related to the α and β chains of inhibin and activin is follistatin. This peptide, as the name implies, is inhibitory to FSH. In

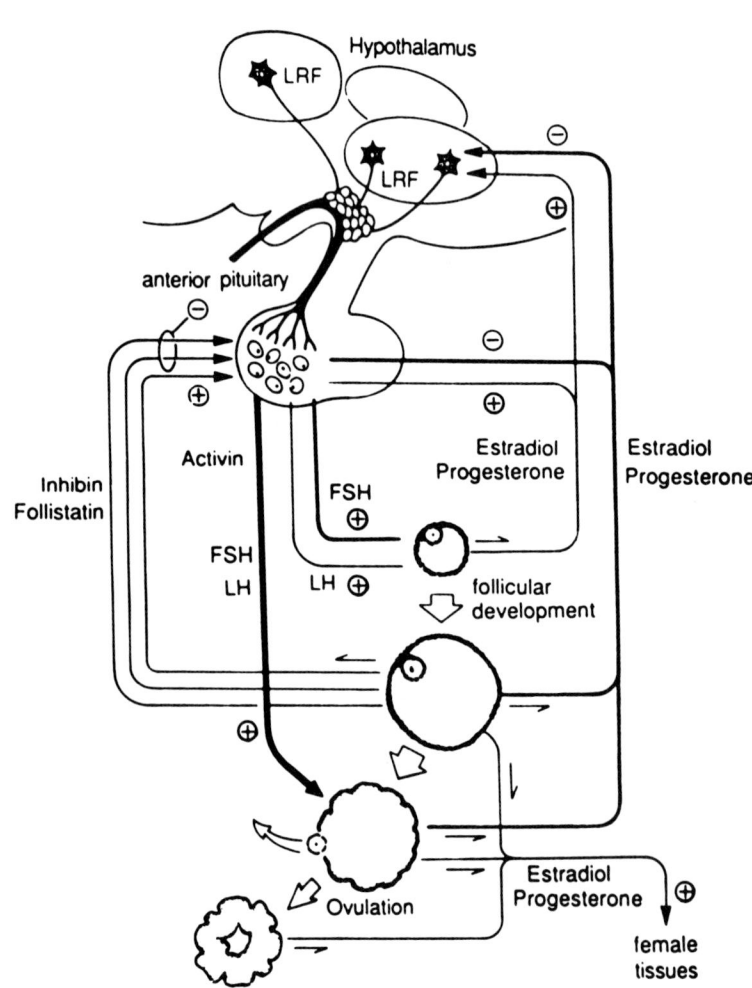

Figure 8–1. Inhibins, activins, and follistatins: Gonadal proteins modulating the secretion of follicle-stimulating hormone (FSH). LH = luteinizing hormone. LRF = luteinizing hormone releasing factor. (From Ying S. Inhibins, activins, and follistatins: Gonadal proteins modulating the secretion of follicle-stimulating hormone. *Endocrine Rev* 9:267, 1988.)

addition, inhibin, activin, follistatin, and a related peptide, transforming growth factor β, may also play a role in follicular E_2 production, exerting an autocrine function on granulosa cell steroidogenesis (1). Because inhibin is the secretory product of granulosa cells, levels in peripheral blood reflect the functional development of the follicle and parallel E_2 levels. In particular, inhibin is secreted in larger quantities after ovulation by luteinized granulosa cells (2) (Fig. 8–2).

We now understand that the ovary is not merely passive in its response to gonadotropin stimulation but has an active role in determining its own fate. In addition, multiple hormonal and growth factors produced by the theca and granulosa cells exert a paracrine and autocrine effect that influences development and steroidogenesis. Apart from the inhibin family of peptides, the pro-opiomelanocortin family, prostaglandins, renin, oxytocin, vasopressin, insulin-like growth factors, and binding protein(s) are all known to be involved, and this list is by no means complete. The oocyte within the antrum of the developing follicle is also nurtured in ways that are as yet incompletely understood. Granulosa cells apparently produce an oocyte maturation inhibitor. Small follicles may secrete factors that inhibit their luteinization, and larger follicles may be able to promote luteinization.

Androgens contribute to ovarian follicular E_2 production through aromatization. Both ovarian and adrenal androgens have the capacity to do this, but by far the predominant substrate is ovarian androstenedione and testosterone, which are produced by the theca cell. Although ovarian aromatization is under FSH control and is modified by the intraovarian factors discussed above (activin and transforming growth factor β produce positive effects; follistatin and inhibin produce inhibitory

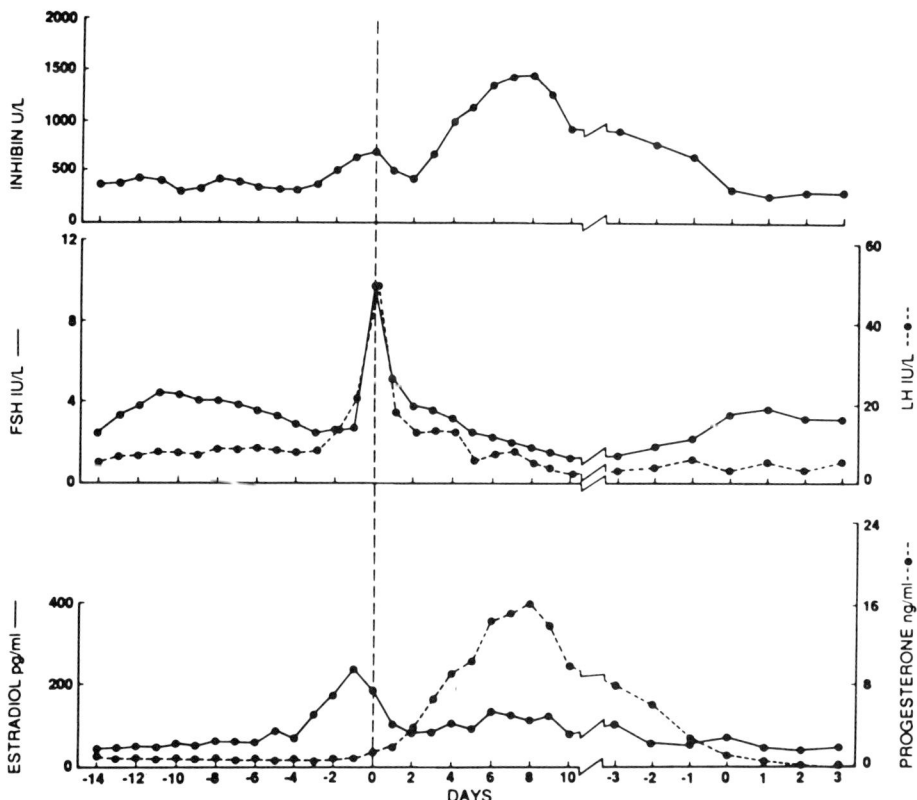

Figure 8–2. Serum inhibin, follicle-stimulating hormone, luteinizing hormone (LH), estradiol, and progesterone concentrations during the normal menstrual cycle. Data were normalized around the day of the LH surge (dotted line). The data are expressed as the geometric mean and 67% confidence limits with between four and six observations per point. The factors for conversion of values of SI units are estradiol (pg/mL × 3.671 = pmol/L) and progesterone (ng/mL × 3.180 = nmol/L). (Adapted from McLachlan RI, Robertson DM, Healy DL, et al. Circulating immunoreactive inhibin levels during the normal human menstrual cycle. *J Clin Endocrinol Metab* 65:954, 1987.)

effects), peripheral aromatization in adipose tissue is not under FSH control. As will be discussed below, the stromal cell of adipose tissue readily converts androstenedione to estrone (E_1), and E_1 is the predominant estrogen in PM women.

A discussion of the circulating levels of reproductive hormones achieved during the menstrual cycle is the key to our understanding of the physiologic actions of these hormones on the CV system as well as of what constitutes rational "replacement" therapy. Figure 8–2 depicts the menstrual cycle changes brought about by LH, FSH, E_2, and progesterone. Serum E_2 concentrations rise from less than 50 pg/mL in the early follicular phase to a midcycle (preovulatory) peak ranging from 200 to 500 pg/mL. Concentrations fall rapidly thereafter and rise again to a smaller but broader luteal phase serum E_2 peak of about 100 to 150 pg/mL. E_1 levels (not depicted) are always less than those of E_2 in ovulatory women and range from 30 to 150 pg/mL throughout the cycle. Progesterone levels are well below 1 ng/mL during the follicular phase, begin to rise at the onset of the midcycle LH surge, and reach about 10 to 20 ng/mL during the midluteal phase.

Androgen levels vary very little during the menstrual cycle, but small midcycle rises in androstenedione and testosterone have been reported. Levels of serum testosterone and androstenedione average 20 to 70 ng/dL and 0.5 to 2.8 ng/mL, respectively. Serum dehydroepiandrosterone sulfate is the predominant circulating adrenal androgen, and values ranging from 0.5 to 2.8 µg/mL do not change during the menstrual cycle.

THE PERIMENOPAUSAL TRANSITION

As the ovary fails, a more rapid decline occurs in the number of healthy follicles containing oocytes than the decline in hormonal secretion. As the total number of healthy granulosa cells declines, inhibin levels decrease, and since inhibin is a major inhibitor of FSH secretion, a monotropic FSH increase occurs as the earliest sign of impending ovarian failure. The elevation of FSH in women of older reproductive age is negatively correlated with the chance of achieving pregnancy (3). Although values of FSH above 40 mIU/mL usually signify a menopausal state, even "normal" values of around 20 mIU/mL may be associated with decreased fertility. Sherman and colleagues first described this monotropic FSH rise during the menopausal transition (4). Although menstrual cycles of normal length continue, cycles exhibit decreased total estrogen secretion, and FSH levels are elevated.

Although the perimenopausal period can span 5 or more years, this is a biologic variable that is not predictable on the basis of chronologic age. Although most women exhibit at least an episodic monotropic FSH rise in their early forties, some women show evidence of this rise prior to age 40. The average age of menopause (51.4 years) has not changed during the last 200 years. This age of menopause demonstrates a Gaussian distribution with a range from 40 to 58.

Consequences of the Menopausal Transition

Because of the episodic nature of FSH secretion, a single FSH level cannot be relied upon to signify the complete cessation of ovarian function. Typically, values wax and wane for some time before a sustained increase in FSH occurs. During this time, when fluctuating FSH values are often accompanied by some changes in the pattern of menstrual bleeding, a gradual increase in the rate of bone loss occurs (5). This bone loss is highly correlated with a reduction in total estrogen production. Although it is not the place of this review to discuss in any detail the effects of estrogen deprivation on bone loss, an analogy can be made here between these effects and the impact of estrogen deprivation on CV function. Just as it has been discovered that there are estrogen receptors in bone (6), arteries, including coronary vessels, have been found to contain sex steroid receptors (7, 8).

Other very early changes include symptoms of vasomotor instability, and this symptom may be a significant problem for some women. Vulvovaginal complaints tend to occur later in the postmenopausal period. The early vasomotor changes, which are the result of subtle but real decreases in estrogen production (often in the presence of FSH levels that are < 40 mIU/mL), demonstrate how estrogen influences vascular and catecholaminergic tone throughout the body. How these changes specifically relate to the occurrence of CV disease is still a matter of speculation.

HORMONAL CHANGES WITH ESTABLISHED MENOPAUSE

Figure 8–3 depicts the typical hormonal changes of PM women compared with those of ovulatory women in the early follicular phase. The most significant findings are the marked reductions in E_2 and E_1. Serum E_2 is reduced to a greater extent than E_1 because it is dependent on ovarian secretion, which has ceased. Serum E_1, on the other hand, is produced primarily by peripheral aromatization from androgens, which are not affected as dramatically. Levels of E_2 average 15 pg/mL and range from 10 to 25 pg/mL. In oophorectomized women, values are usually 10 pg/mL or less. Serum E_1 values average 30 pg/mL but may be higher in obese women because aromatization increases as a function of the mass of adipose tissue (9). Estrone sulfate (E_1S) is a stable circulating reservoir of estrogen, and its levels are the highest of any estrogen. In premenopausal women values are usually above 1000 pg/mL, and in PM women they average 350 pg/mL. A discussion of the interconversions between E_2, E_1, and E_1S may be found elsewhere (10).

Apart from elevations in FSH and LH, pituitary hormones are not affected. Specifically, growth hormone, thyroid-stimulating hormone, and adrenocorticotropic hormone levels are normal. Serum prolactin levels may be very slightly decreased because prolactin is somewhat influenced by estrogen status.

Both the postmenopausal ovary and the adrenal gland continue to produce androgen. That the ovary continues to produce androstenedione and testosterone but not E_2 has been documented (11), and this production has been shown to be at least partially dependent on gonadotropin (12). Androstenedione and testosterone levels are lower in women who have experienced bilateral oophorectomy, with values averaging 0.8 ng/mL and 10 ng/dL, respectively.

The adrenal also continues to produce androstenedione and dehydroepiandrosterone sulfate, and, primarily as a function of aging, these values decrease somewhat (adrenopause), although cortisol secretion remains unaffected. Although some controversy exists about the positive influence of estrogen on adrenal androgens (13), the predominant factor influencing the decreased levels of adrenal androgens is age. Androgens play an important role in providing substrate for aromatization and estrogen production as described.

THE EFFECTS OF ESTROGEN DEPRIVATION

It appears clear that estrogen deprivation increases the risk of CV disease in women. Data from the Framingham Study have been used to compare the incidence of CV disease in men and women as they age. Although the incidence is three times lower in women than in men prior to the menopause (3.1/1000 per year in women aged 45 to 49), it is approximately equal in men and women aged 75 to 79, being 53 and 50.4/1000 per year, respec-

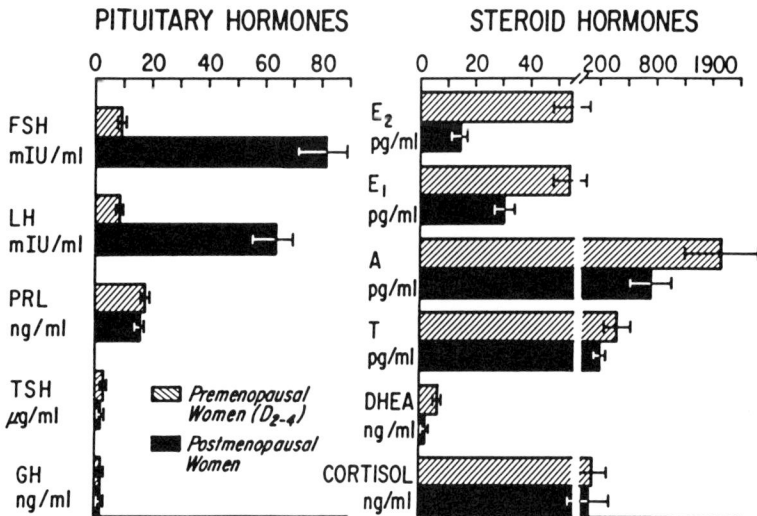

Figure 8–3. Circulating levels of pituitary and steroid hormones in postmenopausal women compared with levels in premenopausal women studied during the first week (days 2 to 4 [D_{2-4}]) of the menstrual cycle. FSH = follicle-stimulating hormone; LH = luteinizing hormone; PRL = prolactin; TSH = thyroid-stimulating hormone; GH = growth hormone; E_2 = estradiol; E_1 = estrogen; A = androstenedione; T = testosterone; DHEA = dehydroepiandrosterone. (From Yen SSC. The biology of menopause. *J Reprod Med* 18:287, 1977.)

tively (14). This trend also pertains to gender differences in mortality due to CV disease.

Although CV disease becomes more prevalent only in later years following a natural menopause, premature cessation of ovarian function (prior to menopause) constitutes an additional risk (15, 16). Premature menopause, occurring before age 35, was shown to increase the risk of myocardial infarction two- to threefold, and premature oophorectomy (prior to age 35) increased the risk sevenfold (15). What causes this increased risk?

When the possible reasons for gender differences in the increase in CV disease as a function of age are examined, the most relevant finding appears to be that total cholesterol rises at an accelerated rate in PM women. Although changes with age, weight, blood pressure, and blood glucose levels are not thought to be substantially different in men and women, the rate of rise in total cholesterol after menopause is significantly different (17) (Table 8–1). This increase in total cholesterol is explained by increases in levels of low-density lipoprotein cholesterol (LDL-C).

In the Framingham cross-sectional study, high-density lipoprotein cholesterol (HDL-C) was not found to decrease after menopause, although total cholesterol, LDL-C, and very low-density lipoprotein (VLDL) did increase. However, in a short-term longitudinal study (18), it was observed that after natural menopause, HDL-C did decrease with time. This is also in keeping with studies showing a decrease in HDL-C after the abrupt cessation of ovarian function such as occurs with oophorectomy or, as shown in some studies, after the use of a gonadotropin-releasing hormone analog (19).

Much significance has been attached to the changes that occur in HDL-C, specifically on the benefits achieved by raising HDL-C with estrogen "replacement" therapy in PM women. This effect, which is largely due to the increase in HDL_2-C with oral estrogen, will be reviewed below. Nevertheless, the changes in HDL-C after a natural menopause may not be marked, and HDL-C levels, for the most part, remain in the normal range. Curiously, in the Pittsburgh study (18), there were no changes in HDL_2-C and no HDL-C changes with estrogen treatment. It is my view, therefore, that although HDL-C changes are important, the increases that occur with estrogen (the raising of "normal" levels by up to 15%) may be viewed as pharmacologic and may not be as important as previously thought. Moreover, these alterations may merely be markers of other more important changes occurring in cholesterol transport. More data are clearly needed on the effects of estrogen deprivation and estrogen "replacement" on subspecies of LDL-C, oxidized forms of LDL-C, and lipoprotein(a) (Lp[a]). Our recent data suggest that some minor but important changes may occur in Lp(a) with estrogen (20).

Apart from the lipid hypothesis as reviewed briefly above, there is good reason to believe that estrogen has direct arterial effects. Therefore, the lack of arterial estrogen receptor activation in a state of estrogen deprivation may affect the endothelium in such a small way that atherosclerotic plaque formation is accelerated and vascular tone is similarly compromised. These effects will be discussed more specifically below.

THE EFFECTS OF SEX STEROIDS ON THE CV SYSTEM

Estrogens and progestins of various types have been prescribed alone and in various

Table 8–1. FRAMINGHAM STUDY: AVERAGES OF SOME CARDIOVASCULAR RISK FACTORS FOR MEN AND WOMEN, AGES 30 to 59 YEARS

	Blood Pressure				Serum Cholesterol		Blood Glucose	
	Systolic		Diastolic					
Age	Men	Women	Men	Women	Men	Women	Men	Women
30–34	125.2	116.7	79.3	73.5	210.0	198.0	80.0	78.1
35–39	127.6	119.6	81.6	76.0	223.8	204.8	79.2	79.7
40–44	131.1	125.6	84.0	79.7	228.6	219.2	81.5	80.6
45–49	130.9	133.9	84.2	83.2	229.7	230.4	84.7	82.4
50–54	135.6	144.7	85.7	87.5	229.9	247.4	84.9	84.1
55–59	140.7	151.5	85.3	88.0	229.2	257.1	84.1	86.8

From Kannel WB, Gordon T. Cardiovascular effects of the menopause. In Mishell DR Jr (Ed), *Menopause: Physiology and Pharmacology*. Chicago, Year Book, 1987, p. 91.

combinations for a variety of disorders. Since not all of these therapies and uses of sex steroids can be discussed, the primary focus here will be on the use of oral contraceptives and the noncontraceptive use of estrogen and progestins for "replacement" therapy in PM women. Specifically, the various types and potencies of the sex steroids will be described as well as their known effects on the CV system.

Oral Contraceptives

Oral contraceptives (OCs) currently contain a synthetic estrogen, ethinyl estradiol (EE_2), and a synthetic 19-nor progestin. The structure of these steroids together with native progesterone and E_2 is depicted in Figure 8–4.

The synthetic steroids are manyfold more potent than their naturally occurring counterparts, progesterone and E_2. In addition, because they are easy to manufacture and are orally efficacious, they have been used in OCs.

The primary mode of action of the OC is a negative feedback exerted on the hypothalamic-pituitary axis that results in inhibition of the ovulatory LH surge. Doses of both EE_2 and the progestins have been lowered substantially in the last 10 years. Now minimum combination doses of 30 to 35 μg of EE_2 with 0.4 or 0.5 mg of norethindrone or a similar 19-nor progestin are standard and are sufficient to inhibit ovulation. These fixed doses are combined in single tablets that are ingested for 21 days of a 28-day cycle. In contrast to these monophasic preparations, the alteration of the steroid content of the pills on different cycle days has led to the marketing of biphasic and triphasic OCs. The intent is to mimic the changes that occur during the menstrual cycle. However, since these are truly pharmacologic agents, in essence the net result is the same, and all the various formulations result in similar total doses of both EE_2 and progestin.

Assessment of the individual effects of either the estrogen or progestin component of OCs has been difficult because they are prescribed

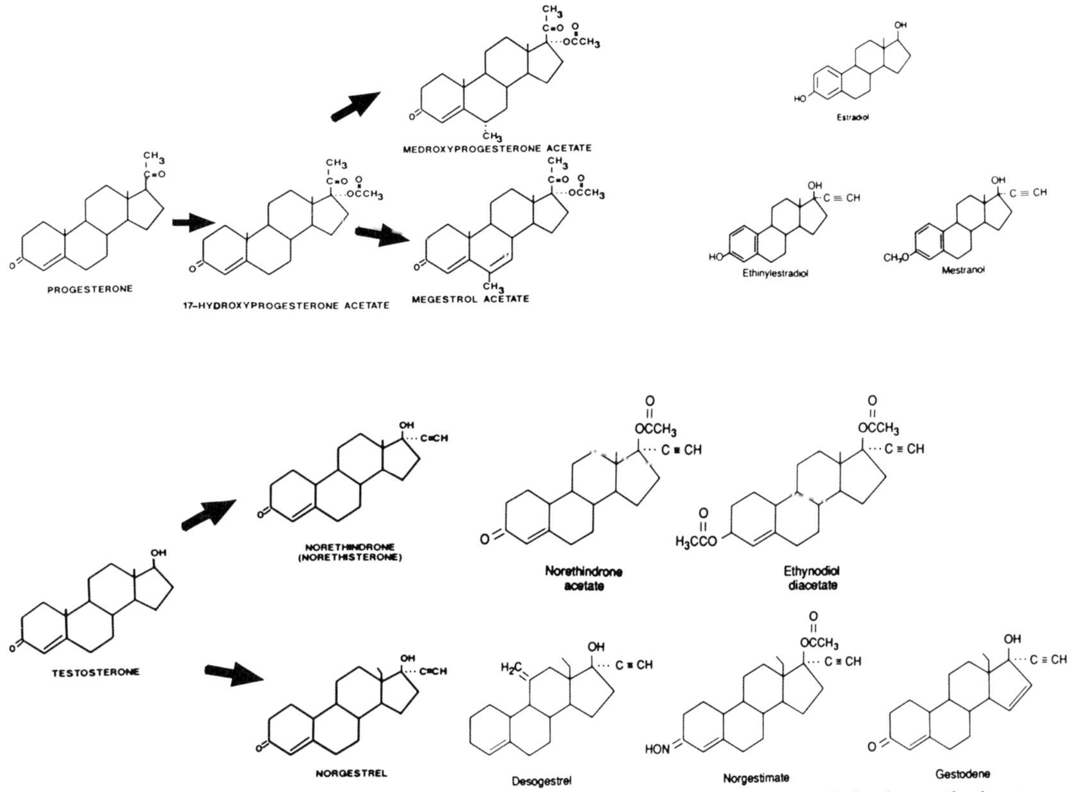

Figure 8–4. Sex steroid hormones. Progestins related to natural progesterone are at upper left, the synthetic estrogens ethinyl estradiol and mestranol are at upper right, and the 19-nor progestins, which are structurally more related to testosterone, are on the bottom. The newest progestins are desogestrel, norgestimate, and gestodene and are derivatives of norgestrel.

in combination and because they often have divergent effects on the same parameter. Thus, the balance or ratio between EE_2 and the progestin component of the pill is extremely important in understanding the metabolic and potential CV effects of OCs. A discussion of the relative potency of these compounds is therefore warranted.

With oral ingestion, the "first passage" effect of estrogen stimulates hepatic globulin production. Our studies have suggested that in this regard, EE_2 is 200- to 1000-fold more potent than native E_2 (21). Thus, 35 µg of EE_2 in combination OCs is at least equivalent to 7 mg of oral estrogen, more than 10 times the "replacement" doses of estrogen used routinely by PM women. This difference in potency helps to explain why certain risk factors associated with estrogen use (e.g., coagulopathy and hypertension, which are discussed below) are not relevant in terms of estrogen replacement doses used for PM women.

The 19-nor progestins, because they are derived from 19-nor ethinyl testosterone (see Fig. 8–4), have inherent androgenic properties in addition to being extremely potent progestins. The "androgenicity" of these compounds, which is somewhat offset by the estrogen component, is largely responsible for the potential metabolic disturbances associated with OC use.

The progestational activity of norethindrone is 300 to 500 times greater than that of progesterone. Although norethindrone, norethindrone acetate, and ethynodiol acetate are clinically equipotent, norgestrel is 3 to 5 times more potent, and levonorgestrel, the active component of norgestrel, is 6 to 10 times more potent. In terms of androgenicity, again, although progesterone is essentially devoid of androgen receptor binding, norethindrone and norethindrone acetate and ethynodiol diacetate are all moderately androgenic and are essentially equal in this regard. Even 1 mg of norethindrone taken orally decreases HDL-C, whereas doses as high as 200 to 300 mg of progesterone are devoid of this effect. The most androgenic 19-nor progestins are norgestrel and levonorgestrel, which are 5 to 9 times more potent than norethindrone (22).

A new generation of 19-nor progestins for oral contraceptive use has emerged. These progestins (see Fig. 8–4) are metabolites of norgestrel and have increased progestational potency without a commensurate increase in androgenic potency. Because of this, very low (microgram) doses can be used in OCs, resulting in very low, if any, androgenic effects. Thus, with doses of 30 to 35 µg of EE_2, these combination OCs result in very favorable metabolic profiles.

What Are the CV Concerns of OCs?

Current low-dose OCs are extremely safe, and there are no real concerns regarding CV safety. The potential concerns discussed below include hypertension, coagulopathy, stroke, carbohydrate intolerance, and myocardial infarction.

Hypertension

Elevations in blood pressure with OCs occur in approximately 5% of cases. This effect can be viewed as an idiosyncratic reaction in much the same way that hypertension has been described in PM women using conjugated equine estrogens (see below). Although it has been suggested that this situation might arise because of estrogen-induced elevations in renin substrate, this elevation occurs in both normotensive and hypertensive pill users. Although it was thought to be related to the dose of estrogen, it occurs even with the lower dose estrogen formulations (23). Some evidence has suggested that a high molecular weight moiety of renin substrate may be increased in patients who develop hypertension (24).

There are no good ways of determining whether a women is at risk for developing hypertension while taking OCs. Although pregnancy-induced hypertension is not a risk factor, women with OC-induced hypertension are more predisposed to develop hypertension in pregnancy. In general, women who have existing hypertension are not candidates for OCs. However, in treated and well-controlled hypertensives, low-dose OCs may be prescribed with close patient monitoring if maximal contraceptive efficacy is desired.

The Risk of Venous Thrombosis

Because estrogen increases various procoagulant factors in blood (factors II, VII, IX, and X), it has been generally assumed that estrogen increases the risk of venous thrombosis. High-dose formulations have been linked to an increased risk of venous thrombosis (two- to fourfold increased risk for superficial and deep vein thrombophlebitis, respectively). However, this risk occurs only during OC use and disappears within 6 weeks upon discontinuation. Lower dose formulations (30 μg EE_2) are essentially devoid of this risk, and recent studies have confirmed the declining rate of venous thrombosis with the lower dose formulations (25).

There is some evidence that venous thrombosis in OC users has been overreported and that these reports may not have been accurate (26). Much of the associated risk is known to be magnified by smoking. This qualification pertains to the risk of arterial thrombosis as well, which will be discussed below. In nonsmoking women, the risk of thrombosis appears to be very small.

With low-dose OCs, there is an increase in fibrinolytic activity, and this may offset the increase in procoagulant factors (27). Most recently, it was shown that with a new low-dose formulation, plasminogen levels and fibrinolytic activity were markedly increased, platelet aggregation was decreased, and the prothrombin and partial thromboplastin times were unchanged (28).

Carbohydrate Intolerance

It has generally been accepted that it is the progestin component of the OC formulation that contributes to a diabetogenic state. Indeed, high-dose progestin formulations have led to abnormal responses to the glucose tolerance test in 4–16% of women (29, 30). This effect has also been thought to be related to the androgenicity of the progestin, with pills containing levonorgestrel having the greatest incidence of hyperinsulinemia and glucose intolerance.

However, with the lowering of the progestin component of OCs in monophasic and triphasic formulations, including those containing levonorgestrel, only minimal effects have been noted on glucose tolerance (31). Recently, the degree of impairment has been assessed in postpartum gestational diabetics (32). The conclusions suggest that even in this susceptible population, low-dose OCs appear to be safe.

Mechanistically, recent data have challenged the concept that it is the 19-nor progestin component that causes insulin resistance. Using computer modeling data obtained from a cross-sectional study employing the intravenous glucose tolerance test, it has been suggested that it is the potent estrogen (EE_2) that explains insulin resistance and that the progestin component merely modifies this response by altering insulin half-life (33). More data are needed to clarify this issue.

Although use of OCs in the gestational or mild type II diabetic may be justified, more controversy surrounds the use of OCs in those with type I or juvenile diabetes because of the known rampant progression of vascular disease. Since it is now generally accepted that OCs are not atherogenic, they may be considered if close assessment of other risk factors (blood pressure, triglyceride levels) is done and close monitoring (renal, ophthalmologic, etc.) is maintained. This is particularly relevant when the risk of pregnancy may be greater than the theoretical concerns associated with OC use in this setting.

Arterial Thrombosis and Myocardial Infarction

Substantial energy has been exerted to determine the risks associated with altered lipoprotein profiles in OC users, particularly as these pertain to the risk of atherosclerosis. Indeed, although older formulations containing high progestin doses were found to reduce HDL-C and to raise LDL-C and triglyceride levels, the newer low-dose formulations are essentially lipid neutral. At least two lines of evidence suggest that OCs are not atherogenic. The first line derives from epidemiologic data, and the second is based on data extrapolated from experiments in the cynomolgus monkey.

Data from Croft and Hannaford (34) and Stampfer et al. (35) have shown definitively that there is no increased risk of myocardial infarction with present or past use of OCs. In the study of the Royal College of General Practitioners (36), previous and current use relative risks (RRs) were 1 and 1.8, respectively. A summary of the RRs for major coronary disease from the Stampfer data is depicted in Table 8–2. Further, deaths due to ischemic heart disease and cerebrovascular dis-

Table 8–2. RELATIVE RISK OF MAJOR CORONARY DISEASE AMONG PAST USERS OF ORAL CONTRACEPTIVES BASED ON DURATION OF USE

Duration of Use (Yr)	No. Cases	Relative Risk	95% Confidence Interval
None	339	1.0	—
<1	45	1.0	0.7–1.4
1–3	32	1.0	0.7–1.4
3–5	20	1.0	0.6–1.7
5–10	25	0.8	0.5–1.2
<10	10	0.7	0.4–1.2

From Stampfer MJ, Willett WC, Colditz GA, et al. A prospective study of past use of oral contraceptive agents and risk of cardiovascular diseases. *N Engl J Med* 319:1313, 1988.

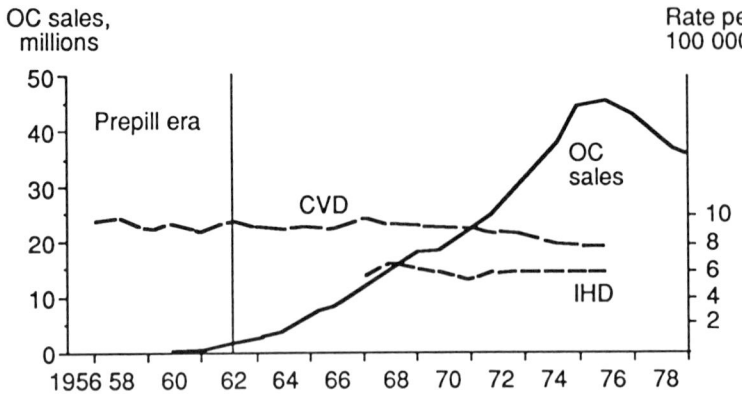

Figure 8–5. Mortality rates in women taking oral contraceptives (OCs), aged 15 to 44 years inclusive, per 100,000 population in England and Wales for cerebrovascular disease (CVD) and ischemic heart disease (IHD). (From Wiseman RA, MacRae KD. Oral contraceptives and the decline in mortality from circulatory disease. *Fertil Steril* 35:277, 1981.)

ease in England and Wales have remained constant or declined while the use of OCs has increased (37) (Fig. 8–5). Finally, in an angiographic study of 76 young women post myocardial infarction, significant atherosclerosis was twice as high in women not using OCs (38). The mechanism, therefore, of myocardial infarction in women taking OCs is *not* atherosclerosis but appears to be related to arterial thrombosis. This condition in turn is almost entirely confined to women who smoke.

The second line of evidence comes from data obtained from the cynomolgus monkey model. Here, Adams and coworkers (39) showed definitively that despite lowered HDL-C levels due to high doses of progestin and a high-fat diet, the OC users had reduced atherosclerosis at necropsy. This "protection" was apparently afforded by the high EE_2 content of the formulation and was not found when the progestin levonorgestrel with its HDL-C–lowering effects was combined with only physiologic amounts of E_2–17β (Fig. 8–6). The effects of estrogen on arteries will be described in greater detail below.

The risks, therefore, of arterial thrombosis and myocardial infarction in OC users occur in women who smoke, particularly if they are over the age of 35. Also, the history of pregnancy-induced hypertension, diabetes, or essential hypertension in this setting magnifies this risk (40). Thus, in nonsmokers, the risk of OCs is low for all CV diseases, including stroke. The RR of stroke with OC use as a function of the duration of use in nonsmokers is not significantly increased, and the RR was found to range from 0.8 to 1.4 (35).

A major harmful interaction, therefore, apparently occurs when a woman who receives OCs also smokes. Data from our group have suggested that this effect might be related to a reduction in prostacyclin and an increase in platelet-derived thromboxane in this setting (41) (Fig. 8–7).

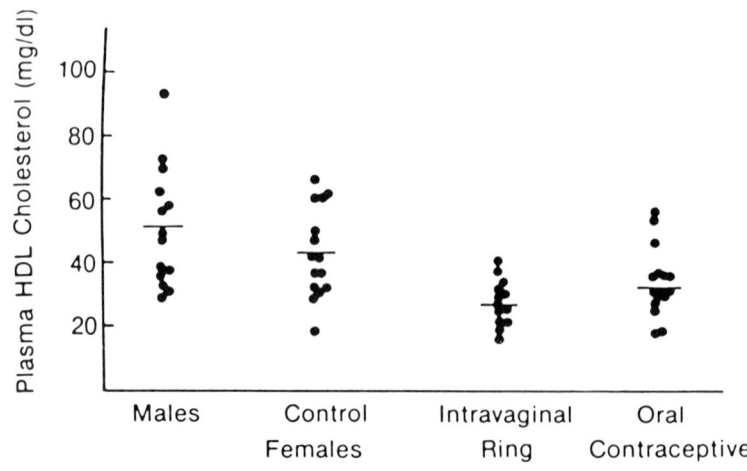

Figure 8–6. Plasma high-density lipoprotein (HDL) cholesterol concentrations among four experimental groups. Females using intravaginal rings and oral contraceptives show no differences (p > .2); both have lower plasma HDL cholesterol than males (p < .02) and control females (p < .02). Males and control females show no differences (p > .2). (From Adams MR, Clarkson TB, Koritnik DR, et al. Contraceptive steroids and coronary artery atherosclerosis in cynomolgus macaques. *Fertil Steril* 47:1010, 1987.)

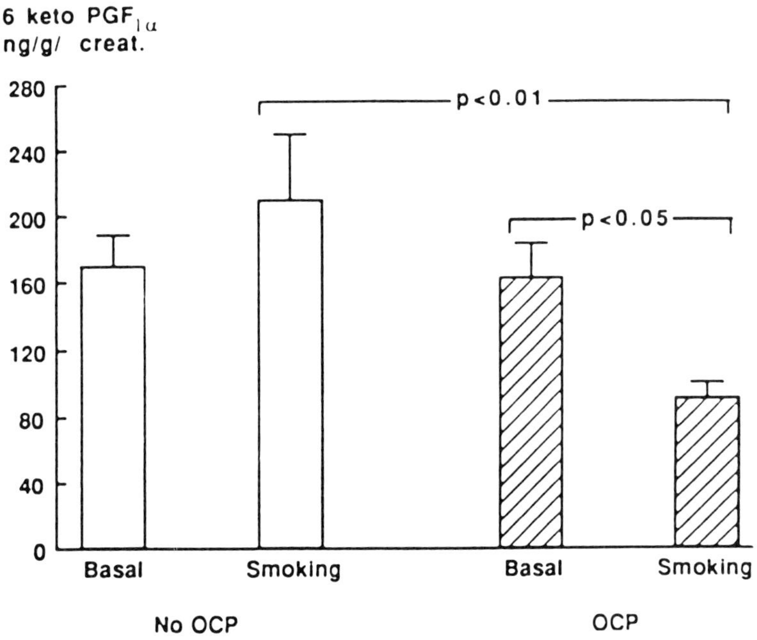

Figure 8–7. Comparison of 6-keto-prostaglandin $F_1\alpha$ (6-keto-$PGF_1\alpha$) excretion while abstaining from smoking (basal) and inhaling cigarette smoke (smoking) in women not using (open bars) or using (solid bars) oral contraceptives (OCP). (Adapted from Mileikowsky GN, Nadler JL, Huey F, et al. Evidence that smoking alters prostacyclin formation and platelet aggregation in women who use oral contraceptives. *Am J Obstet Gynecol* 159:1547, 1988.)

Hormonal Replacement Therapy for PM Women

As stated earlier, there are vast differences between the potencies of the native or natural estrogens, E_2 and E_1, and EE_2 (21). Therefore, many of the concerns regarding OCs and CV disease, which may not even be relevant as described above, are really not concerns at all for women taking natural replacement estrogens.

In terms of relative potency and the stimulation of hepatic globulins, E_1 and E_2 are equipotent, and conjugated equine estrogens are approximately three times more potent because of the equine components. The principal equine component (25%) is equilin sulfate, which has direct and independent hepatic effects (42). Even so, only minor changes in hepatic globulins occur with conjugated equine estrogens.

Depicted in Figure 8–8 are the pharmacokinetic effects of orally administered E_1S and micronized E_2 in PM women. Peak levels are achieved 4 to 6 hours later, and regardless of whether E_1 or E_2 is administered, E_1 circulates in serum predominantly. Table 8–3 depicts the serum concentrations of various estrogens, including conjugated equine estrogens (43), but note that the serum levels of the equine component in conjugated equine estrogens have not been measured. In terms of "physiologic" replacement, using the earlier described hormonal events of the menstrual cycle, oral E_1S doses of 0.625 and 1.25 mg, E_2 doses of 1 and 2 mg, and conjugated equine estrogen doses of 0.625 mg and perhaps 0.9 mg fit into this category. Achieving these levels of hormones should expose a woman to no more steroid than would occur endogenously during the normal menstrual cycle. For transdermal estrogens, both the 0.05- and 0.1-mg E_2 patch achieve "physiologic" replacement averaging

Table 8–3. APPROXIMATE SERUM ESTRONE AND ESTRADIOL LEVELS AFTER VARIOUS DOSES AND TYPES OF ORAL ESTROGEN REPLACEMENT

	Estrone (pg/mL)	Estradiol (pg/mL)
Conjugated equine estrogen (mg)		
0.3	76	19
0.625	153	40
1.25	200	60
Piperazine estrone sulfate (mg)		
0.6	125	34
1.2	200	42
Micronized estradiol (mg)		
1	150	40
2	250	60
Estradiol valerate (mg)		
1	160	50
2	300	60

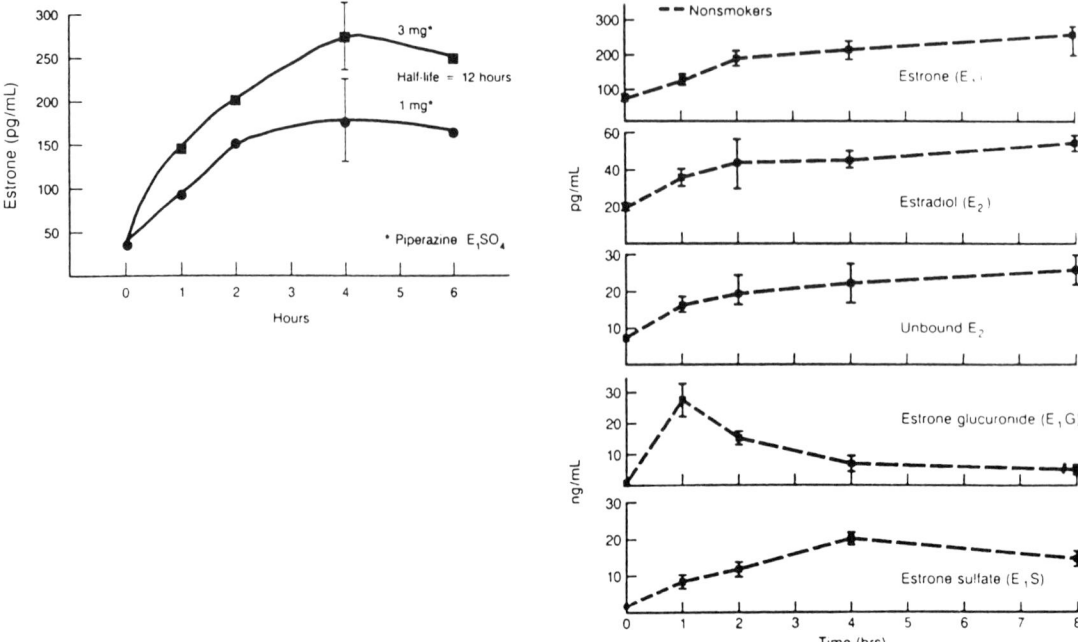

Figure 8–8. Serum estrogen levels after oral estrone sulfate (*left* [from Anderson ABM, Sklovsky E, Sayers K, et al. *Br Med J* 1:140, 1978]) and after 1 mg of oral 17β-estradiol (*right* [from Lobo RA, Cassidenti DL. Pharmacokinetics of oral 17β-estradiol. *J Reprod Med* 37:77, 1992.])

40 to 50 and 70 to 80 pg/mL, respectively (44). A wider range than this, however, can occur. Unlike oral estrogens, with transdermal E_2 delivery, serum E_2 is the predominant circulating estrogen, and E_1 levels are less. A more in-depth review of the pharmacokinetics of various preparations may be found elsewhere (43).

Postmenopausal estrogen use substantially reduces the risk of CV disease and reduces both CV mortality as well as all-cause mortality (45, 46, 47). Although this statement will be reviewed in greater detail below, a brief discussion of the manner in which estrogen affects various aspects of CV function will be reviewed first. This discussion includes the effects of estrogen on blood pressure, carbohydrate tolerance, coagulation, and lipids and lipoproteins. In marked contrast to the previously reviewed effects of OCs, which are minimal but potentially deleterious, many of the effects of natural estrogen on these parameters are beneficial.

Blood Pressure

Natural estrogens either impart no change in blood pressure or lower it in the majority of both normotensive and hypertensive women so treated. As stated above, in approximately 5% of PM women, an idiosyncratic elevation of blood pressure has been observed with the use of conjugated equine estrogens (48). However, the occurrence of sensitivity to this estrogen is rare and does not contraindicate other forms of estrogen replacement. Figure 8–9 illustrates the lowering of blood pressure in both hypertensive and normotensive women receiving two doses of micronized E_2 (49). These changes are compatible with data showing a vasodilatory effect of estrogen resulting in increased blood flow.

Carbohydrate Intolerance

As stated above, OCs may contribute to glucose intolerance in some women. However, there does not appear to be any deleterious effect of natural estrogen replacement on carbohydrate metabolism in PM women. Postmenopausal estrogen users have been found to have a reduced frequency of diabetes. Indeed, there is evidence that estrogen used alone may be beneficial in that estrogen may improve insulin action (50). Recent cross-sectional data have shown that estrogen may improve glucose

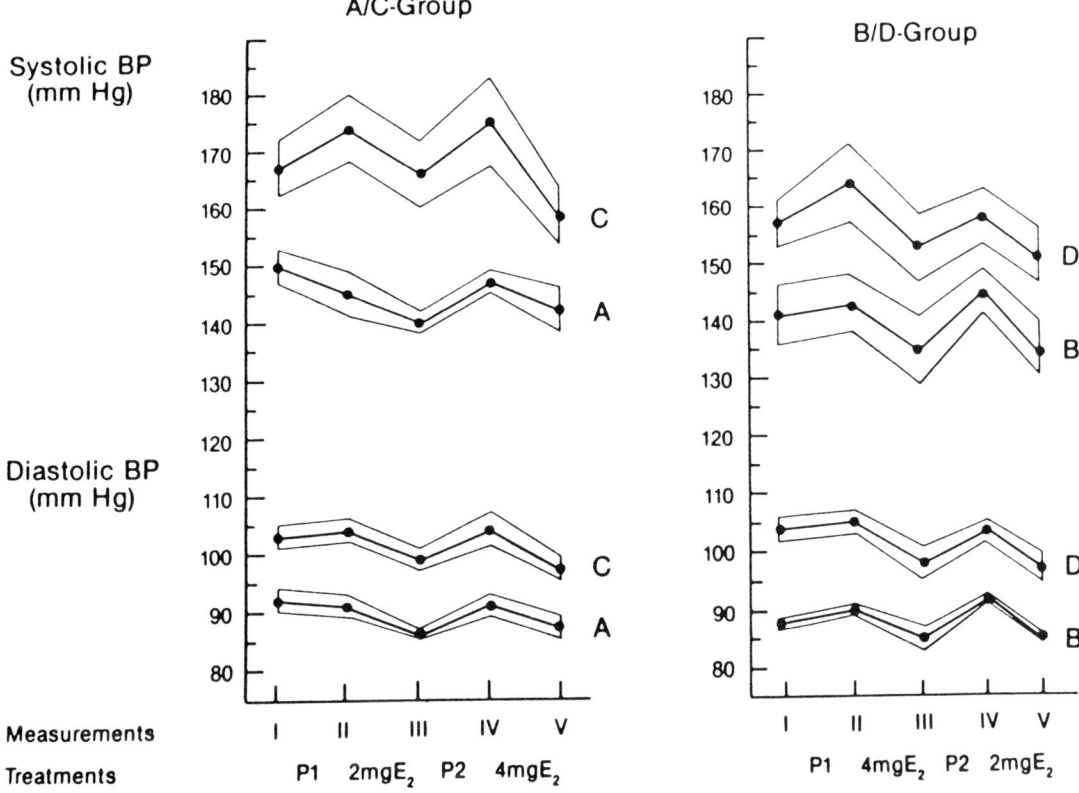

Figure 8–9. The effect of micronized estradiol (E_2) on diastolic and systolic blood pressure in normotensive women (A and B groups) and hypertensive women (C and D groups). Shown are mean values ± standard error of the mean (SEM) for blood pressure in the supine position. P = placebo. (From Luotola H. Blood pressure and hemodynamics in postmenopausal women during estradiol-17β substitution. *Ann Clin Res* 15:1, 1983.)

tolerance in PM women (51). Our own prospective data have shown that doses of 0.625 mg of conjugated equine estrogens may decrease insulin resistance and increase insulin sensitivity in PM women. This effect may be attenuated somewhat by added progestin (52).

Coagulation

Although the EE_2 content of OCs has been implicated in thromboembolic risk because of increases in levels of procoagulant factors produced by the liver, this does not occur with natural estrogen replacement. Figure 8–10 shows a similar effect of oral E_1S and placebo on factor X activity, whereas 30 μg of the 3-methyl ether of EE_2 (mestranol) has a potentially deleterious effect. Conjugated equine estrogens administered with and without progestin, in doses of 0.625 and 1.25 mg daily, have been shown not to have a deleterious effect on procoagulant factors (53, 54). A recent case control study has confirmed that there is no increased risk of thromboembolic phenomena occurring with estrogen replacement (55). In the editorial accompanying this report (56), it was suggested that although the risk of coagulopathy in "normal" PM women is not increased, there are women who are more susceptible to the effects of estrogen. These women are difficult to identify by routine blood tests. In patients with a history of coagulation problems associated with exposure to increased levels of estrogen (pregnancy, OCs) or even with routine replacement therapy, great caution should be exercised. In this setting, "physiologic" replacement with transdermal E_2 might be considered, thus bypassing the hepatic "first passage" effect. Monitoring serum E_2 levels would ensure that an acceptable range of estrogen is achieved.

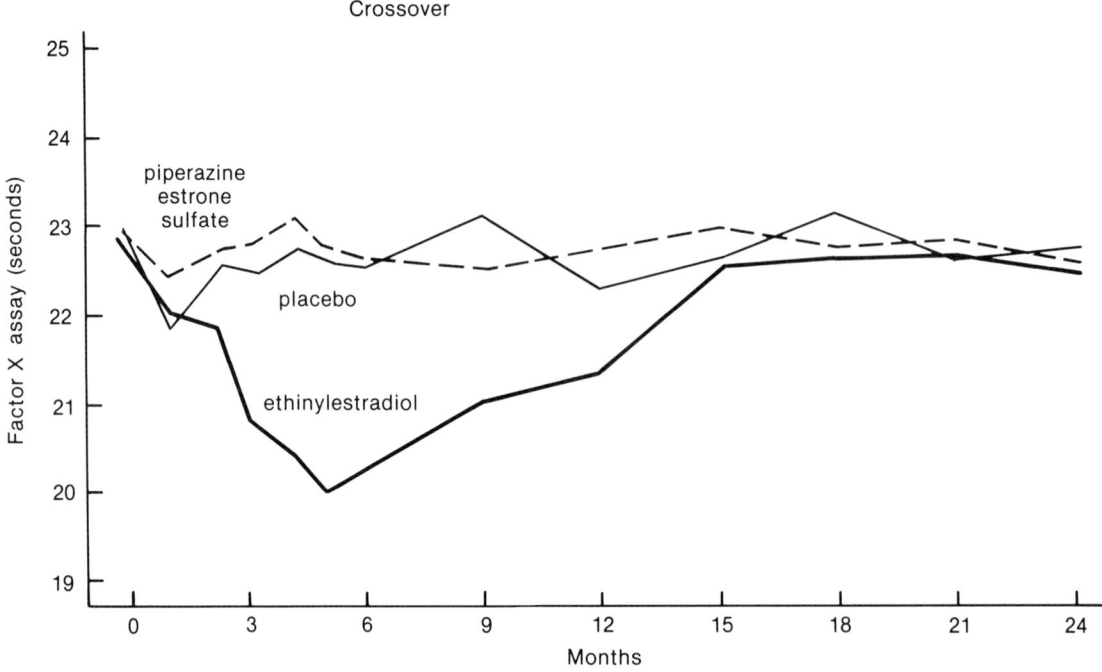

Figure 8–10. Factor X assays during an initial 6-month comparative trial and during the following 18 months after crossover to piperazine estrone sulfate (3 mg/day). (From Aylward M, Maddock J, Lewis PA, et al. Oestrogen replacement therapy and blood clotting. *Curr Med Res Opin* [Suppl. 3]:83, 1977.)

Lipids and Lipoproteins

The effects of estrogen on lipids and lipoproteins are not considered to be a risk factor; in fact, the reverse is the case. These effects have been thought to be the primary cardioprotective feature of estrogen replacement therapy. Details of this interaction have been reviewed recently (57) and may be found in Chapter 9 of this volume. Figure 8–11 depicts a summary of the changes expected with oral estrogen use (the equivalent of 0.625 mg of conjugated equine estrogens). The principal cardioprotective benefit is thought to be related to the increase in HDL-C (specifically, HDL_2-C) and the lowering of LDL-C, which is more variable.

The only potential cause for concern with

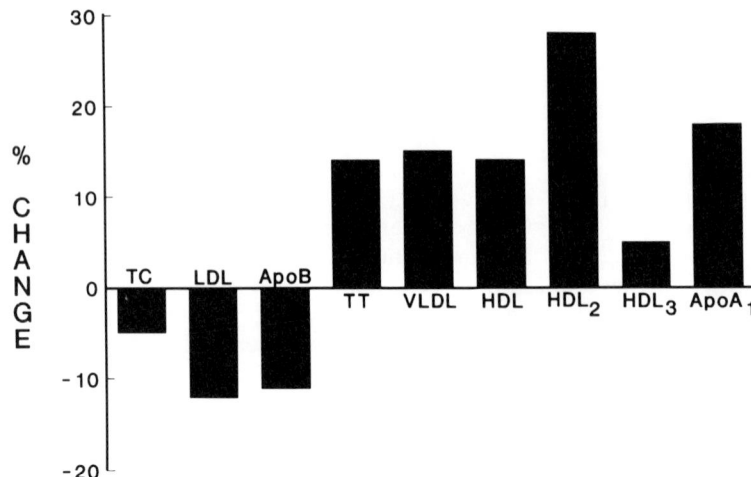

Figure 8–11. Percentage of changes in lipids and lipoproteins with the use of oral estrogen (equivalent to 0.625 mg for at least 3 months). TC = total cholesterol; TT = total triglycerides; LDL = low-density lipoproteins. HDL = high-density lipoproteins. VLDL = very low density lipoproteins; Apo B = apoprotein B. (From Lobo RA. Effects of hormonal replacement on lipids and lipoproteins in postmenopausal women. *J Clin Endocrinol Metab* 73:925, 1991.)

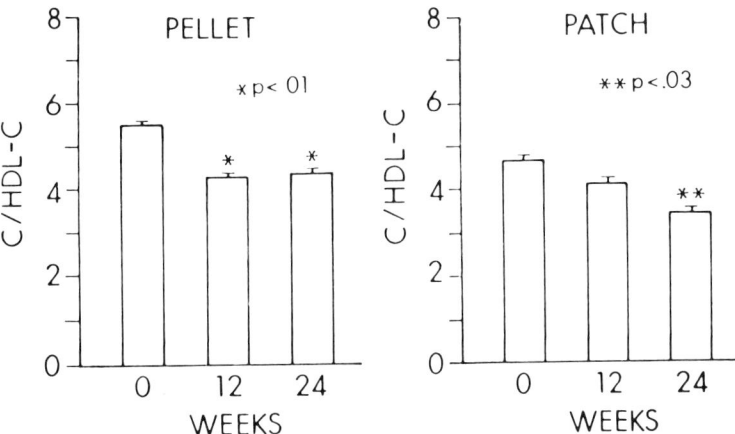

Figure 8–12. Mean (± SE) serum total cholesterol (C), high-density lipoprotein cholesterol (HDL-C) ratio before and during 12 and 24 weeks of subdermal (pellet) and transdermal (patch) estradiol treatment. The significance of difference in the comparison of the C/HDL-C ratios at 12 and 24 weeks with the baseline value is represented as *p < .01 and **p < .03. (From Stanczyk FZ, Shoupe D, Nunez V, et al. A randomized comparison of nonoral estradiol delivery in postmenopausal women. *Am J Obstet Gynecol* 159:1540, 1988.)

oral estrogen use is hypertriglyceridemia. This change is highly variable, with some women showing very small changes with oral estrogen and others showing a dramatic increase. Indeed, in these rare patients, oral estrogen may not be the preferable route of administration. The changes in all lipoproteins are thought to be dose dependent, but it has been suggested that by keeping doses of conjugated equine estrogens to 0.625 mg, total triglycerides and the triglyceride content of lipoproteins will be kept to a low percentage (58). Although it is generally thought that there is an important dose response increase in HDL-C with oral estrogen, a saturation effect does occur, and near maximum benefit is thought to be achieved with doses of 0.625 mg of conjugated equine estrogens (57, 58).

Nonoral forms of estrogen replacement do not achieve the same degree of stimulation of HDL-C and HDL_2-C, but sufficient doses of estrogen, prescribed for at least 6 months, have resulted in significant elevations in HDL-C and a lowering of the C/HDL ratio (44) (Fig. 8–12). With nonoral routes of administration, as illustrated in this figure, triglyceride levels are not increased.

The Cardioprotective Effects of Estrogens

At least 15 cohort (prospective) studies on postmenopausal estrogen use have shown that there is a significantly reduced risk of CV disease when either fatal or nonfatal myocardial infarction was used as an end point (RR range: 0.3 to 0.7). Two recent meta-analyses have been carried out by Bush and Stampfer (45, 46) to evaluate the effect of estrogen on coronary heart disease risk, and both have come to nearly identical conclusions. The calculated RR for all studies taken together was 0.56 (0.5 to 0.61) (46); by including only those studies that were angiographic, prospective, and internally controlled, the RR was 0.5 (0.43 to 0.56). For mortality specifically, the RR was also similar. This CV effect has been demonstrated to occur in all age and socioeconomic groups but does not appear to be dose related. In the United States the data have been derived virtually exclusively with the use of conjugated equine estrogens (0.625 or 1.25 mg). Mortality from stroke in one study (59) was also shown to be reduced by 40–50%, and here a small trend toward a dose response relationship was found. The effect of estrogen in reducing stroke mortality has not been confirmed by other studies.

Because of the high fatality rate attributable to ischemic heart disease, an RR of 0.5 translates into many lives saved among estrogen users. This number has been estimated to be 5250 for every 100,000 estrogen users in the age range 50 to 75 years (60) (Table 8–4) or 333 lives annually (for ischemic heart disease and stroke) per 100,000 estrogen users in the age group 65 to 74 years. This change in mortality is greater than that for any other disease potentially influenced by estrogen, including endometrial cancer and breast cancer.

That postmenopausal estrogen use retards the progression of atherosclerosis is now becoming more widely accepted. Estrogen use has been associated with a reduction in angiographically defined coronary artery disease among women with chest pain as well as a reduction in the probability of finding severe

Table 8–4. ESTIMATED CHANGES IN MORTALITY INDUCED BY DAILY ESTROGEN REPLACEMENT THERAPY (0.625 mg) IN WOMEN AGED 50 to 75 YEARS

Condition	Relative Risk	Cumulative Change in Mortality/100,000
Osteoporotic fractures	0.4	− 563
Gallbladder disease	1.5	+ 2
Endometrial cancer	2.0	+ 63[a]
Breast cancer	1.1	+ 187
Ischemic heart disease	0.5	− 5250
	Net change	− 5561
	Net % change	− 41%

[a]Case fatality rate estimate at 0.05
From Henderson BE, Ross RK, Paganini-Hill A, et al. Estrogen use and cardiovascular disease. *Am J Obstet Gynecol* 154:1181, 1986.

occlusive disease (odds ratio: 0.4) (61, 62). Among women with greater than 70% coronary artery occlusion, the 10-year survival is significantly greater (97%) in estrogen users and is only 65% in nonusers of estrogen (63). The benefit of estrogen also appears to be related to the duration of use. In the Leisure World cohort study (47), all-cause mortality was reduced by 40% with 15 or more years of estrogen use. Although this improvement in mortality was primarily due to a reduction in deaths due to CV disease, other causes, including cancer, were also reduced.

The mechanisms of the cardioprotective effect of estrogen in PM women are not clear. Epidemiologic evidence has suggested that this effect is "substantially" mediated by the increase in HDL-C with the use of oral estrogen (45). However, it is clear that there are other important effects of estrogen. The raising of HDL-C may be responsible for no more than 30–40% of the ascribed benefit of estrogen replacement therapy. The raising of normal HDL-C levels may be viewed as a pharmacologic yet beneficial response. However, this change in HDL-C may be merely a marker of other changes in lipoprotein metabolism that includes reverse cholesterol transport.

A growing body of data supports the notion that the cardioprotective effects of estrogen are mediated directly by the effects of estrogen on the arterial wall. Whether the mechanism is related primarily to direct changes in arterial tone or to changes in lipoprotein metabolism in the arterial wall is not clear, and there is evidence that both mechanisms are operative. The uptake of LDL-C by the arterial wall has been shown to be enhanced by estrogen (64).

Studies in the macaque monkey have shown that coronary atherosclerosis is significantly reduced in monkeys fed a high-fat diet even when HDL-C has been reduced, as reviewed earlier (39) (see Fig. 8–6). This effect has been ascribed to the potent effects of EE_2. In a postmenopausal macaque model, oophorectomized monkeys developed significant coronary atherosclerosis but were protected from this effect if they received nonoral estrogen replacement or estrogen with progesterone (65) (Fig. 8–13). With this nonoral hormonal regimen, HDL-C levels were not affected. When these monkeys were challenged with acetylcholine, the coronary arteries of the nontreated monkeys demonstrated a constriction response characteristic of endothelial damage due to atherosclerosis, whereas the monkeys with estrogen replacement did not (66) (Fig. 8–14). These and other data suggest that estrogen affects the endothelium and causes the production of factors such as endothelial-derived relaxing factor.

Another mechanism that may be operative is a more favorable prostacyclin-thromboxane balance with estrogen. We have shown that

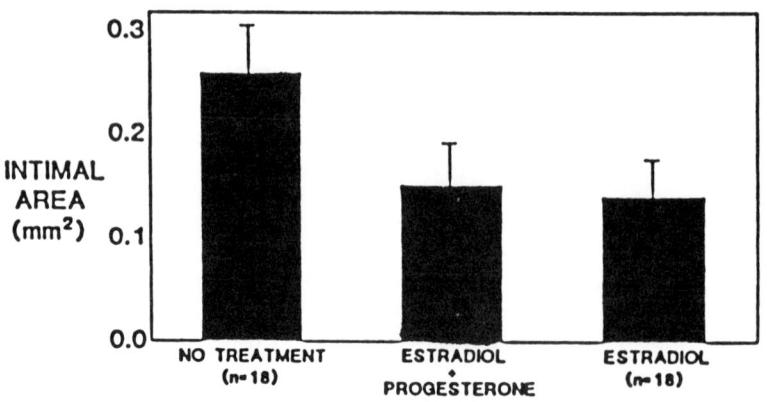

Figure 8–13. Effect of ovariectomy and sex hormone replacement on extent of atherosclerosis expressed as mean intimal area + SEM. (From Williams JK, Adams MR, Klopfenstein HS. Estrogen modulates responses of atherosclerotic coronary arteries. *Circulation* 81:1680, 1990.)

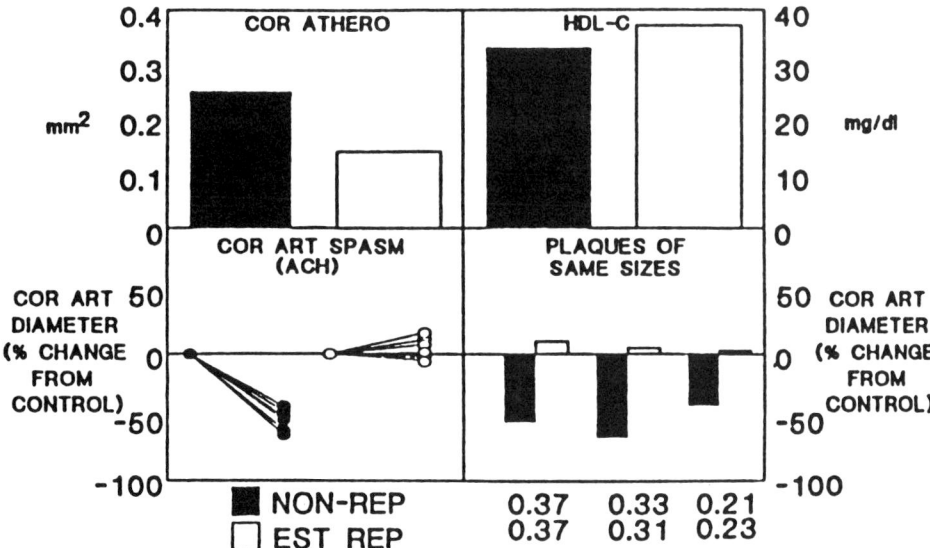

Figure 8–14. Effect of estrogen replacement (EST REP) and no estrogen replacement (NON-REP) on coronary artery plaque size (cross-sectional area in square millimeters), plasma high-density lipoprotein (HDL) cholesterol concentrations, and the response of coronary arteries to acetylcholine (ACH) injection. (From Williams JR, Adams MR, Herrington DM, et al. The effects of short-term estrogen treatment on vascular responses of coronary arteries. *Circulation* 84 [Suppl. II]:II-272, 1991.)

prostacyclin production is reduced in postmenopausal uterine arteries (67) (Fig. 8–15). Other in vitro data (68) and our own preliminary prospective clinical data have shown that estrogen increases 6-keto-prostaglandin $F_1\alpha$ production. These data are also compatible with other human data showing that estrogen increases blood flow. Uterine artery, aortic, and carotid blood flow have been shown to increase with estrogen use (69, 70, 71). The reduction in the pulsatility index of carotid vessels with estrogen is depicted in Figure 8–16.

The Impact of Progestins

All the epidemiologic data for PM women reviewed above pertain to the CV effects of estrogen alone and have not yet been analyzed for the addition of progestins. On a theoretical

Figure 8–15. Effect of 17β-estradiol on total steady state in vitro 6-keto-prostaglandin $F_1\alpha$ (6-keto-$PGF_1\alpha$) production by uterine arteries from pre- and postmenopausal women. (From Steinleitner A, Stanczyk FZ, Levin JH, et al. Decreased in vitro production of 6-keto-prostaglandin $F_1\alpha$ by uterine arteries from postmenopausal women. *Am J Obstet Gynecol* 161:1677, 1989.)

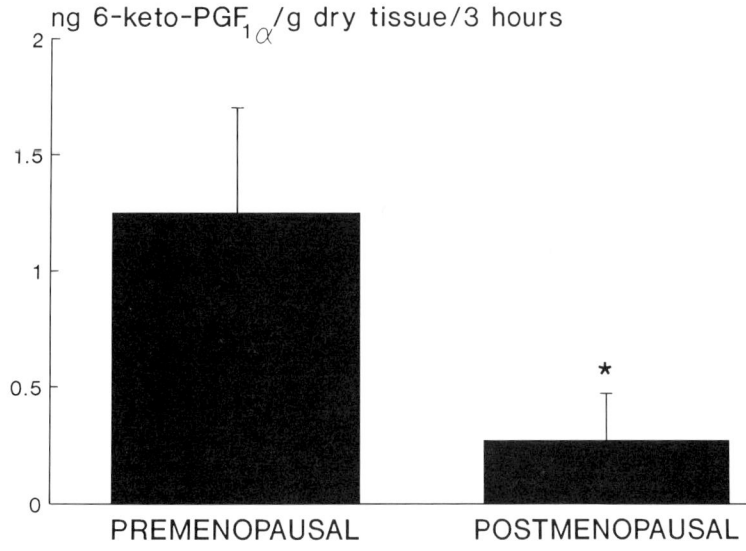

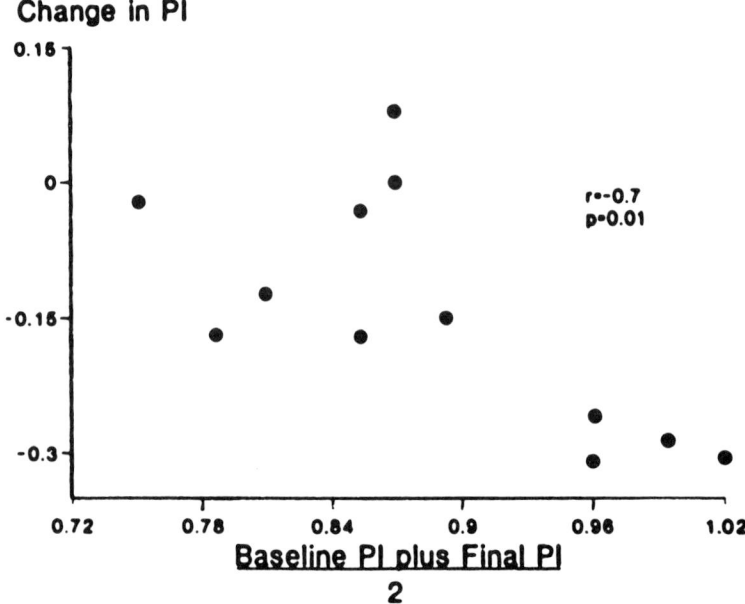

Figure 8–16. Correlation between change in pulsatility index (PI) (between end of study and baseline) and mean of baseline and final PI values. (From Gangar KF, Vyas S, Whitehead M, et al. Pulsatility index in internal carotid artery in relation to transdermal oestradiol and time since menopause. *Lancet* 338:839, 1991.)

basis, progestins may have a negative impact on CV function and can also lead to mood changes and patient discomfort. Therefore, the addition of a progestin is indicated only in women with a uterus in whom endometrial protection is needed.

Progestins have a number of potential adverse effects on the CV system, although there are still no published epidemiologic data. Some data are, nevertheless, of concern. In one study of mentally retarded women (aged 35 to 51 years) treated with a continuous synthetic progestin, lynoestrenol, to induce amenorrhea, 8 of 19 (42%) showed evidence of arterial disease at autopsy compared with only 1 of 15 (7%) untreated women. Several factors might account for the detrimental effects of progestin on CV function. The first is the lipid hypothesis, which postulates a reduction in HDL-C and HDL_2-C during progestin exposure. Second, the potential down-regulation of estrogen receptors in all tissues, including coronary vessels, may be important. Third, the inhibition of endothelial prostacyclin may be a factor. Fourth, a decrease or attenuation in estrogen-mediated blood flow may affect CV function. Fifth, a dose-related progestational effect may adversely influence carbohydrate tolerance. Finally, there may be a change in the quality of life because mood disturbances may occur or increase in patients receiving progestins (72).

Most progestin-mediated effects on lipoproteins are dose and duration related. High doses of progestins are likely to cause a reduction in HDL-C and even an increase in LDL-C, although triglycerides are usually lowered. However, the balance or ratio between the estrogen and progestin doses is extremely important. A high estrogen dose may overcome any harmful progestin effects. The greater the progestin's androgenic potency, the greater its propensity to cause adverse metabolic effects.

The inhibition of HDL-C is largely dose related. However, even 10 mg of medroxyprogesterone acetate, a 17-hydroxyprogesterone derivative, attenuates HDL-C by about 8% and HDL_2-C by about 17%. Sherwin (72) showed that the beneficial effects of conjugated equine estrogens (0.625 to 1.25 mg) on HDL-C and LDL-C may be attenuated by the addition of as little as 5 mg of medroxyprogesterone acetate. The overall effects of various progestins on lipoproteins (57) are listed in Table 8–5.

Even natural progesterone, which is more metabolically inert, has been shown to completely abolish the estrogen-induced changes in prostacyclin in human umbilical arteries in vitro (68). Similarly, several studies have shown that progestins decrease uterine blood flow. Taken together, these data suggest that all progestins influence various parameters of CV function to some extent. Interestingly, however, in the monkey data reviewed above (Fig. 8–13), physiologic levels of progesterone,

Table 8–5. PERCENTAGE CHANGE IN LIPOPROTEINS WITH VARIOUS PROGESTINS DURING SEQUENTIAL ADMINISTRATION COMPARED WITH THE EFFECTS OF UNOPPOSED ESTROGEN

	Micronized P (200 mg)	MPA (5 mg)	MPA (10 mg)	NET (1 ng)	dl-NG (.15)	dl-NG (.25)
HDL	−2	−6	−6%	−10	−14	−18%
HDL_2	0	−11	−19%	−27	−23	−25
HDL_3	0	0	−2%	−1%	0	−8
LDL	0	+3	+7%	+10%	+6	+8
Apo A_1	+1	−5	−11%	−11%	−15	−15
Apo B	0	0	+3%	+10%	+8	+10

Micronized P = micronized progesterone; MPA = medroxyprogesterone acetate; NET = norethindrone; dl-NG = norgestrel.

administered systemically, did not attenuate the beneficial effects of estrogen in reducing coronary atherosclerosis. Clearly, the type of progestin, its dose, and the route of administration are all extremely important in this interaction. It appears, therefore, that although progestins have potentially adverse effects on CV function, if they are administered in lower doses and in a more metabolically inert form, preferably progesterone itself, these effects can be minimized or eliminated.

Dosage Regimens for Hormonal Replacement

Most clinicians currently favor daily estrogen administration, although it is also routine to administer estrogen for 25 days each month. If required, progestins are administered for 10 to 14 days, either on a calendar basis if estrogen is prescribed daily, or on the last 10 to 14 days of a sequential 25-day regimen. An emerging, very popular regimen is the "continuous combined" regimen, in which both estrogen and progestin are taken daily. Although this regimen was originally prescribed for each day of the year, some now are suggesting that it be used for 5 days of the week or for 25 days each month.

Because of the potential deleterious effects of the progestins, my preference is to administer progestins sequentially for 10 days per cycle. Suitable progestins include medroxyprogesterone acetate (5 mg), norethindrone (1 mg), and micronized progesterone (200 mg). Even lower doses may be prescribed if side effects are encountered. Although these and larger doses are known to cause secretory transformation of the endometrium, this occurrence is probably not necessary to avoid endometrial hyperplasia.

Amenorrhea due to an atrophic endometrium may occur in women receiving continuous combined therapy. Although bleeding (spotting) may occur in the first few months, amenorrhea usually ensues. Depending on the combination, a continuous combined regimen may adversely affect the lipid profile. However, the magnitude of these changes and their significance have varied considerably between various studies because of marked differences in patient population and study design. Because of the unknown long-term CV effects of continuous progestogen exposure, it is my preference not to use this regimen as a first-line treatment. However, on balance, if an adequate amount of estrogen is used, the progestogen effect is likely to be minimized.

If treatment with a progestogen is to be successful, the biochemical processes that cause hyperplasia must be reduced or blocked and mitotic activity diminished. It is unnecessary to induce a full range of secretory changes with large progestin doses. These larger doses generally lead to an increased amount of withdrawal bleeding. Prevention of hyperplasia necessitates a reduction in mitotic activity. This and a reduction in bleeding should be the principal aim of an effective regimen (72). With this approach, it is estimated that the maximal inhibitory effect on CV function (including arterial and lipoprotein effects) would be a 15% reduction in benefit for the 10 days of exposure to progestogen (73). This is not likely to affect RR estimates of the cardioprotective effects of hormonal replacement. Nevertheless, it is important to reiterate that only in women with a uterus is any progestin therapy indicated (74).

References

1. Ying S. Inhibins, activins, and follistatins: Gonadal proteins modulating the secretion of follicle-stimulating hormone. *Endocrine Rev* 9:267, 1988.
2. McLachlan RI, Robertson DM, Healy DL, et al. Circulating immunoreactive inhibin levels during the normal human menstrual cycle. *J Clin Endocrinol Metab* 65:954, 1987.
3. Buckler HM, Evans CA, Mamtora H, et al. Gonadotropin, steroid, and inhibin levels in women with incipient ovarian failure during anovulatory and ovulatory rebound cycles. *J Clin Endocrinol Metab* 72:116, 1991.
4. Sherman BM, West JH, Korenman SG. The menopausal transition: Analysis of LH, FSH, estradiol and progesterone concentrations during menstrual cycles of older women. *J Clin Endocrinol Metab* 42:629, 1976.
5. Johnston CC Jr, Hui SL, Witt RM, et al. Early menopausal changes in bone mass and sex steroids. *J Clin Endocrinol Metab* 61:905, 1985.
6. Eriksen EF, Colvard DS, Berg NJ, et al. Evidence of estrogen receptors in normal human osteoblast-like cells. *Science* 241:84, 1988.
7. Lin AL, Gonzalez R Jr, Carey KD, et al. Estradiol-17β affects estrogen receptor content in baboon aorta. *Arteriosclerosis* 6:495, 1986.
8. Ingegno MD, Money SR, Thelmo W, et al. Progesterone receptors in the human heart and great vessels. *Lab Invest* 59:353, 1988.
9. Grodin JM, Siiteri PK, MacDonald PC. Source of estrogen production in postmenopausal women. *J Clin Endocrinol Metab* 36:207, 1973.
10. Lobo RA, Cassidenti DL. Pharmacokinetics of oral 17β-estradiol. *J Reprod Med* 37:77, 1992.
11. Judd HL, Lucas WE, Yen SSC. Effect of oophorectomy on circulating testosterone and androstenedione levels in patients with endometrial cancer. *Am J Obstet Gynecol* 118:793, 1974.
12. Dowsett M, Cantwell B, Anshumala LAL, et al. Suppression of postmenopausal ovarian steroidogenesis with the luteinizing hormone-releasing hormone agonist goserelin. *J Clin Endocrinol Metab* 66:672, 1988.
13. Lobo RA, March CM, Goebelsmann U, et al. The modulating role of obesity and 17β-estradiol (E_2) on bound and unbound E_2 and adrenal androgens in oophorectomized women. *J Clin Endocrinol Metab* 54:320, 1982.
14. Kannel WB, Hjortland MC, McNamara PM, et al. Menopause and the risk of cardiovascular disease: The Framingham Study. *Ann Intern Med* 85:447, 1976.
15. Rosenberg L, Hennekens CH, Rosner B, et al. Early menopause and the risk of myocardial infarction. *Am J Obstet Gynecol* 139:47, 1981.
16. Centerwall BS. Premenopausal hysterectomy and cardiovascular disease. *Am J Obstet Gynecol* 139:58, 1981.
17. Kannel WB, Gordon T. Cardiovascular effects of the menopause. In Mishell DR, Jr (Ed.), *Menopause: Physiology and Pharmacology*. Chicago, Year Book, 1987, p. 91.
18. Matthews KA, Meilahn E, Kuller LH, et al. Menopause and risk factors for coronary heart disease. *N Engl J Med* 321:641, 1989.
19. Jensen J, Nilas L, Christiansen C. Influence of menopause on serum lipids and lipoproteins. *Maturitas* 12:321, 1990.
20. Lobo RA, Notelovitz M, Bernstein L, et al. Lp(a) lipoprotein: Relationship to cardiovascular disease risk factors, exercise and estrogen. *Am J Obstet Gynecol* 166:1182, 1992.
21. Mashchak CA, Lobo RA, Dozono-Takano R, et al. Comparison of pharmacodynamic properties of various estrogen formulations. *Am J Obstet Gynecol* 144:511, 1982.
22. Lobo RA. The androgenicity of progestational agents. *Int J Fertil* 33:6, 1988.
23. Kovacs L, Bartfai G, Apro G, et al. The effect of the contraceptive pill on blood pressure: A randomized controlled trial of three progestogen-oestrogen combinations in Szeged, Hungary. *Contraception* 33:69, 1986.
24. Shionoiri H, Eggena P, Barrett JD, et al. An increase in high-molecular-weight renin substrate associated with estrogenic hypertension. *Biochem Med* 29:14, 1983.
25. Bottinger LE, Boman G, Eklund G, et al. Oral contraceptives and thromboembolic disease; effects of lowering oestrogen content. *Lancet* 1:1097, 1980.
26. Barnes RW, Krapf T, Hoak JC. Erroneous clinical diagnosis of leg vein thrombosis in women on oral contraceptives. *Obstet Gynecol* 51:556, 1978.
27. Bonnar J. Coagulation effects of oral contraception. *Am J Obstet Gynecol* 157:1042, 1987.
28. Daly L, Bonnar J. Comparative studies of 30 μg ethinyl estradiol combined with gestodene and desogestrel on blood coagulation, fibrinolysis, and platelets. *Am J Obstet Gynecol* 163:430, 1990.
29. Kalkhoff RK. Relative sensitivity of postpartum gestational diabetic women to oral contraceptive agents and other metabolic stress. *Diabetes Care* 3:421, 1980.
30. Perlman JA, Russell-Briefel R, Ezzati T, et al. Oral glucose tolerance and the potency of contraceptive progestins. *J Chronic Dis* 38:857, 1985.
31. Notelovitz M, Feldman EB, Gillespy M, et al. Lipid and lipoprotein changes in women taking low-dose, triphasic oral contraceptives: A controlled, comparative, 12-month clinical trial. *Am J Obstet Gynecol* 160:1269, 1989.
32. Kjos SL, Shoupe D, Douyan S, et al. Effect of low-dose oral contraceptives on carbohydrate and lipid metabolism in women with recent gestational diabetes: Results of a controlled, randomized, prospective study. *Am J Obstet Gynecol* 163:1822, 1990.
33. Godsland IF, Walton C, Felton C, et al. Insulin resistance, secretion, and metabolism in users of oral contraceptives. *J Clin Endocrinol Metab* 74:64, 1991.
34. Croft P, Hannaford PC. Risk factors for acute myocardial infarction in women: Evidence from the Royal College of General Practitioners' oral contraception study. *Br Med J* 298:165, 1989.
35. Stampfer MJ, Willett WC, Colditz GA, et al. A prospective study of past use of oral contraceptive agents and risk of cardiovascular diseases. *N Engl J Med* 319:1313, 1988.
36. Royal College of General Practitioners' oral contraceptive users. *Lancet* 1:541, 1981.
37. Wiseman RA, MacRae KD. Oral contraceptives and the decline in mortality from circulatory disease. *Fertil Steril* 35:277, 1981.
38. Engel H-J, Engel E, Lichtlen PR. Coronary athero-

sclerosis and myocardial infarction in young women—role of oral contraceptives. *Eur Heart J* 4:1, 1983.
39. Adams MR, Clarkson TB, Koritnik DR, et al. Contraceptive steroids and coronary artery atherosclerosis in cynomolgus macaques. *Fertil Steril* 47:1010, 1987.
40. Mann JI, Doll R, Thorogood M, et al. Risk factors for myocardial infarction in young women. *Br J Prev Soc Med* 30:94, 1986.
41. Mileikowsky GN, Nadler JL, Huey F, et al. Evidence that smoking alters prostacyclin formation and platelet aggregation in women who use oral contraceptives. *Am J Obstet Gynecol* 159:1547, 1988.
42. Lobo RA, Nguyen HN, Eggena P, et al. Biologic effects of equilin sulfate in postmenopausal women. *Fertil Steril* 49:234, 1988.
43. Lobo RA. Absorption and metabolic effects of different types of estrogens and progesterones. *Clin Obstet Gynecol North Am* 14:143, 1987.
44. Stanczyk FZ, Shoupe D, Nunez V, et al. A randomized comparison of nonoral estradiol delivery in postmenopausal women. *Am J Obstet Gynecol* 159:1540, 1988.
45. Bush TL. Noncontraceptive estrogen use and risk of cardiovascular disease: An overview and critique of the literature. In Korenman SG (Ed.), *The Menopause. Biological and Clinical Consequences of Ovarian Failure: Evolution and Management.* Norwell, MA, Serono Symposium, 1990, p. 211.
46. Stampfer MJ, Willett WC, Colditz GA, et al. Past use of oral contraceptives and cardiovascular disease: A meta-analysis in the context of the Nurses' Health Study. *Am J Obstet Gynecol* 163:285, 1990.
47. Henderson BE, Paganini-Hill A, Ross RK. Decreased mortality in users of estrogen replacement therapy. *Arch Intern Med* 151:75, 1991.
48. Mashchak CA, Lobo RA. Estrogen replacement therapy and hypertension. *J Repro Med* 30 (Suppl. 10):805, 1985.
49. Luotola H. Blood pressure and hemodynamics in postmenopausal women during estradiol-17β substitution. *Ann Clin Res* 15:1, 1983.
50. Ballejo G, Saleem TH, Khan-Dawood FS, et al. The effect of sex steroids on insulin binding by target tissues in the rat. *Contraception* 28:413, 1983.
51. Barrett-Connor E, Laakso M. Ischemic heart disease risk in postmenopausal women. Effects of estrogen use on glucose and insulin levels. *Arteriosclerosis* 10:531, 1990.
52. Lindheim SR, Ditkoff EC, Presser SC, et al. A biomodal effect of estrogen on insulin resistance in postmenopausal women and a potential attenuating effect of progestin. Presented at the 40th Annual Meeting of the Pacific Coast Fertility Society, April 8–12, 1992, Indian Wells, California.
53. Notelovitz M, Ware M. Coagulation risks with postmenopausal oestrogen therapy. In Studd J (Ed.), *Progress in Obstetrics and Gynecology,* Vol. 2. Edinburgh, Churchill Livingstone, 1982.
54. Notelovitz M, Kitchens C, Ware MD, et al. Combination estrogen and progestogen replacement therapy does not adversely affect coagulation. *Obstet Gynecol* 62:596, 1983.
55. Devor M, Barrett-Connor E, Renvall M, et al. Estrogen replacement therapy and the risk of venous thrombosis. *Am J Med* 92:275, 1992.
56. Lobo RA. Estrogen and the risk of coagulopathy. *Am J Med* 92:283, 1992.
57. Lobo RA. Effects of hormonal replacement on lipids and lipoproteins in postmenopausal women. *J Clin Endocrinol Metab* 73:925, 1991.
58. Walsh BW, Schiff I, Rosner B, et al. Effects of postmenopausal estrogen replacement on the concentrations and metabolism of plasma lipoproteins. *N Engl J Med* 325:1196, 1991.
59. Paganini-Hill A, Ross RK, Henderson BE. Postmenopausal oestrogen treatment and stroke: A prospective study. *Br Med J* 297:519, 1988.
60. Henderson BE, Ross RK, Paganini-Hill A, et al. Estrogen use and cardiovascular disease. *Am J Obstet Gynecol* 154:1181, 1986.
61. Sullivan JM, Vander Zwaag R, Lemp GF, et al. Postmenopausal estrogen use and coronary atherosclerosis. *Ann Intern Med* 108:358, 1988.
62. Gruchow HW, Anderson AJ, Barboriak JJ, et al. Postmenopausal use of estrogen and occlusion of coronary arteries. *Am Heart J* 115:954, 1988.
63. Sullivan JM, Vander Zwaag R, Hughes JP, et al. Estrogen replacement and coronary artery disease. *Arch Intern Med* 150:2557, 1990.
64. Wagner JD, Clarkson TB, Adams MR, et al. The effects of oral contraceptives on coronary artery LDL metabolism in female cynomolgus monkeys. *Circulation* 84 (Suppl. II):II-602, 1991.
65. Williams JK, Adams MR, Klopfenstein HS. Estrogen modulates responses of atherosclerotic coronary arteries. *Circulation* 81:1680, 1990.
66. Williams JR, Adams MR, Herrington DM, et al. The effects of short-term estrogen treatment on vascular responses of coronary arteries. *Circulation* 84 (Suppl. II):II-272, 1991.
67. Steinleitner A, Stanczyk FZ, Levin JH, et al. Decreased in vitro production of 6-keto-prostaglandin $F_1\alpha$ by uterine arteries from postmenopausal women. *Am J Obstet Gynecol* 161:1677, 1989.
68. Makila UM, Wahlberg L, Vlinikka L, et al. Regulation of prostacyclin and thromboxane production by human umbilical vessels. The effect of estradiol and progesterone in a superfusion model. *Prostaglandins Leukot Med* 8:115, 1982.
69. Bourne T, Hillard TC, Whitehead MI, et al. Oestrogens, arterial status, and postmenopausal women. *Lancet* 335:1470, 1990.
70. Pines A, Fisman EZ, Levo Y, et al. The effects of hormone replacement therapy in normal postmenopausal women: Measurement of Doppler-derived parameters of aortic flow. *Am J Obstet Gynecol* 64:806, 1991.
71. Gangar KF, Vyas S, Whitehead M, et al. Pulsatility index in internal carotid artery in relation to transdermal oestradiol and time since menopause. *Lancet* 338:839, 1991.
72. Sherwin BB, Gelfand MM. A prospective one-year study of estrogen and progestin in postmenopausal women: Effects on clinical symptoms and lipoprotein lipids. Obstet Gynecol 73:759, 1989.
73. Moyer DL, de Lignieres B, Drigues P, et al. Prevention of endometrial hyperplasia: No correlation with secretory changes and cyclical bleeding. *Fertil Steril* (in press, 1993).
74. Lobo RA. Which progestogen? What dosage? In Proceedings of the International Novo Nordisk Symposium, February 1–2, 1991. *Cardiovascular Effects of Hormone Replacement Therapy.* Copenhagen, Novo Dordisk A/S, 1991, p. 97.
75. Whitehead M, Lobo RA. Progestin use in postmenopausal women. *Lancet* 2:1243, 1988.

CHAPTER 9

Lipoproteins and Lipid Disorders

JOHN C. LAROSA, M.D.

BACKGROUND

Lipoproteins

Lipoproteins are large, spherical, macromolecules with a core of insoluble neutral lipid, triglyceride, and esterified cholesterol, surrounded by a shell of more soluble protein, phospholipid, and unesterified cholesterol. Their major function is the transport of lipids in the plasma for a variety of metabolic purposes (1).

Lipoproteins are traditionally subdivided into several classes based on their hydrated density (Fig. 9–1). All lipoproteins contain the same four basic ingredients: triglycerides, esterified and unesterified cholesterol, phospholipid, and protein. They differ in size, density, and the relative quantities of these four ingredients. Chylomicrons and very low density lipoproteins (VLDL)* are large in diameter and are relatively light lipoproteins that carry most of the plasma triglyceride. Low-density lipoproteins (LDL)* and high-density lipoproteins (HDL)* are smaller, more dense, and carry more cholesterol and protein and much less triglyceride.

Apoproteins

The proteins that form part of the lipoprotein outer shell are called apolipoproteins,

---

*In the clinical context, HDL, LDL, and VLDL are shorthand for the *cholesterol* content of each of these species, i.e., clinical measurements of HDL are really measures of HDL-cholesterol. This is sometimes abbreviated to HDL-C. For simplicity, only the notation HDL, LDL, and VLDL will be used in this text.

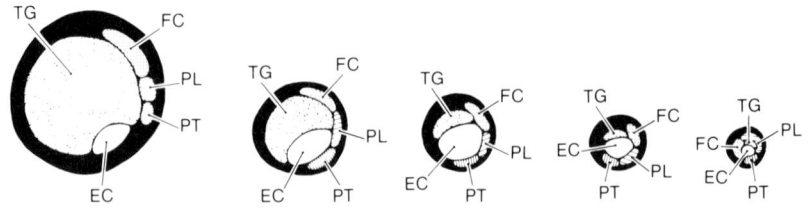

	CHYLOMICRONS	VLDL	IDL	LDL	HDL
Electrophoretic Mobility	Origin	Pre-Beta (Alpha-2) Globulin Region	Beta to Pre-Beta	Beta	Alpha
Hydrated Density	<1.006	<1.006	1.006-1.109	1.019-1.063	1.063-1.21
Diameter (A°)	750-12,000	500-700	300-500	225	100-150
Lipids (%)					
Cholesterol	5	20	40	50	25
Triglycerides	90	60	20	7	5
Phospholipids	3	14	22	22	26
Protein	2	6	18	21	44
Apoprotein	A,B,C,E	A,B,C,E	B,E	B	A,C

FC - Free cholesterol
PL - Phospholipid
PT - Protein
TG - Triglycerides
EC - Esterified cholesterol

VLDL - Very low density lipoproteins
IDL - Intermediate density lipoproteins
LDL - Low density lipoproteins
HDL - High density lipoproteins

Figure 9–1. Plasma lipoproteins. (From LaRosa, JC *Lipoproteins: Their Role in Atherosclerosis and Its Prevention.* Needham Heights, MA, Damon Clinical Laboratories, 1988 and 1990, 19 pages.)

commonly shortened to apoproteins or apos. In addition to their structural functions, apoproteins serve as the activators or inhibitors of the enzymes that catalyze lipoprotein metabolism and as ligands or recognition sites for cell surface receptors that bind circulating lipoproteins (2).

Apoproteins are named by somewhat arbitrary alphabetical nomenclature (Table 9–1). Apoproteins are found in more than one lipoprotein species and, like lipids, may exchange between lipoproteins. ApoA-I and A-II, for example, are found in both HDL and VLDL. ApoB-100 is found in both LDL and VLDL, and the apoCs are found in all lipoprotein species.

OVERVIEW OF LIPOPROTEIN METABOLISM

General Comment

A complete discussion of lipoprotein metabolism is beyond the scope of this chapter. For that, the reader is referred to other sources (1–3). What follows is a brief synopsis.

Lipid transport can be thought of as beginning in the intestine and the liver. Both organs produce large amounts of triglyceride that must be transported for storage in adipose tissue sites. In the intestine, triglyceride accumulates in enterocytes as a result of dietary fat ingestion. In the liver, the triglyceride is synthesized from circulating carbohydrate and free fatty acids, which may be thought of as unused cellular fuel and which cannot be stored without first being transformed into triglyceride.

Chylomicrons and Very Low Density Lipoproteins

Both intestinal and hepatic triglycerides are incorporated into large triglyceride-carrying lipoproteins. In the intestines, these lipoproteins are called chylomicrons; in the liver, they are called VLDL. Both of these lipoproteins are secreted in the peripheral circulation (Fig. 9–2).

Table 9-1. CHARACTERISTICS OF THE MAJOR APOPROTEINS

Apoprotein	MW	Lipoproteins	Metabolic Functions
Apo A-I	28,016	HDL, chylomicrons	Structural component of HDL; LCAT activator
Apo A-II	17,414	HDL, chylomicrons	Unknown
Apo A-IV	46,465	HDL, chylomicrons	Unknown: possibly facilitates transfer of other apos between HDL and chylomicrons
Apo (a)	400–800,000	Lipoprotein (a)	
Apo B-48	264,000	Chylomicrons	Necessary for assembly and secretion of chylomicrons from the small intestine
Apo B-100	512,000	VLDL, IDL, LDL	Necessary for assembly and secretion of VLDL from the liver; structural protein of VLDL, IDL, LDL; ligand for LDL receptor
Apo C-I	6630	All major lipoproteins	
Apo C-II	8900	All major lipoproteins	Activator of lipoprotein lipase
Apo C-III	8800	All major lipoproteins	Inhibitor of lipoprotein lipase; may inhibit hepatic uptake of chylomicron and VLDL remnants
Apo D	22,000	Mainly HDL	Possibly involved in reverse cholesterol transport
Apo E	34,145	All major lipoproteins	Ligand for binding of several lipoproteins to the LDL receptor and possibly to a separate hepatic apo E receptor

From Ginsberg HN. Lipoprotein physiology and its relationship to atherogenesis. Endocrinol Metab Clin North Am 19:211–228, 1990.

TRIGLYCERIDE TRANSPORT

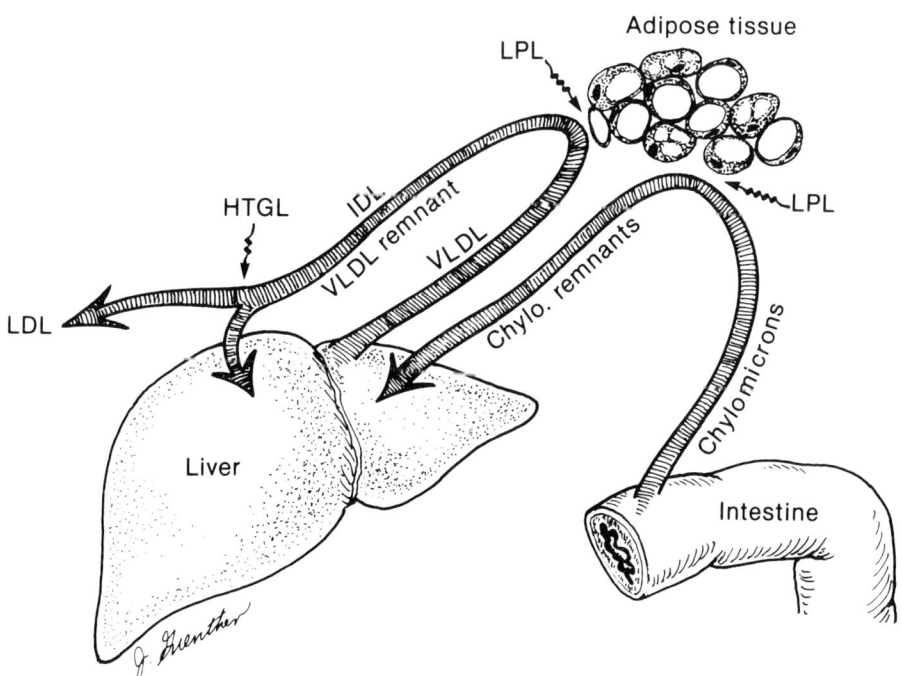

Figure 9-2. Triglyceride transport. HTGL = hepatic triglyceride lipase, LPL = lipoprotein lipase, LDL = low density lipoproteins; VLDL = very low density lipoproteins; IDL = intermediate density lipoproteins, see text for further explanation.

Chylomicrons are *not* transported in the portal circulation but are taken up by intestinal lymphatics and enter the bloodstream via the thoracic duct. In adipose tissue and skeletal muscle, both chylomicrons and VLDL are acted upon by lipoprotein lipase (LPL), a noncirculating enzyme found on the surface of endothelial cells. ApoC-II, present on both chylomicrons and VLDL, is a cofactor that enhances the activity of this enzyme. As a result of this lipolytic reaction, 70–80% of the core triglyceride is converted to free fatty acids, glycerol, and monoglyceride, all of which traverse the cell membrane, are resynthesized into triglyceride, and stored.

As these large triglyceride-carrying lipoprotein particles lose their core triglyceride (but not, for the most part, their core cholesterol), they diminish in size. The redundant constituents of the outer shell (i.e., apoproteins, phospholipid, and free cholesterol) break away and join the HDL fraction. Shell reforms around the smaller cholesterol-enriched core. The resulting smaller lipoproteins are referred to as remnants.

Remnant Metabolism

Chylomicron remnants are removed from circulation by the liver by binding to cell surface receptor proteins, called remnant receptors, apoE receptors, or lipoprotein-related protein (LRP). VLDL remnants are taken up mainly by another cell-surface receptor protein, the apoB-100 or LDL receptor. VLDL remnants also may be recognized by the remnant receptor. Binding to the LDL receptor requires the presence of a form of apoprotein called apoB-100 (Table 9–1), which is present on the surface of VLDL and its remnant. Chylomicron remnants, in contrast, contain another form of apoB, apoB-48 (Table 9–1), which is not recognized by the LDL receptor. Both chylomicron and VLDL remnants contain apoE, however, which facilitates binding to the remnant receptor.

When chylomicron remnants are taken up by the liver, they deliver their cholesterol to that organ. As a result, dietary triglyceride is stored mainly in adipose tissue, while dietary cholesterol is stored in the liver.

VLDL remnants may, however, depending on their size, be metabolized differently. Catabolism of large VLDL, like chylomicrons, results in remnants that are removed from the circulation by the liver. Smaller VLDL, however, lead to remnants that are smaller, called intermediate density lipoproteins (IDL). Smaller VLDL may be acted on in the liver by another noncirculating lipolytic enzyme, hepatic triglyceride lipase (HTGL). These smaller remnants are then converted to LDL, the major carrier of cholesterol in the plasma.

LDL Metabolism

LDL is a smaller lipoprotein than chylomicron and VLDL, with a single apoB-100 molecule on its surface. It carries about 75% of the circulating cholesterol but relatively little triglyceride (Table 9–1). Most human cells contain LDL cell surface receptors, and LDL is thought to be the main external source of cholesterol for cells. About 60% of circulating LDL is removed by the liver, the rest by peripheral tissues. Once bound to the LDL surface receptor, the LDL receptor complex is internalized, and the cholesterol is either stored or used to make cell membranes, bile cells, or gonadal hormones, depending on the tissue involved. As intracellular cholesterol accumulates, it also inhibits cellular cholesterol synthesis as well as the synthesis of LDL receptors.

Only the liver has the ability to convert cholesterol to bile salts and excrete them. Other cells must rely on the presence of HDL to rid themselves of excess cholesterol.

HDL Metabolism

HDL is the smallest, most dense lipoprotein with the least amount of triglyceride. Some nascent forms of HDL are not spherical but rather disc-shaped. These may be thought of as a lipoprotein shell lacking a lipid core. HDL may be synthesized de novo in both the liver and intestine. Some HDL components come directly from the excess surface material produced as chylomicrons, and VLDL are converted to remnants.

It is probable that cholesterol-poor HDL binds to a specific cell surface receptor, picks up free cholesterol from the cell membrane, and adds it to its own surface. In the plasma, in the presence of a protein called apoprotein D (apoD), the free cholesterol in the lipoprotein surface is esterified by accepting a fatty acid molecule from circulating lecithin and interacting with an enzyme called lecithin-cholesterol-acetyl-transferase (LCAT).

Apoprotein A-I on the surface of HDL acts as a cofactor for LCAT. The cholesterol ester formed is then transferred into the HDL core and transported to the liver for excretion or passed onto other lipoproteins by combining with a circulating protein called cholesterol-ester-transfer-protein (CETP). In this way, excess cholesterol is eventually transported to the liver, the only organ from which it can be excreted.

HDL can be subdivided into fractions, depending on the degree of cholesterol saturation. HDL_3 has relatively little cholesterol compared to HDL_2. The HDL that actually may deliver cholesterol to the liver also has on its surface apoE, which can be recognized by both LDL and remnant receptors and thus may be an efficient form for allowing HDL uptake by the liver (1).

DISORDERS OF LIPOPROTEIN TRANSPORT

Genetic Disorders

The number of genetic variances that can affect these lipoprotein pathways is quite large and is beyond the scope of this chapter. For more detailed review, the reader is referred to other sources (3).

Not surprisingly, genetic variation in the enzymes, apoproteins, and receptors that direct the process of lipoprotein metabolism are responsible for most of the inherited abnormalities. For example, chylomicrons may accumulate when LPL is deficient. This occurs in *familial type I or familial lipoprotein lipase deficiency*, a rare, recessively inherited abnormality. *Familial deficiency of apoprotein C-II*, a necessary lipoprotein lipase cofactor, is also a recessive disorder and produces the same result. On the other hand, chylomicrons, VLDL, IDL, and LDL may be quantitatively and qualitatively deficient in *abetalipoproteinemia*, a disorder in which apoprotein B (apoB), a necessary constituent of all of these lipoproteins, is missing or deficient.

VLDL may accumulate in *familial hypertriglyceridemia*, a poorly characterized disorder, in which VLDL is overproduced. VLDL accumulation may also occur. This disorder is thought to be primarily an overproduction of apoB-100, resulting in overproduction of the VLDL, IDL, LDL cascade.

IDL as well as chylomicron remnants may accumulate in *familial dysbetalipoproteinemia* (or *familial type III hyperlipoproteinemia*), a disorder in which normal apoE-III is absent and is replaced with apoE-II, a variant that binds poorly to hepatic apoE receptors. Clinical expression of this disorder requires the presence of another, as yet undefined, genetic abnormality to result in IDL accumulation. Remnants may also accumulate in *familial hepatic triglyceride lipase deficiency*, in which HTGL, necessary for the conversion of IDL to LDL, is deficient.

LDL may accumulate in *familial hypercholesterolemia*, a dominantly inherited deficiency of LDL receptors or LDL receptor activity. In homozygotes, this disorder may lead to severe atherosclerosis in adolescence and early childhood.

HDL may accumulate in *familial hyperalphalipoproteinemia*. Whether this is a discrete single gene disorder and, if so, how it is inherited, is unknown. HDL may be deficient in a variety of rare conditions in which apoA-I is abnormal, including Tangier disease and familial apoA-I C-III deficiency.

The most common forms of HDL deficiency, which result in HDL levels that are low (in the 20 to 30 mg/dL range), however, are not well characterized. The genetics of these disorders are not described despite the fact that HDL levels in this low range may occur in 2–4% of the white male population in the United States (4).

There is no information at present to indicate that common genetic lipoprotein abnormalities are different in women than in men. Indeed, virtually all of the major genetic abnormalities thus far described have occurred in both men and women. The fact that women have higher HDL and higher levels of circulating estrogen, however, may mean that the impact of genetic abnormalities that result in elevations of LDL may be less severe in women than in men.

Secondary Dyslipoproteinemia

In addition to genetic abnormalities directly affecting lipoprotein metabolism, there are a number of diseases that may disturb lipoprotein metabolism in an otherwise normal individual. These so-called secondary causes of dyslipoproteinemia are summarized in Table 9–2 and include such common disorders as diabetes mellitus, chronic renal failure, nephrosis, and hypothyroidism. For a more detailed discussion of these disorders, the reader is referred to other sources (5, 6).

Genotypes and Phenotypes

At one time, disorders in which lipoproteins accumulated were organized into lipoprotein "phenotypes," which really represented a shorthand method of describing which lipoprotein species was elevated. Although the proponents of this system never claimed that these phenotypes were discrete genetic disorders, they were widely assumed to be so. This phenotyping classification has little usefulness today, given our ability to measure HDL, LDL, and apoprotein levels directly. Nevertheless, the phenotyping system has persisted in the names given to some of the common genetic disorders (for example, familial type I and familial type III). A "conversion" schema for relating these phenotypes to currently described genetic abnormalities as well as to secondary dyslipoproteinemias is summarized in Table 9–2.

Lipoproteins and Atherogenesis

At least three lipoprotein species, oxidized or chemically altered LDL, IDL, and chylomicron remnants, can be shown in vitro to convert scavenger cells to foam cells, that is, cells laden with cholesterol ester in their cytoplasm (1). Clinical states in which these three lipoproteins accumulate are associated with an increased risk of clinical atherosclerosis. The mechanisms by which the process of atherosclerosis proceed are incompletely understood. The role of oxidized but not native LDL in producing foam cells is of particular interest because there is evidence in animal models that the lipid-lowering drug probucol, an antioxidant, may prevent atherosclerosis by preventing LDL oxidation (7).

HDL can be shown in vitro to clear cholesterol from foam cells and, presumably, by the process of reverse cholesterol transport, it accumulates and transports cholesterol ester to the liver, where it can be metabolized (2, 8). It is reasonable to presume, then, that diet, exercise, weight control, and drug interventions that lead to lower LDL, IDL, and chylomicron levels and to higher HDL levels will lower the risk of clinical atherosclerosis. Clinical trials to date indicate that this is indeed the case.

EFFECT OF GENDER ON LIPOPROTEIN PHYSIOLOGY

Distribution of Lipoproteins in Males and Females

Lipoprotein levels are not identical in males and females of the same age. This is largely related to the effect of differences in endogenous, gonadal hormone levels, although other, still undefined factors may also play a role. In general, estrogens raise HDL and triglyceride levels and lower LDL levels. Androgens, on the other hand, lower HDL and triglyceride levels and raise LDL cholesterol levels (9). Throughout most of the life cycle, females have higher HDL levels than males (Fig. 9–3).

Table 9–2. GENOTYPES AND PHENOTYPES

Phenotype	Lipoprotein Abnormality	Genetic Abnormality	Secondary Causes
I	Chylomicrons in fasting blood	Familial LPL deficiency (familial type I)	Insulinopenic diabetes Dysgammaglobulinemia
II	Elevated LDL (IIa) or elevated LDL (IIb) + VLDL	Familial hypercholesterolemia Familial combined hyperlipidemia	Hypothyroidism Nephrosis
III	Elevated remnants	Familial dysbetalipoproteinemia Familial HTGL deficiency	Hypothyroidism Hyperinsulinemic diabetes
IV	Elevated VLDL	Familial hypertriglyceridemia	Renal failure Nephrosis Hyperinsulinenic diabetes
V	Elevated VLDL + fasting chylomicronemia	Familial hypertriglyceridemia	Renal failure Insulinopenic diabetes

Age Trends in Lipoprotein-Cholesterol Fractions

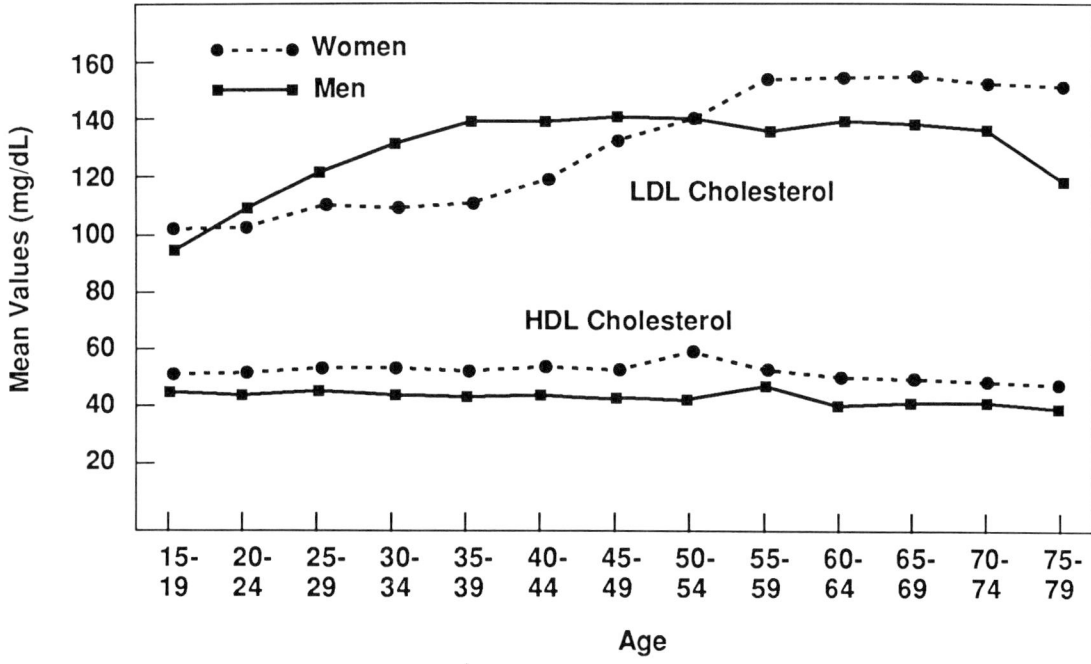

Figure 9-3. Age trends in lipoprotein-cholesterol fractions.(Adapted from Kannel WB. Nutrition and the occurrence and prevention of cardiovascular disease in the elderly. *Nutr Rev* 48:68–78, 1988.)

This is true even after menopause, when it might be expected that estrogen deficiency would produce a significant decline in HDL and equivalency in women and men (10). In fact, a longitudinal study of a cohort of women progressing through menopause does demonstrate a small fall in HDL after menopause, although not of the degree that might be expected and not to levels that are below average in men of the same age (11).

LDL levels, on the other hand, are lower in women than in men until about the age of 55 and beyond. After that, women have considerably higher levels than men of the same age. Longitudinal follow-up of the perimenopausal cohort mentioned above confirms this rise in LDL after menopause. The higher LDL in older women compared to men may also be related to the higher coronary mortality in younger, hypercholesterolemic men, leaving only men with lower cholesterol levels to progress into older age groups.

Lipoproteins and the Female Life Cycle

Circulating lipoprotein levels may be affected in females at points in the life cycle other than menopause. At puberty, HDL levels fall in males, probably as the result of rising circulating androgen levels. Such a decline in HDL is not, however, apparent in females, presumably because of the rising estrogen levels that prevent it. As a result, females have higher HDL levels than males from early adolescence on (12).

During the monthly menstrual cycle estrogen appears to be the dominant influence on lipoprotein levels. LDL levels decline early in the first portion of the cycle and remain low even through the estrogen-dominated second half of the cycle. HDL levels remain unchanged (13). The lack of any progesterone effect on circulating lipoproteins during the menstrual cycle is perhaps not surprising. Studies of exogenously micronized progesterone demonstrate no estrogen-opposing effect with regard to lipoprotein levels (14). The failure of increasing estrogen levels to increase HDL during the first half of the cycle is puzzling and requires further study.

During pregnancy, both LDL and HDL levels rise. Presumably this is related to increasing levels of endogenous estrogen and progesterone. LDL levels, however, stay elevated until several weeks after delivery (15), whereas HDL levels fall at about the twenty-fourth week of pregnancy and are only a little above nonpregnant levels at the time of delivery. Triglyceride levels also rise during pregnancy but fall more rapidly after delivery than do LDL levels (16).

It might be expected that because the sustained increase in LDL is potentially atherogenic, multiple pregnancies would predict an increased risk of coronary heart disease (CHD) in later life. The bulk of epidemiologic evidence, however, indicates that multiparity is not a risk factor for CHD (17).

Lipoproteins as Risk Factors for Atherosclerosis in Women

As in men, circulating lipoproteins are important predictors of coronary disease risk in women. Coronary risk rises with increases in LDL levels and falls with increases in HDL levels (18). Although these relationships are qualitatively similar in women and men, there do appear to be some quantitative differences. HDL, for example, is a more potent predictor of risk in women than in men, implying that HDL may function differently in women (19). Not only are total HDL levels higher in women, there is a greater difference in CHD risk per milligram of difference in HDL.

On the other hand, LDL does not appear to be as strong a predictor of risk in women as in men (18). Reasons for this are not clear. Studies in female primates, however, indicate that the presence of circulating estrogen interferes with LDL uptake in the arterial wall (20). Thus, at a given level, LDL may be less atherogenic in women than in men.

Triglycerides, too, are different in men than in women. In men and in younger women, triglyceride levels are not a statistically independent predictor of coronary risk when HDL and LDL are considered in multivariate analysis (21). In older, postmenopausal women, however, triglycerides do represent an independent predictor of coronary risk (22). Whether this is a direct effect of triglycerides themselves, or whether triglycerides are markers for the presence of other atherogenic lipoproteins is not entirely clear. Support for the latter theory comes from the observation that, as women age, the percentage of smaller, more dense LDL rises (23). Recurrence of such small, dense LDL has been associated with hypertriglyceridemia. Recent evidence suggests that small, dense LDL may be more atherogenic, perhaps because they are more susceptible to oxidation (24). The association of small, dense LDL with triglycerides may explain their predictive power in some older women.

Lipoprotein A (Lp(a)) is a peculiar lipoprotein whose potential significance is only now coming into clearer focus. It is composed of one LDL molecule, including a full complement of lipids, and one molecule of apoB-100 linked by a disulfide bond to a large protein of variable size, called apo(a). Apo(a) is about 80% analogous to plasminogen. Thus, Lp(a) is a molecule with both lipoprotein and clotting potential. Its physiologic function, if any, is unknown (25).

Little is known about the metabolism of Lp(a). Apo(a) is synthesized in the liver. Lp(a) can be bound by LDL receptors and apparently by plasminogen receptors (26).

Several cross-sectional studies have strongly demonstrated that Lp(a) is a cardiovascular risk factor in both men and women (27–28). One cross-sectional study has also indicated that Lp(a) levels are higher in women than in men throughout most of the life span, particularly in the postmenopausal period (28).

Little is known about the effect of diet or drugs on Lp(a) levels, although current studies indicate that diet has little effect on Lp(a) levels (29). Only one commonly used lipid-lowering agent, niacin, has been shown to lower Lp(a) levels (30). Most importantly, there is no evidence that changing Lp(a) levels has any effect on changing the risk of CHD. Until more information is available about Lp(a), it represents an interesting scientific phenomenon but one with few current clinical applications.

ENVIRONMENTAL MODIFIERS OF LIPOPROTEINS IN WOMEN

Diet

In most public health recommendations that address dietary change there is an assumption that men and women will respond in an equivalent fashion. As a result, there is little distinction between recommendations made for women and men. Small studies of mostly premenopausal women, however, suggest that this may not be appropriate. These studies indicate that women (particularly premenopausal women) experience less lowering of *both* LDL and HDL on a low-cholesterol, low-saturated fat diet compared to men of the same age (31–33). It is important to emphasize that these studies generally involve small numbers of subjects and should be considered preliminary. Nevertheless, they raise the possibility that a low-cholesterol, low-saturated fat diet may not be as effective in lowering LDL levels in women as in men.

In one large study of 2000 *postmenopausal* women compared with men of comparable age, a very low fat diet was associated with a greater decline in LDL and triglyceride levels in men than in women and a greater decline in HDL levels in women than in men (34). Overall, there is little evidence to suggest that low saturated fat diets are harmful in women. It may be, however, that their effect is less dramatic than it is in men of the same age.

Weight

Weight loss, too, appears to be less effective in women than in men in lowering LDL and raising HDL levels. Again, the studies involve small numbers of subjects and should be regarded as preliminary. However, like those involving diet, they support the notion that, at least in some women, weight loss may not necessarily be associated with favorable changes in circulating lipoproteins. Indeed, in one study, women actually lowered HDL with the same degree of weight loss that, in the male subjects in the study, was associated with an increase in HDL levels (35).

Body Fat Distribution

Some of these differences in diet and weight loss may be related to the differences in body fat distribution in men and women. In men, fat tends to accumulate around the trunk, increasing the waist-to-hip ratio in the so-called android pattern of obesity. In the majority of women, on the other hand, body fat is more likely to accumulate in the buttocks and thighs, in the so-called gynecoid pattern. In both men and women, truncal fat is correlated with increases in LDL and decreases in HDL (36), and in both men and women, increases in truncal fat are associated with an increased risk of coronary disease and indeed, with an increased risk of mortality (37).

The mechanisms for these differences in the effects of fat, depending on its distribution, are unclear. In men, there is evidence that truncal fat may be associated with increased insulin resistance and hyperinsulinemia. This is not as well demonstrated in women (38), even though women with a tendency to distribute fat in the male pattern have demonstrated higher levels of circulating testosterone (39).

The level of endogenous estrogens may also be of importance. For example, adipose tissue in postmenopausal women can serve as a source of estrogen, synthesizing it from androstenedione (40). It may be that to some extent the benefits of weight reduction in women are offset by the loss of estrogen-producing adipose tissue, with the result that the expected increases in HDL and declines in LDL are not observed or are less prominent than those seen in men. The relationships between total body fat, body fat distribution, and endogenous hormones remain to be delineated, but it is clear that this is a fertile area for defining differences in lipoprotein physiology in men and women.

Exercise

As with diet and weight, exercise, too, appears to be more effective in raising HDL and lowering LDL in men than in women (41). These differences, again, are particularly pronounced in comparisons of younger women and men. In addition, premenopausal women respond to exercise with lipoprotein changes that are less consistent than they are in older, postmenopausal women (42). Again, the relationships between exercise, changes in total body fat and body fat distribution, and changes in endogenous hormone levels are still poorly delineated. Nevertheless, taken together, these observations imply that endogenous estrogen may, particularly in younger women, act as a physiologic buffer, maintaining lipoprotein levels in the face of changes in diet and body fat. Clearly, this is an area that requires considerable further investigation in the future.

Diabetes

In nondiabetic men and women, CHD rates are measurably different until men and women

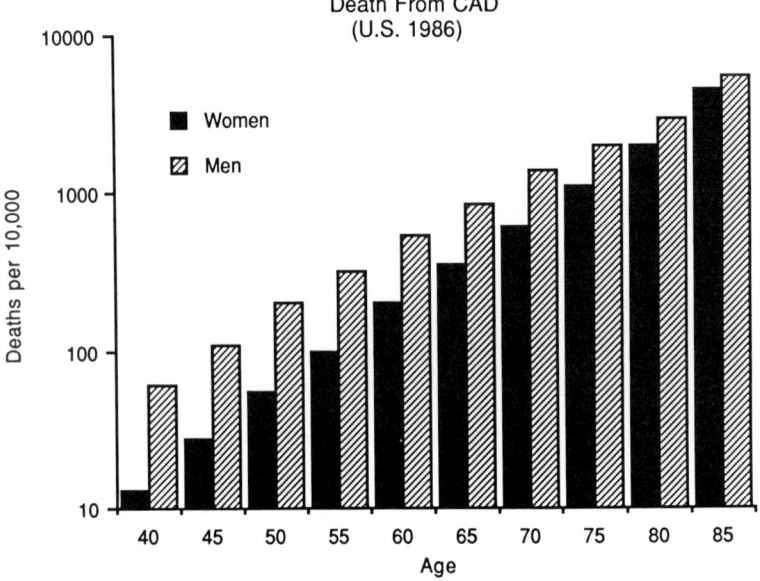

Figure 9–4. Death from CAD in the United States, 1986. (From Bush TL. The epidemiology of cardiovascular disease in postmenopausal women. *Ann NY Acad Sci* 592:263–271, 1990.)

reach their late sixties and early seventies, at which point they become more or less equal. At every age group until that point is reached, men have a higher risk of coronary disease than women (Fig. 9–4) (43). In the presence of diabetes, however, that is not the case. Diabetic men and women have virtually the same rate of coronary disease (Fig. 9–5). The explanation for this is not immediately apparent. One explanation that has been put for-

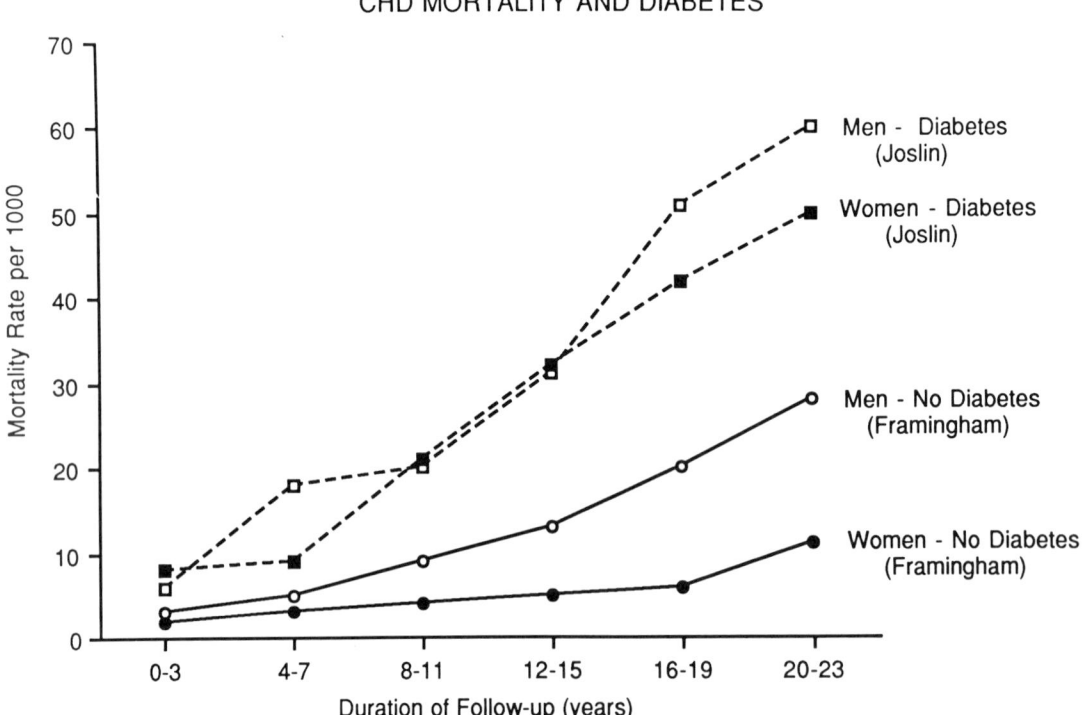

Figure 9–5. CHD mortality and diabetes. (Adapted from Krolewski AS, Warram JF, Valsania P, et al. Evolving natural history of coronary artery disease in diabetes mellitus. *Am J Med* (Suppl. 2A):56S–61S, 1991.)

ward is that diabetic women have greater and more adverse changes in lipoprotein levels than do diabetic men. Although this is, in fact, the case, diabetic women, nevertheless, continue to have more favorable lipoprotein levels than diabetic men (44). HDL levels are higher and LDL levels are lower, even in diabetic women, compared to diabetic men. Thus, while changes in circulating lipoprotein levels may be part of the explanation for the equalization of coronary risk in diabetic men and women, it is undoubtedly not the whole explanation.

Exogenous Gonadal Hormones

The effect of exogenous gonadal hormones in the form of oral contraceptives (OC) or hormone replacement therapy (HRT) is the subject of Chapter 8 in this text. As a general comment, it should be pointed out, however, that these regimens affect circulating lipoprotein levels depending on their relative potency as androgens or estrogens. Since most of the regimens currently in use involve a combination of exogenously administered estrogen and progestin (most of which have some androgenic properties), the net effect of a given preparation on circulating lipoproteins is not always predictable but is the result of these two opposing constituents.

Even modern low-dose OCs have somewhat adverse effects on lipoproteins, raising LDL and lowering HDL levels, particularly in the so-called HDL_2 fraction, which is thought to be the fraction most protective against coronary disease (45). Less is known about the effects of estrogen-progestin combinations used in postmenopausal HRT regimens. As a general comment, however, those regimens that involve the addition of a progestin to the exogenously administered estrogen generally also compromise the beneficial effects of estrogen in raising HDL and lowering LDL levels.

TREATMENT OF LIPOPROTEIN DISORDERS IN WOMEN

Evidence of Benefit in Women

Given the differences in lipoprotein metabolism in women and men, it is not unreasonable to ask whether lowering cholesterol is of the same importance in preventing CHD in women. Most of the recently reported trials of cholesterol lowering have excluded women and have concentrated instead on middle-aged men. The original rationale for this concentrated attention on middle-aged men was related to the fact that it was this age group that was most at risk of "premature" CHD. As more data have accumulated and this question has been reexamined, however, it has been realized that coronary disease is the most common cause of death and disability in both women and men, although coronary disease is generally clinically manifest in women about 5 to 10 years later than it is in men (Fig. 9–4).

Concern is sometimes expressed that there are insufficient clinical trial data to justify cholesterol-lowering interventions in women and that extrapolations of the evidence of benefits of cholesterol lowering for men to women are unjustified. Although this argument is not totally without merit, it is important to recognize that what data exist are strongly supportive of the idea that cholesterol lowering is an important intervention in both women and men. In the Newcastle (46), Edinburgh (47), and Finnish (48) Mental Hospital studies, all done in Europe in the late 1960s and early 1970s, both men and women were included in the data, and the two genders were analyzed separately. A recent meta-analysis of these three studies (49) demonstrated that equivalent cholesterol lowering in women and men was associated with equivalent reductions in coronary death rates.

In addition, a recent study of the effects of aggressive cholesterol lowering and HDL increase, induced by a combination of diet and multidrug therapy, was recently completed in severely hypercholesterolemic men and women (50). This study, utilizing serial coronary angiography, is particularly instructive because it demonstrated that progression of CHD and even regression of that disease could be induced in both sexes. Interestingly, the effect was more pronounced in the women in the study than in the men, even though the degree of LDL decrease and HDL increase was virtually identical in both sexes. Thus, although the mass of evidence that cholesterol lowering is of benefit is greater in men than in women, what evidence does exist in women indicates that the benefits of intervention are operative in both sexes.

Current Guidelines for Treatment of Lipoprotein Disorders

Guidelines for the detection, evaluation, and treatment of hypercholesterolemia and related disorders have been developed by the National Cholesterol Education Program (NCEP) (51). They have generally recommended that LDL be the primary target of intervention but that the total cholesterol level, which is more widely available and better standardized, be the primary screening parameter. Table 9–3 lists NCEP definitions of normal total and LDL cholesterol levels. These were not considered to be different in women than in men. HDL, in these guidelines, is not considered a primary target for intervention. Individuals with low HDL levels (defined in the guidelines as less than 35 mg/dL [0.9 meq/L]) are treated as having an additional risk factor.

Triglycerides are not addressed in depth in these guidelines. When triglyceride levels are over 250 mg/dL (2.8 meq/L), however, they are recommended as targets for therapeutic intervention. Drugs that lower triglycerides, however, are suggested only if LDL levels are also high, if HDL is low, if triglycerides are very high [over 1000 mg/dL (11.4 meq/L)], or if there is a personal or family history of CHD or other manifestations of atherosclerosis.

Selection of both male and female subjects for further screening is limited to those with cholesterol levels of greater than 240 mg/dL (6.2 meq/L) or those whose screening cholesterol levels are in the 200 to 239 mg/dL (5.2–6.2 meq/dL) range and who also have established coronary disease or other risk factors. Similarly, subjects with LDL levels of over 190 mg/dL (4.9 meq/L) or between 160 and 190 mg/dL (4.1–4.9 meq/L) in the presence of established disease or other risk factors are candidates for drug therapy.

Other risk factors include male sex, cigarette smoking, hypertension, diabetes, obesity, HDL of less than 35 mg/dL (0.9 meq/L), and a family history of coronary disease.

The major difference in applying these guidelines to men and women lies in the recommendation that men need only have one risk factor (since male sex is itself considered to be a risk factor) in order to be candidates for earlier and more intense intervention. For example, a cigarette smoking man with a total cholesterol level in the 200 to 239 mg/dL (5.2–6.2 meq/dL) range should, according to the guidelines, have an LDL measurement. A woman who is a smoker, however, would require one other risk factor before triggering an LDL measurement. In similar fashion, a man with an LDL between 160 and 190 mg/dL (4.1–4.9 meq/dL) who was a smoker would become a candidate for drug therapy, whereas a woman with the same LDL would require another risk factor before drugs were considered.

In this way, the guidelines attempted to account for the fact that the risk of coronary disease is lower in women than in men through most of the life span, and that drug intervention, in particular, should be more limited in women than in men.

Coronary disease, on the other hand, is the most common form of death and disability in women as well as in men, and an argument can be made that these distinctions should, in view of the evidence that cholesterol lowering is of benefit in both men and women, not be maintained. Diabetic women, moreover, have the *same* risk of CHD as diabetic men. Resolution of such issues will await further studies of cholesterol lowering in women and further

Table 9–3. NCEP CUT-OFF POINTS FOR TOTAL AND LDL CHOLESTEROL LEVELS

	Total Cholesterol		LDL Cholesterol
Normal	<200 mg/dL (5.2 meq/L)	Normal	<130 mg/dL (3.4 meq/L)
Borderline	200–239 mg/dL (5.2–6.2 meq/L)	Borderline	130–159 mg/dL (3.4–4.1 meq/L)
High	>240 mg/dL (>6.2 meq/L)	High risk	>160 mg/dL (>4.1 meq/L)

Drug Therapy Guidelines

Those with LDL >190 (4.9 meq/L) after trial of diet

Those with LDL >160 (4.1 meq/L) after trial of diet if CHD is present or in the presence of two other risk factors (women) or one other risk factor (men)

evidence of the particular benefits of lowering LDL and raising HDL.

As noted above, there may be reason to expect a lesser response to diet in women than in men. There is no reason to expect that drug therapy will be less effective in women than in men. Indeed, in the regression study involving hypercholesterolemic men and women noted above (50), LDL decreases and HDL increases were virtually identical in women and men.

It has sometimes been suggested that estrogen replacement therapy (ERT) itself might be viewed as a first line of therapy for hypercholesterolemic women, since estrogen tends to lower LDL and raise HDL levels. In addition, it is important to remember that estrogen may have beneficial protective effects on the arterial wall that are not reflected in circulating lipoprotein levels. What is lacking in all of this are clinical trials clearly demonstrating the benefits (and perhaps the drawbacks) of ERT on coronary morbidity and mortality, and indicating the correct drug regimen(s). Until such studies are completed, decisions about estrogen intervention will have to rely on the available epidemiologic observational data that indicate that unopposed estrogen lowers both coronary and all-cause mortality rates in postmenopausal women (52). This issue is discussed in detail in Chapter 8.

SUMMARY

Lipoprotein disorders occur in women as well as in men. In both men and women, observational studies indicate that the same relationships exist between coronary atherosclerosis and lipoprotein abnormalities. Clinical evidence of the benefits of favorable alterations in circulating lipoproteins are less abundant in women than in men but are not completely absent. Clinical trials indicate that, whether the end points are coronary death or changes in coronary anatomy, the benefits of lowering total or LDL cholesterol levels or increasing HDL are present in women as well as in men. LDL appears to be a less important risk factor in women, perhaps because estrogen itself protects the arterial wall against LDL deposition. HDL is a better predictor of risk in women than in men. Triglyceride appears to be a better independent predictor of coronary risk in postmenopausal women than in men of the same age.

As women pass through the life cycle, unique changes in circulating lipoproteins occur. As girls pass through puberty, HDL levels do not fall as they do in boys of the same age. In pregnancy, LDL, HDL, and triglyceride levels all rise, although only LDL levels stay elevated until well after delivery. After menopause, LDL levels rise sharply while HDL levels decline modestly. All of these effects probably reflect, at least in part, the impact of endogenous gonadal hormones.

Other life-style changes have different effects on lipoproteins in women than in men. Based on incomplete and preliminary studies, diet, weight loss, and exercise all appear to be less effective in producing favorable alterations in circulating lipoprotein levels in women than in men. The reasons for this difference are unclear, although it is tempting to speculate that endogenous gonadal hormone levels may play a role. Pharmaceutical therapy, on the other hand, seems to be as effective in women as in men, not only in producing favorable changes in lipoproteins but also affecting the coronary anatomy. Finally, exogenous gonadal hormones are potentially important in modifying lipoprotein levels and therefore coronary risk in women. This topic is covered in depth in Chapter 8.

Current guidelines for lipoprotein abnormalities in women differ in subtle ways from those recommended for men. Basically, these guidelines set higher thresholds for lipoprotein evaluations in hypercholesterolemic women and higher thresholds for drug treatment in women who are found to have elevations of LDL.

Better understanding of the interaction between lipoprotein abnormalities, life-style factors, and coronary atherosclerosis will almost surely await clarification of the inter-relationships between circulating lipoproteins, endogenous gonadal hormones, body weight and body fat distribution, and perhaps even circulating insulin levels. Based on current knowledge, there is every reason to feel comfortable in intervening to lower LDL levels in women as well as in men. It is important, however, not to lose sight of the fact that lipoprotein levels and function in women and men are not identical and may not have the same relationship to coronary atherosclerosis. It is entirely likely that, as our knowledge about the differences in gender becomes more sophisticated, unique guidelines for women, separate from those for men, may be required.

References

1. Ginsberg HN. Lipoprotein physiology and its relationship to atherogenesis. *Endocrinol Metab Clin North Am* 19:211–228, 1990.
2. Mahley RW, Innerarity TL, Rall SC Jr, et al: Plasma lipoproteins: Apolipoprotein structure and function. *J Lipid Res* 25:1277–1294, 1984.
3. Schonfeld G. Inherited disorders of lipid transport. *Endocrinol Metab Clin North Am* 19:229–257, 1990.
4. LaRosa JC, Chambless LE, Criqui MH, et al. Patterns of dyslipoproteinemia in selected North American populations: The Lipid Research Clinics Program Prevalence Study. *Circulation* 73 (Suppl. I) I-12–I-29, 1986.
5. LaRosa JC. Dyslipoproteinemia secondary to common clinical disorders. Mechanisms and treatment. *Cardiovasc Risk Factors* 1:52–60, 1990.
6. LaRosa JC. Secondary hyperlipoproteinemia. In Rifkind BM, Levy RI (Eds.), *Hyperlipidemia: Diagnosis and Therapy*. New York, Grune & Stratton, 1977, pp. 205–216.
7. Steinberg D, Parthasarathy S, Carew TE, et al. Beyond cholesterol. Modifications of low-density lipoprotein that increase its atherogenicity. *N Engl J Med* 320:915–924, 1989.
8. Brown MS, Goldstein JL. Lipoprotein metabolism in the macrophage: Implications for cholesterol deposition in atherosclerosis. *Annu Rev Biochem* 52:223–261, 1983.
9. Seed M. Sex hormones, lipoproteins, and cardiovascular risk. *Atherosclerosis* 90:1–7, 1991.
10. Kannel WB. Nutrition and the occurrence and prevention of cardiovascular disease in the elderly. *Nutr Rev* 46:68–78, 1984.
11. Matthews KA, Meilahn E, Kuller LH, et al. Menopause and risk factors for coronary heart disease. *N Engl J Med* 321:641–646, 1989.
12. Rifkind BM, Segal P. Lipid Resource Clinics reference values for hyperlipidemia and hypolipidemia. *JAMA* 250:1869–1872, 1983.
13. Kim HJ, Kalkhoff RK. Changes in lipoprotein composition during the menstrual cycle. *Metabolism* 28:663–668, 1979.
14. Ottosson UB, Johansson BG, von Schoulz B. Subfractions of high-density lipoprotein cholesterol during estrogen replacement therapy: A comparison between progestogens and natural progesterone. *Am J Obstet Gynecol* 151:746–750, 1985.
15. Fahraeus L, Larsson-Cohn U, Wallentin L. Plasma lipoproteins including high density lipoprotein subfractions during normal pregnancy. *Obstet Gynecol* 66:468–472, 1985.
16. Desoye G, Schweditsch MO, Pfeiffer KP, et al. Correlations of hormones with lipid and lipoprotein levels during normal pregnancy and postpartum. *J Clin Endocrinol Metab* 64:704–712, 1987.
17. Oliver MF. Ischaemic heart disease in young women. *Br Med J* 4:253–259, 1974.
18. Eaker ED, Castelli WP. Coronary heart disease and its risk factors among women in the Framingham Study. In Eaker ED, Packard B, Wenger N, et al. (Eds.), *Coronary Heart Disease in Women*. New York, Haymarket Doyma, 1987, pp. 122–130.
19. Gordon DJ, Probstfield JL, Garrison RF, et al. High-density lipoprotein cholesterol and cardiovascular disease: Four prospective studies. *Circulation* 79:8–15, 1989.
20. Wagner JD, Clarkson TB, St. Clair RW, et al. Estrogen replacement therapy (ERT) and coronary artery (CA) atherogenesis in surgically postmenopausal cynomologus monkeys (abstract). *Circulation* 80 (Suppl. II):331, 1989.
21. Austin MA. Epidemiologic associations between hypertriglyceridemia and coronary heart disease. *Semin Thromb Hemost* 14:137–142, 1988.
22. Castelli WP. The triglyceride issue: A view from Framingham. *Am Heart J* 112:432–437, 1986.
23. Campos H, McNamara JR, Wilson PWF, et al. Differences in low density lipoprotein subfractions and apolipoproteins in premenopausal and postmenopausal women. *J Clin Endocrinol Metab* 67:30–35, 1988.
24. de Graaf J, Hak-Lemmers HLM, Hectors MPC, et al. Enhanced susceptibility to in vitro oxidation of the dense low density lipoprotein subfraction in healthy subjects. *Arteriosclerosis* 11:298–306, 1991.
25. Scanu AM, Fless GM. Lipoprotein(a): Heterogeneity and biological relevance. *J Clin Invest* 85:1709–1715, 1990.
26. Utermann G. The mysteries of lipoprotein(a). *Science* 246:904–910, 1989.
27. Dahlen GH. Incidence of Lp(a) lipoprotein among populations. In Scanu AM (Ed.), *Lipoprotein(a)*. New York, Academic Press, 1990, pp. 151–173.
28. Sandkamp M, Assmann G. Lipoprotein(a) in PROCAM participants and young myocardial infarction survivors. In Scanu AM (Ed.), *Lipoprotein(a)*. New York, Academic Press, 1990, pp. 205–209.
29. Brewer HB. Effectiveness of diet and drugs in the treatment of patients with elevated Lp(a) levels. In Scanu AM (Ed.), *Lipoprotein(a)*. New York, Academic Press, 1990, pp. 211–220.
30. Carlson LA, Hamsten A, Asplund A. Pronounced lowering of serum levels of lipoprotein(a) in hyperlipidaemic subjects treated with nicotinic acid. *J Int Med* 226:271–276, 1989.
31. Mensink RP, Katan MB. Effect of monounsaturated fatty acids versus complex carbohydrates on high-density lipoproteins in healthy men and women. *Lancet* 8525:122–125, 1987.
32. Masarei JRL, Rouse IL, Lynch WJ, et al. Effects of a lacto-ovo vegetarian diet on serum concentration of cholesterol, triglyceride, HDL-C, HDL$_2$-C, HDL$_3$-C, apoprotein-B, and Lp(a). *Am J Clin Nutr* 40:468–478, 1984.
33. Ernst N, Bowen P, Fisher M, et al. Changes in plasma lipids and lipoproteins after a modified fat diet. *Lancet* 1:111–113, 1980.
34. Barnard RJ. Effects of life-style modification on serum lipids. *Arch Intern Med* 151:1389–1394, 1991.
35. Brownell KD. Differential changes in plasma high-density lipoprotein-cholesterol levels in obese men and women during weight reduction. *Arch Intern Med* 141:1142–1146, 1981.
36. Soler JT, Folsom AR, Kushi LH, et al. Association of body fat distribution with plasma lipids, lipoproteins, apolipoproteins AI and B in postmenopausal women. *J Clin Epidemiol* 41:1075–1081, 1988.
37. Lapidus L, Bengtsson C, Larsson B, et al. Distribution of adipose tissue and risk of cardiovascular disease and death: A 12 year follow up of participants in the population study of women in Gothenburg, Sweden. *Br Med J* 289:1257–1261, 1984.
38. Donahue RP, Orchard TJ, Becker DJ, et al. Physical activity, insulin sensitivity, and the lipoprotein profile

in young adults: The Beaver County study. *Am J Epidemiol* 127:95–103, 1988.
39. Hauner H, Ditschuneit HH, Pal SB, et al. Fat distribution, endocrine and metabolic profile in obese women with and without hirsutism. *Metabolism* 37:281–286, 1988.
40. Grodin JM, Siiteri PK, MacDonald PC. Source of estrogen production in postmenopausal women. *J Clin Endocrinol Metab* 36:207–214, 1973.
41. Lokey EA, Tran ZV. Effects of exercise training on serum lipid and lipoprotein concentrations in women: A meta-analysis. *Int J Sports Med* 10:424–429, 1989.
42. Hartung GH, Moore CE, Mitchell R, et al. Relationship of menopausal status and exercise level to HDL cholesterol in women. *Exp Aging Res* 10:13–18, 1984.
43. Bush TL. The epidemiology of cardiovascular disease in postmenopausal women. *Ann NY Acad Sci* 592:263–271, 1990.
44. Krolewski AS, Warram JH, Valsania P, et al. Evolving natural history of coronary artery disease in diabetes mellitus. *Am J Med* 90: (2A)56S–61S, 1991.
45. Notelovitz M, Feldman EB, Gillespy M, et al. Lipid and lipoprotein changes in women taking low-dose, triphasic oral contraceptives: A controlled, comparative, 12-month clinical trial. *Am J Obstet Gynecol* 160:1269–1280, 1989.
46. Group of Physicians of the Newcastle upon Tyne Region. Trial of clofibrate in the treatment of ischaemic heart disease. *Br Med J* 4:767–775, 1971.
47. Research Committee of the Scottish Society of Physicians: Ischaemic heart disease: A secondary prevention trial using clofibrate. *Br Med J* 4:775–784, 1971.
48. Miettinen M, Karvonen MJ, Turpeinen O, et al. Effect of cholesterol-lowering diet on mortality from coronary heart-disease and other causes. *Lancet* 2:835–838, 1972.
49. Rossouw JF. International trials (abstract). Presented at *Cholesterol and Heart Disease in Older Persons and in Women*, June 18–19, 1990. National Heart, Lung, and Blood Institute, National Institutes of Health, Bethesda, MD.
50. Kane JP, Malloy MJ, Ports TA, et al. Regression of coronary atherosclerosis during treatment of familial hypercholesterolemia with combined drug regimens. *JAMA* 264:3007–3012, 1990.
51. Report of the National Cholesterol Education Program Expert Panel on detection, evaluation, and treatment of high blood cholesterol in adults. *Arch Intern Med* 148:36–69, 1988.
52. Barrett-Connor E. Estrogen and coronary heart disease in women. *JAMA* 265:1861–1867, 1991.

CHAPTER 10

Carbohydrate Metabolism, Obesity, and Diabetes

ANGELA SPELSBERG, M.D., M.Sc.
PAUL M. RIDKER, M.D., M.P.H.
JOANN E. MANSON, M.D., Dr.P.H.

Abnormalities of carbohydrate metabolism play a major role in influencing the cardiovascular health of women. In particular, women with diabetes mellitus or obesity often have a substantially elevated risk of cardiovascular disease. In this chapter the physiology of carbohydrate metabolism is reviewed as well as the unique epidemiologic and clinical aspects of caring for female patients with diabetes and obesity.

CARBOHYDRATE METABOLISM

Normal Physiology

The maintenance of normal blood sugar levels represents one of the major biochemical tasks of the human organism, requiring a delicately balanced interaction of glycogenesis,

Table 10-1. MAINTENANCE OF PLASMA GLUCOSE DURING FASTING

Length of Fast	Source of Plasma Glucose	Mechanisms	Tissues Using Glucose	Primary Fuel of Brain
3-4 hr	Diet	Intestinal absorption	All	Glucose
4-16 hr	Liver	Glycogenolysis	All except liver (↓ rates in muscle and adipose tissue)	Glucose
16-48 hr	Liver	Gluconeogenesis (± glycogenolysis)	All except liver (further ↓ rates in muscle and adipose tissue)	Glucose
2-24 days	Liver, kidney	Gluconeogenesis	Brain, RBC, renal medulla	Glucose Ketones
>4 weeks	Liver, kidney	Gluconeogenesis	Brain, RBC, renal medulla (↓ rates)	Ketones Glucose

From Ruderman NB, et al. Gluconeogenesis and its disorders in man. In Hanson RW, Mehlman MA (Eds.), *Gluconeogenesis: Its Regulation in Mammalian Species*. New York, Wiley, 1976, pp. 515-532.

glycogenolysis, glycolysis, and gluconeogenesis (Table 10-1). Insulin and glucagon play a predominant role in the regulation of these processes, particularly in liver and muscle cells.

Ingested complex carbohydrates of different dietary origins are split during the digestive process into three absorbable simple sugars: glucose, fructose, and galactose. Glucose, the most important saccharide, is rapidly taken up by the different organ tissues and used as the main energy provider through four major metabolic pathways. These pathways include the storage of glucose as glycogen in liver and muscle cells, anaerobic glycolysis to pyruvate and lactate, aerobic oxidation, and lipogenesis by triglyceride formation (1).

Gluconeogenesis, which involves the formation of glucose from noncarbohydrate sources such as pyruvate, lactate, glycerol, and amino acids, occurs primarily in the liver. Gluconeogenesis is primarily stimulated by glucagon, although thyroid and glucocorticoid hormones can also play major regulatory roles (1). A comparison of hepatic glucose output through gluconeogenesis and glycogenolysis in nondiabetic and diabetic metabolism is presented in Figure 10-1.

In large part, normal carbohydrate metabolism is regulated by the interaction of insulin, catecholamines, glucagon, and the glucocorticoid hormones (Table 10-2). Secretion of insulin (which is synthesized in the pancreatic beta cells) depends on several conditions, with glucose availability being the most important one. Secretion appears to be biphasic, with a rapid, high-peaked first secretory phase lasting for a few minutes after glucose exposure, followed by a continuous (up to 1 hour) lower-peaked second secretory phase.

Catecholamines interfere with both insulin secretion and insulin effectiveness. Catecholamines also influence glucose metabolism through direct stimulation of glycogenolysis and gluconeogenesis. The hyperglycemic ef-

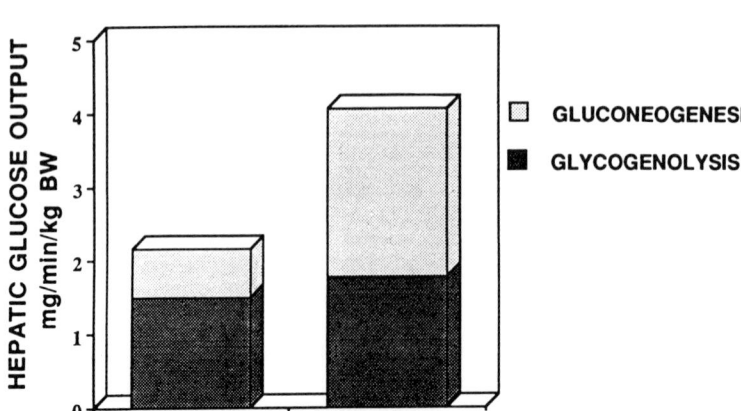

Figure 10-1. Components (glycogenolysis and gluconeogenesis) of hepatic glucose output in controls and type II diabetic persons. (From Consoli A, Nurjhan N, Capani F, et al: Predominant role of gluconeogenesis in increased hepatic glucose production in NIDDM. *Diabetes* 38:550, 1989).

Table 10-2. THE DEFENSE OF BLOOD SUGAR

Process	Hormones Involved
Glucose intake and absorption	Cortisol ← ACTH ← CRF Thyroxine ← TSH ← TRH
Glycogenolysis	Glucagon (between meals) Epinephrine (in emergencies) (insulin suppression) Cortisol Thyroxine
Gluconeogenesis	Cortisol GH Glucagon (insulin suppression) Epinephrine
Use of alternative energy sources	Epinephrine GH (insulin suppression)

ACTH = Adrenocorticotropic hormone; CRF = corticotropin-releasing factor; TSH = thyroid-stimulating hormone; TRH = thyrotropin-releasing hormone; GH = growth hormone.

fects of epinephrine and norepinephrine are intensified by the sympathetic stimulation of glucagon secretion and lipolysis (2).

Glucagon, which is produced in the pancreatic alpha cells, is released in healthy subjects predominantly in response to ingestion or infusion of proteins or amino acids and prolonged physical activity. Simultaneous secretion of insulin and glucagon avoids postprandial hypoglycemia due to high insulin concentrations (1).

Glucocorticoid hormones interfere with carbohydrate metabolism by increasing gluconeogenesis and glycogenesis in combination with enhanced protein breakdown. Glucocorticoids antagonize insulin binding to its receptors, thereby reducing cellular glucose uptake. Hyperinsulinemia, insulin resistance, and hyperglycemia are characteristic features of prolonged exposure to elevated glucocorticoid concentrations (2).

Although less important than insulin, glucagon, catecholamines, and glucocorticoids, other hormones such as the sex steroids and growth-regulating hormones also affect carbohydrate metabolism. It has been hypothesized that these factors rather than insulin secretion interfere with insulin effectiveness. Possible diabetogenic actions of sex steroid hormones include direct insulin-antagonistic effects, associations with elevated levels of contrainsulin hormones, and alterations of intestinal glucose absorption (3, 4). Polycystic ovarian disease and other hyperandrogenic conditions in women are frequently associated with hyperinsulinemia. With oral contraceptive use, both estrogens and progestins have been shown to promote insulin resistance and glucose intolerance (3). Exogenous estrogens have been demonstrated to cause greater elevations in blood glucose levels and higher insulin requirements than progestins (5). The influence of postmenopausal estrogens on glucose tolerance remains uncertain; the use of these hormones does not appear to increase the risk of clinical noninsulin-dependent diabetes mellitus (NIDDM) among current or past users (6).

Pregnancy profoundly influences carbohydrate metabolism and insulin sensitivity, including increasing a tendency to develop fasting hypoglycemia and hyperketonemia as well as postprandial hyperglycemia. After an overnight fast, pregnant women have lower plasma glucose and insulin levels and higher ketone body and free fatty acid (FFA) concentrations than nonpregnant women (1). During the second half of pregnancy, the insulin response to glucose or protein intake markedly exceeds nonpregnant values, whereas glucose levels tend to be normal to high, suggesting insulin resistance that is probably due to hormonal changes. Proposed diabetogenic hormones include human placental lactogen (HPL), estrogen, progesterone, and prolactin. HPL, progesterone, and estrogen seem to augment insulin secretion, but their influence on tissue insulin resistance remains controversial. Prolactin also appears to induce hyperinsulinemia as well as tissue resistance to insulin; it may also suppress glucagon secretion (1).

Abnormal Physiology

Insulin Resistance

Insulin resistance is defined as a normal or elevated blood sugar concentration in the presence of hyperinsulinemia. The causal mechanisms of insulin resistance are not fully understood but have been related to reduced tissue sensitivity or reduced effectiveness of insulin. From a clinical perspective, a close interaction clearly exists between obesity, diabetes, and insulin resistance (7).

In patients with NIDDM, a 30-40% reduction in response to exogenous insulin has been measured (8). Both immunologic and nonimmunologic processes are involved in the development of insulin resistance. For example, insulin antibodies have been identified that neutralize exogenous insulin. Nonimmunologic mechanisms of insulin resistance include nonspecific protein binding of circulating insulin, lower tissue sensitivity related to insulin receptor disorders, and the effect of increased concentrations of counterregulatory hormones such as glucagon, growth hormone, catecholamines, and thyroid hormone (9). Recently, two rare insulin-resistant conditions have been described in women. One condition (type A) occurs in young women with acanthosis nigricans and polycystic ovaries who have abnormal or absent insulin receptors. The other abnormality (type B) is found in older women with autoimmune disorders in whom immunologic blocking of insulin receptors can be detected. In both syndromes hyperinsulinemia is not related to obesity and does not cause diabetes (10).

Impaired Glucose Tolerance

The response to an ingested or infused glucose load should be investigated if the fasting glucose concentration in venous plasma is elevated but does not exceed the diagnostic threshold value for overt diabetes ($\geq$ 140 mg/dL or 7.8 mmol/L). Impaired glucose tolerance (IGT) is diagnosed if one of the plasma glucose concentrations at 30, 60, or 90 minutes after glucose loading exceeds 200 mg/dL (11.1 mmol/L) and if the 2-hour value is $\geq$ 140 mg/dL but < 200 mg/dL (11) (Table 10–3). From a clinical standpoint, the predictive importance of IGT has not been fully elucidated, although data suggest that 1–5% per year of IGT patients will ultimately develop diabetes (12).

Gestational Diabetes

The diagnosis of gestational diabetes is reserved exclusively for those women who develop impaired glucose tolerance or manifest diabetes during pregnancy with resolution after parturition. The criteria for an abnormal oral glucose tolerance test in pregnant women must take into account the metabolic changes of pregnancy, which include a tendency to develop fasting hypoglycemia and hyperketonemia as well as postprandial hyperglycemia. Fasting venous plasma glucose values above 105 mg/dL (5.8 mmol/L) and a 60-minute value of 190 mg/dL (10.6 mmol/L) or above *or* a 120-minute value of 165 mg/dL (9.2 mmol/L) or above *or* a 180-minute value of 145 mg/dL (8.1 mmol/L) or above suggest gestational diabetes (12) (Table 10–3). The probability that a woman with gestational diabetes will develop manifest diabetes within a timespan of 16 years

Table 10–3. CRITERIA FOR THE DIAGNOSIS OF DIABETES MELLITUS, IMPAIRED GLUCOSE TOLERANCE, AND GESTATIONAL DIABETES

	NDDG Criteria[a]	WHO Criteria[b]
	Venous Plasma Glucose[c]	*Venous Plasma Glucose*[c]
Diabetes Mellitus		
Fasting	$\geq$140	$\geq$140
OGTT[d] (2-hour value)	$\geq$200 (11.1) *and* one other value $\geq$200 11.1) between 0 and 2 hours	$\geq$200 (11.1) (values between 0 and 2 hours are not included in the criteria)
Random	"Gross and unequivocal elevation" of glucose levels with classic symptoms of uncontrolled diabetes	$\geq$200 (11.1)
Impaired Glucose Tolerance		
Fasting	<140 (7.8)	<140 (7.8)
OGTT (2-hour value)	140–199 (7.8–11.1)	140–199 (7.8–11.1)
OGTT (½, 1, or 1½ hour value)	$\geq$200 (11.1)	(not included in the criteria)
Gestational Diabetes[e]		
Fasting	$\geq$105 (5.8)	
1 hour	$\geq$190 (10.6)	
2 hours	$\geq$165 (9.2)	
3 hours	$\geq$145 (8.1)	

[a] National Diabetes Data Group. *Diabetes* 28:1039, 1979.
[b] World Health Organization. WHO Tech Rep Series 646. Geneva, 1980.
[c] mg/dL (mM/L).
[d] OGTT = oral glucose tolerance test.
[e] Two or more elevated values are required to make the diagnosis.

is approximately 35%. Women with high fasting glucose levels (> 130 mg/dL or 7.2 mmol/L) prior to delivery are at greatest risk (13).

Insulin-Dependent Diabetes Mellitus

Insulin-dependent diabetes mellitus (IDDM) has been recognized to occur usually, but not always, in nonobese subjects below 30 years of age. It is associated with a high tendency for ketosis and high levels of circulating islet cell antibodies in the majority of patients. Insulin treatment is essential to avoid ketoacidosis. The diagnosis of IDDM is usually obvious after almost complete autoimmune destruction of beta islet cells leads to typical symptoms. The pathogenetic mechanism is believed to include genetic susceptibility to environmental hazards (e.g., viral infections that lead to inflammatory changes of the islet cell surface). The altered cell surface provokes autoimmune attack by islet cell antibodies and lymphocytes, which finally destroys the beta cells and leads to irreversible diabetes (9). Criteria for the diagnosis of diabetes mellitus are presented in Table 10–3.

Noninsulin-Dependent Diabetes Mellitus

NIDDM patients are generally over 40 years old and obese (14). In contrast to patients suffering from IDDM, individuals who develop NIDDM are not prone to become ketoacidotic even with severe hyperglycemia. Therefore, it is the risk of ketoacidosis rather than treatment with insulin that is the central difference between these two disease entities.

The pathogenesis of NIDDM is not fully understood. In particular, the time sequence of the characteristic abnormalities in insulin secretion and the resistance to insulin is an issue of controversy (Fig. 10–2). Obesity plays a major role in NIDDM, leading to the hypothesis that obesity-induced insulin resistance represents the causal mechanism of insulin hypersecretion and final exhaustion of the beta cell. However, not every obese subject develops NIDDM; there seems to be an additional susceptibility of beta cells responsible for the insulin secretion abnormalities leading to hyperglycemia. Plasma insulin levels are normal to elevated and responsiveness to exogenous insulin may be substantially decreased. Rarely, a ketosis-resistant and noninsulin-dependent diabetes occurs in young patients (maturity-onset diabetes of the young [MODY]). This disease has an autosomal dominant transmission and is more benign than the other diabetic conditions with respect to course and outcome (15). Clinically, NIDDM and IDDM do not differ substantially in terms of chronicity and outcome; both forms of diabetes lead to progressive vascular and neurologic damage, impairing the quality of life and life expectancy in women and men.

Secondary Diabetes

A variety of systemic diseases that interfere with glucose metabolism can cause secondary diabetes, including hormone-producing tumors, inborn errors of metabolism, insulin receptor abnormalities, insulin-resistant syndromes, and hereditary neuromuscular disorders. Isolated pancreatic disease, surgical removal or toxic damage of the pancreas, and drug side effects (diuretics, corticosteroids and other contrainsulin hormones, antidepressants, phenytoin, streptozotocin) are possible other causes of diabetes that have to be considered in the differential diagnosis (9).

Obesity

Although not strictly considered an abnormality of carbohydrate metabolism, obesity is currently regarded as a heterogeneous disorder of multifactorial origin (16). Variables implicated in its etiology include genetic predisposition, hypothalamic disturbances, metabolic or endocrine imbalances, nutritional variation, physical inactivity, and emotional disorders (14).

Obesity is defined as an excess of body fat associated with an increased fat cell size (17). Unfortunately, distinctions between normal and abnormal body fat mass are based on somewhat arbitrary cutoff points. Normal body fat content is considered to lie between 15 and 20% of body weight in men and between 20 and 25% of body weight in women (18). Several measures of adiposity have been used to estimate body fat content in epidemiologic studies, including determinations of skinfold thickness at different body sites (18–21), rela-

Pathogenesis of NIDDM

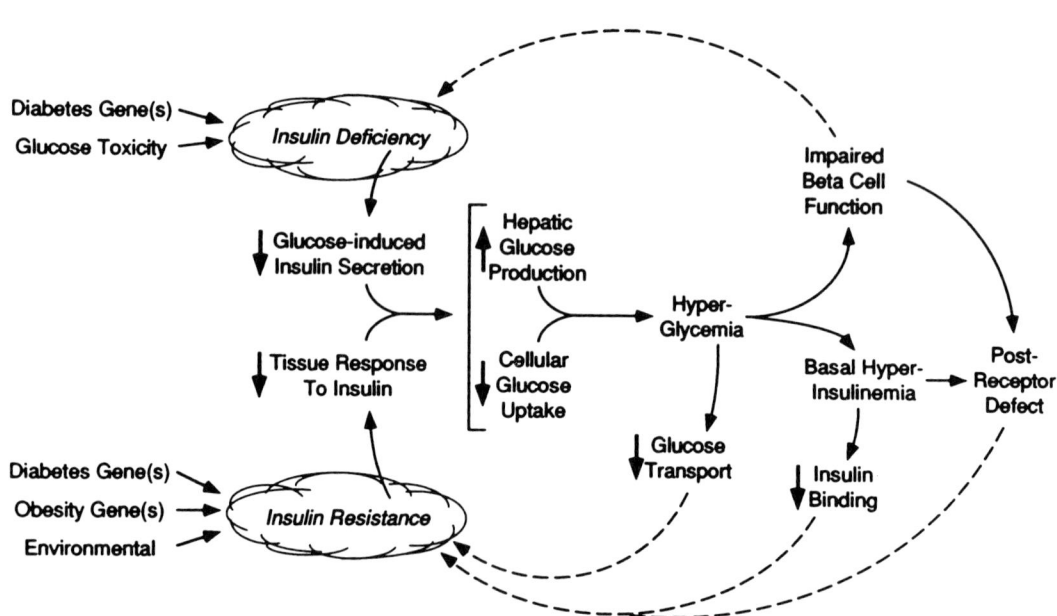

Figure 10–2. Pathogenetic sequence of events leading to the development of glucose intolerance, insulin resistance, and impaired insulin secretion in noninsulin-dependent diabetes. Note that whether the primary defect that initiates the glucose intolerance resides in the β-cell or in peripheral/hepatic tissues, development of insulin resistance eventually will ensue or become aggravated, respectively. By the time that overt fasting hyperglycemia (>140 mg/dL) develops, both impaired insulin secretion and severe insulin resistance are present. Broken arrows represent positive feedback loops, which result in self-perpetuation of primary defects. (Reprinted with permission from DeFronzo RA, Deibert D, Felig P, et al. Insulin sensitivity and insulin binding to monocytes in maturity onset diabetes. *J Clin Invest* 63:939–944, 1979. © by the American Diabetes Association.)

Table 10-4. BODY MASS INDEX (BMI) AT SPECIFIED RELATIVE WEIGHTS IN ADULTS

Metropolitan Relative Weight	BMI	
	Men	Women
Desirable		
1959	22.0	21.5
1983	22.7	22.4
20% overweight		
1959	26.4	25.8
1983	27.2	26.9
40% overweight		
1959	30.8	30.1
1983	31.1	32.3 approx
NCHS NHANES II		
Overweight[a]	27.8	27.3
Severely overweight[b]	31.1	32.3

During the period of growth, obesity is defined by weights, specific for height, age, and sex, that exceed the median weight plus 2 SD, derived from a reference population. (From Epstein FH, Higgins M. Epidemiology of obesity. In: Bjorntorp P, Brodoff BN, eds. Obesity. Philadelphia, JB Lippincott Co, 1992, pp 330-342.)
[a] ≥85th percentile for ages 20-29 years.
[b] ≥95th percentile for ages 20-29 years.

these indices, however, has limitations. For example, skinfold thicknesses are of limited value in patients with nonuniform distributions of body fat (20, 21), and relative weight tables have generally been confounded by cigarette smoking, preexisting disease, and "over-control" for physiologic effects of obesity such as hypertension and diabetes (24, 25). In this regard, the BMI (or Quetelet index) has the advantage of being relatively constant for subjects of the same degree of fatness regardless of height, and thus provides a reliable measure of obesity. Using the BMI, obesity is defined as equal to or greater than 27.3 kg/m^2 for women and 27.8 kg/m^2 for men based on data that relate this level with substantial risk elevation (16). The BMI values corresponding to desirable weights and specified levels of obesity are presented in Table 10-4. A comparison of average U.S. weights with Metropolitan Life Insurance Reference Tables for Weight recommended weights and the recent weight guidelines from the U.S. Department of Agriculture are shown in Table 10-5.

The distribution of body fat also influences cardiovascular health. Fat accumulation in the waist, abdomen, and upper body is more metabolically active than that in the hip, thigh, or buttocks (16). Abdominal fat accumulation is

tive weight tables corrected for height and sex (22, 23), and the body mass index (BMI, defined as the weight [kilograms] divided by the square of the height [meters]). Each of

Table 10-5. COMPARISON OF AVERAGE WEIGHTS IN THE NATIONAL HEALTH AND NUTRITION EXAMINATION SURVEY (NHANES I) (35) WITH METROPOLITAN REFERENCE TABLES (30, 31) AND U.S. DEPARTMENT OF AGRICULTURE GUIDELINES (32)

Height (Ft In)	Metropolitan Tables[a] (Medium Frame) (Weight in Pounds)		U.S. Department of Agriculture Guidelines[b] for Age Groups (1989) (Weight in Pounds)		National Health and Nutrition Examination Survey I Average Weight 40-49 years (1971-1974) (Weight in Pounds)
	(1959)	(1983)	19-34 years (1989)	≥35 years	
4 9	94-106	106-118			127
4 10	97-109	106-120			131
4 11	100-112	110-123			136
5 0	103-115	112-126	97-128	108-138	141
5 1	106-118	115-129	101-132	111-143	138
5 2	109-122	118-132	104-137	115-148	141
5 3	112-126	121-135	107-141	119-152	148
5 4	116-131	124-138	111-146	122-157	151
5 5	120-135	127-141	114-150	126-162	156
5 6	124-139	130-144	125-164	138-178	156
5 7	128-143	133-147	129-169	142-183	158
5 8	132-147	136-150	132-174	146-188	172
5 9	136-151	139-153	136-179	151-194	—
5 10	140-155	142-156	140-184	155-199	—

[a] Not age-specific (1959 tables for ages ≥25 years, 1983 tables for ages 25-59 years).
[b] The higher weights in the ranges generally apply to men, the lower weights more often apply to women, who have less muscle and bone.
Modified from Manson JE, et al. Body weight and longevity: A reassessment. *JAMA* 257:353-358, 1987; and U.S. Department of Agriculture. *Nutrition and Your Health: Dietary Guidelines for Americans*. Washington, D.C., U.S. Government Printing Office, 1990.

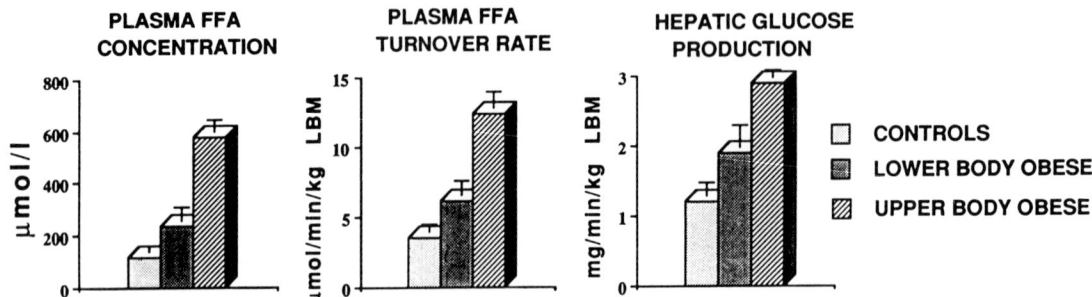

Figure 10–3. Plasma FFA concentration and turnover and hepatic glucose production in controls and obese individuals of different body fat distribution, at plasma insulin concentration of mU/liter and euglycemia. (From Jensen MD, Haymond MW, Rizza RA, et al. Influence of body fat distribution on free fatty acid metabolism in obesity. Reproduced from the *Journal of Clinical Investigation*, 1989, *83*, 1168, by copyright permission of the American Society for Clinical Investigation.)

an important predictor of NIDDM, hypertriglyceridemia, hypertension, and CHD in women as well as in men (26). The increased sensitivity of abdominal fat cells to lipolytic stimuli and the subsequent direct delivery of fatty acids and glycerol to the liver, thus inducing insulin resistance, are possible pathophysiologic explanations for these observed associations (Fig. 10–3). The waist circumference and waist-to-hip ratio are often used to estimate abdominal obesity. A waist-to-hip ratio higher than 0.80 in women or 0.95 in men is predictive of a substantially increased risk of cardiovascular disease. The impact of body fat distribution on the risk of cardiovascular disease and NIDDM will be discussed in detail in later sections of this chapter.

CARDIOVASCULAR HEALTH AND OBESITY

Demographics

Data on the prevalence of obesity in American women are mainly derived from the National Health Examination Surveys (NHANES) (27, 21) (Fig. 10–4). In general, women have a higher prevalence of obesity than men, with approximately 23.8% of all American women considered overweight (BMI > 27.2 kg/m^2) (7). Demographic trends among black women are particularly worrisome; in American black women, obesity is twice as prevalent as in American white women. Further, the average weight gain for black women after the age of 18 is double that of whites (28). Women of lower socioeconomic classes have the highest probability of being obese, the prevalence being inversely related to the level of education (29). Finally, Americans with eastern European ancestry tend to have higher rates of obesity than those of western European origin (29).

Smoking also appears to play an important

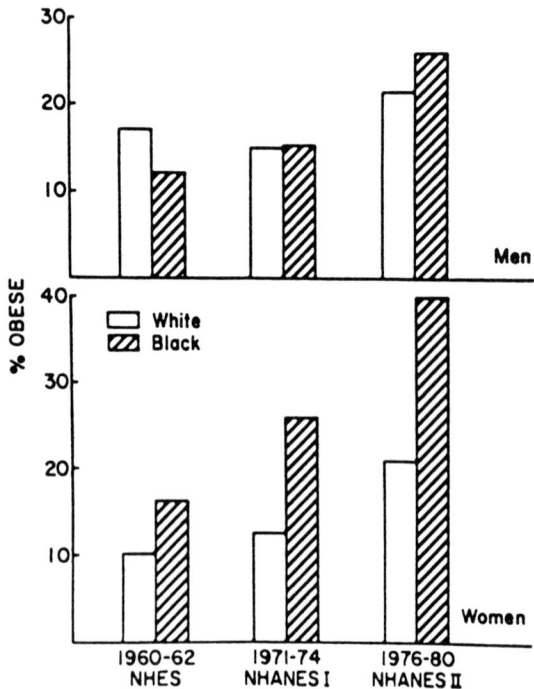

Figure 10–4. Percentage of population classified as obese in three surveys of representative samples of the United States population. NHES = National Health Examination Survey; NHANES = National Health and Nutrition Examination Survey. (Data adapted from Wong FL, Trowbridge FL. *Clin Nutr* 3:94–99, 1984. From Barrett-Connor EL. Obesity, atherosclerosis and coronary artery disease. *Ann Intern Med* 103:1010–1015, 1985.)

role in determining demographic trends in obesity. Smoking is inversely related to body weight in both men and women (30). Smoking cessation, however, has consistently been found to be associated with weight gain (31). For example, during 3 years of follow-up in the Finnmark Study, a mean weight increase of 2.7 kg was observed among women who quit smoking cigarettes (32).

Role of Genetics, Diet, and Physical Activity

The role of genetic factors in human obesity has not been fully elucidated. Familial clustering of obesity and high correlations of biologic parent-children weights have been observed (33). A large Danish study in adopted versus natural children showed a clear relationship between hereditary factors and obesity. Body weights of adopted children were more highly correlated with body weights of natural parents (in particular mothers) than with the weights of adoptive parents (33). Although the genetic influences on obesity are appreciable, environmental factors also appear to be important in the expression of the severity of the condition. Recent investigations have shown a significant correlation of weight with total fat intake and saturated fat intake (34).

Physical inactivity is also a major determinant of obesity in women. Exercise increases energy expenditure, lowers blood pressure, has a favorable influence on blood lipids, and increases the basal metabolic rate (35). Decreased physical activity leads to positive energy balance, storage of triglycerides in adipose cells, and enlargement of adipose tissue mass. Although obese subjects tend to be less physically active than nonobese people (36, 37), the causal relationship may be bidirectional because obesity is both a cause and a consequence of physical inactivity (16).

Obesity and Hypertension

A consistently positive association between obesity and hypertension has been demonstrated in cross-sectional and longitudinal studies of both men and women (16). The NHANES II data showed a 2.6 times higher prevalence of hypertension in obese white women compared with nonobese women (2.5 times higher in white males). In younger age groups (20 to 44 years), the association was even stronger (5.6 times higher prevalence of hypertension [blood pressure ≥ 160/95 mmHg] in the obese women) (38). In black men and women, the risk of hypertension among the obese was less pronounced (2.0 and 1.5 times, respectively), indicating that factors other than obesity may play a more important role in the development of hypertension in blacks compared with whites (38).

Epidemiologic data describing the positive relationship between blood pressure (BP) and relative weight are remarkably consistent. The Chicago Heart Association Detection Project (39) and the Chicago Health Department Study (40), which together examined the health status of nearly 30,000 women, each found blood pressure to be highly correlated with relative weight, although the gradient was more pronounced in black women than in white women. The Lipid Research Clinics cross-sectional data (41) showed a high correlation between weight gain from adolescence (15 to 18 years) into adulthood (30 to 54 years) and blood pressure increase in white men and white women. Similarly, in the Princeton-LRC substudy (28), systolic and diastolic BPs were significantly higher for those in the upper quartile of weight gain compared with those in the lowest quartile, a relationship that was evident in both sexes among blacks and whites. Finally, the Framingham cohort showed a strong impact of relative weight on systolic BP, with every 10% increase in relative weight leading to an elevation of systolic BP by 6.5 mmHg (42). Overweight women (≥ 114% recommended weight) in the age groups of 30 to 39, 40 to 49, and 50 to 59 years experienced a two- to threefold increased prevalence of hypertension in all age groups compared with their leaner peers (43, 44).

Fat distribution patterns have also been found to predict hypertension and diabetes. Specifically, the risk for individuals with abdominal fat accumulation is greater than that for those with peripheral fat (45–47). For example, in the Framingham Offspring Study (48), the relative risk (RR) of developing hypertension in overweight women (BMI ≥ 23 kg/m^2) compared with women of normal weight was 3.16. If subscapular skinfold thickness (≥ 1.00 cm) was used to define obesity, the association was even stronger (RR = 3.35), with obesity accounting for 64.4% of cases of hypertension among the obese (48).

Currently, the mechanism linking obesity

and hypertension remains controversial. It has been hypothesized that hyperinsulinemia secondary to insulin resistance in the obese is responsible for the observed blood pressure elevations. Plausible pathophysiologic actions of hyperinsulinemia include increased renal tubular sodium reabsorption and increased sympathetic nervous system stimulation (49).

Obesity and Blood Lipids

Obesity is commonly associated with hypertriglyceridemia and, to a lesser extent, hypercholesterolemia and decreased levels of high-density lipoprotein (HDL) (16, 50). Although evidence linking hypertriglyceridemia to coronary artery disease is controversial, data from the Framingham Study suggest that hypertriglyceridemia ($\geq$ 150 mg/dL) is associated with decreased levels of HDL ($\leq$ 40 mg/dL) in a subgroup of women and men with increased CHD risk (51). The evidence of an atherogenic effect of hypertriglyceridemia in these data is stronger in women than in men.

The Framingham data also demonstrate a 12 mg/dL rise in serum cholesterol for every 10% increase in relative weight (42). For women with predominantly abdominal fat distribution, such relative weight increases can compound lipid abnormalities (52). Intra-abdominal body fat is more metabolically responsive to adrenergic stimulation of lipolysis (53) and can lead to further elevations of plasma free fatty acids and triglycerides.

Obesity, Insulin Resistance, and Glucose Intolerance

Abdominal and upper body obesity have both been shown to be associated with insulin resistance and glucose intolerance (54, 55) (Fig. 10–5). Pancreatic insulin secretion and plasma insulin levels are generally elevated in the obese. It is hypothesized that hyperinsulinemia occurs secondary to an increase in peripheral insulin resistance (56).

The higher plasma insulin levels associated with upper body obesity can be explained by high pancreatic secretion and an additional impairment of hepatic degradation of insulin (54). Increased free fatty acid concentrations due to enhanced lipolysis in abdominal fat interfere with hepatic insulin and glucose metabolism, thereby elevating plasma insulin lev-

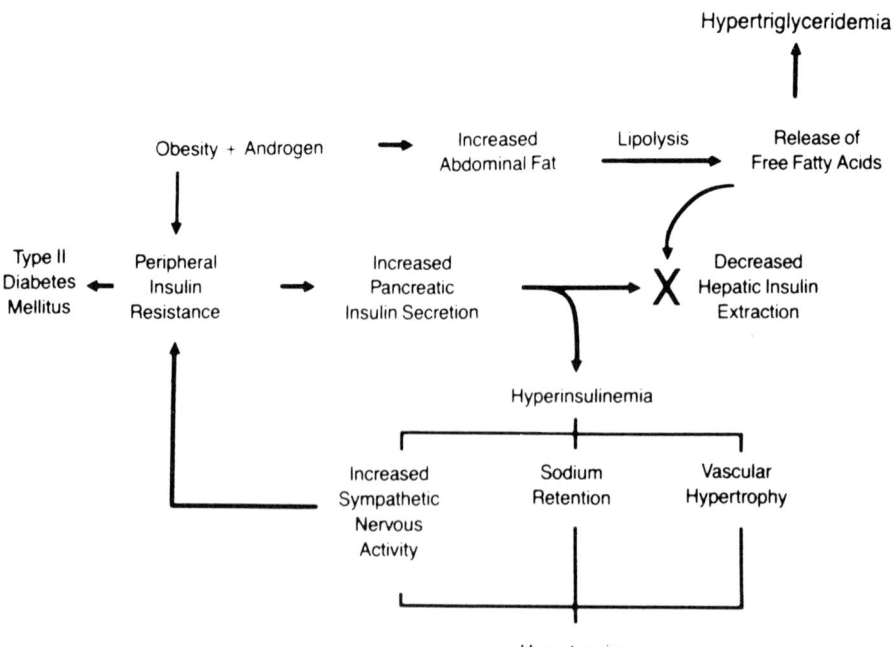

Figure 10–5. Possible link of upper body obesity and hyperinsulinemia. An overall scheme of the mechanism by which upper body obesity could promote glucose intolerance, hypertriglyceridemia, and hypertension via hyperinsulinemia. (From Kaplan NM. The deadly quartet. Upper body obesity, glucose intolerance, hypertriglyceridemia, and hypertension. *Arch Intern Med* 149:1514–1520, 1989.)

els (53, 57). Increased free fatty acids also stimulate hepatic gluconeogenesis and inhibit insulin-stimulated glucose uptake, leading to substantial hyperglycemia in the presence of normal to elevated insulin levels (57) (see Fig. 10–3).

Obesity, Hyperinsulinemia, and Syndrome X

The apparent atherogenicity of hyperinsulinemia was first observed in clinical studies in nondiabetic men after myocardial infarction; men with myocardial infarction had significantly higher insulin levels after oral glucose tolerance testing than noninfarction controls (58). In the prospective Helsinki Policemen Study (59), hyperinsulinemia was found to be an independent risk factor for CHD (nonfatal myocardial infarction). Men with the highest fasting and 2-hour insulin concentrations after an oral glucose load had the highest incidence of CHD death and of nonfatal myocardial infarction.

More recent studies have continued to show a strong relationship between hyperinsulinemia and increased risk of coronary artery disease. A significant association between 1-hour serum insulin concentrations and CHD mortality was observed in the Busselton Study in Australia; this effect was independent of other risk factors, although it was not statistically significant in women (60). The Paris Prospective Study (61) of 7246 nondiabetic men also demonstrated that fasting insulin and fasting insulin-to-glucose ratios were independently related to CHD mortality and incidence of nonfatal myocardial infarction. Finally, a Finnish case-control study (62) investigated the relationship between fasting plasma insulin levels and serum lipid and lipoproteins in 119 men and 106 women with NIDDM (case group) and 65 nondiabetic men and 59 nondiabetic women (control group). Fasting plasma insulin levels correlated significantly with elevated triglycerides and decreased total HDL-cholesterol and HDL_2 levels in diabetic and nondiabetic men and women. The associations between total triglycerides, HDL, and insulin concentration remained significant in diabetic and nondiabetic women after adjustment for other factors (BMI, alcohol intake, smoking, physical activity, and fasting glucose levels) (62).

The constellation or "clustering" of hyperinsulinemia, hypertriglyceridemia, abdominal obesity, decreased HDL-cholesterol, and hypertension has been observed frequently in patients with CHD. It has been suggested that this specific risk factor constellation constitutes a separate disease entity, syndrome X (57). Each individual factor contributing to the syndrome has been classified as an independent risk factor for CHD. The rationale for describing syndrome X as a distinct disease entity derives from the hypothesis that each of these risk factors occurs secondary to a common underlying cause, insulin resistance (see Fig. 10–5).

Currently, the causal link between hyperinsulinemia, dyslipidemias, and hypertension has not been fully clarified (54) and several epidemiologic studies have shown conflicting results. In women, four population-based studies (49, 63, 64, 65) found a positive association between fasting or postchallenge insulin concentrations and blood pressure. The Beaver County (63) and the CARDIA Study (65) were carried out in young adults, and insulin levels were found to be independently related to systolic BP in women but not in men. A positive relationship in obese women was found in the Israel Study (49) and the Pittsburgh Healthy Women Study (64). In contrast, the Rancho Bernardo Study (66) investigated 784 women aged 50 to 93 years and found no significant relationship between fasting or postchallenge insulin and hypertension levels after control for age, glucose tolerance, and BMI.

At present, the evidence of a link between obesity, hyperinsulinemia, and hypertension is compelling for younger adults and children. In addition, a causal association between hyperinsulinemia and chest pain in patients with microvascular angina and no structural changes of the coronary artery walls has been hypothesized in women and men (67). Further investigation of these associations among adults, particularly among women, is needed.

Obesity and Atherosclerosis

The role of obesity as a risk factor for CHD remains controversial. In general, the impact of obesity on mortality has been underestimated (24) due to the failure of most studies to control for cigarette smoking, disease-induced weight loss, and other potential confounding variables (24). The Manitoba Study (68) and the Los Angeles Heart Study (69) showed an independent, although small, effect of relative weight on the incidence of myocardial infarction in white men that was restricted to younger age groups (20 to 40 and 40 to 49 years of age, respectively). A combined analysis of the divergent results found in the eight cohorts of the Pooling Project (70) revealed an overall consistent positive relationship between relative weight and CHD in white men; each substudy, however, came to different results, ranging from no association to U-shaped curves (16). In contrast, the Framingham Study (71) and the recently published Seventh-day Adventist Study (72) have demonstrated a linear independent relationship between relative weight and CHD mortality in white men. Lean men in the lowest BMI quintile group of the Seventh-day Adventist Study had a significantly decreased risk across all age groups, compared with the highest BMI quintile group (RR = 0.32 at age 50 to RR = 0.71 at age 90). Both studies controlled for potential confounding by cigarette smoking.

Few prospective studies have been conducted to investigate the association between obesity and CHD in women. The Gothenborg Study (73) followed 1462 middle-aged Swedish women over a 10-year period and revealed only a small increase in CHD incidence with increasing body mass, which was not statistically significant. The American Cancer Society study (74) showed a positive association between self-reported weight and CHD mortality. In that study, grossly obese women (> 140% above the average for the cohort) had a twofold increase in CHD mortality compared with lean women. This relationship was particularly pronounced in women between 40 and 60 years of age, showing a 3 to 3.5 times elevated risk of CHD death compared to women of average weight in the cohort. In the Framingham Study, as previously stated, relative weight was directly related to risk of cardiovascular disease in both women and men (Fig. 10–6). Finally, the Nurses' Health Study

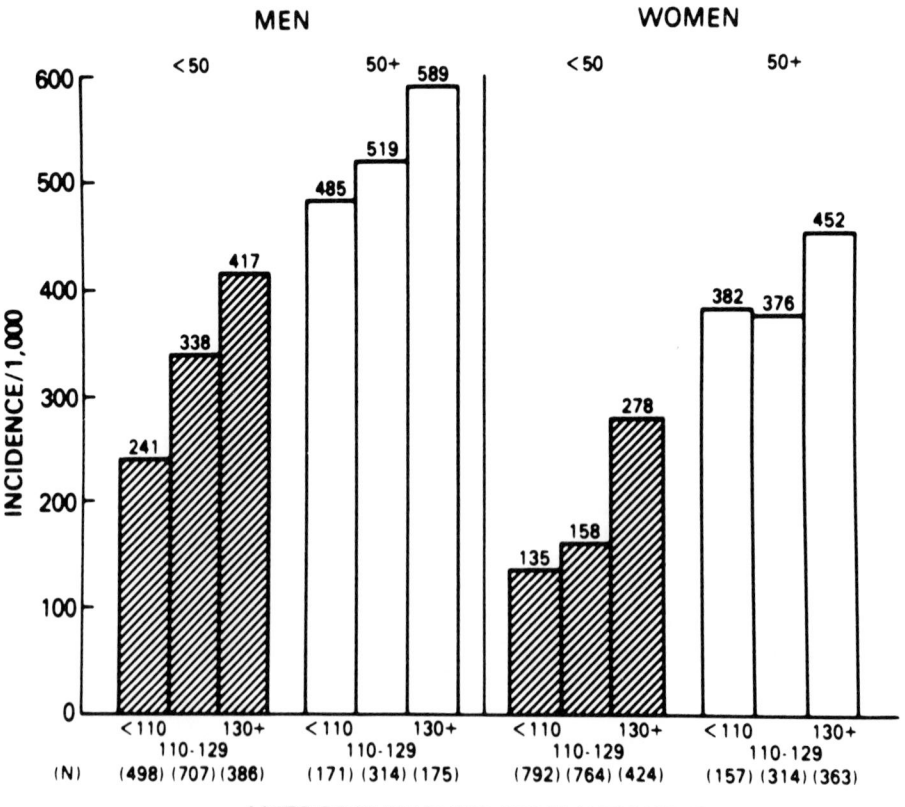

Figure 10–6. Correlation between the 26-year incidence of cardiovascular disease by MRW at entry among Framingham patients younger/older than age 50. N = the number at risk for an event. Numbers above the bars give the actual incidence rates per 1000. (From Hubert HB, Feinleib M, McNamara PM, et al. Obesity as an independent risk factor for cardiovascular disease: A 26-year follow-up of participants in the Framingham Heart Study. *Circulation* 67:970, 1983.)

(NHS) (75), a large-scale prospective cohort study comprising 121,700 female registered nurses aged 30 to 55 years, showed a linear increase in risk of nonfatal and fatal CHD events with increasing self-reported weight category (Figs. 10–7 and 10–8). In this study, which also controlled for confounding by smoking, 70% of the coronary events in the heaviest BMI category ($\geq$ 29 kg/m^2) were attributable to obesity, and the rates of CHD were 3.3 times those in the leanest category. In addition, women with mild to moderate overweight (25 $\leq$ BMI < 29 kg/m^2) had an 80% higher risk of CHD than their leaner peers.

Clinical Manifestations of Cardiovascular Disease in Obesity

Obesity and the Heart

The pathologic effects of obesity on myocardial cells and vascular function have long been appreciated. Postmortem studies of chronically obese patients demonstrate marked increases in left ventricular mass that, in contrast to that seen in hypertension, tend to occur in an eccentric distribution (76–78). Diastolic dysfunction appears to be relatively common among obese patients both with and without hypertension.

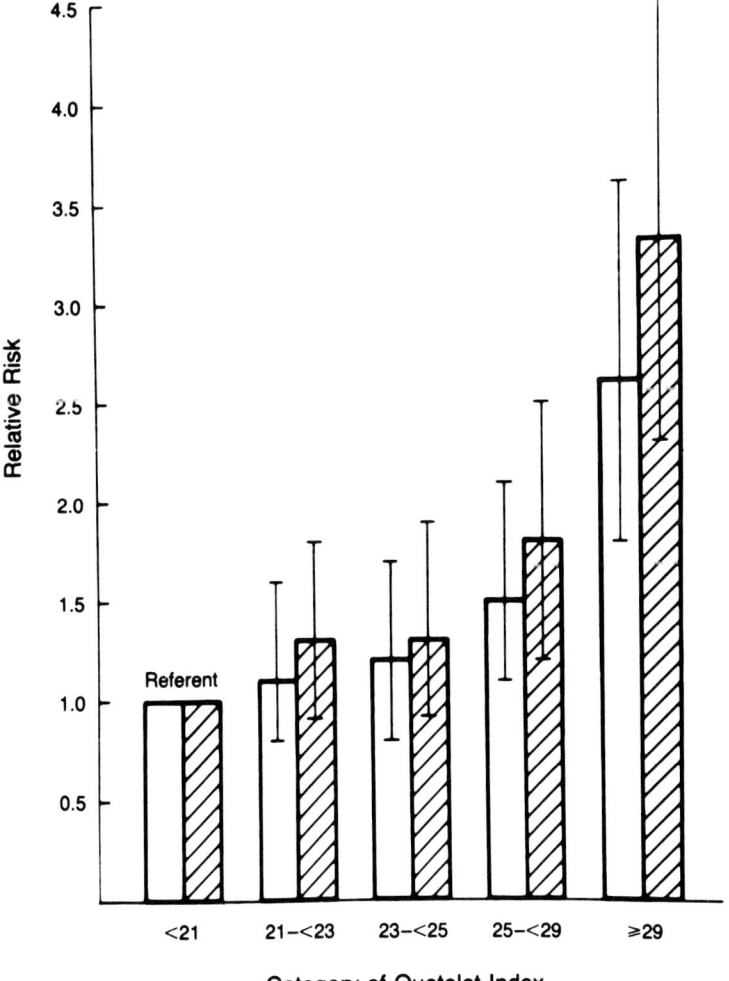

Figure 10–7. Relative risks of nonfatal myocardial infarction and fatal coronary heart disease (combined) according to category of Quetelet index in a cohort of U.S. women 30 to 55 years of age in 1976. The reference category was that with an index under 21. For the other categories, open bars show the relative risks as adjusted for age, and hatched bars show the relative risks as adjusted for both age and smoking. The vertical lines represent 95% confidence limits. (From Manson JE, Colditz GA, Stampfer MJ, et al. A prospective study of obesity and risk of coronary heart disease in women. *N Engl J Med* 32:882–889, 1990.)

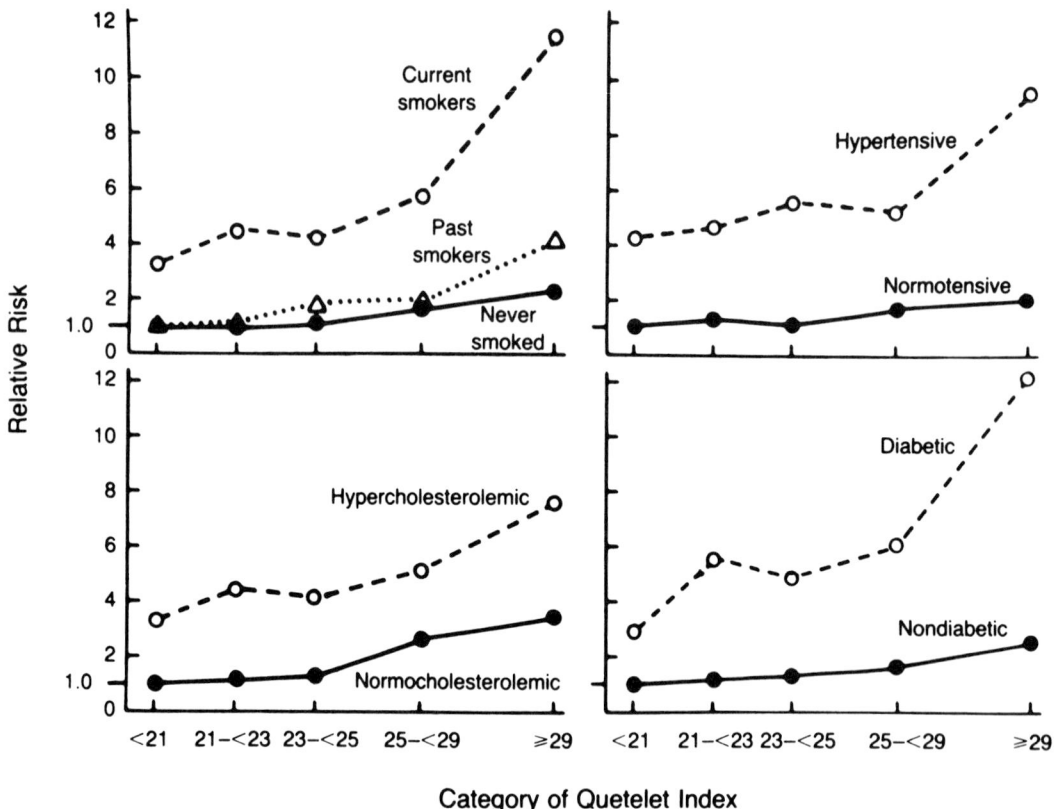

Figure 10–8. Relative risks of nonfatal myocardial infarction and fatal coronary heart disease (combined), according to category of Quetelet index and coronary risk-factor status, after adjustment for age and smoking. The reference group in each panel comprised the women in the leanest Quetelet index category who did not have the specified coronary risk factor. The diabetic group included women who received their diagnoses at $\geq$ 30 years of age. In all strata, the relative risk in the heaviest Quetelet category was at least twice that in the leanest. (From Manson JE, Colditz GA, Stampfer MJ, et al. A prospective study of obesity and risk of coronary heart disease in women *N Engl J Med* 32:882–889, 1990.)

At the circulatory level, chronic obesity is associated with elevations of cardiac preload, marked increases in cardiac output, and an expansion of the plasma volume (79). Stroke volumes and left ventricular filling pressures are higher in obese patients at rest and increase further as demands on cardiac output elevate. Not surprisingly, these changes can lead to substantial increases in peripheral edema even among obese patients without evidence of overt right heart failure.

Weight loss can improve cardiac hemodynamics by reducing overall cardiac demand. Reversibility of eccentric hypertrophy has been documented among obese individuals able to maintain weight reduction (80), as have improvements in ventricular chamber size, ejection fraction, and ventricular filling pressures (81, 82). From a functional standpoint, weight loss among obese individuals generally improves exercise tolerance, although success in maintaining weight loss is often limited. Of equal importance, even modest weight loss among obese subjects appears to reduce blood pressure, most likely secondary to reduced sympathetic stimulation (83, 84). It is important that major weight reduction be undertaken with the care and supervision of a knowledgeable physician; case reports suggest that sudden death can occur with rapid weight reduction, usually the result of QT prolongation and electrolyte disturbances (85–87).

The extent to which obesity modifies the clinical spectrum of cardiovascular disease among women compared with men is unclear. Several studies indicate that women fare worse than men following a first acute myocardial infarction (88, 89) and that mortality among obese diabetic women is exceptionally high (90). However, this relationship is difficult to quantify because women tend to suffer their first infarction 10 years later in life than men.

Thus, age-related weight gain may confound the relationship between obesity itself and acute cardiovascular risk.

Obesity unfavorably alters the risk-to-benefit ratio for all patients undergoing revascularization procedures. For women, who have been demonstrated to have significantly smaller coronary arteries than men (91), obesity is likely to play an even greater role. For example, in the National Heart Lung and Blood Institute registry of percutaneous transluminal coronary angioplasty (PTCA), women were far more likely to sustain procedure-related complications or suffer acute fatalities than were men, even after adjusting for age (92). In fact, the relative risk of death for women undergoing PTCA in this registry remained fivefold higher for women than for men after adjusting for all available baseline characteristics. Similarly, women undergoing coronary bypass surgery appear to have higher operative mortalities than men (93), at least in part because of higher baseline risk (94, 95). Thus, the avoidance of obesity is particularly critical for women because their risks of procedure-related complications are already greater than those of men.

Prevention and Treatment of Obesity

The prevention and treatment of obesity requires a thorough evaluation of several possible etiologic factors including eating disorders, family history of obesity, abuse of laxatives or diuretics, and level of physical activity as well as consideration of the presence or absence of abdominal obesity, hypertension, glucose intolerance, and lipid disorders. In general, the decision to treat depends on the amount of excessive body weight, the distribution of fat, and accompanying risk factors. Dietary restriction is the first line of therapy in most cases, although for grossly obese patients (BMI > 40), especially when obesity is associated with insulin resistance and its complications, surgical treatment or pharmacotherapy should be considered (96).

Weight loss leads to favorable changes in other cardiovascular risk factors including improvements in glucose tolerance, blood pressure, and lipid abnormalities. In particular, hypertriglyceridemia and hypercholesterolemia are improved with weight loss and increased physical activity (97–99). However, obesity is a chronic condition in which recidivism is common. Critical factors associated with maintenance of appropriate body fat content include reductions in dietary fat as well as regular exercise programs (100, 101). Behavioral modification is crucial for successful treatment of obesity (102). At present, four guiding principles underlie the treatment of obesity: self-monitoring of daily food intake, physical activity, and mood states; contingency management plans including rewards for appropriate behavior; stress management; and cognitive-behavioral strategies designed to improve self-control and attitude. Maintenance of weight reduction also appears essential because weight cycling (phases of rapid weight loss and subsequent weight regain) has been shown to be related to an increased risk of coronary heart disease morbidity and mortality (103).

Patient education about the cardiovascular and other health effects of obesity must become a public health priority. Recent data suggest that the prevalence of obesity in children and adolescents is steadily increasing (16) and that these trends continue into adulthood. Sex and race differences related to degree of obesity have also become apparent and indicate that black women and women with central fat accumulation should be primary targets for such interventional programs. However, long-term benefits of weight loss or reduction of regional fat depositions on cardiovascular mortality and all-cause mortality in women and men are still controversial. The lack of standardization and quality control of the different weight loss programs poses a particular threat to the correct assessment of the long-term consequences of weight loss. Further studies are needed to address this issue.

CARDIOVASCULAR HEALTH AND DIABETES MELLITUS

Demographics

Although diabetes mellitus is one of the most common chronic diseases and represents the seventh leading cause of death in the United States, epidemiologic studies of the frequency, determinants, and outcomes of IDDM and NIDDM are scant. The incidence of IDDM peaks in the 10- to 14-year age group and reaches 21/100,000 new cases per year in boys and 24/100,000 new cases per year in girls in this age group. In general, males tend to have higher incidence rates of IDDM than females (104). Race and social class also seem to be determinants of IDDM, with white children showing higher incidence rates than nonwhites. However, the true impact of racial or socioeconomic differences cannot be inferred from the data currently available (104).

In contrast to IDDM, NIDDM and IGT represent widespread chronic conditions affecting predominantly obese persons older than 40 years of age. IGT and NIDDM together affect approximately 11% of the U.S. adult population (105), although it has been estimated that nearly half of all NIDDM patients are unaware of their condition or are not properly diagnosed (106). In both sexes and in all age groups, blacks have a higher prevalence of NIDDM than whites (Table 10-6). Above age 54, one in every four black women has diabetes. White women show slightly lower prevalences than white men below age 65 but exceed male prevalences thereafter (106). Incidence data reveal a strong age relationship with a 34-fold increase of NIDDM between ages 25 and 74 (104).

Ethnicity is associated with the development of NIDDM. However, methodologic differences make comparisons between countries difficult. As with IDDM, the prevalence of NIDDM is low in Japan compared to northern European countries and the United States. Interestingly, migrant studies have shown an increasing prevalence and incidence of NIDDM in Japanese and Pacific Indian migrants to westernized countries (107, 108). Several Indian tribes in the United States and in the Pacific show extremely wide ranges of NIDDM prevalence. For example, the prevalence of NIDDM is only 1.5% in rural Melanesians but is as high as 30% in urbanized Nauruans (107) and 25% in Pima Indians (109).

Role of Genetics, Obesity, Diet, and Physical Activity

In IDDM, viral infections have been hypothesized to cause inflammatory changes of beta cells leading to autoimmune destruction; genetic factors have been implicated in susceptibility to this process. It is clear that familial clustering plays an important role in IDDM, since siblings of IDDM patients experience risks of developing the disease that are 5 to 20 times higher than those in the general population (104). Also, the concordance rate (approximately 50%) in monozygotic twin studies provides evidence of a genetic transmission pattern in IDDM (104). Although an association between HLA-DR3 and HLA-DR4 antigens and IDDM has been observed consistently in different population-based studies, it is uncertain whether these antigens are directly involved in the pathogenetic process of IDDM or are markers of other etiologic factors (104).

NIDDM is most likely of polygenic origin (1). Studies in homozygous twins have demonstrated a 95–100% concordance rate, whereas offspring of diabetic parents have the

Table 10–6. AGE-STANDARDIZED[a] PREVALENCE OF DIAGNOSED DIABETES AND TOTAL DIABETES IN BLACK WOMEN, AND MEN AND WHITE WOMEN AND MEN IN THE U.S. POPULATION AGED 20–74 YEARS

	National Health Interview Surveys, 1979–1981				National Health and Nutrition Examination Survey I, 1976–1980			
	White Women (%)	White Men (%)	Black Women (%)	Black Men (%)	White Women (%)	White Men (%)	Black Women (%)	Black Men (%)
Diagnosed[b] Diabetes	3.4	3.4	7.1	5.5	3.1[c]	5.3[d]		
Total[e] Diabetes	NA	NA	NA	NA	6.7	5.2	10.2	8.9

[a] Standardized to U.S. 1980 population.
[b] Self-reported diagnosis of diabetes by a physician during the preceding 12 months.
[c] Data for white women and black women combined.
[d] Data for white men and black men combined.
[e] Impaired glucose tolerance and diabetes (National Diabetes Data Group Criteria) according to oral glucose tolerance testing after 75 g oral glucose load.
NA = Not available.
From Harris MI. Noninsulin-dependent diabetes mellitus in black and white Americans. *Diabetes Metab Rev* 6:71–90, 1990.

disease in 30–50% of cases (1). For MODY diabetes, an autosomal dominant transmission is assumed. Although no HLA antigen association with NIDDM has been identified (1, 9), a family history of diabetes is a strong risk factor.

Cross-cultural, migrant, and correlational studies have all demonstrated that obesity is a well-established risk factor for NIDDM and IGT (110, 111). Unfortunately, prospective studies that have investigated the relationship of obesity and NIDDM are rare and generally include only small numbers of women. A cross-sectional analysis of 32,662 white women in a weight loss program (112) showed an increasing prevalence of NIDDM with increasing relative weight. The Framingham cohort (113) showed a more than twofold increase in the prevalence of NIDDM in women who weighed ≥ 140% of relative weight (prevalence of NIDDM 17.3%) compared to women in lower weight categories (prevalence of NIDDM 8.3% and 7.8%). The Nurses' Health Study (114) investigated the relation of BMI to the risk of clinical NIDDM among 113,861 U.S. women during an 8-year follow-up period; an increased risk of NIDDM in women with a BMI of greater than 22 kg/m^2 and a markedly increased risk of NIDDM in women with a BMI of more than 25 kg/m^2 were observed. The age-adjusted relative risk was 5.5 in the 25- to 25.9-kg/m^2 BMI category and increased almost exponentially to an RR estimate of 60.9 in the over 35 kg/m^2 BMI category. Within the total cohort, 90.4% of NIDDM diagnoses were attributable to a BMI of greater than 22 kg/m^2 (114). Women who gained more than 3 kg from age 18 to the time of the study were at substantially higher risk for developing NIDDM than women with stable weights.

Fat distribution also is a risk factor for NIDDM. As the Gothenborg Study (115) revealed, subjects in the lowest waist-to-hip ratio (WHR) category did not show an elevation of NIDDM incidence despite increasing BMI values. In the middle and upper thirds of WHR, NIDDM risk increased with increasing BMI (115). A cross-sectional analysis of the TOPS cohort (116) also found a positive relation between upper body fat accumulation (indicated by upper tertiles of WHR, or neck and bust girth values) and risk of NIDDM.

The association between dietary factors and NIDDM has been controversial. After controlling for BMI and weight change, no consistent association between NIDDM and dietary intake of carbohydrates, fat, fiber, or other nutrients has been observed (117).

The potential benefits of physical activity in preventing NIDDM have been investigated in a few epidemiological studies, mostly involving men (110). Support for a benefit of exercise is provided by descriptive comparisons of active rural and inactive urban populations as well as cross-sectional studies of sedentary individuals compared to more active individuals in Pacific populations (118–121). Two studies (122, 123) did not, however, show any significant association between glucose tolerance and physical activity. A retrospective study among college alumnae showed a relative risk of 3.41 in female nonathletes compared with athletes (124). The Nurses' Health study, to our knowledge the only prospective large-scale investigation of physical activity and incidence of NIDDM in women, detected a significant reduction in NIDDM incidence among women who engaged in vigorous exercise at least once per week compared with women who did not exercise weekly (125). Risk reductions were seen in obese and nonobese women.

Diabetes and Blood Lipids

The interrelationship of IDDM, NIDDM, and IGT with cardiovascular disease is complex (126). At least in part, these increases in risk are related to changes in lipid patterns among diabetic patients.

From a clinical standpoint, diabetic dyslipoproteinemia includes elevated total triglycerides, elevated VLDL-triglycerides, and decreased HDL-cholesterol (HDL-C). In general, these effects are more pronounced in women than men (127). The response of dyslipoproteinemia to treatment with insulin in NIDDM is variable (128). In adequately treated IDDM, triglycerides, total cholesterol, and HDL-C blood levels do not seem to be adversely altered compared to levels in nondiabetics (127). As indicated earlier, the impact of hypertriglyceridemia as an independent risk factor for CHD is controversial (129). However, recent data from the Framingham cohort identified a subgroup of nondiabetic men and women with elevated triglyceride levels (≥ 150 mg/dL) and low HDL-C levels (≤ 40 mg/dL) who experienced an increased risk of CHD (51).

In well-controlled IDDM, HDL-C levels are normal to elevated (128). Cross-sectional studies have consistently demonstrated an inverse relation between HDL-C levels and CHD risk in NIDDM patients (127). In the Framingham cohort (130), diabetic women had significantly lower HDL-C levels than nondiabetics. However, in a comparison of CHD risk of diabetic versus nondiabetic women and men, low HDL-C levels could not fully explain the increased CHD risk of individuals with NIDDM (129). Total cholesterol and LDL levels have not been shown to be different between diabetic and nondiabetic males and females and have not been related to an increased risk of CHD in diabetic patients (106, 127, 131).

Diabetes and Hypertension

IDDM, NIDDM, and IGT are all associated with an increased prevalence of hypertension (127). Prevalence of hypertension in the NHANES II data was higher in black diabetics than in whites in each age group below age 65 (106). The overall prevalence of hypertension among diabetics was 63–70%; in the general population (aged 10 to 74) the prevalence of hypertension was 40%. The Bedford (132), Whitehall (133), Israeli (134), and Framingham (131) studies all showed significantly higher mean systolic BP and diastolic BP values in male and female diabetics compared with nondiabetic subjects.

Diabetes and Atherosclerosis

Diabetic women and men have more adverse coronary risk factor profiles than nondiabetic individuals. In the Framingham Study, diabetic women were more obese and hypertensive and had substantially lower HDL-C values than their nondiabetic peers (131). Multivariate analyses of the prospective data from Framingham indicate that the excess risk of CHD was particularly pronounced in diabetic women and could not be explained by conventional risk factors alone. After adjusting for these risk factors, the relative risk of total cardiovascular (CVD) events for diabetic women aged 45 to 74 was 2.0 compared with nondiabetic women, 3.3 for CVD mortality, 2.1 for CHD, and 5.0 for peripheral artery disease (130). The relative impact of diabetes was greater for diabetic women than diabetic men, completely eliminating the usual female advantage with respect to CVD mortality. Similarly, analyses from the Nurses' Health Study showed a three- to sevenfold increase in CVD events among diabetic women; a total of 13.8% of coronary events and 14.8% of CVD deaths in the cohort were attributable to diabetes (126).

Sex differences in cardiovascular mortality among diabetics have been studied in several prospective cohorts both in the United States and abroad (Table 10-7). In general, these studies have found that the incidence of myocardial infarction and total mortality observed

Table 10-7. SEX DIFFERENCES IN CORONARY HEART DISEASE AMONG DIABETICS IN FIVE U.S. COHORT STUDIES

Study Location	Years of Study	Age (Years)	Multiply[a] Adjusted Risk Among Diabetics	
			Men	Women
Rancho Bernardo	1972–1980	40–79	2.4	3.5
Framingham	1948–1968	45–74	1.7	3.3
Evans[b] County	1967–1974	≥22	1.0	2.8
Tecumseh	1959–1978	40–54	7.9	7.7
		55–69	2.6	0.6
		≥70	1.9	5.3
Nurses' Health Study	1976–1984	30–55	—	3.0

[a] Multiply adjusted risks control for blood pressure, cholesterol, and cigarette smoking with other covariates in some studies. Rancho Bernardo and Tecumseh used the Cox standardized risk ratio; Framingham, relative risks; and Evans County, a standardized mortality ratio.
[b] Risk estimates are crude.

Modified from Barrett-Connor E, Orchard T. Diabetes and heart disease. In National Diabetes Group. *Diabetes in America.* U.S. PHS 85-1468, XVI, 1–41, Bethesda, MD, National Institutes of Health, 1985; and Manson JE, et al. A prospective study of maturity onset diabetes mellitus and risk of coronary heart disease and stroke in women. *Arch Intern Med* 151:1141–1147, 1991.

in diabetic women could not be explained by the presence of other traditional coronary risk factors (135). In an additional study that also addressed the risks of IGT (132), the relative odds of dying from CHD were 5.16 times higher for females with IGT than for control women, whereas women with NIDDM had a 2.12 times higher risk than those with IGT. Moreover, women with IGT and NIDDM had a relatively greater increase in mortality risk than men with these conditions. The underlying mechanisms responsible for these differences remain unclear.

Overall, the increased risk of premature atherosclerosis among diabetics is considerable (136). In one study of juvenile onset diabetes in which patients were followed for 20 to 40 years, nearly 25% died of coronary artery disease compared to 8% of a comparable group without diabetes (137). Cross-sectional studies among diabetic patients demonstrate differing rates of coronary atherosclerosis in different geographic locations, with rates particularly elevated in regions where the background incidence of cardiovascular disease was high. These data suggest that environmental factors may be related to the initiation and promotion of early atherosclerosis in patients with diabetes (138).

Clinical Manifestations of Cardiovascular Disease in Diabetics

Coronary Artery Disease

Patients with long-standing diabetes typically demonstrate nonspecific atherosclerosis in the large epicardial and peripheral arteries as well as microangiopathic changes and diffuse endothelial proliferation in the small arteriolar beds. Compared to nondiabetics, patients with glucose intolerance have more extensive coronary atherosclerosis (139), particularly if they require insulin therapy to maintain normoglycemia (140). These anatomic changes, however, are unlikely to represent the only pathologic process predisposing diabetics to increased risks of acute thrombosis.

In recent years, it has become apparent that hemostatic risk factors for acute thrombosis exist (141) and are highly prevalent among diabetics. For example, diabetics appear to have hyperaggregable platelets (142) in comparison to nondiabetics as well as impaired fibrinolytic function as measured by plasma levels of endogenous tissue plasminogen activator and plasminogen activator inhibitor (143, 144). Further, elevated levels of fibrinogen, a well-documented independent risk factor for coronary heart disease (145, 146, 147) are known to correlate with increasing blood sugar concentration. Data from the Framingham cohort suggest that abnormalities of fibrinogen may prove particularly important among diabetic women (130).

The clinical impact of accelerated atherosclerosis, platelet abnormalities, endothelial dysfunction, and impaired fibrinolysis is immense among diabetic patients. Not only is the incidence of acute myocardial infarction markedly increased among diabetics, but the rate of major complications including congestive heart failure, shock, metabolic acidosis, arrhythmias, and myocardial rupture are elevated, as is the risk of in-hospital mortality (148–151). For those diabetics who survive the early phase of infarction, the long-term prognosis is significantly poorer than it is in nondiabetics (152, 153), at least in part because of the larger initial infarct size and subsequent reductions in ejection fraction (154). The high incidence of complications associated with cardiovascular disease in diabetes is further compounded by the fact that silent myocardial ischemia is common among diabetics (155), making the diagnosis of angina and exertional ischemia more difficult in these patients (156, 157). Although the use of ambulatory ST-segment monitoring for the detection of asymptomatic ischemia among diabetic patients is promising, little prospective data supporting the use of this screening technique is currently available (158).

Postinfarction management of diabetic patients must take into account the high incidence of cardiac autonomic dysfunction, which can alter anginal thresholds and directly affect cardiac performance, and may be associated with an increased risk of sudden death due to a slowing of the heart rate and subsequent prolongation of the QT interval (159–162). In addition, enthusiasm for performing invasive cardiac interventions in postinfarction diabetic patients must be tempered by the increased complication and restenosis rates suffered by these patients. In particular, long-term survival following coronary artery bypass surgery is reduced among diabetic patients, although graft patency rates and improvements in angina appear to be similar to those found in nondiabetic patients (163, 164).

The higher prevalence of diabetes mellitus among women may explain at least part of the difference in cardiovascular mortality experienced by women compared to men. For example, in a recent study examining the causes of increased in-hospital and 1-year mortality among women after myocardial infarction, a history of diabetes emerged as a highly significant predictor of outcome for women (RR = 1.7, 95% CI 1.10–2.53) but not for men (RR = 0.96, 95% CI 0.69–1.34) (89). In that study, the age-adjusted prevalence of diabetes was 29.1% for women compared to only 18.0% for men, a highly significant difference ($p < 0.0005$). Such findings do not appear to be isolated; in the Multicenter Investigation of Limitation of Infarct Size (MILIS) study, in which in-hospital mortality for women exceeded that of men by 6%, the major independent predictors of outcome for women were age, hypertension, presence of clinical congestive heart failure, and a history of diabetes (165). Similarly, among women hospitalized for acute infarction in the Survival and Ventricular Enlargement Trial (SAVE) study, 31.6% had diabetes compared to only 19.9% of men, a factor that may have led to sex differences in the management of patients with acute coronary disease (166). These findings, together with those of several other registry studies (167), suggest that women with diabetes comprise a high-risk subset of patients in need of particularly aggressive in-hospital and postdischarge care.

For women surviving infarction who are being considered for revascularization procedures, the presence of diabetes considerably adds to the expected risks. Compared to men undergoing bypass surgery (168) or angioplasty (92), women are far more likely to suffer from diabetes and diabetic vascular complications. In fact, sex-related differences in the prevalence of diabetes have been considered a major factor determining both the safety and efficacy of cardiovascular intervention. For example, in the Coronary Artery Surgery Study (CASS) registry, diabetes mellitus was present in 15% of the women but only 10% of the men. The presence of diabetes does not, however, explain all of the apparent differences in revascularization rates experienced by women. In a major study evaluating discharge abstracts from over 80,000 admissions for coronary heart disease in Massachusetts and Maryland, the odds of undergoing angiography and revascularization were substantially lower for women, even after adjusting for age, race, insurance status, and the presence of congestive heart failure and diabetes (169).

Because of their increased risk of coronary occlusion and the high prevalence of silent myocardial ischemia, diabetic patients should be counseled directly about risk reduction strategies to prevent coronary disease. Currently, there are insufficient data to determine whether strict control of hyperglycemia can retard the progression of atherosclerosis among diabetic patients. Thus, primary prevention efforts must be directed toward the avoidance and treatment of other cardiovascular risk factors, in particular obesity, hypertension, hyperlipidemia, and smoking.

Diabetic Cardiomyopathy

Diabetic patients without evidence of epicardial atherosclerosis, valvular heart disease, or hypertension may nonetheless suffer from congestive heart failure (170). In fact, in the Framingham Study, diabetic men were found to have a risk of congestive heart failure twice that of nondiabetics, and the risk among diabetic women was increased fivefold (171). This excess risk persisted after control for other established coronary risk factors and the presence of known coronary disease. Of all groups examined, the risk of nonischemic congestive heart failure was highest among female diabetics who required daily insulin therapy. Overall, diabetes appears to promote heart failure to a significantly greater extent in women than in men, for both ischemic and nonischemic causes (172).

The pathologic changes underlying diabetic cardiomyopathy remain controversial. Abnormalities of glycoprotein deposition, subendothelial proliferation, intimal hyaline deposition, and capillary microaneurysms all have been found among diabetic patients (173–175). These changes appear important; noninvasive cardiac studies have demonstrated that abnormalities of both systolic and diastolic function are common among diabetics, including those free of hypertension and coronary disease (170). These changes appear to occur early in the course of disease well before any evidence of significant epicardial atherosclerosis. In two studies employing exercise radionuclide ventriculography, ejection fractions were found to be normal among young diabetic men aged 35 or less but failed to increase appropriately as demands on left ventricular output were made (176, 177).

The management of diabetic patients with

congestive heart failure must include aggressive treatment of hypertension and dyslipoproteinemias because these factors are often present and may exacerbate the direct effects of glucose intolerance on myocardial function. Avoidance of excess alcohol intake and smoking remain essential for all patients. The use of beta-blocking agents may mask symptoms of hypoglycemia, whereas afterload-reducing vasodilators may cause symptomatic hypotension among diabetics with autonomic dysfunction. These agents should therefore be used with appropriate clinical caution.

Prevention and Treatment of NIDDM

The evidence of an aggregation of risk factors in diabetic women directs primary prevention of NIDDM toward changes in life style including weight reduction, diet, and physical activity. Once diabetes develops, serious complications including retinopathy, nephropathy, and the high risk of cardiovascular disease require major therapeutic efforts.

Good adherence to therapy and meticulous control of other coronary risk factors and of blood sugar levels are thought to be protective against late sequelae (16). However, at present, there is no firm evidence that atherosclerotic complications of diabetes can be prevented or reversed by normalization of glucose concentrations. Little is known about the actual benefits of physical activity or dietary modifications in relation to the risk of cardiovascular disease in diabetic individuals. Weight loss has been shown to improve glucose tolerance in NIDDM patients (178, 179). However, the success rates of weight loss and subsequent maintenance of reduced body weight are low (7). Studies in patients with mild NIDDM have demonstrated a benefit of exercise in increasing insulin sensitivity and glucose tolerance as well as inducing favorable changes in blood lipid levels (180–182).

References

1. Shafir E, Bergman M, Felig P. Fuel metabolism. The endocrine pancreas: Diabetes mellitus. In Felig P, Baxter JD, Broadus AE, Frohman LA (Eds.), *Endocrinology and Metabolism*. New York, McGraw-Hill, 1986, pp. 1043–1165.
2. Hamburg S, Hendler R, Sherwin RS. Epinephrine: Exquisite sensitivity to its diabetogenic effects in normal men. *Clin Res* 27:252A–257, 1979.
3. Porte D, Halter JB. The endocrine pancreas and diabetes mellitus. In Williams RH (Ed.), *Textbook of Endocrinology* (6th ed.). Philadelphia, W.B. Saunders, 1981, pp. 716–843.
4. Kalkhoff, RK. Effects of oral contraceptive agents and sex steroids on carbohydrate metabolism. *Annu Rev Med* 23:429–438, 1972.
5. Blum M, Rusecky Y, Gelernter I. Glycohemoglobin (Hb A1) levels in oral contraceptive users. *Eur J Obstet Gynecol Reprod Biol* 15:97–101, 1983.
6. Manson JE, Rimm EB, Colditz GA, et al. A prospective study of postmenopausal estrogen therapy and subsequent incidence of noninsulin-dependent diabetes mellitus. *Ann Epidemiol* 2:665–673, 1992.
7. Cooppan R, Flood TM. Obesity and diabetes. In Marble A, Krall LP, Bradley RF, Christlieb AR, Soeldner JS (Eds.), *Joslin's Diabetes Mellitus*. Philadelphia, Lea & Febiger, 1985, pp. 373–379.
8. De Fronzo RA, Deibert D, Felig P, et al. Insulin sensitivity and insulin binding to monocytes in maturity onset diabetes. *J Clin Invest* 63:939–944, 1979.
9. Foster DW. Diabetes mellitus. In Wilson JD, Braunwald E, Isselbacher KJ, et al. (Eds.), *Harrison's Principles of Internal Medicine*. New York, McGraw-Hill, 1991, pp. 1739–1759.
10. Flier JS, Eastman RC, Minaker KL, et al. Acanthosis nigricans in obese women with hyperandrogenism. Characterization of an insulin-resistance state distinct from the type A and B syndrome. *Diabetes* 34:101–108, 1985.
11. National Diabetes Data Group. Classification and diagnosis of diabetes and other categories of glucose intolerance. *Diabetes* 28:1039, 1979.
12. Marble A, Ferguson BD. Diagnosis and classification of diabetes mellitus and nondiabetic melliturias. In Marble A, Krall LP, Bradley RF, Christlieb AR, Soeldner JS (Eds.), *Joslin's Diabetes Mellitus* (12th ed.). Philadelphia, Lea & Febiger, 1985, pp. 332–352.
13. Metzger BE, Bybee DE, Freinkel N, et al. Gestational diabetes mellitus: Correlations between the phenotypic and genotypic characteristics of the mother and abnormal glucose tolerance testing during the first year postpartum. *Diabetes* 34(Suppl.):111–117, 1985.
14. Salans LB. Fuel metabolism. The obesities. In Felig P, Baxter JD, Broadus AE, Frohman LA (Eds.), *Endocrinology and Metabolism*. New York, McGraw-Hill, 1986, pp. 1203–1244.
15. Fajans S, Floyd JC, Taylor CI, et al. Heterogeneity of insulin responses in latent diabetes. *Trans Assoc Am Physicians* 87:83–89, 1974.
16. National Institutes of Health Consensus Development Panel on the Health Implications of Obesity. Health implications of obesity: National Institutes of Health consensus development conference statement. *Ann Intern Med* 103:1073–1077, 1985.
17. Durnin JVGA, Wormesly J. Body fat assessed from total body density and its estimation from skinfold thickness: Measurements of 481 men and women aged 17 to 72 years. *Br J Nutr* 32:77–82, 1974.
18. Keys A. Overweight, obesity, coronary heart disease and mortality. *Nutr Rev* 38:297–307, 1980.
19. Keys A, Fidanza F, Karvonen MJ, et al. Indices of relative weight and obesity. *J Chron Dis* 25:329–343, 1972.

20. Abraham S, Carroll M, Naijar MF. Trends in obesity and overweight among adults age 20–74 years: United States 1960–62, 1971–1974, 1976–1980. In National Center for Health Statistics, *Vital and Health Statistics*, Series 11. Hyattsville, MD, National Center for Health Statistics, 1985.
21. Borkan GA, Hults, DE, Gerzof SG, et al. Age changes in body composition revealed by computed tomography. *J Gerontol* 38:673–677, 1983.
22. New weight standards for men and women. *Stat Bull NY Metropolitan Life Insurance Co.* 40:1–4, 1959.
23. 1983 Metropolitan height and weight tables. *Stat Bull NY Metropolitan Life Insurance Co.* 64:2–9, 1983.
24. Manson JE, Stampfer MJ, Hennekens CH, et al. Body weight and longevity. A reassessment. *JAMA* 257:353–358, 1987.
25. Willett WC, Stampfer MJ, Manson JE, et al. New weight guidelines for Americans: Justified or injudicious? *Am J Clin Nutr* 53:1102–1103, 1991.
26. Kissebah AH, Vydelingum N, Murray R, et al. Relation of body fat distribution to metabolic consequences of obesity. *J Clin Endocrinol Metab* 54:254–260, 1982.
27. Abraham S. Weight by height and age for adults 18–74 years: United States, 1971–74. U.S. Department of Health, Education, and Welfare Publication PHS 79-1656. Hyattsville, MD, National Center for Health Statistics, 1979.
28. Khoury P, Morrison JA, Mellies MJ, et al. Weight change since age 18 years in 30- to 55-year-old whites and blacks. Associations with lipid values, lipoprotein levels, and blood pressure. *JAMA* 250:3179–3187, 1983.
29. Stunkard AJ. Obesity and the social environment: Current status, future prospects. In Bray G (Ed.), *Obesity in America*. U.S. DHEW Publication NIH 79-359. Washington, D.C., U.S. Government Printing Office, 1979, p. 206.
30. Carney RM, Goldberg AP. Weight gain after cessation of cigarette smoking. A possible role for adipose-tissue lipoprotein lipase. *N Engl J Med* 310:614–616, 1984.
31. Mann GV. The influence of obesity on health. *N Engl J Med* 291:178–232, 1974.
32. Lund-Larsen PG, Tretli S. Changes in smoking habits and body weight after a three-year period—the Cardiovascular Disease Study in Finnmark. *J Chron Dis* 35:773–780, 1982.
33. Stunkard AJ, Thorkild MD, Sorenson TIA, et al. An adoption study of human obesity. *N Engl J Med* 314:193–198, 1986.
34. Romieu I, Willett WC, Stampfer MJ, et al. Energy intake and other determinants of relative weight. *Am J Clin Nutr* 47:406–412, 1988.
35. Brownell KD. The psychology and physiology of obesity: Implications for screening and treatment. *J Am Diet Assoc* 84:406–414, 1984.
36. Bullen BA, Reed RB, Mayer J. Physical activity of obese and nonobese adolescent girls appraised by motion picture sampling. *Am J Clin Nutr* 14:211–216, 1964.
37. Brownell KD, Stunkard AJ. Physical activity in the development and control of obesity. In Stunkard AJ (Ed.), *Obesity*, Philadelphia, W.B. Saunders, 1980, p. 300.
38. Van Itallie TB. Health implications of overweight and obesity in the United States. *Ann Intern Med* 103:983–988, 1985.
39. Stamler J, Rhomberg P, Schoenberger J, et al. Multivariate analysis of the relationship of seven variables to blood pressure: Findings of the Chicago Heart Association Detection Project in Industry, 1967–1972. *J Chron Dis* 28:527–544, 1975.
40. Stamler J, Stamler R, Rhomberg P, et al. Multivariate analysis of the relationship of six variables to blood pressure: Findings from the Chicago Community Surveys, 1965–1972. *J Chron Dis* 28:499–526, 1975.
41. The Lipid Research Clinics Population Studies Data Book. I. *The Prevalence Study*. U.S. Department of Health, Education, and Welfare Publication (NIH) 80–1527. Bethesda, MD, National Institutes of Health, 1980.
42. Van Itallie TB. Obesity: Adverse effects on health and longevity. *Am J Clin Nutr* 32:2723–2733, 1979.
43. Kannel WB, Gordon T. Physiological and medical concomittants of obesity: The Framingham Study. In Bray G (Ed.), *Obesity in America*. U.S. DHEW Publication NIH 79-359. Washington, D.C., U.S. Government Printing Office; 1979, pp. 125–163.
44. Kannel WB, Brand N, Skinner JJ, et al. The relation of adiposity to blood pressure and development of hypertension. The Framingham Study. *Ann Intern Med* 67:48–54, 1967.
45. Kannel WB, LeBauer EJ, Dawber TR, et al. Relation of body weight to development of coronary heart disease. *Circulation* 35:734–744, 1969.
46. Wilson PF, Kannel WB, Anderson KM. Lipids, glucose intolerance and vascular disease: The Framingham Study. *Monogr Atheroscler* 13:1–11, 1985.
47. Kannel WB. Metabolic risk factors for coronary heart disease in women: Perspective from the Framingham Study. *Am Heart J* 114:413–419, 1987.
48. Garrison RJ, Kannel WB, Stokes J, et al. Incidence and prevalence of hypertension in young adults: The Framingham Offspring Study. *Prev Med* 16:235–251, 1987.
49. Modan M, Halkin H, Almog S, et al. Hyperinsulinemia—a link between hypertension, obesity, and glucose intolerance. *J Clin Invest* 75:809–817, 1985.
50. Wood PD, Stefanick MI, Williams PT, et al. The effects of plasma lipoproteins of a prudent weight-reducing diet, with or without exercise, in overweight men and women. *N Engl J Med* 325:461–466, 1991.
51. Levy D, Kannel WB. Cardiovascular risks: New insights from Framingham. *Am Heart J* 116:2664–2667, 1988.
52. Nestel PJ, Whyte HM, Goodman DW. Distribution and turnover of cholesterol in humans. *J Clin Invest* 48:982–986, 1969.
53. Richelsen B. Increased alpha$_2$ but similar β-adrenergic receptor activities in subcutaneous gluteal adipocytes from females compared with males. *Eur J Clin Invest* 16:302–309, 1986.
54. Kaplan NM. The deadly quartet. Upper-body obesity, glucose intolerance, hypertriglyceridemia, and hypertension. *Arch Intern Med* 149:1514–1520, 1989.
55. Krotkiewski M, Björntorp P, Sjöström L, et al. Impact of obesity on metabolism in men and women: importance of regional adipose tissue distribution. *J Clin Invest* 72:1150–1162, 1983.
56. Olefsky JM, Koltermann OG, Scarlett JA. Insulin action and resistance in obesity and non-insulin dependent type II diabetes mellitus. *Am J Physiol* 243:E15–30, 1982.
57. Reaven GM. Role of insulin resistance in human

disease. Banting Lecture 1988. *Diabetes* 37:1595–1607, 1988.
58. Martin DB. Atherogenicity of insulin. *Diabetes Res Clin Pract* (Suppl.) :58–61, 1988.
59. Pyoeraelae K. Relationship of glucose tolerance and plasma insulin to the incidence of coronary heart disease: Results from two population studies in Finland. *Diabetes Care* 2:131–141, 1979.
60. Wellborn TA, Wearne K. Coronary heart disease incidence and cardiovascular mortality in Busselton with reference to glucose and insulin concentrations. *Diabetes Care* 2:154–160, 1979.
61. Ducimetiere P, Eschwege E, Papoz L, et al. Relationship of plasma insulin levels to the incidence of myocardial infarction and coronary heart disease mortality in a middle-aged population. *Diabetologia* 19:205–210, 1980.
62. Laakso M, Pyoeraelae K, Voutilainen E, et al. Plasma insulin levels and serum lipids and lipoproteins in middle-aged non-insulin dependent diabetic and non-diabetic subjects. *Am J Epidemiol* 123:611–621, 1987.
63. Donahue RP, Orchard TJ, Becker DJ, et al. Sex differences in the coronary heart disease risk profile: A possible role for insulin. The Beaver County Study. *Am J Epidemiol* 125:650–657, 1987.
64. Wing RR, Bunker CH, Kuller LH, et al. Insulin, body mass index, and cardiovascular risk factors in premenopausal women. *Arteriosclerosis* 9:479–484, 1989.
65. Manolio TA, Savage PJ, Burke GL, et al. Association of fasting insulin with blood pressure and lipids in young adults. The CARDIA Study. *Arteriosclerosis* 10:430–435, 1990.
66. Asch S, Wingard DL, Barrett-Connor E. Are insulin and hypertension independently related? *Ann Epidemiol* 1:231–244, 1991.
67. Dean JD, Jones CHJ, Hutchison SJ, et al. Hyperinsulinemia and macrovascular angina ("syndrome X"). *Lancet* 337:456–457, 1991.
68. Rabkin SW, Mathweson FA, Hsu PH. Relation of body weight to development of ischemic heart disease in a cohort of young North American men after a 26 year observation period: The Manitoba Study. *Am J Cardiol* 39:452–458, 1977.
69. Chapman JM, Massey FJ. The interrelationship of serum cholesterol, hypertension, body weight, and risk of coronary disease: Results of the first 10 years' follow-up in the Los Angeles Heart Study. *J Chron Dis* 17:933–949, 1964.
70. Pooling Project Research Group. Relation of blood pressure, cholesterol, smoking habit, relative weight, and ECG abnormalities to incidence of major coronary events: Final report of the Pooling Project. *J Chron Dis* 31:201–306, 1978.
71. Hubert HB, Feinlieb M, McNamara PM, et al. Obesity as an independent risk factor for cardiovascular disease: A 26-year follow-up of participants in the Framingham Heart Study. *Circulation* 249:2199–2203, 1983.
72. Lindstedt K, Tonstad S, Kuzma J. Body mass index and patterns of mortality among Seventh-day Adventist men. *Int J Obes* 15:397–406, 1991.
73. Noppa H, Bengtsson C, Wedel H, et al. Obesity in relation to morbidity and mortality from cardiovascular disease. *Am J Epidemiol* 111:682–692, 1980.
74. Lew EA, Gaefinkel L. Variations in mortality by weight among 750,000 men and women. *J Chron Dis* 32:563–576, 1979.
75. Manson JE, Colditz GA, Stampfer MJ, et al. A prospective study of obesity and risk of coronary heart disease in women. *N Engl J Med* 32:882–889, 1990.
76. Amad KH, Brennan JC, Alexander JK. The cardiac pathology of obesity. *Circulation* 32:740–745, 1965.
77. Safer ME, Dimitriv VM. Asymmetric septal hypertrophy and the early phase of hypertension. In: Messerli FH (ed), *The Heart and Hypertension*. New York, Yorke Medical Books, 1987, pp 209–218.
78. Warnes CA, Roberts WC. The heart in massive (more than 300 pounds or 136 kilograms) obesity: Analysis of 12 patients studied at necropsy. *Am J Cardiol* 54:1087, 1984.
79. De Devitiis O, Fazio S, Petitto M, Maddalena G, Contaldo F, Mancini M. Obesity and cardiac function. *Circulation* 64:477–482, 1981.
80. MacMahon SW, Wilcken DEL, Macdonald GJ. The effect of weight reduction on left ventricular mass: A randomized controlled trial in young, overweight hypertensive patients. *N Engl J Med* 314:334, 1986.
81. Alpert MA, Terry BE, Kelly DL. Effect of weight loss on cardiac chamber size, wall thickness and left ventricular function in morbid obesity. *Am J Cardiol* 55:783, 1985.
82. Reisin E, Frohlich ED, Messerli FH, et al. Cardiovascular changes after weight reduction in obesity hypertension. *Ann Intern Med* 98:315, 1983.
83. Young JB, Landsberg L. Weight loss and reduction in blood pressure. *N Engl J Med* 298:1033, 1978.
84. DeHaven J, Sherwin R, Hendler R, Felig P. Nitrogen and sodium balance and sympathetic nervous system activity in obese subjects treated with a low calorie protein or mixed diet. *N Engl J Med* 302:477–482, 1980.
85. Pringle TH, Scobie IN, Murray RG, et al. Prolongation of the QT interval during therapeutic starvation: A substrate for malignant arrhythmias. *Int J Obes* 7:253, 1982.
86. Sandhofer F, Dienstl F, Bolzano K, Schwingshackl H. Severe cardiovascular complication associated with prolonged starvation. *Br Med J* 1:462–463, 1973.
87. Spencer IOB. Death during therapeutic starvation for obesity. *Lancet* 1:1288–1290, 1986.
88. Wenger NK. Coronary disease in women. *Annu Rev Med* 36:285–294, 1985.
89. Greenland P, Reicher-Reiss H, Goldbourt U, Behar S, Israeli SPRINT Investigators. In-hospital and 1-year mortality in 1,524 women after myocardial infarction: Comparison with 4,315 men. *Circulation* 83:484–491, 1991.
90. Tansey MJB, Opie LH, Kennelly BM. High mortality in obese women diabetics with acute myocardial infarction. *Br Med J* 1:1624–1626, 1977.
91. O'Connor GT, Olmstead EM, Coffin LH, Maloney CT, Morton JR, Plume SK, Malenka DJ, Diehl MJ, for the Northern New England Cardiovascular Disease Study Group. Gender and in-hospital mortality associated with coronary artery bypass grafting. *Circulation* 83:723A, 1991.
92. Holmes DR, Holubkov R, Vliestra RE, et al. Comparison of complications during percutaneous transluminal coronary angioplasty from 1977 to 1981 and from 1985 to 1986: The National Heart, Lung, and Blood Institute PTCA registry. *J Am Coll Cardiol* 12:1149–1155, 1988.

93. Loop FD, Golding LR, MacMillan JP, Cosgrove DM, Lytle BW, Sheldon WC. Coronary artery surgery in women compared to men: Analysis of risks and long term results. *J Am Coll Cardiol* 1:383–390, 1983.
94. Khan SK, Nessim S, Gray R, Czer LS, Chaux A, Matloff J. Increased mortality of women in coronary artery bypass surgery: Evidence for referral bias. *Ann Intern Med* 112:561–567, 1990.
95. Tobin JN, Wassertheil-Smoller S, Wexler JP, Steingart RM, Budner N, Lense L, Wachspress J. Sex bias in considering coronary bypass surgery. *Ann Intern Med* 107:19–25, 1987.
96. Blackburn GL, Kanelers BS. Medical evaluation and treatment of the obese patient with cardiovascular disease. 60:g55–g58, 1987.
97. Olefsky JM, Reaven GM, Farquhar JW. Effects of weight reduction in obesity: Studies of carbohydrate and lipid metabolism. *J Clin Invest* 41:53:64–76, 1974.
98. Reisin E, Abel R, Modan M, et al. Effect of weight loss without salt restriction on the reduction of blood pressure in overweight hypertensive patients. *N Engl J Med* 298:1–6, 1978.
99. Tuck ML, Sowers J, Dornfield L, et al. The effect of weight reduction on blood pressure, plasma renin activity, and plasma aldosterone levels in obese patients. *N Engl J Med* 304:930–933, 1981.
100. Meredith CN, Frontera WR, Hughes LA, et al. Peripheral effects of endurance training in young and old subjects. *J Appl Physiol* 66:2844–2849, 1989.
101. Pavlou KN, Krey S, Steffee WP. Exercise as an adjunct to weight loss and maintenance in moderately obese patients. *Am J Clin Nutr* 49:1115–1123, 1989.
102. Foreyt JP, Gododrick GK. Health maintenance through exercise and nutrition. In Blechman, EA (ed), *Behavior Modification with Women*. New York, Guilford Press, 1984, pp. 221–244.
103. Lissner L, Odell PM, D'Agostino RB, et al. Variability of body weight and health outcomes in the Framingham population. *N Engl J Med* 324:1839–1843, 1991.
104. Krolewski AS, Warram JH. Epidemiology of diabetes mellitus. In Marble A, Krall LP, Bradley RF, Christlieb AR, Soeldner JS (Eds.), *Joslin's Diabetes Mellitus* (12th ed.) Philadelphia, Lea & Febiger, 1985, pp. 12–42.
105. Harlan LC, Harlan WR, Landis JR, et al. Factors associated with glucose tolerance in adults in the United States. *Am J Epidemiol* 126:674–684, 1987.
106. Harris MI. Noninsulin-dependent diabetes mellitus in black and white Americans. *Diabetes Metab Rev* 6:71–90, 1990.
107. Ostbye T, Welby TJ, Prior IAM, et al. Type 2 (non-insulin-dependent) diabetes mellitus, migration and westernisation: The Tokelau Island Migrant study. *Diabetologia* 32:585–590, 1989.
108. Kawate R, Yamakido M, Nishimoto Y, et al. Diabetes mellitus and its vascular complications in Japanese migrants on the island of Hawaii. *Diabetes Care* 2:161–167, 1979.
109. WHO Study Group on Diabetes Mellitus. *Technical Report Series 727*. Geneva, WHO, 1985.
110. Barrett-Connor E. Epidemiology, obesity, and non-insulin-dependent diabetes mellitus. *Epidemiol Rev* 11:172–181, 1989.
111. Jarrett RJ. Epidemiology and public health aspects of non-insulin-dependent diabetes mellitus. *Epidemiol Rev* 11:151–171, 1989.
112. Morris RD, Rimm DL, Hartz AJ, et al. Obesity and heredity in the etiology of non-insulin-dependent diabetes mellitus in 32,662 white women. *Am J Epidemiol* 130:112–121, 1989.
113. Wilson PWF, Anderson KM, Kannel WB. Epidemiology of diabetes mellitus in the elderly. *Am J Med* 80:3–9, 1986.
114. Colditz GA, Willett WC, Stampfer MJ, et al. Weight as a risk factor for clinical diabetes in women. *Am J Epidemiol* 132:501–513, 1990.
115. Ohlson LO, Larsson B, Svardsudd K, et al. The influence of body fat distribution on the incidence of diabetes mellitus. 13.5 years of follow-up of the participants in the study of men born in 1913. *Diabetes* 34:1055–1058, 1985.
116. Freedman DS, Rimm AA. The relation of body fat distribution, as assessed by six girth measurements, to diabetes mellitus in women. *Am J Public Health* 79:715–720, 1989.
117. Colditz GA, Manson JE, Willett WC, et al. Diet and the risk of diabetes. *Am J Clin Nutr* 55:1018–1023, 1992.
118. Zimmet P, Dowse G, Finch C, et al. The epidemiology and natural history of NIDDM—lessons from the South Pacific. *Diabetes Metab Rev* 6:91–124, 1990.
119. Taylor R, Ram P, Zimmet P, et al. Physical activity and prevalence of diabetes in Melanesian and Indian men in Fiji. *Diabetologia* 27:578–582, 1984.
120. King H, Zimmet P, Raper LR, et al. Risk factors for diabetes in three Pacific populations. *Am J Epidemiol* 119:396–409, 1984.
121. Dowse GK, Zimmet P, Gareboo H, et al. Abdominal obesity and physical inactivity as risk factors for NIDDM and impaired glucose tolerance in Indians, Creole, and Chinese Mauritians. *Diabetes Care* 14:271–282, 1991.
122. Jarrett, RJ, Shipley MJ, Hunt R. Physical activity, glucose intolerance, and diabetes mellitus: The Whitehall study. *Diabetic Med* 3:549–551, 1986.
123. Montoye HJ, Block WD, Metzner H, et al. Physical activity and glucose tolerance: Males age 16–64 in a total community. *Diabetes* 26:172–177, 1977.
124. Frisch RE, Wyshak G, Albright TE, et al. Lower prevalence of diabetes in female former college athletes compared with nonathletes. *Diabetes* 35:1101–1105, 1986.
125. Manson JE, Rimm EB, Stampfer MJ, et al. Physical activity and incidence of non-insulin dependent diabetes mellitus in women. *Lancet* 338:774–778, 1991.
126. Manson JE, Colditz GA, Stampfer MJ, et al. A prospective study on maturity-onset diabetes mellitus and risk of coronary heart disease and stroke in women. *Arch Intern Med* 151:1141–1147, 1991.
127. Pyörälä K, Laakso M, Uusitupa M. Diabetes and atherosclerosis: An epidemiologic view. *Diabetes Metab Rev* 3:463–524, 1987.
128. Goldberg RB. Lipid disorders in diabetes. *Diabetes Care* 4:561–672, 1981.
129. Barrett-Connor E, Orchard T. Diabetes and heart disease. In National Diabetes Data Group. *Diabetes in America*. Diabetes data compiled 1984. U.S. Department of Health and Human Services Publication PHS 85-1468: XVI, 1–41. Bethesda, MD, National Institutes of Health, 1985.
130. Kannel WB, D'Agostino RB, Wilson PWF, et al.

130. Diabetes fibrinogen, and risk of cardiovascular disease: The Framingham experience. *Am Heart J* 120:672–676, 1990.
131. Gordon T, Castelli WP, Hjortland MC, et al. Diabetes, blood lipids, and the role of obesity in CHD risk for women. The Framingham study. *Ann Intern Med* 87:393–397, 1977.
132. Jarrett RJ, McCartney P, Keen H. The Bedford survey: Ten year mortality rates in newly diagnosed diabetics, borderline diabetics and normoglycaemic controls and risk indices for coronary heart disease in borderline diabetics. *Diabetologia* 22:79–84, 1982.
133. Jarrett RJ, Keen H, McCartney M, et al. Glucose tolerance and blood pressure in two population samples: Their relation to diabetes mellitus and hypertension. *Int J Epidemiol* 63:54–64, 1978.
134. Herman JB, Medalie JH, Goldbourt U. Differences in cardiovascular morbidity and mortality between previously known and newly diagnosed adult diabetics. *Diabetologia* 13:229–234, 1977.
135. Lapidus L, Bengtsson C, Blohmé G, et al. Blood glucose, glucose tolerance and manifest diabetes in relation to cardiovascular disease and death in women. A 12-year follow-up of participants in the population study of women in Gothenburg, Sweden. *Acta Med Scand* 218:455–462, 1985.
136. Krolewski AS, Warram JH, Rand LI, et al. Epidemiologic approach to the etiology of type I diabetes mellitus and its complications. *N Engl J Med* 317:1390–1398, 1987.
137. Krolewski AS, Kosinski EJ, Warram JH, et al. Magnitude and determinants of coronary artery disease in juvenile-onset, insulin-dependent diabetes mellitus. *Am J Cardiol* 59:750–755, 1987.
138. World Health Organization Multinational Study of Vascular Disease in Diabetes. Prevalence of small vessel and large vessel disease in diabetic patients from 14 centers. *Diabetologia* 28:615–640, 1985.
139. Waller BF, Palumbo, PJ, Lie JT, et al. Status of the coronary arteries at necropsy in diabetes mellitus with onset after age 30 years: Analysis of 229 diabetic patients with and without clinical evidence of coronary heart disease and comparison of 183 control subjects. *Am J Med* 69:498–506, 1980.
140. Lemp GF, et al. Association between the severity of diabetes mellitus and coronary arterial atherosclerosis. *Am J Cardiol* 60:1015–1019, 1987.
141. Ridker PM, Hennekens CH. Hemostatic risk factors for coronary heart disease. *Circulation* 83:1098–1100, 1991.
142. Halushka PV, Lurie D, Colwell JA. Increased synthesis of prostaglandin E-like material by platelets from patients with diabetes mellitus. *N Engl J Med* 297:1306, 1977.
143. Juhan-Vague I, Vague PH, Alessi MC, et al. Relationships between plasma insulin, triglyceride, body mass index, and plasminogen activator inhibitor 1. *Diabetes Metab* 13:331–336, 1987.
144. Vague P, Juhan-Vague I, Chabert V, et al. Fat distribution and plasminogen activator inhibitor activity in non-diabetic obese women. *Metabolism* 38:913–915, 1989.
145. Kannel WB, Wolf PA, Castelli WP, et al. Fibrinogen and risk of cardiovascular disease: The Framingham Study. *JAMA* 258:1183–1186, 1987.
146. Wilhelmsen L, Svardsudd K, Korsan-Bengtsen K, et al. Fibrinogen as a risk factor for stroke and myocardial infarction. *N Engl J Med* 311:501–505, 1984.
147. Meade TW, Chakrabarti R, Haines AP, et al. Hemostatic function and cardiovascular death: Early results of a prospective study. *Lancet* 1:1050–1054, 1980.
148. Herlitz J, Malmberg K, Karlson BW, et al. Mortality and morbidity during a five-year follow-up of diabetics with myocardial infarction. *Acta Med Scand* 224:31, 1988.
149. Stone PH, Muller JE, Hartwell T, et al. The effect of diabetes mellitus on prognosis and serial left ventricular function after acute myocardial infarction: Contribution of both coronary disease and diastolic left ventricular dysfunction to the adverse prognosis. *J Am Coll Cardiol* 14:49, 1989.
150. Abbott RD, Donahue RP, Kannel WB, et al. The impact of diabetes on survival following myocardial infarction in men vs women. The Framingham Study. *JAMA* 260:3456, 1988.
151. Smith JW, Buckels LJ, Carlson K, et al. Clinical characteristics and results of noninvasive tests in 60 diabetic patients after acute myocardial infarction. *Am J Med* 75:217, 1983.
152. Smith JW, et al. Prognosis of patients with diabetes mellitus after acute myocardial infarction. *Am J Cardiol* 54:718–721, 1984.
153. Ulvenstam G, Aberg A, Bergstrand R, et al. Long-term prognosis after myocardial infarction in men with diabetes. *Diabetes* 34:787, 1985.
154. Gwilt DJ, Petri M, Lewis PW, et al. Myocardial infarct size and mortality in diabetic patients. *Br Heart J* 54:466, 1985.
155. Chipkin SR, Frid D, Alpert JS, et al. Frequency of painless myocardial ischemia during exercise tolerance testing in patients with and without diabetes mellitus. *Am J Cardiol* 59:61, 1987.
156. Felsher J, Meissner MD, Hakki AH, et al. Exercise thallium imaging in patients with diabetes mellitus: prognostic implications. *Arch Intern Med* 147:313, 1987.
157. Nesto RW, Phillips RT, Kett KG, et al. Angina and exertional myocardial ischemia in diabetic and non-diabetic patients: Assessment by exercise thallium scintigraphy. *Ann Intern Med* 108:170, 1988.
158. Nesto RW, Roland TP. Asymptomatic myocardial ischemia in diabetic patients. *Am J Med* 80:40–47, 1986.
159. Lloyd-Mostyn RH, Watkins PJ. Defective innervation of heart in diabetic autonomic neuropathy. *Br Med J* 3:15, 1975.
160. Roy TM, Peterson HR, Snider HL, et al. Autonomic influence on cardiovascular performance in diabetic subjects. *Am J Med* 87:382, 1989.
161. Zola B, Kahn JK, Juni JE, et al. Abnormal cardiac function in diabetic patients with autonomic neuropathy in the absence of ischemic heart disease. *J Clin Endocrinol Metab* 63:208, 1986.
162. Kahn JK, Sisson JC, Vinik AI. QT interval prolongation and sudden cardiac death in diabetic autonomic neuropathy. *J Clin Endocrinol Metab* 64:751, 1987.
163. Salomon NW, Page US, Okies JE, et al. Diabetes mellitus and coronary artery bypass: Short-term risk and long-term prognosis. *J Thorac Cardiovasc Surg* 85:264, 1983.
164. Lawrie GM, Morris GC, Glaeser DH. Influence of diabetes mellitus on the results of coronary bypass surgery: Follow-up of 212 diabetic patients 10 to 15 years after surgery. *JAMA* 256:2967–2971, 1986.

165. Tofler GH, Stone PH, Muller JE, et al. Effects of gender and race on prognosis after myocardial infarction: adverse prognosis for women, particularly black women. *J Am Coll Cardiol* 9:473–482, 1987.
166. Steingart RM, Packer M, Hamm P, et al. Sex differences in the management of coronary artery disease. *N Engl J Med* 325:226–230, 1991.
167. Varma VK, Murphy PL, Hood WP, et al. Are women with acute myocardial infarction managed differently from men? *J Am Coll Cardiol* 19:20A, 1992.
168. Eaker ED, Kronmal B, Kennedy JW, Davis K. Comparison of the long-term, post-surgical survival of women and men in the Coronary Artery Surgery Study (CASS). Am Heart J 117:71–81, 1989.
169. Ayanian JZ, Epstein AM. Differences in the use of procedures between women and men hospitalized for coronary heart disease. *N Engl J Med* 325:221–225, 1991.
170. Zarich SW, Nesto RW. Diabetic cardiomyopathy. *Am Heart J* 118:1000–1012, 1989.
171. Kannel WB, Hjortland M, Castelli WP. Role of diabetes in congestive heart failure: The Framingham Study. *Am J Cardiol* 34:29–34, 1974.
172. Kimmelsteil C, Goldberg GJ. Congestive heart failure in women: Focus on heart failure due to coronary artery disease and diabetes. *Cardiology* 77 (Suppl. 2):71–79, 1990.
173. Zoneraich S, Silverman G, Zoneraich O. Primary myocardial disease, diabetes mellitus, and small vessel disease. *Am Heart J* 5:754–755, 1980.
174. Factor SM, Minase T, Sonnenblick EH. Clinical and morphological features of human hypertensive-diabetic cardiomyopathy. *Am Heart J* 74:446–458, 1980.
175. Factor SM, Okun Em, Ninase T. Capillary microaneurysms in the human diabetic heart. *N Engl J Med* 302:384–388, 1980.
176. Vered Z, Battler A, Segal P, et al. Exercise-induced left ventricular dysfunction in young men with asymptomatic diabetes mellitus (diabetic cardiomyopathy). *Am J Cardiol* 54:633–637, 1984.
177. Mildenberger RR, Bar-Shlomi B, Druck MN, et al. Clinically unrecognized ventricular dysfunction in young diabetic patients. *J Am Coll Cardiol* 4:234–238, 1984.
178. Doar JWH, Thompson ME, Wilde CE, et al. Influence of treatment with diet alone on oral glucose tolerance test and plasma sugar and insulin levels in patients with maturity onset diabetes mellitus. *Lancet* 1:1263–1268, 1975.
179. Berger M, Baumhoff EE, Gries FA. Weight reduction and glucose intolerance in obesity (in German). *Deutsch Med Wochenschr* 101:307–311, 1976.
180. Ruderman NB, Ganda OP, Johansen K. The effect of physical training on glucose tolerance and plasma lipids in maturity-onset diabetes. *Diabetes* 28 (Suppl.):89–94, 1979.
181. Saltin B, Lindgärde F, Houston M, et al. Physical training and glucose tolerance in middle-aged men with chemical diabetes. *Diabetes* 28 (Suppl.):30–37, 1979.
182. Ruderman NB, Apelian AZ, Schneider SH. Exercise in therapy and prevention of type II diabetes: Implication for blacks. *Diabetes Care* 13 (Suppl.):1163–1168, 1990.

CHAPTER 11

Smoking and Cardiovascular Disease

LINDA P. FRIED, M.D., M.P.H.
DIANE M. BECKER, Sc.D.

The role of smoking in causing cardiovascular disease in women has, until recently, been unclear. Early studies suggested either a weak association at best, or no association between smoking and cardiovascular disease in women, whereas the association was strong for middle-aged men (1–2). Such data contributed to what the Surgeon General has described as "the fallacy of women's apparent immunity" to smoking (3). *The Surgeon General's Report on the Health Consequences of Smoking for Women* (3) concludes:

In (the) studies conducted during the past three decades, relative mortality risks among female smokers appeared to be less than those of male smokers. It is now clear, however, that these studies were comparing the death rates of a generation of established, lifelong male smokers with a generation of women who had not yet taken up smoking with full intensity.

Even these older women who reported smoking a large number of cigarettes per day had not smoked cigarettes in the same way as their male counterparts. Now that the cigarette smoking characteristics of women and men are becoming increasingly similar, their relative risks of smoking-related illness will become increasingly similar.

The weight of current evidence has now clearly established that smoking is an independent and important risk factor for coronary heart disease, peripheral vascular disease, stroke, and subarachnoid hemorrhage in women. Many recent studies have assessed women who have smoked from younger ages, for longer periods, and more heavily than was the case in earlier studies. They have shown elevated risks of cardiovascular disease in women due to smoking that are comparable to those for male smokers. This chapter will

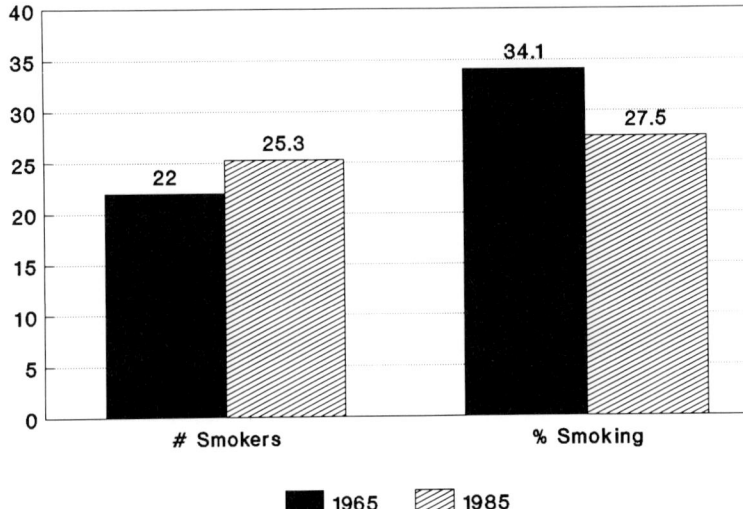

Figure 11-1. The numbers and proportion of women 18 years and older who smoked cigarettes in the United States, 1965 and 1985. (From United States Department of Health and Human Services. Reducing the health consequences of smoking: 25 years of progress. A report of the Surgeon General. DHHS Pub. No. (CDC) 89-8411. Washington, D.C., U.S. Government Printing Office, 1989, pp. 133–136.)

review the scientific bases for this conclusion, its implications for the cardiovascular health status of women, the characteristics of women smokers, and the opportunities and approaches taken to promoting smoking cessation in women.

EPIDEMIOLOGY OF SMOKING IN WOMEN

Since 1965, the numbers of women who smoke has increased, and women have started smoking at younger ages and more heavily than was the case previously. As seen in Figure 11–1, 22 million women aged 18 and older in the United States smoked in 1965; by 1985, the number of women smoking had risen to 25.3 million (3). At the same time, the overall percentage of women who smoke decreased from 34.0% in 1965 to 27.5% in 1985 (3). This recent proportion is still substantially higher than the 18% of adult women who smoked in 1935 (53% of men smoked in 1935) (3). Overall, the proportion of women smoking has decreased only 6% since the 1964 issuance of the first Surgeon General's report on smoking and health, while the proportion of men smoking has decreased 21% (5).

In 1965 only 12% of older women smokers, those born before 1906, had started smoking in their teens. Between 1965 and 1985, the number of women aged 60 years or older who had started smoking in their teens increased tenfold (4). As a result, the cumulative impact of many years of smoking is now seen in this cohort. The trend of women beginning to smoke in their teens has persisted and in fact has increased in recent years. As seen in Table 11–1, the average age at initiation of smoking in women has decreased from 23 years among women born between 1910 and 1919 to 18 years among those born between 1950 and

Table 11-1. AVERAGE AGE AT INITIATION OF REGULAR[a] SMOKING AMONG WOMEN, BY RACE AND BIRTH COHORT—UNITED STATES

	1910–1919		1920–1929		1930–1939		1940–1949		1950–1959	
	Age (yr)	*95% CI*[b]	*Age (yr)*	*95% CI*[b]	*Age (yr)*	*95% CI*[b]	*Age (yr)*	*95% CI*[b]	*Age (yr)*	*95% CI*[b]
White	22.9	(±0.5)	21.0	(±0.3)	19.4	(±0.2)	18.6	(±0.2)	17.5	(±0.1)
Black	23.0	(±1.8)	21.8	(±0.9)	20.4	(±0.9)	19.5	(±0.4)	18.4	(±0.3)

[a]Regular was self-defined.
[b]Confidence interval.
From Centers for Disease Control. Differences in the age of smoking initiation between blacks and whites. *MMWR* 40(44):755, 1991.

1959 (6). More than 86% of women smokers born between 1950 and 1959 began smoking before the age of 21 (6).

The intensity of smoking by women has changed in addition to frequency and age at onset. Among women smokers from 1965 to 1985, the proportion who smoked more than 25 cigarettes per day rose from 14% to 21% (4). In addition, the way women smoke has changed. As reported by Doll and colleagues, women physicians who began smoking before World War I reported inhaling much less frequently than men; specifically, in 1980, among subjects 65 to 74 years of age, 54% of male physicians who smoked said they inhaled, compared with 18% of female physicians (7). This disparity has decreased since World War II. Recent data indicate that these changes in cigarette smoking habits are strongly associated with risk of cardiovascular disease in women, as discussed below.

For women, smoking rates are strongly associated with education. Among women with less than 12 years of education, 37% smoke cigarettes compared with 26% of women with 16 or more years of education. When stratifying by race, this trend holds for white women but is not clearly present for blacks (8). Associations with other indices of socioeconomic status, including occupation, are less strong.

Thus, more women are smoking now than in 1965; they are also smoking more heavily, and are quitting less frequently than men. These changed patterns of smoking are of significant import in assessing the risk of cardiovascular disease for women.

SMOKING AS A RISK FACTOR FOR CARDIOVASCULAR DISEASE IN WOMEN

Coronary Heart Disease

The preponderance of data from studies conducted in women since the 1970s indicates that cigarette smoking is a strong independent risk factor for coronary heart disease in women. Smoking confers a two- to sixfold increased risk of both fatal coronary heart disease and nonfatal myocardial infarction, compared to never smoking, in numerous prospective studies of women across the entire adult age range with 3 to 22 years of follow-up (7, 9–13). Data from the Nurses' Health Study show that, overall, half of all cases of fatal and nonfatal coronary heart disease in women aged 30 to 55 years is attributable to cigarette smoking (9).

Recent studies generally indicate that the risks of smoking in women are comparable to those in men across the adult age spectrum. For younger women, case-control studies show that risks for women under age 50 range from a 1.4- to 14-fold increase among smokers compared to those who never smoke (14–16), which is comparable to the risks in men of similar age (16, 17). In the Nurses' Health Study, women who were current smokers, aged 30 to 55 at baseline, had a three-fold increased risk of myocardial infarction compared to nonsmokers. Heavy smokers ($\geq$ two packs per day) had a fivefold increased risk (9). In the Framingham Study, the relative risks of smoking for fatal and nonfatal coronary heart disease (excluding angina) in people 50 to 59 years were 1.9 for women and 1.8 for men, based on 10 years of follow-up (18). In the Established Populations for Epidemiologic Study of the Elderly (EPESE) of people 65 and older, the relative risk of cardiovascular mortality associated with smoking was 1.6 for women and 2.0 for men in a 5-year follow-up (11).

Although there has been a high concordance among recent studies regarding the association of smoking with fatal coronary heart disease and nonfatal myocardial infarction in women, findings in relation to angina have been less consistent. The Nurses' Health Study found that smoking 15 or more cigarettes per day was associated with a 2.6-fold increased risk of incident angina compared with women who had never smoked (9). This study used a stringent definition of angina pectoris. Subjects with a positive response to the Rose angina questionnaire (19) also had to have medical record verification through either documented evidence of coronary artery bypass surgery, coronary angiography showing more than 70% obstruction of any coronary artery, or ST-segment depression of more than 1 mm on exercise stress testing. In addition, the study excluded women with angina pectoris who also had a history of congenital heart disease, mitral valve prolapse, or rheumatic heart disease. Seventy-five percent of the cases of angina were confirmed by coronary arteriography.

In contrast, two studies finding no association of smoking with angina used more standardized clinical definitions. For example, in the Framingham Study, cigarette smoking was not significantly associated with coronary heart disease in women 50 to 59 years of age when a history of angina was included in the definition but was associated when angina was excluded, as above, adjusting for systolic blood pressure, relative weight, serum cholesterol, and glucose intolerance in two separate multivariate logistic regression models (18). For women aged 65 and older in the Framingham Study there was no significant association of smoking 20 or more cigarettes per day with coronary heart disease, including all incident angina, coronary insufficiency, myocardial infarctions, and fatal coronary heart disease (20). Angina was defined here based on a typical history of chest pain using standardized criteria.

The difference in findings between studies of the relationship between smoking and angina in women may thus result from differences in criteria for the definition of angina. This marked effect of case definition may be associated with the fact that the history of angina in women, especially mild or moderate angina, carries a substantially higher false positive rate compared with arteriographic diagnosis than it does in men (21). In addition, secular changes in rates of smoking–particularly heavy smoking—may play a role in the disparity of the findings. Most women who smoked in the Framingham Study smoked lightly. In only 7% of the biannual examinations did women 45 to 54 years old report smoking more than 20 cigarettes per day (22). In contrast, 23% of the person-years of follow-up in the Nurses' Health Study were of women who reported smoking 15 or more cigarettes per day (9). Although the Framingham Study reported the results of a cohort that was middle-aged in 1948 to 1952, the Nurses' Health Study described the experience of women who were 30 to 55 years of age in 1976. Thus, disparity in findings in these major studies likely reflects secular trends in smoking habits in women and differences in the case definition of angina, as well as the power of the studies to detect associations in women.

A consistent finding in all these studies is that the risk of coronary heart disease in women increases with the number of cigarettes smoked, and that even a few cigarettes smoked per day confers increased risk. Risk of total coronary heart disease (excluding angina) or first myocardial infarction is elevated twofold among women smoking as few as one to four cigarettes per day, compared to women who have never smoked. Risk increases in a stepwise fashion with increasing consumption, with a sevenfold increased risk for women smoking 35 or more cigarettes per day (9, 14–16, 23–25). For women 30 to 55 years of age in the Nurses' Health Study, 58% of the coronary heart disease among the lightest smokers was attributable to cigarette use, compared to 91% among the heaviest smokers (9).

Notably, there appears to be little or no increased risk of coronary heart disease in women who have stopped smoking for 2 or more years. Former smokers have the same rates of both fatal coronary heart disease and nonfatal myocardial infarction as do women who never smoked (9, 11, 14, 15, 24, 25). This consistent finding suggests that the preeminent mechanisms by which smoking causes coronary heart disease are relatively acute ones. The major exception to this statement is one study that showed an association of past smoking history with sudden death for women 25 to 44 years, in a 12-year follow-up of white women in Washington County, Maryland (12).

Low-Yield Cigarettes

A significant clinical and public health question is whether smoking so-called low-yield cigarettes alters the risk of coronary heart disease for women. Cigarettes that have lower yields of nicotine and carbon monoxide have been marketed with the strong suggestion that they are less hazardous to health. Women make up the largest proportion of smokers of low-yield cigarettes (26), and it has been suggested that the advent of a presumeably safer cigarette has contributed to the slower decline in smoking rates among women compared to men (27). Recent data do not support this presumption. Studies concur in their findings that women who smoke low-yield cigarettes have higher risk of coronary heart disease than do nonsmokers (28, 29). In addition, there is no decrease in risk of a first nonfatal myocardial infarction in women smoking low-yield cigarettes compared to higher yield brands (27). Relative risks for low-yield cigarettes were comparable to those in other studies that evaluated all smokers together. There was no significant difference in risk when smokers were evaluated by either machine-determined nicotine levels or carbon monoxide levels. Thus, smoking low-yield cigarettes does not appear to decrease the risk of coronary artery disease in women significantly.

Stroke

In general, recent studies show a strong association between cigarette smoking and cerebrovascular disease in women. In both case-control and longitudinal studies, women who were current smokers had a two- to threefold increased risk of fatal and nonfatal stroke compared to those who never smoked (26–28). All of these studies adjusted for the effects of hypertension in these risk estimates. Prospective studies that have looked at stroke subtypes find that smoking by women confers a two- to threefold increased risk of thromboembolic stroke (27, 28) and a fivefold increased risk of subarachnoid hemorrhage (27, 29). Conflicting findings have been reported regarding a possible interaction of smoking with hypertension, causing a combined higher risk of stroke in women (26, 27).

As with the risk of coronary heart disease, the risk of stroke increases in a dose-response relationship with increasing numbers of cigarettes smoked per day. For example, in the Nurses' Health Study of women 30 to 55 years old at baseline, the relative risk of stroke was 2.2 for women smoking 1 to 14 cigarettes per day, and 3.7 for women smoking 25 or more cigarettes per day (27). Risk of subarachnoid hemorrhage also increased among women who smoked 25 or more cigarettes per day, to a relative risk of 10 (27).

Thus, recent studies show a strong independent association of smoking with both stroke and subarachnoid hemorrhage in women. This risk increases with the number of cigarettes smoked per day. It is noteworthy, however, that the risk of stroke is increased for women smoking only a few cigarettes a day (27, 28). Finally, smoking cessation appears to lead, after a 2-year period of not smoking, to a decrease in risk of stroke in women down to the levels seen in women who have never smoked (27).

Peripheral Vascular Disease

It is well recognized that cigarette smoking is associated with the development of peripheral arterial disease as well as with the severity of symptoms resulting from this. This finding has been consistent for women and men. In the Framingham Heart Study, smoking was a comparably strong risk factor for both women and men, with a threefold increased risk of incident peripheral vascular disease in heavy smokers (30). Data from the Rancho Bernardo Study indicate that the association of smoking appears to be with large-vessel, not small-vessel, peripheral vascular disease (31). A smaller study of 245 women with arteriosclerotic peripheral vascular disease suggested that the association is primarily with proximal (aortoiliac) disease, with a lesser association found with distal (femoropopliteal) disease; in this study, relative risks with smoking were 30 and 6, respectively (32). Finally, as with other cardiovascular diseases, the risk diminishes with smoking cessation, reaching the level of risk of those who never smoked after a 5-year period of no cigarette smoking (32).

MECHANISMS OF THE RELATIONSHIP OF SMOKING TO CORONARY HEART DISEASE

There is considerable evidence linking cigarette smoking to cardiovascular disease through both chronic and acute atherogenic effects. In terms of the chronic effects, autopsy studies have consistently shown an association between cigarette smoking and the degree of atherosclerosis in coronary, cerebral, and peripheral vessels (33, 34). Animal models and human studies have also demonstrated arterial injury related to increased levels of blood nicotine and carbon monoxide (35, 36). Cigarette smokers also have significantly lower levels of high density lipoprotein cholesterol, the potentially protective lipoprotein subfraction. This usually increases modestly with smoking cessation (37–39).

In terms of possible acute effects of smoking, it has been noted that increased platelet aggregability and clotting factors such as fibrinogen, which are known to predispose to thrombus formation and endothelial dysfunction, occur with exposure to carbon monoxide and nicotine as well as other gas and vapor-phase components of cigarette smoke (40–44). Natural thrombolytic substances such as plasminogen are lower in smokers (45) and increase with smoking cessation (46). Cigarette smoking has also been associated with increased blood pressure and heart rate acutely and may result in increased myocardial oxygen demands (39). Cigarette smoking in women is also associated with increased levels of adrenal androgens (DHEA and androstenedione) (47) and with a natural menopause that occurs 1 to 2 years earlier than that in nonsmokers (48). Whether earlier menopause is associated with risk of coronary heart disease in women remains unclear (49).

Thus, the observed relationship between cigarette smoking and cardiovascular disease probably results from multiple mechanisms that interact to cause atherosclerosis, vascular injury, and thrombotic occlusion of vessels. The marked decline in risk associated with smoking cessation (50) suggests, however, that the acute effects of smoking are of primary importance.

ORAL CONTRACEPTIVES AND CARDIOVASCULAR DISEASE IN WOMEN

Early studies of oral contraceptive use demonstrated a significant increase in fatal and nonfatal cardiovascular disease events in women who were current users of oral contraceptives (51). Past use of oral contraceptives has little or no impact on cardiovascular risk. There is a marked increase in the relative risk of myocardial infarction and stroke in persons who are both current smokers and current users of oral contraceptives, the relative risks reaching 20 to 30 times those of nonsmoking, noncontraceptive users of the same age (15, 24). Risk is especially high for heavy smokers and older premenopausal women.

The primary mechanism by which oral contraceptives are associated with cardiovascular disease appears to be thromboembolic (52). Both oral contraceptives and smoking have a marked effect on coagulation and on platelet activity (53); this is consonant with thrombogenesis. It is not surprising that the combination of these two factors leads to such a marked interactive excess risk. Although the early studies showing this relationship involved the use of agents with higher doses of hormones than are currently used and are thought to be more atherogenic, the current use of oral contraceptive agents in smokers or the continuance of smoking in women using oral contraceptives is strongly discouraged.

TRENDS IN SMOKING CESSATION IN WOMEN

Although the prevalence of cigarette smoking has until recently been lower in women than in men in the United States, women who smoke have consistently demonstrated lower quit rates than men. This has been the case in both the general population, as reflected in spontaneous quit rates, and in smoking cessation programs. Women are also thought to be less likely than men to stop smoking following a myocardial infarction. In 1965, 32% of women and 50% of men were current smokers, whereas in 1987, 27% of women and 32% of men were smokers, indicating a decline in absolute percentage of almost 20% in men and only 5% in women. This is largely accounted for by a considerably slower rate of cessation in women smokers than in men. In the general population, the percentage of former smokers among those who ever smoked is now approximately 49% among men but only 40% among women (54). However, the difference may not be so great when one considers that many men take up alternative forms of tobacco use, whereas few women do the same. This is important in estimating risk, because it has been shown that former cigarette smokers who use cigars or pipes as a nicotine delivery system after stopping cigarette smoking continue to inhale. Thus, when quit rates are adjusted for use of other forms of tobacco after smoking cessation, primarily pipe and cigar smoking, the respective prevalences of former smokers fall to 45% among men and 40% among women. Further, when snuff and chewing tobacco were reclassified among former smokers, the former smoking prevalences among those who ever smoked fell to 42% among men and 40% among women (55).

Although reclassification of other forms of tobacco reduces the apparent smoking cessation differences between men and women, women who have smoked in their lifetime still remain less likely to become former smokers. Women appear to be quitting smoking at a rate of only 0.33 percentage points per year, whereas the decline has been approximately 0.84 percentage points per year for men over a 12-year period, even when adjusted for the switch to other forms of tobacco use after cigarette cessation (56).

Although there have been a number of hypotheses as to why women fail to quit at the same rates as men, none have been empirically supported. Explanations range from a shift in women's societal roles and increased participation of women in high-stress work environments to biologic differences, many of which remain to be determined. Recent observations suggest that cigarette smoking may be more addictive for women, leading to increased difficulty with smoking cessation compared to men. Still others have suggested that women have been differentially targeted by the tobacco industry and have been continually exhorted to smoke cigarettes, using persuasive communication techniques that tout a new role for women in today's society, one that includes cigarette smoking as a symbol of power. The issue remains unresolved, but given the fact that women do not escape the risk of smoking-related diseases, it is important to develop and implement strategies to shift the paradigm in favor of markedly higher cessation rates among women who already smoke and lower smoking adoption rates in the younger cohorts of women at high risk for starting to smoke.

SMOKING CESSATION STRATEGIES IN WOMEN

At present, more than 95% of smokers who ultimately become successful quitters do so without the assistance of any formal program. However, spontaneous smoking cessation rates are lower for women than for men. During the past two decades, approximately 26% of women smokers indicated that they had *never* tried to quit smoking, whereas only 22% of men had never tried (54). Women do present to formal treatment programs in approximately equal numbers as men. However, in this context, far fewer women than men are successful in achieving cessation. In many studies of participants in smoking cessation interventions, women in general have been found to have lower success in sustained cessation than men. There does not appear to be any specific explanation for this, nor does there appear to be any specific smoking cessation strategy that markedly improves quit rates in women. It has been hypothesized that weight gain may account for some of the failures seen in smoking cessation programs, and some authors have hypothesized a potential biologic explanation related to differentially severe withdrawal syndromes, a hypothesis for which no empirical evidence exists. More recently, preliminary data on the response of women to nicotine replacement suggests that women are less likely to quit in such programs than with other methods. Some investigators have also shown modest improvements in women's cessation rates in intervention programs in which strong social support is included (57, 58).

Thus, the issue of how best to achieve smoking cessation in women remains unresolved. In general, the most successful smoking cessation strategies are those that are multimodal, combining cognitive, behavioral, social, and pharmacologic components (59). Pharmacologic treatment alone, specifically nicotine replacement, has only a modest impact on cessation rates. It appears critical that supportive and behavioral components be included in intervention programs to optimize the success rates for women. Although the evidence is modest, at least two studies suggest that strong social support from significant others and the social environment are particularly important for women (57, 58).

WEIGHT GAIN AND THE IMPACT ON CESSATION IN WOMEN

It has long been noted that cigarette smoking is associated with lower body weight and that smoking cessation may be associated with significant weight gain, particularly in women (60). Almost 80% of successful quitters gain weight, with an average weight gain of 4 to 6 pounds, although 3.5% of successful quitters may suffer weight gains that exceed 20 pounds. Women appear to be more likely to suffer higher weight gains after cessation, although this has not been a consistent finding (61). There is some evidence that this different propensity toward increased weight gain in women may be at least partially mediated through gender differences in postcessation diet (60). However, although increases in food intake, particularly carbohydrates, are often observed, decreases in resting metabolic rate are also noted in people quitting smoking. This suggests that weight gain may be only partially accounted for by eating behaviors (61, 62).

Physical activity does not appear to play either a positive or a negative role in weight change.

The weight gain attributed to smoking cessation does not appear to be accompanied by any increase in cardiovascular risk or attendant risk factors in women (63, 64). In fact, it appears that in spite of weighing less in general, smokers have a greater propensity toward central obesity as measured by waist-to-hip ratio and may actually bear an excess cardiovascular disease risk (65).

The major problem associated with body weight and cigarette smoking in women appears to be related to the social implications of weight in women, particularly young women (66). Many women who return to smoking after stopping report doing so with the deliberate intention of controlling weight. Unfortunately, successful strategies to ameliorate the weight gain experienced by many women who stop smoking have not been determined. Randomized trials of diet and physical activity have suggested that such regimens either have no impact or that a modest reduction in weight gain may be achieved with intensive interventions after cessation. In all studies, persons randomized to the intervention gained weight (67). Recently, there has been some evidence that nicotine replacement therapy may at least partially ameliorate or delay the weight gain associated with cessation (68–70). The development of effective ways to reduce postcessation weight gain is important for sustained smoking cessation in women who fear the weight gain that occurs postcessation.

SMOKING CESSATION

Nonpharmacologic Interventions

Between 95% and 99% of successful quitters, male and female, have done so "on their own" without the assistance of formal or commercial programs (71). However, as discussed above, a relatively small proportion of women have quit compared to men. This argues for increased attention to recommendations to quit by clinicians, and for more participation by women smokers in smoking cessation programs. From a clinical practice perspective, it is important to recognize that state-of-the-art interventions are the same for men as for women. Because we have increasingly documented the important role of nicotine withdrawal syndromes, pharmacologic measures are becoming a more important strategy for cessation. Behavioral, cognitive, psychological, and educational strategies have been used successfully to bring about smoking cessation and may be used alone or in combination with pharmacologic therapy. There is no clearly superior method. Programs that offer combinations of methods have consistently been shown to be superior to single-method strategies for smoking cessation. As mentioned above, there are at present no identifiable ways in which women respond differently to smoking cessation interventions.

Behavioral Strategies

Behavioral approaches, either in groups or with individuals, have remained the core of smoking cessation programs. Programs are available throughout the United States from the American Lung Association (Freedom from Smoking), The American Cancer Society (Fresh Start), and the Seventh-Day Adventist Church (Five-Day Plan). The American Heart Association offers a self-help program, Calling It Quits. Most programs use a combination of methods and offer self-help materials. Commercial programs exist both nationally and locally. These programs are approximately equal in their success rate to noncommercial ventures.

Pharmacologic Interventions

Nicotine Replacement Therapy

The goal of nicotine replacement is to provide smokers with the primary pharmacologic reinforcer of smoking, nicotine, in an effort to diminish serious physical withdrawal symptoms after cessation of smoking. Several studies have shown that nicotine replacement reduces anxiety, irritability, and restlessness, and may partially ameliorate the weight gain associated with cessation (72). Nicotine replacement is available only by physician's prescription in eight packets of twelve 2-mg pieces of gum (96 pieces per box). Replacement systems are designed to minimize reinforcement of the many other features of cigarette smoking and to remove exposure to the other noxious compounds.

Although nicotine Polacrilex gum has been

available for some time, a nicotine transdermal delivery system has recently emerged as a potentially better way to deliver a consistent dose of nicotine. Nasal aerosols and solutions are all under investigation but have not yet been released for general use. The transdermal nicotine delivery system is available in 24-hour patches of progressively decreasing doses, usually starting at 21 mg/day and decreasing over 2 to 3 months to 7 mg/day. Problems associated with gum use include oral ulcers, excess salivation, and jaw ache related to chewing, all of which diminish with time. The risk of oral ulcers can be reduced if individuals are instructed to move the gum around in their mouths when they chew. The major side effect of the nicotine patch is skin irritation, which can be minimized by relocating the patch to a new site every day and returning to the original site only after a minimum of 7 days. Nicotine replacement should be used with caution in persons with severe hypertension, arrhythmias, unstable angina, or recent myocardial infarction because it has been shown to increase both heart rate and blood pressure. When using the gum, weaning should occur gradually over a month or two. This may be done by using a fixed tapering schedule, or the individual may choose to reduce the amount slowly according to symptoms. The transdermal patch has a natural tapering system built into its use. In both instances, addiction to the replacement system has been observed in small numbers of people.

Use of a Psychosocial Model to Guide Clinical Practice

To better understand the overall process of quitting smoking and the probability of success of treatment, it is helpful to have a conceptual view of how people quit smoking. One of the most helpful of the psychosocial models of smoking cessation is the Prochaska Readiness for Change Model. In this model, smoking cessation is viewed as a dynamic process. There are at least four distinct stages of the smoking cessation continuum that are useful for practitioners working with a smoking patient (73, 74). The *precontemplation* stage is one in which the individual is not even thinking about stopping smoking; in fact, she may not view it as a problem at all. It has been suggested that persons in this stage may be defensive, unwilling to discuss cessation, or even to entertain the notion. The *contemplation* stage represents recognition of smoking as a problem but with no commitment to stop smoking. Individuals in this stage appear to talk readily about smoking as a problem but will not commit to a quit date. The *action* stage is the period in which smokers will take action. Action may include quitting as well as attempts to change smoking behavior by brand switching, reducing the number of cigarettes smoked, purchasing cigarettes by the pack instead of carton, or avoiding social situations where smoking is a problem. The *maintenance* phase is the period when people have actually quit and are striving to remain smoke-free. The fear of relapse is strong initially and diminishes with time. *Relapse* is, unfortunately, a very common process for most quitters. Only 4% of smokers maintain cessation without any relapses at all. Relapsers may return to any stage on the continuum, but, if they do, they usually approach action again sometime in the future. It is important to recognize that the probability of being a successful quitter is increased with each quit attempt. Few people quit on the first attempt and most studies suggest that it takes an average of three to four attempts to maintain quit status (71). This model, diagrammed in Figure 11-2, has important therapeutic implications. The stage of readiness may focus the dialogue about smoking that occurs between patients and health care providers. It may be possible in a single clinical encounter only to attempt to move a smoker from the precontemplation to the contemplation stage. The action approach suggested in Figure 11-2 may only be possible if it can be ascertained that a smoker is contemplating quitting. Smokers in the action stage may be particularly amenable to both non-pharmacologic and pharmacologic interventions.

THE SOCIAL CONTEXT OF SMOKING IN WOMEN

The media has played an undeniably powerful role in smoking behavior of both women and men, although it has been difficult to develop an empirical knowledge base that proves this contention. Tobacco advertising and promotion of sales of tobacco to women have escalated in recent years (75). Women's magazines still retain a high proportion of

ALGORITHM FOR PHYSICIAN INTERVENTIONS FOR SMOKING CESSATION

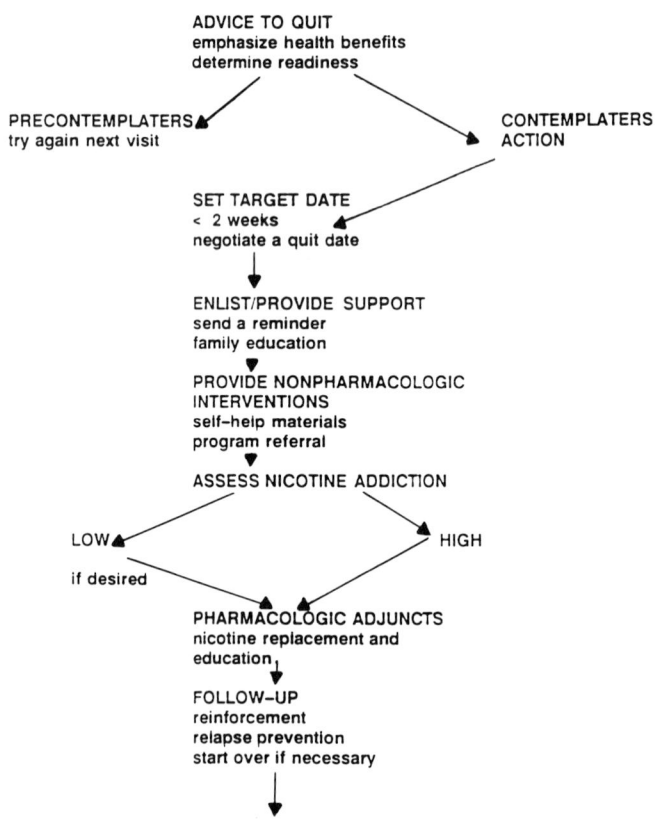

Figure 11-2. Algorithm for clinical intervention to effect smoking cessation.

cigarette advertising, which often project positive images associated with attractiveness and new roles for women in today's society (76). Further, it appears that the media may underreport the health hazards of smoking when a significant portion of the advertising is related to smoking, particularly in media targeted to women (77). Women's national sports events have been frequently sponsored by the tobacco industry, where cigarettes designed specifically for women have been highly visible and associated with images of health and athletic prowess (76). During the twentieth century, cigarette smoking has been viewed as a rite of passage from adolescence to adulthood, and some smoking policy experts have proposed that a similar social-psychological construct may exist as women take on leadership roles in today's workplace. Thus, at least among certain groups of women, the social context of cigarette smoking remains reinforcing, and persuasive marketing techniques continue to exhort women to smoke as a symbol of the rights women have gained in the latter part of this century (77, 78).

In summary, smoking is a strong, independent risk factor for cardiovascular disease in women. Enhanced clinical educational efforts to prevent young women, in particular, from starting to smoke are needed to decrease the risk of cardiovascular disease. In addition, women at high risk as a result of smoking are likely to benefit from clinical assistance in smoking cessation.

References

1. Kannel WB, Castelli WP, McNamara PM. Cigarette smoking and risk of coronary heart disease. Epide-

miologic clues to pathogenesis. The Framingham Study. In Wynder EL, Hoffman D (Eds.), *Toward a Less Harmful Cigarette*. National Cancer Institute Monograph No. 28. Washington, D.C., U.S. Department of Health, Education and Welfare, Public Health Service, National Cancer Institute, 1968, pp. 9–20.
2. Epstein FH. Some uses of prospective observations in the Tecumseh Community Health Study. *Proc R Soc Med* 60 (1):56–60, 1967.
3. U.S. Department of Health and Human Services. *The Health Consequences of Smoking for Women: A Report of the Surgeon General*. Washington D.C., U.S. Government Printing Office, 1980, pp. 133–136.
4. U.S. Department of Health and Human Services. *Reducing the Health Consequences of Smoking: 25 Years of Progress. A Report of the Surgeon General*. DHHS Publication No. (CDC) 89-8411, Washington D.C., U.S. Government Printing Office, 1989.
5. Centers for Disease Control. Cigarette smoking in the United States, 1986. *MMWR* 36:581–585, 1987.
6. Centers for Disease Control. Differences in the age of smoking initiation between blacks and whites. *MMWR* 40:755–756, 1991.
7. Doll R, Gray R, Hafner B, et al.: Mortality in relation to smoking: 22 years' observations on female British doctors. *Br Med J* 280:967–971, 1980.
8. National Center for Health Statistics. *Health, United States, 1990*. Hyattsville, MD, Public Health Service, 1991.
9. Willett WC, Green A, Stampfer MJ, et al. Relative and absolute excess risks of coronary heart disease among women who smoke cigarettes. *N Engl J Med* 317:1303–1309, 1987.
10. LaCroix AZ, Guralnik JM, Curb JD, et al. Chest pain and coronary heart disease mortality among older men and women in three communities. *Circulation* 81:437–446, 1990.
11. LaCroix AZ, Lang J, Scherr P, et al. Smoking and mortality among older men and women in three communities. *N Engl J Med* 324:1619–1625, 1991.
12. Bush TL, Comstock GW. Smoking and cardiovascular mortality in women. *Am J Epidemiol* 118:480–488, 1983.
13. Aronow WS, Herzig AH, Etienne F, et al. 41-month follow-up of risk factors correlated with new coronary events in 708 elderly patients. *J Am Geriatr Soc* 37:501–506, 1989.
14. Slone D, Shapiro S, Rosenberg L, et al. Relation of cigarette smoking to myocardial infarction in young women. *N Engl J Med* 298:1273–1276, 1978.
15. Rosenberg L, Kaufman DW, Helmrich SP, et al. Myocardial infarction and cigarette smoking in women younger than 50 years of age. *JAMA* 253:2965–2969, 1985.
16. Mietinnin OS, Neff RK, Jick H. Cigarette smoking and non-fatal myocardial infarction: Rate ratio in relation to age, sex and predisposing condition. *Am J Epidemiol* 103:30–36, 1976.
17. Doll R, Peto R. Mortality in relation to smoking: 20 years' observations on male British doctors. *Br Med J* 2:1525–1536, 1976.
18. Eaker E, Packard B, Thoma TJ. Epidemiology and risk factors for coronary heart disease in women. In Douglas PS (Ed.), *Heart Disease in Women*. (Cardiovascular Clinics). Philadelphia, F.A. Davis, 1989, pp. 120–145.
19. Harris T, Cook EF, Kannel WB, et al. Proportional hazards analysis of risk factors for coronary heart disease in individuals aged 65 and older. The Framingham Heart Study. *J Am Geriatr Soc* 36:1023–1928, 1988.
20. Pearson TA. Coronary arteriography in the study of the epidemiology of coronary artery disease. *Epidemiol Rev* 6:140–166, 1984.
21. Kuller LH, Meilahn E. Dissent to the negative association in women between cigarette smoking and uncomplicated angina pectoris in the Framingham Heart Study data. *J Clin Epidemiol* 44:877–878, 1991.
22. Mann JI, Doll R, Thorogood M, et al. Risk factors for myocardial infarction in young women. *Br J Prev Soc Med* 30:94–100, 1976.
23. Rosenberg L, Shapiro S, Kaufman DW, et al. Cigarette smoking in relation to the risk of myocardial infarction in young women. Modifying influence of age and predisposing factors. *Int J Epidemiol* 9:57–63, 1980.
24. Croft P. Hannaford PC. Risk factors for myocardial infarction in women: Evidence from the Royal College of General Practitioners' Oral Contraception Study. *Br Med J* 298:165–168, 1989.
25. Wynder EL, Goodman MT, Hoffman D. Demographic aspects of the low-yield cigarette: considerations in the evaluation of health risk. *J Nat Cancer Inst* 72:817–822, 1984.
26. Bonita R, Scragg R, Stewart A, et al. Cigarette smoking and risk of premature stroke in men and women. *Br Med J* 293:6–8, 1986.
27. Colditz GA, Bonita R, Stampfer MJ, et al. Cigarette smoking and risk of stroke in middle-aged women. *N Engl J Med* 318:937–941, 1988.
28. Wolf PA, D'Agostino RB, Kannel WB, et al. Cigarette smoking as a risk factor for stroke. The Framingham Study. *JAMA* 259:1025–1029, 1988.
29. Sacco RL, Wolf PA, Bharucher NE, et al. Subarachnoid and intracerebral hemorrhage: Natural history, progress, and precursive factors in the Framingham Study. *Neurology* 34:847–854, 1984.
30. Kannel WB. Epidemiologic studies on smoking in cerebral and peripheral vascular disease. In Wynder EL, Hoffman D, Gori GB (Eds.), *Proceedings of the Third World Conference on Smoking and Health*, New York, June 2–5, 1975. Vol. I. *Modifying the Risk for the Smoker*. U.S. Department of Health, Education, and Welfare, Public Health Service, National Institutes of Health, National Cancer Institute. DHEW Publication No. (NIH) 76-1221, 1976, pp. 257–274.
31. Criqui MH, Browner D, Fronek A, et al. Peripheral arterial disease in large vessels is epidemiologically distinct from small vessel disease. An analysis of risk factors. *Am J Epidemiol* 129:1110–1119, 1989.
32. Weiss NS. Cigarette smoking and arteriosclerosis obliterans: An epidemiologic approach. *Am J Epidemiol* 95:17–25, 1972.
33. U.S. Department of Health and Human Services. *The Health Consequences of Smoking: Cardiovascular Disease. A Report of the Surgeon General*. U.S. DHHS Publication (PHS) 94-50204. Washington, D.C., U.S. Government Printing Office, 1983.
34. Sackett DK, Gibson RW, Bross IDJ, et al. Relation between aortic atherosclerosis and the use of cigarettes and alcohol. An autopsy study. *N Engl J Med* 279:1413–1420, 1968.
35. Sarma JSM, Tillmanns H, Ikeda S, et al. The effect of carbon monoxide on lipid metabolism of human coronary arteries. *Atherosclerosis* 22:193–198, 1975.
36. Zimmerman M, McGeachie J. The effect of nicotine

on aortic endothelium. A quantitative ultrastructural study. *Atherosclerosis* 63:33–41, 1987.
37. Willett W, Hennekens CH, Castelli W, et al. Effects of cigarette smoking on fasting triglyceride, total cholesterol, and HDL-cholesterol in women. *Am Heart J* 105:417–421, 1983.
38. Fortman SP, Haskell WL, Williams PT. Changes in high density lipoprotein cholesterol after changes in cigarette use. *Am J Epidemiol* 124:706–710, 1986.
39. Klein LW. Cigarette smoking, atherosclerosis, and the hemodynamic coronary response. A unifying hypothesis. *J Am Coll Cardiol* 4:972–974, 1984.
40. Hawkins RI. Smoking, platelets and thrombosis. *Nature* 236:450–452, 1972.
41. Renaud S, Blache D, Dumont E, et al. Platelet function after cigarette smoking in relation to nicotine and carbon monoxide. *Clin Pharmacol Ther* 36:389–395, 1984.
42. Markowe JLJ, Marmot MG, Shipley MJ, et al. Fibrinogen: A possible link between social class and coronary heart disease. *Br Med J* 291:1312–1314, 1985.
43. Rival J, Riddle JM, Stein PD. Effects of chronic smoking on platelet function. *Thromb Res* 45:75–85, 1987.
44. Meade TW, Imeson J, Stirling Y. Effects of changes in smoking and other characteristics on clotting factors and the risk of ischemic heart disease. *Lancet* 2:986–988, 1987.
45. Dotevall A, Khutti J, Teger-Nilsson A, et al. Platelet reactivity, fibrinogen and smoking. *Eur J Haematol* 38:55–59, 1987.
46. Ernst E, Matrai A. Abstention from chronic cigarette smoking normalizes blood rheology. *Atherosclerosis* 64:75–77, 1987.
47. Khaw K-T, Chir MBB, Tazuke S, et al. Cigarette smoking and levels of adrenal androgens in postmenopausal women. *N Engl J Med* 318:1705–1709, 1988.
48. McKinlay SM, Bifano NL, McKinlay JB. Smoking and age at menopause in women. *Ann Intern Med* 103:350–356, 1985.
49. Barrett-Connor E, Bush TL. Estrogen and coronary heart disease in women. *JAMA* 265:1861–1867, 1991.
50. Hermanson B, Omenn GS, Kronmal RA, et al. Beneficial six-year outcome of smoking cessation in older men and women with coronary artery disease. Results from the CASS Registry. *N Engl J Med* 319:1365–1369, 1988.
51. Stampfer MJ, Willett WC, Colditz GA, et al. Past use of oral contraceptives and cardiovascular disease: a meta-analysis in the context of the Nurses' Health Study. *Am J Obstet Gynecol* 163:285–291, 1990.
52. Stadel BV. Oral contraceptives and cardiovascular disease. *N Engl J Med* 305:672–677, 1981.
53. Mileikowsky GN, Nadler JL, Huey F, et al. Evidence that smoking alters protacyclin formation and platelet aggregation in women who use oral contraceptives. *Am J Obstet Gynecol* 1598:1547–1552, 1988.
54. Massey JT, Moore TF, Parsons VL, et al. *Design and Estimation for the National Health Interview Survey, 1985–1994.* Series II, No. 110, Hyattsville, MD, August, 1989.
55. Schoenborn CA, Boyd GM. Smoking and other tobacco use: United States 1987. *Vital and Health Statistics, National Center for Health Statistics,* Hyattsville, MD, Series 10, No. 169, September 1989.
56. Fiore MC, Novotney TE, Pierce JP, et al. Trends in cigarette smoking in the United States: The changing influence of gender and race. *JAMA* 261:49–55, 1989.
57. Gritz ER. The female smoker: Research and intervention targets. In Cohen J, et al. (Eds.), *Psychosocial Aspects of Cancer.* New York, Raven Press, 1982.
58. Fisher EB, Bishop DB. Sex-roles, social support, and smoking cessation. Presented at the Society of Behavioral Medicine, San Francisco, March, 1989.
59. Schwartz JL. *Review and Evaluation of Smoking Cessation Methods: The United States and Canada 1978–1985.* NIH Publication No. 87-2940. Bethesda, MD, U.S. Department of Health and Human Services, 1987.
60. Klesges RC, Eck LH, Clark E. The effects of smoking cessation and gender on dietary intake, physical activity, and weight gain. *Int J Eat Dis* 435–446, 1990.
61. U.S. Department of Health and Human Services. *The Health Consequences of Smoking: Nicotine Addiction.* A Report of the Surgeon General. 1988, U.S. DHHS Publication (CDC) 88-8406. Washington, D.C., 1988.
62. Hall SM, McGee R, Tunstall C, et al. Changes in food intake and activity after quitting smoking. *J Consult Clin Psychol* 57:81–86, 1989.
63. Tuomilheto J, Nissinen A, Pusks P, et al. Long-term effects of cessation of smoking on body weight, blood pressure, and serum cholesterol in the middle-aged population with high blood pressure. *Addictive Behaviors* 11:1–9, 1986.
64. Stamford BA, Matter S, Fell RD, et al. Effects of smoking cessation. *Am J Clin Nut* 43:486–494, 1986.
65. Shimokata H, Muller DC, Andres R. Studies in the distribution of body fat. III. Effects of cigarette smoking. *JAMA* 261:1169–1173, 1989.
66. Klesges RC, Klesges LM. Cigarette smoking as a dieting strategy in a university population. *Intl J Eat Dis* 7:413–419, 1988.
67. Mermelstein R. Preventing weight gain following smoking cessation. Presented at the Society of Behavioral Medicine, Washington, D.C., 1987.
68. Gross J, Stitzer ML, Maldonado J. Nicotine replacement: Effects of postcessation weigh gain. *J Consult Clin Psychol* 57:87–92, 1989.
69. Emont SL, Cummings KM. Weight gain following smoking cessation. A possible role for nicotine replacement in weight management. *Addictive Behaviors* 12:151–155, 1987.
70. Klesges RC, DePue K, Andrain J, et al. Metabolic effects of nicotine gum and cigarette smoking: Potential implication for postcessation weight gain? *J Consult Clin Psychol* 59:749–752, 1991.
71. U.S Department of Health and Human Services. *The Health Benefits of Smoking Cessation. A Report of the Surgeon General.* Centers for Disease Control, Atlanta, GA, US DHHS Publication (CDC), 90-8416, 1990.
72. Hughes JR, Miller SA. Nicotine gum to help stop smoking. *JAMA* 252:2855–2858, 1984.
73. Prochaska JO, DiClemente CC. Stages and processes of self-change of smoking: Toward an integrative model of change. *J Consult Clin Psychol* 51:390–395, 1983.
74. Prochaska JO, Velicer WF, DiClemente CC, et al. Measuring processes of change: Applications to the cessation of smoking. *J Consult Clin Psychol* 56:520–528, 1988.
75. Albright CL, Altman DG, Slater MD, et al. Cigarette advertisements in magazines: Evidence for a differ-

ential focus on women's and youth magazines. *Health Ed Q* 15:225–233, 1988.
76. Cotton P. Tobacco foes attack ads that target women, minorities, teens and the poor. *JAMA* 264:1505–1506, 1990.
77. Warner KE, Goldenhar LM, McLaughlin CG. Cigarette advertising and magazine coverage of the hazards of smoking: A statistical analysis. *N Engl J Med* 326:305–309, 1992.
78. Amos A, Bostock Y. Policy on cigarette advertising and coverage of smoking and health in European women's magazines. *Br Med J* 304:99–100, 1992.

CHAPTER 12

Hemostasis and Thrombosis

BABETTE B. WEKSLER, M.D.

Gender-related differences in hemostasis may contribute to the differences in incidence of cardiovascular disease that have been observed in men and women. Objective studies that compare platelet function and blood coagulation in the two sexes have been few. Both platelet hyperactivity and hypercoagulability contribute to the manifestations of atherosclerosis, whereas the protection of premenopausal women from arteriosclerosis has been appreciated for many years, suggesting that hormonal factors play a role. In contrast, women may experience gender-related venous and arterial occlusive disease as a result of certain hormonal exposures. The major source of information on both the decreased risk of arteriosclerosis and the increased risks of venous thromboembolism comes from evaluation of the hemostatic effects of pregnancy and of hormonal replacement, in terms of both oral contraceptives and postmenopausal estrogen administration.

Women are more likely than men to develop autoimmune phenomena, which may be associated with cytopenias, vasculitis, or circulating anticoagulants. Clinically, these phenomena may be associated with hemorrhage, but they are more likely to predispose the patient to thrombosis, both arterial and venous.

REVIEW OF NORMAL HEMOSTASIS

The hemostatic mechanisms that protect the vascular system after injury are closely linked to the processes of inflammation and wound healing. These mechanisms have evolved from a primitive all-purpose system of repair after injury that is already present in simple multicellular animals. Thus, the activation of hemostasis is enhanced during inflammatory processes and after tissue injury of many types. Normally, there is a balance between prothrombotic and antithrombotic activities that tightly regulates hemostasis. Inappropriate activation of hemostasis, for example, in a situation of altered vascular endothelial function, may produce thrombosis, i.e., pathologic clotting. In many disease states and under special physiologic conditions—for women, specifically, pregnancy—this hemostatic balance may be altered either toward hemorrhage or toward thrombosis.

Hemostasis includes three major phases: *primary hemostasis*, the initial response to vascular injury, which involves platelet activation, platelet plug formation, and initiation of the coagulation cascade; *secondary hemostasis*, in which the fibrin clot is formed and stabilized; and *fibrinolysis*, in which the clot is resolved and tissue repair promoted.

Primary Hemostasis. Platelets, circulating as nonadhesive discs filled with potentially vasoactive materials, do not interact with the normal blood vessel wall but, following vascular injury, rapidly adhere to the exposed vascular subendothelium, aggregate into a primary "hemostatic plug," and release their vasoactive contents locally in the area of damage. Simultaneously, the activated platelet membrane provides a specialized surface on which enzymatically active thrombin is rapidly and efficiently generated, leading to cleavage of fibrinogen. Fibrin is then quickly formed on the platelet plug, which initiates the process of secondary hemostasis, or production of a permanent clot. In a small vessel the process of primary hemostasis takes 3 to 5 minutes and is measured by the bleeding time.

Platelet counts are similar for the two sexes, as are platelet responses to aggregating agents, once the hematocrit has been taken into consideration (see later discussion). During the reproductive years, the platelet count in women may vary during the menstrual cycle within the normal range of 150,000 to 400,000/ μL. Platelet function, however, does not change significantly during the menstrual cycle nor during pregnancy (1, 2) unless the pregnancy is complicated by hypertension (2). The normal bleeding time also varies little with gender; it may be slightly longer in women than in men (3). Specific effects of sex steroids at pharmacologic doses on platelet function will be discussed later.

Secondary Hemostasis. Blood coagulation, involving the production of a stable fibrin clot from soluble plasma fibrinogen, represents the second phase of hemostasis and involves a complex activation cascade of enzymes and cofactors that originate from the blood plasma, from platelets, and from the vessel wall or injured tissues. This process is summarized in Figure 12–1. Activation of either the extrinsic or intrinsic coagulation pathway, which interact, produces a prothrombinase complex that cleaves prothrombin to the active enzyme thrombin. Thrombin then acts on soluble fibrinogen to release small peptides, permitting formation of fibrin monomers that polymerize end-to-end to form fibrin I. The fibrin polymer is further stabilized by side-to side cross-linking of fibrin strands by the transglutaminase, factor XIII. The conversion of coagulation factors from their circulating precursor forms to active enzymes generally takes place on specialized surfaces that accelerate and regulate this process. In addition to providing a catalytic surface for the formation of the prothrombinase complex and contributing factor V, platelets also release factor XIII and induce clot retraction by contraction of platelet actomyosin proteins. Thrombin generation on the platelet surface is

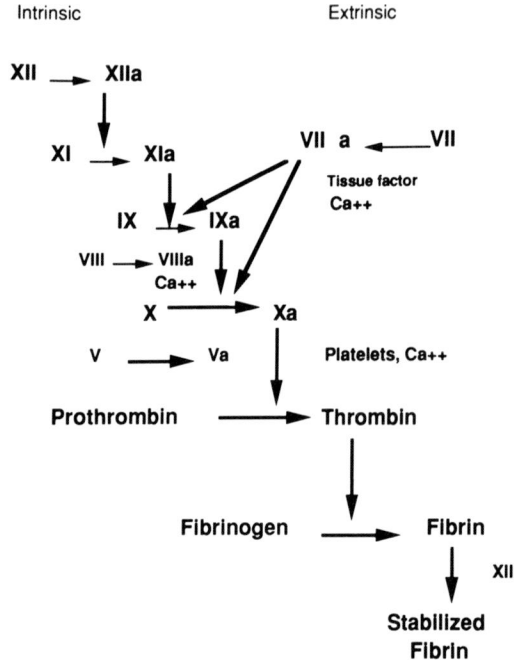

Figure 12–1. Blood coagulation schema. Two pathways, intrinsic and extrinsic (requiring tissue injury), interact and form a final common pathway to produce a prothrombinase complex that cleaves prothrombin to thrombin. Active thrombin then activates soluble fibrinogen to form fibrin monomer, which then polymerizes to form stable fibrin, cross-linked by factor XIII. There is major amplification of the later steps in the pathways, so that the generation of a few molecules of factor Xa, for example, leads to the generation of thousands of molecules of thrombin.

accelerated more than 100,000-fold. In recent years it has been realized that the activated platelet membrane is only one of several possible types of catalytic cell surfaces that promote coagulation. Inflammatory cytokines or microbial products may alter the normally antithrombotic surface of the vascular endothelium, changing it to a prothrombotic surface that binds and activates multiple factors of the coagulation cascade and providing tissue factor, an important cofactor for the activation of the extrinsic coagulation system (4, 5). Activated monocytes also provide a procoagulant surface. Thus, mechanical injury to vessels is not necessary to initiate coagulation, and changes in vascular properties related to inflammatory disease or altered physiology are also important factors in determining the hemostatic balance.

Levels of plasma coagulation factors are similar for the two sexes and are normally present, in proenzyme or procoagulant form, far in excess of the concentrations required for normal hemostasis. Levels of fibrinogen and of factor VII are slightly but significantly higher in women; the fibrinogen level in women increases with age (6). The levels of several plasma coagulation factors increase during pregnancy and during certain types of hormonal therapy as detailed below. Similarly, levels of the major protease inhibitors that serve as regulators of activated coagulation factors do not generally differ between the sexes but may be affected by sex hormones in some instances. Whereas only 10% of the normal level of a coagulation factor protects against severe bleeding (except during surgery or trauma, in which higher levels are required), about 50% of the normal level of a coagulation inhibitor is required to prevent increased risk of thrombosis.

Fibrinolysis. Fibrinolysis, or clot dissolution, displays many parallels to the process of coagulation in terms of circulating proenzymes, activators released by specific stimuli, and regulators (Fig. 12–2). A low level of fibrinolysis probably operates continually at the luminal surface of blood vessels as an important means of maintaining vascular patency. The main fibrinolytic proenzyme of the blood plasma, plasminogen, is most efficiently activated to plasmin, the fibrin-cleaving enzyme, when bound to a surface: The vascular endothelial surface or fibrin itself and regulators of this process are contributed both by platelets and by the vascular endothelium. In particular, endothelium releases not only potent plasminogen activators but also plasminogen activator inhibitor-1 (PAI-1). Men have lower plasma tissue plasminogen activator (tPA) activity and higher PAI-1 levels than women (7). With increasing age, both tPA and PAI-1 levels rise in women, so that by their sixties women have higher levels of PAI-1 than do men (8). The placenta releases a different plasminogen activator inhibitor-2 (PAI-2) (9). Moreover, when thrombin becomes bound to the protein thrombomodulin on the vascular endothelium, it loses its ability to cleave fibrinogen and instead activates the natural anticoagulant protein C (Fig. 12–3). Activated protein C inactivates factors Va and VIIIa and can enhance fibrinolysis. Thus, thrombin itself contributes not only to the limitation of coagulation but also to the stimulation of fibrinolysis. Besides being a potent activator of platelets, thrombin is a comitogen for mesenchymal

Figure 12–2. Fibrinolysis is initiated by the cleavage of plasminogen to plasmin in the presence of a plasminogen activator; plasmin cleaves fibrin with increased efficiency when the process takes place on a surface: the fibrin clot or the vascular wall.

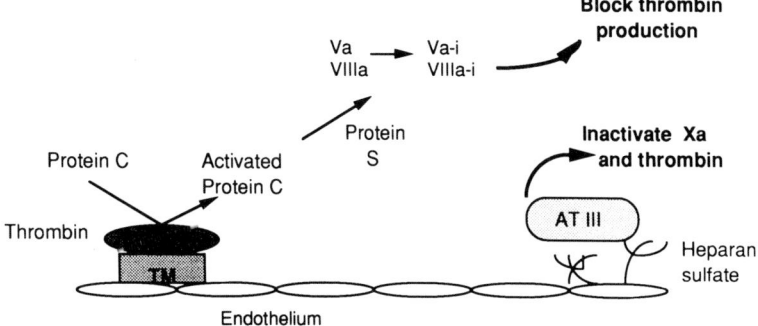

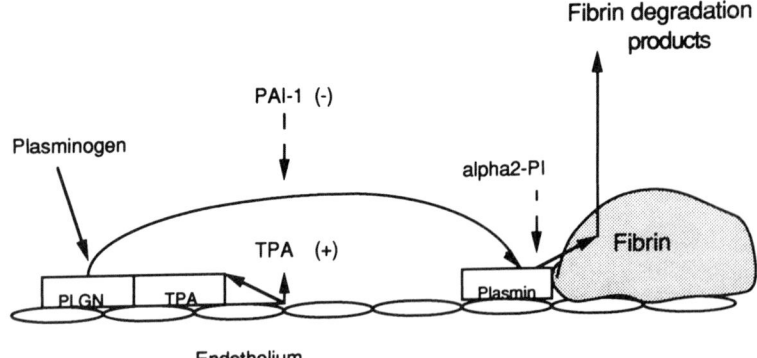

Figure 12–3. The natural anticoagulant systems. Thrombomodulin (TM) on the endothelial surface binds thrombin, inhibiting its coagulant activity and altering its protease specificity so that it activates protein C. Activated protein C, in the presence of its cofactor protein S, inactivates factors Va and VIIIa, downregulating the coagulation process by decreasing the rate of thrombin formation. Antithrombin III (AT III), in a reaction manyfold accelerated by heparan sulfate proteoglycan on the luminal surface of the endothelium, binds to and inhibits activity of all serine protease coagulation factors.

cells involved in wound healing, such as fibroblasts and vascular smooth muscle cells. Surface-bound fibrin is thought to act as a reservoir for active thrombin incorporated into a thrombus; this thrombin may be slowly released to produce delayed effects promoting wound healing or atherogenesis (10).

Vascular Surface and Coagulation. Since both coagulation and fibrinolysis preferentially take place on surfaces, it is crucial to consider the role of the vascular wall in the regulation of these two vital processes (Table 12–1). Normal vascular endothelium is nonthrombogenic and has been termed the ideal blood-compatible container. Numerous properties of endothelial cells contribute actively to its nonthrombogenicity, including the secretion of prostaglandins (PGI_2 and PGE_2) and nitric oxide (the endothelium-derived relaxing factor), which inhibit platelet activation; the presence of heparan sulfate, a heparinlike proteoglycan bound to the endothelial surface; and the action of ecto-ADPases, which break down platelet-activating ADP to platelet-inhibitory adenosine. Specific inhibitors of coagulation factors such as antithrombin III, thrombomodulin, and protein C are also available at the endothelial surface, and tissue plasminogen activator is released from, binds to, and is protected by the endothelium, promoting fibrinolysis at the interface between endothelium and blood.

Activated Endothelium. In marked contrast, endothelium disturbed by interaction with endotoxin, microorganisms (both bacteria and viruses), or inflammatory cytokines presents a prothrombotic surface that promotes blood coagulation (4, 5). Endothelial cells so activated may remain morphologically intact yet support the initiation of coagulation by releasing tissue factor and by presenting binding sites for factors IX and X so that thrombin can be locally generated. Activated endothelium itself produces cytokines and displays surface receptors for leukocytes that activate the latter. Under the same conditions, thrombomodulin expression is down-regulated and PAI-1 release is enhanced, so that thrombin inactivation, protein C activation, and fibrinolysis are all diminished. Moreover, platelets that contact an abnormal vessel wall tend to become activated, in part in response to turbulent blood flow or to minute amounts of locally formed thrombin; therefore, platelets in this

Table 12–1. HEMOSTATIC PROPERTIES OF VASCULAR ENDOTHELIUM

Antithrombotic	Prothrombotic
Prostacyclin	von Willebrand factor
Nitric oxide	Binding or activation of factor
Heparan sulfate	IX or factor X
Antithrombin III	Tissue factor
ADPase	Cytokines (IL-1)
Thrombomodulin	Cell adhesion receptors
Plasminogen activator	Platelet-activating factor
Fibrinolytic assembly	PDGF
Lipoprotein-associated coagulation inhibitor	Plasminogen activator inhibitor-1

setting also tend to favor hemostasis and to promote microvascular clotting.

EFFECTS OF SEX STEROIDS ON HEMOSTASIS

The protection of premenopausal women from the atherosclerosis observed in epidemiologic studies has been interpreted as a suggestion that estrogen and progesterone may be important factors in preventing atherogenesis and its thrombotic complications. The relative contribution to this protection of hormone-induced changes in hemostasis versus changes in lipoprotein profiles or vascular physiology and rheology has not been entirely clarified, but epidemiologic studies of the vascular complications of oral contraception and of the prevention of occlusive vascular disease in postmenopausal women receiving replacement hormonal therapy have led to considerable information about the effects of these hormones on hemostasis.

HEMOSTASIS IN PREGNANCY

It has long been known that during pregnancy marked changes take place in the hemostatic system in terms of both coagulation and fibrinolysis (1, 9, 11, 12). Platelet turnover is faster in pregnancy, plasma β-thromboglobulin levels increase, and platelet life span is slightly reduced in late pregnancy (13). The platelet count normally falls from prepregnancy levels, reaching a nadir by about 30 weeks, although for most women the count remains within the normal range, and counts above 100,000/μL are not associated with complications. Plasma levels of fibrinogen, factor VII, factor VIII, and von Willebrand's factor all increase. Fibrinogen normally rises to a level of 400 to 600 mg/dL by the third trimester and may increase plasma viscosity (11). These changes are believed to protect against hemorrhage during gestation. The fibrinolytic activity of plasma, measured in the euglobulin fraction, has been observed to decrease, but the fibrinolytic activity of whole blood appears to increase, and a higher level of fibrin degradation products is detected during pregnancy, suggesting that fibrin turnover normally increases during pregnancy (14). This suggests that euglobulin lysis times, the major fibrinolytic measurement used in older studies, may not reflect the overall physiologic status of blood fibrinolysis during pregnancy (12, 15). The placenta produces a specific inhibitor of plasminogen activation, PAI-2, that is considered protective against local hemorrhage.

Newer evidence has better established the status of fibrinolysis during pregnancy. Direct measurement of PAI-1, the endothelial-derived inactivator of plasminogen, shows a marked increase in both antigen and activity levels after the twentieth week of pregnancy, reaching three times nonpregnant levels by term (9). In addition, the plasma level of PAI-2 rises from undetectable levels (<10 ng/mL in the nonpregnant state) to 260 ng/mL at term (9). Concomitantly, there is a steady increase in urokinase-type plasminogen activator to more than double baseline values, with a 50% increase in the levels of tissue plasminogen activator. The net effect is a balance between changes in activators and inhibitors, as measured by radioactive fibrin-plate assay of unfractionated pregnancy plasma, so that fibrinolysis remains essentially unchanged during pregnancy and then decreases shortly after delivery (16). In the presence of the marked increases in plasma coagulation factors during pregnancy plus the venous stasis that results from the enlarging uterus, the lack of a concomitant rise in net fibrinolytic activity may contribute to the increased incidence of venous thrombosis observed during pregnancy and the puerperium.

Additional hemostatic changes are seen with complications of pregnancy such as preeclampsia and will be discussed later.

EFFECTS OF ORAL CONTRACEPTIVES ON HEMOSTASIS

Clinical Correlations

Oral contraceptives (OCs) have been widely used for about 30 years. During this time it has become clear, from studies in the United States and Europe of women taking the earlier developed, higher-estrogen OCs, that usage of these OC preparations has untoward vascular effects that include venous thromboembolic disease, myocardial infarction, and stroke, particularly in older patients and those who smoke

(17–22). Data from three major studies involving over 80,000 women suggested a fourfold increase in morbidity from vascular complications, with an increase in deaths from myocardial infarction or stroke concentrated in those who were over 35 years old and in those who were smokers (23). The death rate from vascular complications attributed to oral contraceptives has been estimated as 22 to 24 deaths/100,000 women/year. These studies also revealed a fourfold increase in relative risk of deep vein thrombosis and pulmonary embolism, and a twofold increase in postoperative venous thromboembolism, resulting in an estimated 19 cases of venous thromboembolic disease per 10,000 current users per year (23). It should be emphasized that these data represent studies in women who were using relatively high-estrogen forms of OCs, whereas current users mainly take low-estrogen preparations that have a lesser thrombogenic potential. Data from a long-term study of the vascular complication rate associated with the mini-estrogen pill offering similar contraceptive potency are not yet available.

The risk of overt venous thromboembolism in these studies appears to be related mainly to the estrogen component of the oral contraceptive and is confined to current usage (23–25). In contrast, the pathogenesis of arterial vascular disease associated with oral contraceptives is more complex, probably relates to both the estrogen and progesterone components of the OC, involves not only current users, and seems to involve both increased platelet activity and enhanced fibrin deposition (24). Additional risk factors for atherogenesis such as hypertension, glucose intolerance, and hyperlipidemia also are involved in the increased risk of development of occlusive arterial disease in OC users. The combination of longtime OC use, age over 35 years, and smoking produces the greatest risk; smoking appears to promote pathologic platelet–vessel wall interactions (26).

Hemostatic Effects

Estrogens in OCs are known to increase plasma levels of prothrombin, factors VII, VIII, IX, and X, and fibrinogen in a manner similar to that occurring in pregnancy (6) (Table 12–2). Estrogen administered as OCs also decreases antithrombin III (AT III) levels and, at higher dosages, vascular release of tissue plasminogen activator (23). The advent of low-estrogen (<50 µg mestranol) OC preparations has reduced the excess risk of venous thromboembolism. Low-dose estrogen use has been associated with enhanced fibrinolytic activity involving increased tissue plasminogen activator release after venous occlusion and decreased PAI-1 levels (23, 27, 28). Further studies with low-estrogen preparations have shown that increases in tPA and plasminogen levels occur with a fall in PAI-1 that in sum favor enhanced fibrinolysis (28). The authors of this latter study caution that although low-estrogen OCs produce both procoagulant and profibrinolytic changes in hemostasis that may be mutually compensatory when groups of subjects are investigated, this compensation may not occur in individual subjects.

Another coagulation-related plasma factor that is gender dependent, is altered by OCs, and may affect the incidence of thromboembolic disease is protein S (29). Protein S is a cofactor for the anticoagulant effects of activated protein C. Congenital protein S deficiency, an autosomal trait, is associated with thromboembolic disease. About 40% of protein S circulates free in plasma and is functionally active, whereas 60% is bound to C4b-binding protein, an inhibitor of the complement system, and is not biologically active. During pregnancy there is a decrease in both functional and antigenic protein S (30), and in women taking OCs there is a significantly decreased functional protein S level that reflects lower free protein S antigen (29). Inflammation, which raises C4b-binding protein levels and therefore increases formation of nonfunctional protein S–C4b-binding protein complexes, may further decrease functional

Table 12–2. EFFECT OF FEMALE SEX HORMONES ON COAGULATION

Increased Levels
 Fibrinogen
 Factor XII
 Factor VIII
 von Willebrand factor
 Vitamin K–dependent factors
 Fibrinogen-fibrin degradation products
 Plasminogen activator inhibitor-1 (endothelial)
 Plasminogen activator inhibitor-2 (placental)
 Plasminogen activator

Decreased Levels
 Antithrombin III
 Proteins S

protein S levels independent of hormonal status and may further predispose a woman toward a prothrombotic state.

POSTMENOPAUSAL ESTROGEN REPLACEMENT THERAPY AND HEMOSTASIS

Clinical Correlations

Decreased morbidity and mortality from cardiovascular disease has been reported in several large studies of postmenopausal women taking estrogen replacement therapy. Whether changes in the hemostatic system, in lipid metabolism, or in the arterial wall are more prominently involved in the decreased risk of cardiovascular disease has not been established (31). Reduction of coronary artery disease and peripheral vascular disease has been reported in several prospective studies, but no change in stroke incidence in relation to estrogen replacement has been found in two large studies involving thousands of women (32, 33). Detailed discussion of clinical studies examining the effects of hormone replacement therapy are included in Chapter 8.

Hemostatic Effects

Does hormonal replacement therapy after menopause adversely affect the coagulation system? Estrogen administered by the oral route undergoes a "first pass" clearance in the liver that has numerous effects on hepatic metabolism. Postmenopausal women who receive conjugated estrogens or other oral estrogen formulations or estrogen-progesterone have been shown to have increases in vitamin K-dependent coagulation factors VII, IX, and X for the first few months of treatment with return to baseline values by 4 to 6 months (34). Several other plasma proteins synthesized in the liver, such as fibrinogen and α_2-macroglobulin, do not change or are decreased by replacement estrogens (6); fibrinopeptide A is not increased by estrogen administration, although there is a small rise in plasminogen and α_1-antiprotease at higher doses of conjugated estrogens, and ceruloplasmin, a marker of hepatic estrogen metabolism, is also elevated (35). Stimulation of hepatic lipases leads to a decrease in low-density lipoprotein (LDL) cholesterol levels and a rise in high-density lipoproteins $(HDL)_2$ cholesterol (36).

A decrease in plasma antithrombin III related to oral estrogen treatment has been observed only with mestranol administration and could persist (34). However, administration of conjugated estrogens has been shown to be associated with a significant decrease in factor Xa inhibitory activity of plasma despite stable antithrombin III levels (37). The reduction of factor Xa inhibitory activity was dose-related. Thus, replacement oral estrogen therapy contributes to increases in liver-related procoagulant proteins and plasminogen, the central proenzyme in fibrinolysis. The net clinical effect of these hemostatic changes has been evaluated in epidemiologic studies, which indicate that there is no increase in intravascular clotting episodes, including venous thromboembolism, in postmenopausal women receiving estrogen replacement therapy (38).

Transdermal Estrogen

In contrast to the changes in hemostatic function that are observed with oral replacement estrogen, neither coagulation factors nor fibrinolytic parameters appear to be affected by transdermally administered estrogen, an alternative form of therapy that has been increasing in popularity during the past few years for postmenopausal estrogen replacement. Protracted absorption of slowly released estrogen through the skin avoids much of the hepatic first-pass effects of oral estrogen therapy, as evidenced by the lack of changes in plasma ceruloplasmin or plasma lipoproteins observed with such administration (35, 39). It should be pointed out that transdermal estrogen use does not produce an increase in plasma HDL cholesterol levels (a well-known effect of oral estrogen), a possible factor in the antiatherosclerotic action of estrogen replacement therapy.

HEMOSTATIC CHANGES IN VASCULAR COMPLICATIONS OF PREGNANCY

Preeclampsia and Pregnancy-Associated Hypertension

Coagulation abnormalities have been associated with preeclampsia since the first pathologic description in 1893, which documented small-vessel thrombosis in this condition (13). Whether these vascular changes and thrombi are primary or secondary to the pregnancy-associated hypertension characteristic of preeclampsia has been a matter of controversy (40). Increased consumption of coagulation factors has been observed in preeclampsia, including a marked increase in factor VIII clotting activity, a higher ratio of factor VIII antigen to factor VIII clotting activity than in normal pregnancy (41), an increased fibrinopeptide A level, elevated fibrin split products, and increased circulating thrombin-antithrombin complexes (14, 16). These signs of intravascular thrombin activation and consumption coagulopathy may precede the onset of clinical preeclampsia (11, 16). At the same time, a decrease in antithrombin III levels in women with preeclampsia has been observed (13, 42). This decline may also precede clinical manifestations (13).

In normal pregnancy the plasma fibrinogen concentration increases progressively with time, and fibrin turnover as measured by fibrinopeptide A or fibrin split products is enhanced (12, 14, 16). Normally an increase in fibrinolytic activity appears to balance the enhanced fibrin generation. This can be measured by plasma levels of plasminogen activators or D-dimers (16). D-dimers are fragments of cross-linked fibrin that are specifically liberated during fibrinolysis. In preeclampsia the release of plasminogen activator from the vascular endothelium is impaired and there is a net reduction in fibrinolytic activity. In severe preeclampsia, plasminogen activator inhibitor levels are increased, particularly PAI-1, which may derive in part from platelet activation (43). PAI-2, the placental plasminogen activator, may decrease in preeclamptic pregnancy due to placental damage (9).

Another coagulation-related vascular abnormality associated with pregnancy-induced hypertension is decreased prostacyclin biosynthesis, accompanied by increased thromboxane production (44). Prostacyclin (PGI_2), produced by blood vessels, is a natural antagonist to platelet-derived thromboxane A_2, a potent platelet activator and vasoconstrictor. During normal pregnancy, prostacylin production rises progressively, and this rise is thought to contribute to the regulation of blood pressure in the presence of an expanded plasma volume (45). Prostacyclin synthesis, measured as urinary excretion of the PGI_2 metabolite 2,3-dinor-6-keto-$PGF_{1\alpha}$, increases in hypertensive pregnancies as well as in normotensive pregnancies. However, prospective evaluation of women at risk for development of preeclampsia has shown that their increase in PGI_2 metabolite excretion was significantly less than that seen in normotensive women who did not develop preeclampsia, and that the difference was observable by the twentieth week of gestation, prior to the rise in blood pressure (46). Following delivery, both women who developed preeclampsia and those who had normal pregnancies excreted similar amounts of 2,3-dinor-6-keto $PGF_{1\alpha}$, an indication that the abnormality in prostacyclin metabolism was restricted to pregnancy and was not a chronic underlying vascular difference (46).

Other studies have shown that umbilical blood vessels and placental tissue from patients with preeclampsia have a lower capacity to produce PGI_2 than comparable tissues obtained after normal pregnancy (44, 45). Plasma from preeclamptic women may contain factors that are toxic to endothelium (in vitro) (47), or it may have enhanced mitogenic activity that may derive from damaged endothelial cells or from platelets activated within the circulation (48).

Platelet reactivity may be enhanced in pregnancy-induced hypertension and in pregnancies in diabetics (2). Thrombocytopenia occurs in severe preeclampsia, with about 15% of women experiencing platelet counts of $< 100 \times 10^9$/L (49). A syndrome comprising hemolysis, elevated liver enzymes, and thrombocytopenia (HELLP syndrome) has been described in association with pregnancy-induced hypertension as a variant of preeclampsia (50, 51).

Many attempts to design a laboratory index of hemostatic parameters that could predict the subsequent development of preeclampsia have been unsuccessful. Although tPA antigen, the factor VIII antigen/factor VIII clotting activity ratio, ATIII activity, PAI-1 activity, and platelet count during the last 2 weeks of gestation in women who develop preeclampsia are significantly different from normal (40), each of these tests shows a wide range of values that makes predictive sensitivity inadequate.

Venous Thromboembolism in Pregnancy

Deep venous thrombosis, especially in the lower limbs, is not uncommon in pregnancy (incidence approximately 0.1%), and pulmonary embolism, although rare, continues to be a major cause of maternal mortality (52, 53). The combination of increased levels of coagulation factors and stasis produced by the enlarging uterus, which mechanically obstructs pelvic and leg venous return, provides the clinical setting for an increased risk of thrombosis (11). Women with documented prior venous thrombosis during pregnancy continue to exhibit enhanced values of coagulant activation and should probably receive prophylactic anticoagulation during subsequent pregnancies (54). Diagnosis of thromboembolism in pregnancy is not easily documented because tests with radioactive iodine labeling are strongly contraindicated owing to the concentration of isotope in the fetal thyroid. However, venography can be performed with pelvic shielding, and lung scan with short half-life isotopes should be performed if pulmonary embolism is strongly suspected (11, 52, 55). Patients with life-threatening changes in cardiac output should be treated with embolectomy (52). Thrombolytic treatment is contraindicated. Treatment of patients with documented pulmonary emboli by full-dose heparin is preferred to oral anticoagulation because heparin does not cross the placenta, and its effects can be rapidly reversed (55, 56). Warfarin should be avoided during early pregnancy because of its teratogenic effects, and heparin is now recommended instead of warfarin during the middle trimester as well, in part because of the continuing risk of fetal neuropathy and in part because of the difficulty of reversing the effect of oral anticoagulants should an obstetric emergency arise (55). Prolonged use of heparin may induce osteoporosis in some women, and this possibility must be weighed in an individual case. Heparin-induced thrombocytopenia must also be kept in mind. In women who have deep venous thrombosis, it must be remembered that anticoagulant treatment should be continued for about 6 weeks postpartum until the coagulation mechanism fully returns to the prepregnant state. Warfarin can be used after about the tenth postpartum day if an oral drug is desired because it is not excreted in an active form in breast milk.

Women with known cardiac valvular lesions or prosthetic heart valves may require warfarin use during pregnancy as prophylaxis against arterial thromboembolism, with substitution of heparin after the thirty-sixth week (55, 57).

Thrombotic Microangiopathy in Pregnancy and the Postpartum Period

In addition to preeclampsia, microvascular thrombosis may occur in pregnant women in the form of thrombotic thrombocytopenic purpura (TTP) or the hemolytic uremic syndrome (HUS) (58). The differential diagnosis between TTP and preeclampsia is a difficult one, but it should be remembered that disseminated intravascular coagulation is not a feature of TTP. Management of TTP in late pregnancy is delivery of the infant. Management of TTP in early pregnancy has not been systematically studied, but successful treatment with plasmapheresis and plasma exchange has been reported in a small number of cases (58). Disseminated intravascular coagulation (DIC) occurs in those complications of pregnancy in which products of conception enter the circulation: amniotic fluid embolism, abruptio placentae, fetal death in utero, or clostridial sepsis. Mild, transient DIC has been documented in association with hypertonic saline induction of abortion.

Paroxysmal Nocturnal Hemoglobinuria

This rare acquired disorder is characterized by increased complement-mediated lysis of blood cells, intravascular hemolysis, bone marrow hypoplasia, and thrombotic episodes. Pregnancy is of very high risk in paroxysmal nocturnal hemoglobinuria (PNH), with thrombosis being among the most serious complications, including Budd-Chiari syndrome and cerebral vein thrombosis. Small series of cases have been reported in which patients were successfully managed with transfusion and anticoagulation (59).

HEMOSTATIC ALTERATIONS ASSOCIATED WITH THROMBOEMBOLIC DISEASE

Factor Deficiencies

Thromboembolic phenomena are associated with defects in the fibrinolytic and natural anticoagulant system, such as congenital partial (heterozygous) deficiencies of antithrombin III, protein C, or protein S (Table 12–3). These are usually autosomal recessive conditions exhibiting variable penetrance in heterozygotes, who usually have levels of the specific deficient factor approaching 50% of normal. Affected individuals have an increased risk of venous thromboembolism (rarely, arterial thrombosis) before the age of 40; pregnancy is often the precipitating event for affected women, since pregnancy involves numerous increases in other coagulation factors as well as mechanical factors favoring stasis in pelvic and leg veins. In several studies the incidence of thrombosis related to pregnancy in ATIII-deficient women was 62–68% in the absence of prophylactic anticoagulation, and in protein C-deficient women it was about 25%. In a series of 78 women from 44 families with a deficiency of ATIII, protein C, or protein S, during a total of 155 pregnancies undertaken without anticoagulant treatment, thrombosis was documented in 48 episodes (8 superficial vein thromboses, 39 deep vein thromboses/or pulmonary embolism, and 1 cerebral vein thrombosis, representing thrombotic complications in 18%, 7%, and 0%, respectively) (60). In untreated women in this series who had no thrombosis during pregnancy and no anticoagulation postpartum, venous thrombosis was observed postpartum in 33%, 19%, and 17%, respectively, for the three conditions. Thus, these patients were more likely to incur venous thrombosis postpartum if untreated. Within a given family, the appearance of pregnancy-associated thrombosis is quite variable, however (61). No precise biologic marker is yet available to indicate the degree of risk that can be used to select candidates for anticoagulation. For example, although the prothrombin fragment F_{1+2} is elevated in ATIII deficiency, consistent with increased thrombin activity, the level is no greater in heterozygotes who have had clinical thrombosis than in their asymptomatic relatives who also have the deficiency (62). Therefore, individual histories must be considered when one is prescribing anticoagulation during pregnancy for these patients, but prophylactic postpartum anticoagulants should be given to all women with congenital deficiencies of ATIII, protein C, and protein S for 6 weeks postpartum (i.e., until other coagulation parameters have returned to normal, nonpregnant levels [60]).

In addition to inherited deficiencies of antithrombin III, protein C, and protein S, which are detected in 10–12% of patients with venous thrombosis (uncommonly arterial thrombosis), certain inherited qualitative abnormalities in fibrinogen (dysfibrinogenemias) or plasminogen may be associated with increased thrombotic risk. Some abnormal fibrinogens form clots that resist or impair normal fibrinolysis, and this is considered to cause a thrombotic tendency. These represent rare conditions, but, like homocystinemia, they should be considered when thrombosis occurs at an early age, in patients with a strongly positive family history of thrombosis, or in patients with an unusual location for spontaneous thrombosis.

HEMATOLOGIC RISK FACTORS FOR CARDIOVASCULAR DISEASE

Hematologic risk factors for cardiovascular disease include those related to inherited thrombotic disorders affecting specific, usually single, coagulation factors or natural anticoagulants, and those related to more complex clinical disorders in which thrombosis reflects secondary changes in blood cells or vascular surfaces and is often multifactorial. Thus, smoking, diabetes, hypertension, hyperlipidemias, high-dose estrogen, immobility, and inflammation may all have prothrombotic effects on hemostatic mechanisms and on the vessel wall. Although the incidence of cardiovascular disease in women in the Framingham Study increased with age from 3 to 6/1000 women at menopause to 50.4/1000 women aged 75 to 79, only in the latter period did the

Table 12–3. RISK FACTORS FOR THROMBOEMBOLISM IN WOMEN

Smoking
Smoking plus oral contraceptives
Oral contraceptives
Pregnancy
Obesity
Venous stasis
Surgery
Congenital deficiency of antithrombin III, protein C, or protein S
Inflammation
Antiphospholipid syndrome
Connective tissue disease
Homocystinuria
Myeloproliferative syndrome with thrombocytosis

incidence equal that in men, and the death rates remained less than those in men (63). Few of the major risk factors are restricted to women, and these have been discussed earlier in this chapter under the topics of changes in hemostatic function related to oral contraceptive use, pregnancy and its complications, and the postpartum period. The antiphospholipid syndrome occurs in both sexes, although it is more common in women and may lead to important vascular complications both related to and unrelated to pregnancy.

HEMOSTATIC IMBALANCE: INCREASED PROCOAGULANTS AND DEFECTIVE FIBRINOLYSIS

Abnormalities of fibrinolysis are currently considered common risks for both venous and arterial thrombotic disease. Because fibrinogen and factor VII levels are independent risk factors for myocardial infarction and stroke (64, 65, 65a), adequate activity of the fibrinolytic system may be a crucial balancing force in preventing thrombosis. Moreover, a direct relationship between factor VII levels and triglyceride levels has been found in patients with atherosclerosis, linking coagulation with lipid metabolism (66); a similar correlation has been observed in healthy populations (6). Although previous studies of these correlations were limited to male subjects, a recent large survey in the United States showed that fibrinogen and factor VII levels are higher in women than in men, and that the fibrinogen level in women increases with age, smoking, obesity, and the menopause (6, 65a). Increased fibrinogen is associated with increased platelet reactivity (65a). Factor VII in women also increases with age. As pointed out earlier, the marked rise in fibrinogen and other plasma procoagulant levels during pregnancy is not matched by a similar rise in fibrinolytic factors, so there is a relative lack of enhanced fibrinolytic capacity during pregnancy and postpartum that is reflected in an increased thrombosis risk at these times.

Plasminogen-Activator Inhibitor

The vascular endothelium releases both tissue plasminogen activator and PAI-1. Indeed, defective synthesis or release of tissue plasminogen activator by the vascular endothelium may enhance thrombosis in either sex. Smoking, for example, decreases fibrinolytic activity and enhances PAI-1 release. Furthermore, the enhanced production of PAI-1 by blood vessels in response to inflammatory stimuli also impairs fibrinolysis. Young survivors of myocardial infarction, both men and women, have been reported to have long-term increased plasma levels of PAI-1 and decreased fibrinolytic activity (67), which also correlated with high plasma triglycerides. PAI-1 activity undergoes a circadian rhythm, and the increased occurrence of both myocardial infarction and stroke in the early morning has been correlated with lower fibrinolytic activity and with enhanced platelet activity on arising (68). Increased PAI-1 levels have also been found in patients with systemic lupus erythematosus and a history of thrombosis (69).

Lipoprotein(a)

Increased levels of a plasma lipid different from low-density lipoprotein cholesterol and triglycerides may alter hemostatic function in a prothrombotic direction by other mechanisms. Lipoprotein(a) (Lp(a)) is an LDL-like molecule that contains not only apolipoprotein B but also apolipoprotein(a) (apo(a)) a moiety that closely resembles part of the plasminogen molecule (70). High levels of Lp(a) have been linked epidemiologically with an increased risk of myocardial infarction, and Lp(a) accumulates in atherosclerotic lesions (71, 72). Unlike other lipoproteins, Lp(a) levels are not influenced by age or sex (36). Apo(a) contains multiple repeats of the "kringle 4" region of plasminogen but lacks the latter's active site and so does not have enzymatic potential. The genes for Lp(a) and for plasminogen are closely linked on chromosome 6 (71). At concentrations found in plasma, Lp(a) can compete with plasminogen for binding sites on the endothelial surface and thus can interfere with the generation of plasmin that normally operates with great efficiency on the endothelial surface, resulting in decreased fibrinolysis (71, 72). This molecular mimicry of plasminogen by Lp(a), which impairs normal fibrinolytic function at the vascular wall, appears to provide an important link between thrombotic and atherosclerotic processes.

Fibrinolytic potential can be increased by

exercise, cessation of smoking, and dietary intervention that lowers serum triglycerides (73). Dietary supplementation by fish oil or niacin can lower triglycerides and Lp(a) levels (74). Lp(a) levels are not affected by endogenous estrogens but may be lowered by danazol (which raises LDL) (36). Of greater interest is a recent report that Lp(a) levels fall significantly in postmenopausal women after treatment with oral estrogen and progestin for 6 to 12 months (75). Elevated levels of PAI-1 and of factor VII may be reduced by physical training and weight loss in men; effects in women have not been studied specifically (76). Postmenopausal estrogen replacement can decrease PAI-1 activity (24).

Abnormal Homocyst(e)ine Metabolism

Elevated plasma levels of homocyst(e)ine associated with cerebral infarction and premature atherosclerosis occur in individuals homozygous for several inborn errors of metabolism including deficiency of cystathionine β-synthase. These syndromes result in accumulation of methionine derivatives in the plasma (> 20 times normal levels) and homocystinuria. Infusion of similar concentrations of homocystine in experimental animals results in endothelial damage.

Recent attention has turned to an association between heterozygosity for homocystinuria and ischemic peripheral vascular (77) or cerebrovascular disease (78). Homocyst(e)ine has been shown to alter endothelial function, promote binding of Lp(a) to vascular cells (79), and decrease thrombin inactivation and fibrinolysis at the endothelial surface (80), all of which are activities that favor atherosclerosis. Elevation of homocyst(e)ine levels after loading with methionine has now been utilized as an independent risk factor for premature vascular disease (77, 78). One study of consecutive patients presenting at less than 50 years of age with angiographically documented occlusive peripheral or cerebral vascular disease in the absence of diabetes, hypertension, or hyperlipidemia showed that 30% were heterozygous for homocystinuria due to cystathionine synthase deficiency (77). In particular, seven of seven women presenting with peripheral vascular disease showed this abnormality. In contrast, none of 25 patients with premature myocardial infarction showed homocystinuria.

In a prospective study of patients with fresh stroke, transient ischemic attacks (TIA), or increased risk factors for cerebrovascular disease compared to age-matched controls, significantly elevated total homocyst(e)ine concentrations were found in up to a third of stroke or TIA patients and those with a high risk of cerebrovascular disease but not in the normal control group (78). The mean value in the patient and at risk groups was about twice that in the control group. There was also a correlation between homocyst(e)ine level and uric acid.

Healthy young women have lower homocyst(e)ine levels than healthy men, the difference diminishing with aging. It has been postulated that a highly efficient metabolism of methionine in premenopausal women protects them against accumulation of these thiol-amino acids (81). At menopause an "abrupt increase" in plasma homocyst(e)ine has been observed, so that the sex difference disappears with aging and the development of atherosclerosis (82). In the study of homocyst(e)ine and stroke detailed above (78), no gender-related difference was found in homocyst(e)ine levels in any subgroup; however, the average age of the study subjects was in the sixties. Thus, a modest elevation of plasma homocyst(e)ine levels alters vascular function and is implicated as an additional risk factor for the development of occlusive vascular disease, with hormonal status acting to protect premenopausal women.

ANTIPHOSPHOLIPID SYNDROME, LUPUS ANTICOAGULANT, AND VASCULAR DISEASE

Diseases characterized by autoimmune phenomena, such as systemic lupus erythematosus (SLE) and the antiphospholipid syndrome, are associated with a high risk of both venous and arterial thrombosis (47, 83). In particular, deep venous thrombosis and cerebral arterial thrombosis are common complications of these syndromes. In the past decade it has become clear that patients with autoantibodies directed against negatively charged phospholipids, two-thirds of whom do not have underlying rheumatic disease or SLE, are also at risk for thrombosis (84, 85). Indeed, the most common coagulation abnormality associated with stroke in young persons is the primary antiphospholipid syndrome (86) (Table 12–4).

Antibodies directed against phospholipids include anticardiolipins (which produce false-positive serologic tests for syphilis) and the lupus anticoagulant. Despite its name, the lupus anticoagulant is present in only a fraction (21–65%) of patients with systemic lupus erythematosus (84, 85, 87). Although these antibodies interfere with coagulation assays that depend upon catalytic phospholipid surfaces, their occurrence is clinically associated with thrombosis rather than with hemorrhage (83). In general, IgG subclass antibodies are more closely linked with thrombosis than are IgM antibodies. Prolonged partial thromboplastin time, positive anticardiolipin titer, prolonged dilute Russell's viper venom time, and positive blood thromboplastin inhibition are typical laboratory findings in this setting. Either type, lupus anticoagulant or anticardiolipin, may be found alone, but frequently both occur together, with concurrence reported in 60–90% of cases studied (83). These antibodies prolong the clotting time in assays by competing for binding of coagulation factors to the phospholipid surface but in different ways; the lupus anticoagulant also recognizes an epitope on prothrombin complexed to lipid, but anticardiolipin does not (88).

These antibodies are more common in women than in men, as are most autoimmune phenomena. Most individuals with antiphospholipid antibodies, including those with SLE and rheumatoid arthritis, do not suffer thrombotic episodes (84). Thus, screening for these antibodies does not help to guide treatment in general. However, women with SLE who have fetal distress during pregnancy or recurrent fetal loss have a high incidence of anticardiolipin antibodies (89). On the other hand, in women with a history of recurrent spontaneous abortion or intrauterine fetal growth retardation, there is an increased incidence of antiphospholipid antibodies (89, 90), and fetal outcome for these women may be improved by low-dose aspirin therapy given throughout the pregnancy, starting at about 20 weeks (89, 91–93). Early reports suggesting that high-dose prednisone given to suppress the autoantibody was beneficial to fetal outcome were not sustained by further studies and tended to induce preeclampsia. However, recent investigation suggests that the presence of antiphospholipid antibodies in a *primipara* is not predictive of these pregnancy complications (94).

In women with recurrent fetal loss, the pathologic findings underlying these complications have been shown to involve microvascular placental thrombosis and fibrin deposition, resulting in compromised placental function. The fact that aspirin therapy during pregnancy results in improved pregnancy outcome and decreased fetal wastage implicates platelet activation and possibly a thromboxane-prostacyclin production imbalance in the pathogenesis of this syndrome, as is believed to occur in preeclampsia (95). Endothelial dysfunction related to the presence of the antibodies has been postulated to underlie the pathology of excess fetal wastage in these women. For example, serum from certain patients with lupus anticoagulants was demonstrated to inhibit prostacyclin production by endothelial cells in vitro (47), but this is far from a universal phenomenon. Thrombocytopenia may also be associated with the presence of antiphospholipid antibodies.

Thromboembolic complications have been observed in about one-third of patients with a positive lupus anticoagulant or anticardiolipin titer (87). The risk of stroke is increased in the presence of a second cardiovascular lesion, for example, valvular heart disease, myocardial infarction, or coronary angioplasty (96–98). Such strokes may be caused by emboli arising from the mitral or aortic valve, and echocardiographic examination of one series of antibody-positive patients with cerebrovascular ischemic events has revealed a high incidence (73%) of valvular abnormalities, including bland vegetations (98). Since anticoagulation or antiplatelet therapy may be beneficial, and untreated patients commonly experience multiple episodes of cerebral ischemia, careful evaluation of cardiac abnormalities in patients with the combination of antiphospholipid antibody and cerebral ischemia is warranted. An increased incidence of anticardiolipin antibodies has been encountered in patients with

Table 12–4. CHARACTERISTICS OF THE ANTIPHOSPHOLIPID SYNDROME

Antiphospholipid antibodies
  Anticardiolipin
  Lupus anticoagulant
Livedo reticularis
Recurrent spontaneous abortion
Fetal growth retardation
Venous and arterial thrombosis
Stroke
Cardiac valvular lesions

known valvular heart disease or a history of myocardial infarction, and this incidence rises further after infarction in the latter group (97). In one series of patients followed prospectively after myocardial infarction or percutaneous transluminal coronary angioplasty (PTCA), positive anticardiolipin titer was associated with increased risk of thrombotic events or postangioplasty reocclusion (96).

Some studies have suggested that thrombosis in these situations is related to reduced vascular production of prostacyclin, but recent studies do not support this hypothesis. Neither have clear data implicating platelet activation per se been obtained. An association between anticardiolipin antibodies, thrombosis, and increased levels of plasminogen activator inhibitor has also been postulated (69, 99); the lupus anticoagulant has been shown to inhibit protein C activation by endothelial cells (100) and might induce PAI-1 release by endothelium (69). That thrombotic complications were more frequent in young survivors—of both sexes—of myocardial infarction who had persistently elevated PAI-1 levels suggests a potential link between biologic activity of antiphospholipid antibodies and arterial thrombosis (67).

PROTHROMBOTIC HEMOSTATIC ABNORMALITIES IN MALIGNANCY

Myeloproliferative Syndromes

Essential thrombocythemia, a clonal myeloproliferative disorder characterized by overproduction of platelets with relatively normal leukocyte and erythrocyte counts, is associated with a thrombotic diathesis, or a combination of thrombosis and hemorrhage, especially in older persons. The platelets are unusually large and of variable size (wide platelet distribution) and are abnormal in function, displaying numerous qualitative defects such as decreased α-adrenergic receptors as well as altered markers of in vivo activation. However, a subset of patients who present at a young age, particularly young women with essential thrombocythemia, have a benign course, tend to be free of thrombohemorrhagic complications, and may require little or no treatment (101). Complications of pregnancy, however, including fetal growth retardation and recurrent abortion, are common in young women with essential thrombocythemia and are associated with multiple placental thrombi and infarctions (102). Low-dose aspirin appears to improve pregnancy outcome in such cases, as it does in the antiphospholipid antibody syndrome (see previous section). In patients who develop either thrombosis or hemorrhage (and the same patient often shows both types of complications at different times), chemotherapy with hydroxyurea, α-interferon, or anagrelide to reduce the platelet count toward the normal range improves the clinical symptoms, although the qualitative platelet abnormalities are not corrected (103). For erythromelalgia (painful episodes of redness and burning of the hands and feet, representing recurrent microcirculatory obstruction by platelet thrombi in patients with essential thrombocythemia or other thrombocytosis in myeloproliferative diseases), low-dose aspirin is strikingly beneficial (104).

In the other myeloproliferative diseases, such as polycythemia vera and chronic myelogenous leukemia, marked thrombocytosis may similarly be present, the platelets may function abnormally, and a mixed picture of thromboses and hemorrhage is common. In these conditions, both sexes have similar clinical pictures, and no subgroup of young patients with a particularly benign course has been identified. Therapy to normalize the blood count often decreases the incidence of thrombohemorrhagic complications, particularly if the platelet count is lowered. The therapies listed above are used. A recently completed, large cooperative study using anagrelide to lower the platelet count suggests that this drug, which decreases megakaryocytic production of platelets but is not leukemogenic, will become an important and safe therapeutic option in the control of thrombocythemia (103).

THROMBOEMBOLISM IN WOMEN RECEIVING CANCER CHEMOTHERAPY

Malignancies of many types, especially abdominal cancers, such as carcinoma of the colon or pancreas, are associated with thromboembolic complications. Trousseau's syndrome of migratory thrombophlebitis represents a chronic disseminated intravascular coagulation in the presence of cancer that may also include a marked thrombocytosis. Thrombogenic effects of anticancer chemotherapy have been described, associated particularly with breast cancer, and many individual case reports have been published implicating particular chemotherapy regimens. A careful prospective study of women with stage II breast cancer who were to receive multidrug chemotherapy for 12 or 36 weeks revealed a 6.8% incidence of documented thrombosis during 979 patient-months of chemotherapy but no thrombotic events during 2413 patient-months without chemotherapy in the same group (105). Thromboses occurred in sites distant from infusion sites and were significantly more common in women older than 50 years. Most of the episodes were deep vein thrombosis or pulmonary embolism and required hospitalization and anticoagulation therapy. The drug regimens included cyclophosphamide, methotrexate, fluorouracil, vincristine, prednisone, and, for the 12-week course, doxorubicin and tamoxifen. The mechanism of the thrombogenic effect of these drugs has not been identified; suggested explanations have included reduction in blood fibrinolytic activity, damage to endothelium leading to release of procoagulants, and decreased antithrombin III due to the estrogenic effects of tamoxifen. In this study the thrombotic episodes requiring hospitalization were as common as infections or neutropenia requiring hospitalization. The findings of this and similar studies suggest that multidrug chemotherapy in older breast cancer patients, even ambulatory patients with a low tumor burden, carries an increased thrombotic risk (105).

SEX DIFFERENCES IN RESPONSE TO ANTITHROMBOTIC THERAPY

Aspirin

Since many of the large clinical trials testing the efficacy of aspirin in the prevention of myocardial infarction or stroke were conducted in exclusively male or largely male populations, less is known about the effectiveness of antithrombotic therapy in women. Overall, the incidence of both myocardial infarction and stroke is greater in men than in women; in some reports a greater decline in stroke mortality was noted for women than for men (18). Earlier trials of aspirin, which have shown clear benefit in secondary prevention of heart attack or stroke in male patients, either failed to demonstrate benefit in women or included too few women for accurate subgroup analysis. In addition, some of these studies demonstrated a better overall prognosis in women that might have obscured potential beneficial effects. Early studies in the 1970s of aspirin given to prevent postoperative pulmonary embolism after hip surgery suggested that women either did not benefit (106) or required much larger doses of aspirin for a beneficial effect.

However, most studies evaluating the effect of aspirin on platelet function have shown little gender-related differences in drug effectiveness or in dose-response curves. Although both gastrointestinal absorption and plasma deacetylation of aspirin vary extensively from subject to subject, very little aspirin is required to produce a full antiplatelet effect (< 100 mg/day). In one small study of patients undergoing hip surgery, women were shown to have significantly higher baseline platelet counts than men and had greater platelet aggregation responses to epinephrine, ADP, and collagen than did men, but after aspirin both sexes showed a similar inhibition of platelet activation (107). The sex difference once reported in aggregation responses to adenosine diphosphate and adrenaline (more sensitive in young women than in age-matched men [108]) has been subsequently shown to reflect differences in effective anticoagulant concentration of blood (109, 110) due to sex differences in hematocrit. Thus, anticoagulants are diluted to a different degree, resulting in hematocrit-dependent differences in plasma free calcium levels. Calcium strongly affects platelet responsiveness. In older subjects, especially those at high risk of cardiovascular disease, platelet aggregation is enhanced similarly in both sexes (108). However, studies of serotonin release from activated platelets suggest that platelets in women release more serotonin than do platelets in men when stimulated with aggregated immunoglobulin but that thrombin induces similar release in both sexes (111). Menopause per se does not affect platelet aggregation responses, nor does in vitro addition of estradiol or progesterone. Addition of testosterone in vitro, however, has been observed to enhance platelet aggregation responses to several stimulating agents (111).

Aspirin inhibits platelet aggregation that depends upon the production of thromboxane A_2, lengthens bleeding time, and blocks thromboxane A_2 synthesis by platelets because the drug covalently and permanently inactivates a key platelet enzyme in prostaglandin synthesis, cyclo-oxygenase (PGH synthase). Because platelets are incapable of protein synthesis and thus cannot produce new, active enzyme, the antiplatelet effect of a single dose of aspirin lasts for the life span of a platelet in the circulation (i.e., about a week). In general, platelets in men and women are similarly inhibited by aspirin, and the sensitivity of platelets in women to inhibitory effects of aspirin is not altered by the administration of oral contraceptives. Spontaneous platelet aggregation in stirred whole blood, monitored by a decrease in the number of single platelets, was more inhibited by aspirin in men than in women; orchiectomized males had a lessening of aspirin effect, and addition of testosterone directly to blood samples increased the aspirin effect (112). These findings suggest that testosterone, but not estradiol, affects the antithrombotic efficacy of aspirin. Ticlopidine, which acts by blocking ADP-receptor function on platelets without affecting prostaglandin synthesis, appears to inhibit platelet aggregation similarly in both sexes (113, 114).

In contrast to the results of these clinical studies, several more recent clinical trials have reported similar prevention of occlusive cardiovascular events in both sexes by antiplatelet therapy with aspirin or ticlopidine. In patients undergoing coronary artery bypass surgery who were given dipyridamole preoperatively with aspirin added within a few hours after surgery, both men and women experienced fewer graft occlusions than did patients receiving placebo (115). Improved outcome was observed both early (within 2 months of surgery) and late (1 year). In the French AICLA study of stroke prevention by dipyridamole and aspirin, both sexes benefited (116). Results were similar in the European Stroke Prevention Study, in which risk reduction was 34.8% for men and 31.8% for women at 2 years for aspirin plus dipyridamole vs. placebo (117). Other studies have discounted the theory that dipyridamole has additional beneficial effects when combined with aspirin. Similar findings of risk reduction independent of gender were obtained in studies of aspirin prophylaxis of patients with nonrheumatic atrial fibrillation (118–120). Several trials have suggested that low doses of aspirin (30 to 160 mg/day) may be as beneficial as larger doses that produce greater gastric irritation. Thus, in the Dutch TIA trial study group of 3131 patients (35% women), the risk of death, stroke, or myocardial infarction was similar in patients receiving 30 mg/day of aspirin and in those receiving 283 mg/day, and no gender differences in outcome were recorded (121).

Ticlopidine

Ticlopidine blocks fibrinogen binding to the fibrinogen receptor or platelets and other cells, thus inhibiting platelet aggregation by numerous agonists, including ADP, epinephrine, and collagen. Ticlopidine may also lower plasma fibrinogen levels. It does not affect thromboxane synthesis, however, and thus has a very different antiplatelet action from that of aspirin. Two large recent studies of ticlopidine versus aspirin in stroke prevention showed benefit in women as well as in men. In the Ticlopidine Aspirin Stroke Study (TASS) in which 35% of patients entered after recent TIA or stroke were women, 500 mg/day of ticlopidine reduced the risk of death or nonfatal stroke at 3 years by 17% compared to 1300 mg/day of aspirin (cumulative event rate 14.3% vs. 17.2%, respectively) (114). Ticlopidine reduced the risk of fatal and nonfatal stroke by 27% compared with aspirin (event rate 7.8% vs. 10.8% for aspirin). The risk reduction for men by ticlopidine in comparison with aspirin was 10% for death or nonfatal stroke and 19% for all strokes. In the Canadian American Ticlopidine Study (CATS), in which the entry criterion was a recently completed atherothrombotic stroke, 38% of patients analyzed were women (113). No gender-related differences in efficacy of ticlopidine were observed (26% risk reduction in women and 23% in men for drug vs. placebo) for prevention of stroke, myocardial infarction, or vascular death. Cumulative event rates at 3 years in women given ticlopidine versus placebo were 26.5% versus 35.7%, and in men, 23.4% versus 30.5% (122).

Another approach to establishing the effect of aspirin on cardiovascular events has been prospective evaluation during a 6-year period of a cohort of 87,000 healthy, registered nurses enrolled in the Nurses' Health Study (123). Women who reported taking one to six aspirin tablets per week incurred an age-adjusted relative risk of first myocardial infarction of 0.68 (p = .005) compared with women who took no aspirin. No risk reduction was observed for women who took more than seven aspirin per week. It should be noted that women in the latter category also had more coronary risk factors, were physically less active, and ingested more alcohol. In multivariate analyses that adjusted for major coronary risk factors, hormone use, diet, and cholesterol, the relative risk of myocardial infarction in women > 50 years of age was 0.68 (p = .02) for those who took one to six aspirins per week. Moreover, risk reduction was greater in aspirin-takers who were current smokers or who had hypercholesterolemia or a history of hypertension.

In contrast to the association between aspirin usage and reduced risk of myocardial infarction, no change in incidence of ischemic stroke was observed in women who took up to 14 aspirin per week; a slight increase of hemorrhagic stroke occurred in women who took more than 15 aspirin. Total mortality was not altered in women who took aspirin, although there was a trend toward a reduction in cardiovascular death among women taking one to six aspirin. The results of this interesting observational study provide a basis for future randomized controlled trials of antiplatelet therapy in women for the prevention of cardiovascular events, although they fall short of permitting establishment of clear guidelines for optimal antiplatelet therapy either for healthy women or for women at increased risk of cardiovascular disease.

Anticoagulation

No gender-related differences in responses to anticoagulants have been described. At one time it appeared that elderly women had more bleeding complications during heparin therapy, but with closer monitoring of heparin dosage, this is no longer considered a problem. Heparin-induced thrombocytopenia, which occurs in a sizeable minority of patients of both sexes treated with heparin, presents in two forms (124). A mild thrombocytopenia, in which the platelet count remains > 100,000/ μL and appears slowly, probably represents a direct platelet-activating effect of heparin and does not require discontinuation of treatment. In contrast, rapid induction of severe thrombocytopenia, occasionally associated with acute arterial thrombosis, represents an antibody-mediated process and can be life-threatening. An immune complex mechanism has been identified, but antibody in the patient's plasma is not easy to demonstrate (125). In this instance, heparin must be discontinued; sometimes heparin from a different animal source can be substituted. In a sensitized patient, miniheparin or even heparin-flushing of an arterial or venous line may induce the thrombocytopenia. Both standard and low-molecular-weight heparin may cause this problem.

With oral anticoagulants, estrogen therapy decreases the anticoagulant effect of coumarins because of its stimulation of liver function, so that the use of hormonal therapy must be taken into account in tailoring the dose of oral anticoagulant. Oral anticoagulants are generally contraindicated during pregnancy because of the teratogenic effects described earlier. Subcutaneous adjusted-dose heparin is used instead during pregnancy as described previously and can be administered by the patient at home. The subject of anticoagulation for valvular heart disease during pregnancy has been discussed previously in the section on complications of pregnancy. Osteoporosis and spontaneous fractures are rare complications of chronic heparin therapy that occur over periods of months (126).

References

1. Yamazaki H, Motomiya T, Kikutani N, et al. Platelet aggregation during menstrual cycle and pregnancy. *Thromb Res* 14:333–340, 1979.
2. Greer IA, Calder AA, Walker JJ, et al. Increased platelet reactivity in pregnancy-induced hypertension and uncomplicated diabetic pregnancy: an indication for antiplatelet therapy. *Br J Obstet Gynecol* 95:1204–1206, 1989.
3. Bain B, Forster T. A sex difference in the bleeding time. *Thromb Haemos* 43:131–132, 1980.
4. Stern DM, Nawroth PP, Handley D, et al. An endothelial cell dependent pathway of coagulation. *Proc Natl Acad Sci USA* 82.2523–2527, 1985.
5. Stern DM, Nawroth PP. Modulation of endothelial cell hemostatic properties by tumor necrosis factor. *J Exp Med* 163:740–745, 1986.
6. Folsom AR, Wu KK, Davis CE, et al. Population correlates of plasma fibrinogen and factor VII, putative cardiovascular risk factors. *Atherosclerosis* 91:191–205, 1991.
7. Koh SC, Yuen R, Viegas OA, et al. Plasminogen activators t-PA, u-PA and its inhibitor (PAI) in normal males and females. *Thromb Haemos* 66:581–585, 1991.
8. Takada Y, Takada A. Plasma levels of t-PA, free PAI-1 and a complex of tPA with PAI-1 in human

males and females at various ages. *Thromb Res* 55:601–609, 1989.
9. Kruithof E, Tran-Thang C, Gudinchet A, et al. Fibrinolysis in pregnancy: A study of plasminogen activator inhibitor. *Blood* 69:460–466, 1987.
10. Weitz JI, Hudoba M, Massel D, et al. Clot-bound thrombin is protected from inhibition by heparin-antithrombin III but is susceptible to inactivation by antithrombin III-independent inhibitors. *J Clin Invest* 86:385–391, 1990.
11. Inglis TC, Stuart J, George AJ, et al. Haemostatic and rheological changes in normal pregnancy and pre-eclampsia. *Br J Haematol* 50:461–465, 1982.
12. Fletcher AP, Alkjerskig NK, Burstein R. The influence of pregnancy upon blood coagulation and plasma fibrinolytic enzyme function. *Am J Obstet Gynecol* 134:743–751, 1979.
13. Weiner CP. Clotting alterations associated with the pre-eclampsia/eclampsia syndrome. Handbook of Hypertension: Hypertension in Pregnancy. Amsterdam, Elsevier, 10:241–256, 1988.
14. deBoer K, ten Cate JW, Sturk A, et al. Enhanced thrombin generation in normal and hypertensive pregnancy. *Am J Obstet Gynecol* 160:95–100, 1989.
15. Jespersen J. Pathophysiology and clinical aspects of fibrinolysis and inhibition of coagulation. Experimental and clinical studies with special reference to women on oral contraceptives and selected groups of thrombosis prone patients. *Dan Med Bull* 35:1–33, 1988.
16. Ballegeer V, Mombaerts P, Declerck PJ, et al. Fibrinolytic response to venous occlusion and fibrin fragment D-dimer levels in normal and complicated pregnancy. *Thromb Haemos* 58:1030–1032, 1987.
17. Mann JI, Doll R, Thorogood M, et al. Risk factors for myocardial infarction in young women. *Br J Prev Soc Med* 30:94–100, 1976.
18. Collaborative Group for the Study of Stroke in Young Women. Oral contraceptives and stroke in young women. Associated risk factors. *JAMA* 231:718–722, 1975.
19. Mann JI, Vessey MP, Thorogood M, Doll R. Myocardial infarction in young women with special reference to oral contraceptive practice. *Br Med J* 2:241–245, 1975.
20. Stadel BV. Oral contraceptives and cardiovascular disease. Parts 1 and 2. *N Engl J Med* 305:612–618, 672–677, 1981.
21. Spain DM, Siegel H, Bradess VA. Women smokers and sudden death: the relationship of cigarette smoking to coronary disease. *JAMA* 224:1005–1007, 1973.
22. Rosenberg L, Kaufman DW, Helmrich SP, et al. Myocardial infarction and cigarette smoking in women younger than 50 years of age. *JAMA* 263:2965–2969, 1985.
23. Bonnar J. Coagulation effects of oral contraception. *Am J Obstet Gynecol* 157:1042–1048, 1987.
24. Jespersen J, Petersen KR, Skouby SO. Effects of newer oral contraceptives on the inhibition of coagulation and fibrinolysis in relation to dosage and type of steroid. *Am J Obstet Gynecol* 163:396–403, 1990.
25. Wilson PW, Garrison RJ, Castelli WP. Postmenopausal estrogen use, cigarette smoking and cardiovascular morbidity in women over 50. *N Engl J Med* 313:1038–1043, 1985.
26. Rangemark C, Wennmalm A. Cigarette smoking and urinary excretion of markers for platelet/vessel wall interaction in healthy women. *Clin Sci* 81:11–15, 1991.
27. Siegbahn A, Ruusuvaara L. Age dependence of blood fibrinolytic components and the effects of low-dose oral contraceptives on coagulation and fibrinolysis in teenagers. *Thromb Haemos* 60:361–364, 1988.
28. Gevers Leuven JA, Kluft C, Bertina RM, et al. Effects of two low-dose oral contraceptives on circulating components of the coagulation and fibrinolytic systems. *J Lab Clin Med* 109:631–636, 1987.
29. Boerger LM, Morris PC, Thurnau GR, et al. Oral contraceptives and gender affect Protein S status. *Blood* 69:692–694, 1987.
30. Comp PC, Thurnau GR, Welsh J, et al. Functional and immunologic Protein S levels are reduced during pregnancy. *Blood* 68:881–885, 1986.
31. Henderson BE, Paganini-Hill A, Ross RK. Decreased mortality in users of estrogen replacement therapy. *Arch Intern Med* 151:75–78, 1991.
32. Stampfer MJ, Willett WC, Colditz GA, et al. A prospective study of postmenopausal estrogen therapy and coronary heart disease. *N Engl J Med* 313:1044–1049, 1985.
33. Stampfer MJ, Colditz GA, Willett WC, et al. Postmenopausal estrogen therapy and cardiovascular disease. Ten year follow-up from the Nurses' Health Study. *N Engl J Med* 325:756–762, 1991.
34. Bonnar J, Haddon M, Hunter DH, et al. Coagulation system changes in post-menopausal women receiving oestrogen preparations. *Postgrad Med J* 52 (Suppl.6):30–34, 1976.
35. Alkjaersig N, Fletcher AP, De Ziegler D, et al. Blood coagulation in postmenopausal women given estrogen treatment: Comparison of transdermal and oral administration. *J Lab Clin Med* 111:224–228, 1988.
36. Seed M. Sex hormones, lipoproteins and cardiovascular risk. *Atherosclerosis* 90:1–7, 1991.
37. Gitel S, Wessler S. Do natural estrogens pose an increased risk of thrombosis in postmenopausal women. *Thromb Res* 13:279–283, 1978.
38. Boston Collaborative Drug Surveillance Program, Surgically confirmed gallbladder disease, venous thromboembolism, and breast tumors in relation to postmenopausal estrogen therapy. *N Engl J Med* 290:15–19, 1974.
39. Chetkowski RJ, Meldrum DR, Steingold KA, et al. Biologic effects of transdermal estradiol. *N Engl J Med* 314:1615–1620, 1986.
40. Caron C, Goudemand J, Marey A, et al. Are haemostatic and fibrinolytic parameters predictors of preeclampsia in pregnancy-associated hypertension? *Thromb Haemos* 66:410–414, 1991.
41. Bergmann F, Rotmensch S, Rosenzweig B, et al. The role of von Willebrand factor in pre-eclampsia. *Thromb Haemos* 66:525–528, 1991.
42. Weiner CP, Kwaan HC, Xu C, et al. Antithrombin III activity in women with hypertension during pregnancy. *Obstet Gynecol* 65:301–306, 1985.
43. Gilabert J, Estelles A, Aznar J, et al. Contribution of platelets to increased plasminogen activator inhibitor type 1 in severe preeclampsia. *Thromb Haemos* 63:361–366, 1990.
44. Walsh SW. Preeclampsia: An imbalance in placental prostacyclin and thromboxane production. *Am J Obstet Gynecol* 152:335–340, 1985.
45. Walsh SW, Behr MJ, Allen NH. Placental prosta-

cyclin production in normal and toxemic pregnancies. *Am J Obstet Gynecol* 151:110–111, 1985.
46. Fitzgerald DJ, Entman SS, Mulloy K, et al. Decreased prostacyclin biosynthesis preceding the clinical manifestation of pregnancy-induced hypertension. *Circulation* 75:956–963, 1987.
47. Carreras LO, Defreyn G, Machin S, et al. Arterial thrombosis, intrauterine death and "lupus" anticoagulant: Detection of immunoglobulin interfering with prostacyclin formation. *Lancet* 1:244–246, 1981.
48. Musci TJ, Roberts JM, Rodgers GM, et al. Mitogenic activity is increased in the sera of preeclamptic women before delivery. *Am J Obstet Gynecol* 159:1446–1451, 1988.
49. Thiagarajah S, Bourgeois FJ, Harbert GM. Thrombocytopenia in preeclampsia. Associated abnormalities and management principles. *Am J Obstet Gynecol* 150:1–7, 1984.
50. Weinstein L. Syndrome of hemolysis, elevated liver enzymes and low platelet count: A severe consequence of hypertension in pregnancy. *Am J Obstet Gynecol* 142:159–167, 1982.
51. Sibai BM, Taslimi MM, El-Nazer A, et al. Maternal-perinatal outcome associated with the syndrome of hemolysis, elevated liver enzymes and low platelets in severe pre-eclampsia/eclampsia. *Am J Obstet Gynecol* 155:501–509, 1986.
52. Letsky EA, de Swiet M. Thromboembolism in pregnancy and its management. *Br J Haematol* 57:543–552, 1984.
53. Koonin LM, Atrash HK, Lawson HW, et al. Maternal mortality surveillance, United States, 1979–1986. *MMWR* 40:13, 1991.
54. Hellgren M, Nygards EB. Blood coagulation and fibrinolysis in fertile women with previous thromboembolic complications and effects of venous occlusion. *Thromb Res* 24:453–465, 1981.
55. Ginsberg JS, Hirsh J. Anticoagulants during pregnancy. *Ann Rev Med* 40:79–86, 1989.
56. Ginsberg JS, Hirsh J. Use of anticoagulants during pregnancy. *Chest* 98:156S–160S, 1989.
57. Sareli P, England MJ, Berk MR, et al. Maternal and fetal sequelae of anticoagulation during pregnancy in patients with mechanical heart valve prostheses. *Am J Cardiol* 63:1462–1465, 1989.
58. Weiner CP. Thrombotic microangiopathy in pregnancy and the postpartum period. *Semin Hematol* 24:119–129, 1987.
59. Solal-Celigny P, Tertian G, Fernandez H, et al. Pregnancy and paroxysmal nocturnal hemoglobinuria. *Arch Intern Med* 148:593–595, 1988.
60. Conard J, Horellou MH, Van Dreden P, et al. Thrombosis and pregnancy in congenital deficiencies of AT III, Protein C or Protein S: Study of 78 women. *Thromb Haemos* 65:319–320, 1990.
61. Mazza JJ. Antithrombin III (AT-III) deficiency spanning four generations. *Thromb Haemos* 66:737–738, 1991.
62. Rosenberg RD, Bauer KA. New insights into hypercoagulable states. *Hosp Prac* 21:131–147, 1986.
63. Lobo RA. Lipids, clotting factors and diabetes: Endogenous risk factors for cardiovascular disease. *Am J Obstet Gynecol* 158:1584–1591, 1988.
64. Meade TW, Mellows S, Brozovic M, et al. Haemostatic function and ischaemic heart disease: Principal results of the Northwick Park Study. *Lancet* 2:533–537, 1986.
65. Wilhelmsen L, Svardsudd K, Korsan-Bengsten K, et al. Fibrinogen as a risk factor for stroke and myocardial infarction. *N Engl J Med* 311:501–508, 1984.
65a. Cook NS, Ubben D. Fibrinogen as a major risk factor in cardiovascular disease. *TIPS Reviews* 11:444–451, 1990.
66. Cortellaro M, Boschetti C, Cofrancesco E, et al. The PLAT study: A multidisciplinary study of hemostatic function and conventional risk factors in vascular disease patients. *Atherosclerosis* 90:109–118, 1991.
67. Hamsten S, Wiman B, de Faire U. Increased plasma levels of a rapid inhibitor of tissue plasminogen activator in young survivors of myocardial infarction. *N Engl J Med* 313:1557–1563, 1985.
68. Ridker PM, Manson JE, Buring JE, et al. Circadian variation of acute myocardial infarction and the effect of low-dose aspirin in a randomized trial of physicians. *Circulation* 82:897–902, 1990.
69. Violi F, Ferro D, Valesini G, et al. Tissue plasminogen activator inhibitor in patients with systemic lupus erythematosus and thrombosis. *Br Med J* 300:1099–1102, 1990.
70. Mbewu AD, Durrington PN. Lipoprotein(a): Structure, properties and possible involvement in thrombogenesis and atherogenesis. *Atherosclerosis* 85:1–14, 1990.
71. Hajjar KA, Gavish D, Breslow JL, et al. Lipoprotein(a) modulation of endothelial cell surface fibrinolysis and its potential role in atherosclerosis. *Nature* 339:303–305, 1989.
72. Miles LA, Fless GM, Levin EG, et al. A potential basis for the thrombotic risks associated with lipoprotein(a). *Nature* 339:301–303, 1989.
73. Andersen P, Nilsen D, Beckmann S, et al. Increased fibrinolytic potential after diet intervention in healthy coronary high-risk individuals. *Acta Med Scand* 223:499–506, 1988.
74. Beil FU, Terres W, Orgass M, et al. Dietary fish oil lowers lipoprotein(a) in primary hypertriglyceridemia. *Atherosclerosis* 90:95–97, 1991.
75. Soma M, Fumagalli R, Paoletti R. Plasma Lp(a) concentration after oestrogen and progestagen in postmenopausal women. *Lancet* 337:612–613, 1991.
76. Gris JC, Schved JF, Feugeas O, et al. Impact of smoking, physical training and weight reduction on FVII, PAI-1 and hemostatic markers in sedentary men. *Thromb Haemost* 64:516–520, 1990.
77. Boers GH, Smals AG, Trijbels FJ, et al. Heterozygosity for homocystinuria in premature peripheral and cerebral occlusive arterial disease. *N Engl J Med* 313:709–715, 1985.
78. Coull BM, Malinow MR, Beamer N, et al. Elevated plasma homocyst(e)ine concentration as a possible independent risk factor for stroke. *Stroke* 21:572–576, 1990.
79. Harpel PC, Chang VT, Borth W. Homocysteine enhances the binding of lipoprotein(a) to plasmin-modified fibrin providing a potential link between thrombosis and atherosclerosis. *Blood* 76(Suppl.1):510a, 1990.
80. Rodgers GM, Conn MT. Homocysteine, an atherogenic stimulus, reduces Protein C activation by arterial and venous endothelial cells. *Blood* 75:895–901, 1990.
81. Boers GH, Smals AG, Trijbels FJ, et al. Unique efficiency of methionine metabolism in premenopausal women may protect against vascular disease in the reproductive years. *J Clin Invest* 72:1976–1981, 1983.

82. Kang SS, Wong PWK, Cook HY, et al. Protein-bound homocyst(e)ine: A possible risk factor for coronary artery disease. *J Clin Invest* 77:1482–1486, 1986.
83. Asherson RA, Khamashta MA, Gil A, et al. Cerebrovascular disease and antiphospholipid antibodies in systemic lupus erythematosus, lupus-like disease and the primary antiphospholipid syndrome. *Am J Med* 86:391–399, 1989.
84. Love PE, Santoro SA. Antiphospholipid antibodies: anticardiolipin and the lupus anticoagulant in systemic lupus erythematosus (SLE) and in non-SLE disorders. *Ann Intern Med* 112:682–698, 1990.
85. Elias M, Eldor A. Thromboembolism in patients with the "lupus"-type circulating anticoagulant. *Arch Intern Med* 144:510–515, 1984.
86. Montalban J, Codina A, Ordi J, et al. Antiphospholipid antibodies in cerebral ischemia. *Stroke* 22:750–753, 1991.
87. Petri M, Rheinschmidt M, Whiting-O'Keefe Q, et al. The frequency of lupus anticoagulant in systemic lupus erythematosus. *Ann Intern Med* 106:524–531, 1987.
88. Bevers EM, Galli M, Barbui T, et al. Lupus anticoagulant IgG's (LA) are not directed to phospholipids only, but to a complex of lipid-bound human prothrombin. *Thromb Haemos* 66:629–632, 1991.
89. Lockshin MD, Druzin ML, Goei S, et al. Antibody to cardiolipin as a predictor of fetal distress or death in pregnant patients with systemic lupus erythematosus. *N Engl J Med* 313:152–156, 1985.
90. Branch DW, Scott JR, Kochenour NK, et al. Obstetric complications associated with the lupus anticoagulant. *N Engl J Med* 313:1322–1326, 1985.
91. Sureau C. Prevention of perinatal consequences of pre-eclampsia with low-dose aspirin: Results of the EPREDA trial. *Eur J Obstet Gynecol Reprod Biol* 41:71–73, 1991.
92. Hadi HA, Treadwell E. Lupus anticoagulant and anticardiolipin antibodies in pregnancy: A review. I. Immunochemistry and clinical implications. *Obstet Gynecol Survey* 45:780–785, 1990.
93. Hadi HA, Treadwell E. Lupus anticoagulant and anticardiolipin antibodies in pregnancy: A review. II. Diagnosis and management. *Obstet Gynecol Survey* 45:786–791, 1990.
94. Infante-Rivard C, David M, Gauthier R, et al. Lupus anticoagulants, anticardiolipin antibodies and fetal loss—a case control study. *N Engl J Med* 325:1063–1066, 1991.
95. Feinstein DI. Lupus anticoagulant, thrombosis and fetal loss (editorial). *N Engl J Med* 313:1348–1349, 1985.
96. Barbut D, Borer JS, Gharavi A, et al. Prevalence of anticardiolipin antibody in isolated mitral or aortic regurgitation, or both, and possible relation to cerebral ischemic events. *Am J Cardiol* 70:901–905, 1992.
97. Hamsten A, Norberg R, Bjorkholm M, et al. Antibodies to cardiolipin in young survivors of myocardial infarction: An association with recurrent cardiovascular events. *Lancet* 1:113–115, 1986.
98. Barbut D, Borer JS, Wallerson D, et al. Anticardiolipin antibody and stroke: Possible relation of valvular heart disease and embolic events. *Cardiology* 79:99–109, 1991.
99. Awada H, Barlowatz-Meimon G, Dougados M, et al. Fibrinolysis abnormalities in systemic lupus erythematosus and their relation to vasculitis. *J Lab Clin Med* 111:229–236, 1988.
100. Cariou R, Tobelem G, Soria C, et al. Inhibition of Protein C activation by endothelial cells in the presence of lupus anticoagulant (letter). *N Engl J Med* 314:1193–1194, 1986.
101. Hoagland HC, Silverstein MN. Primary thrombocythemia in the young patient. *Mayo Clin Proc* 53:578–583, 1978.
102. Jones EC, Mosesson MW, Thomason JL, et al. Essential thrombocythemia in pregnancy. *Obstet Gynecol* 71:501–503, 1988.
103. Anagrelide Study Group. Anagrelide, a therapy for thrombocythemic states. Experience in 577 patients. *Am J Med* 92:69–76, 1992.
104. Michiels JJ, Abels J, Stekette J. Erythromelalgia caused by platelet-mediated arteriolar inflammation and thrombosis in thrombocythemia. *Ann Intern Med* 102:466–472, 1985.
105. Levine MN, Gent M, Hirsh J, et al. The thrombogenic effect of anticancer drug therapy in women with stage II breast cancer. *N Engl J Med* 318:404–407, 1988.
106. Harris WH, Salzman EW, Athanasoulis CA, et al. Aspirin prophylaxis of venous thromboembolism after total hip replacement. *N Engl J Med* 297:1246–1249, 1977.
107. Coppe D, Wessinger SJ, Ransil BJ, et al. Sex differences in the platelet response to aspirin. *Thromb Res* 23:1–21, 1981.
108. Johnson M, Ramey E, Ramwell PW. Sex and age differences in human platelet aggregation. *Nature* 253:355–357, 1975.
109. Kelton JG, Powers P, Julian J, et al. Sex-related differences in platelet aggregation: Influence of hematocrit. *Blood* 56:38–41, 1980.
110. Aspey B, Harrison MJG. Sex difference in effect of aspirin on blood platelet aggregation may be artifact. *Stroke* 22:1089–1090, 1991.
111. Moore A, Weksler BB, Nachman RL. Sex-related platelet release of serotonin. *Thromb Res* 21:469–474, 1981.
112. Spranger M, Aspey BS, Harrison MJG. Sex difference in antithrombotic effect of aspirin. *Stroke* 20:34–37, 1989.
113. Gent M, Easton JD, Hachinski VC, et al. The Canadian-American Ticlopidine study (CATS) in thromboembolic stroke. *Lancet* 1:1215–1220, 1989.
114. Hass WK, Easton JD, Adams HP, et al. A randomized trial comparing ticlopidine hydrochloride with aspirin for the prevention of stroke in high-risk patients. *N Engl J Med* 321:501–507, 1989.
115. Chesebro JH, Clements IP, Fuster V. A platelet-inhibitor-drug trial in coronary-artery bypass operations: Benefit of perioperative dipyridamole and aspirin therapy on early postoperative vein-graft patency. *N Engl J Med* 301:73–78, 1982.
116. Bousser MG, Eschwege E, Haguenau M, et al. "AICLA" controlled trial of aspirin and dipyridamole in the secondary prevention of athero-thrombotic cerebral ischemia. *Stroke* 14:5–14, 1983.
117. ESPS Group. European Stroke Prevention Study. *Stroke* 21:1122–1130, 1990.
118. Stroke Prevention in Atrial Fibrillation Study Group. Preliminary report of the stroke prevention in atrial fibrillation study. *N Engl J Med* 322:863–869, 1990.
119. Stroke Prevention in Atrial Fibrillation Investigators.

Stroke prevention in atrial fibrillation study. Final results. *Circulation* 84:527–539, 1991.
120. Petersen P, Boysen G, Gotfredsen J, et al. Placebo-controlled, randomised trial of warfarin and aspirin for prevention of thromboembolic complications in chronic atrial fibrillation: the Copenhagen AFASAK study. *Lancet* 1:175–179, 1989.
121. The Dutch TIA Trial Study Group. A comparison of two doses of aspirin (30 mg vs. 283 mg a day) in patients after a transient ischemic attack or minor ischemic stroke. *N Engl J Med* 325:1261–1266, 1991.
122. Hershey LA. Stroke prevention in women: Role of aspirin versus ticlopidine. *Am J Med* 91:288–292, 1991.
123. Manson JE, Stampfer MJ, Colditz GA, et al. A prospective study of aspirin use and primary prevention of cardiovascular disease in women. *JAMA* 266:521–527, 1991.
124. Bell WR. Heparin-associated thrombocytopenia and thrombosis. *J Lab Clin Med* 111:600–608, 1988.
125. Kelton JG, Sheridan D, Santos A. Heparin-induced thrombocytopenia. Laboratory studies. *Blood* 77:925–931, 1988.
126. Wise PH, Hall AJ. Heparin-induced osteopenia in pregnancy. *Br Med J* 281:110–113, 1980.

CHAPTER 13

Exercise and Physical Activity

MARY L. O'TOOLE, Ph.D.

Regular physical activity has long been associated by lay and medical personnel with optimal health (1, 2). Although a cause and effect relationship between physical activity and optimal health has not been validated through rigorous scientific study, improved physical fitness does convey benefits to the cardiovascular system that are manifest both during rest and during exercise. Exercise also has a positive effect on known cardiovascular risk factors. Additionally, available evidence suggests that exercise may be a useful adjunct to therapy in the secondary prevention of cardiovascular disease. This chapter will focus on the potential influence of exercise on the lives of apparently healthy women, women with cardiovascular risk factors, and women with known cardiovascular disease.

EXERCISE AND HEALTH
Fitness Assessment in Women

The gold standard for assessing physical fitness is the measurement of aerobic capacity or maximal oxygen uptake ($\dot{V}O_2$ max). $\dot{V}O_2$ max represents the attainment of maximal aerobic energy transfer and requires integration of the respiratory, cardiovascular, and neuromuscular systems. Before puberty, there is no difference in $\dot{V}O_2$ max between boys and girls (3). After puberty, women are unable to attain $\dot{V}O_2$ max values as high as those of men. Based on means from cross-sectional data of varied (in terms of habitual activity) populations, differences can be as large as 50% when $\dot{V}O_2$ is reported as liters/minute, 20–25% when body weight is considered (mL/kg/minute), and 9% when body composition is considered (mL/kg fat-free mass/minute) (3, 4). These differences have been attributed to three physiologic characteristics of women: a higher percentage of body fat, a smaller oxygen-carrying capacity (lower hemoglobin levels, smaller heart, smaller blood volume), and a smaller muscle fiber area (4). The gender difference between similarly trained endurance athletes is usually smaller than that of the general population because of training-induced changes in body composition and blood volume. For example, elite female distance runners (5) have been reported to have a mean $\dot{V}O_2$ max of 67.1 mL/kg/minute compared with 78.8 mL/kg/minute for elite male runners (15% difference). These values can be compared to an expected $\dot{V}O_2$ max of approximately 36 mL/kg/minute in sedentary women and 45 mL/kg/minute in sedentary men (3, 6) of the same age. The relationship of these high levels of cardiovascular and aerobic fitness to optimal health has not been clearly established in women or men.

Effects of Exercise on Cardiovascular Mortality and Morbidity

Despite some evidence that women have increased their leisure-time activity since 1970 (7), a 1985 survey reported that only 7% of U.S. females aged 18 to 65 years are regularly and appropriately active (8, 9). This conclusion is very worrisome because increasing evidence shows that inactivity may be an independent risk factor for cardiovascular disease in both men and women. Few studies have addressed the relationship of physical fitness or habitual activity level to cardiovascular disease in women. Powell et al. (10) found that only 5 of 43 studies examining the relationship between activity and coronary heart disease (CHD) included and reported data on women. Of these, three reported increased relative risk of low activity compared with high activity for the endpoints of angina, myocardial infarction, and CHD death (11–13). However, two large cohort studies (Framingham and Goteburg) failed to find a statistically significant relationship between activity levels and death from CHD in women (14, 15). The latter also did not find a relationship between activity and either angina or myocardial infarction (MI). When only leisure time physical activity was considered, both Marti et al. (16) and Salonen et al. (17) concluded that leisure-time physical activity was only weakly related to risk factors for CHD. Thus, strong evidence for the beneficial effects of exercise on longevity or coronary artery disease in women is lacking.

Blair et al. (18) reported one of the few large (n = 3120 women; 10,224 men) prospective studies of the relationship between fitness (exercise time during a maximal treadmill test) and mortality. The least fit women (lowest quintile) had a 4.7 relative risk for all-cause mortality compared to the most fit (highest quintile). A plateau in death rate was seen for women who had achieved a 9 metabolic equivalent (MET) level of exercise (second lowest quintile) during the treadmill test. One MET is approximately equal to a resting oxygen uptake of 3.5 mL/kg/minute. These relationships remained strong when data were adjusted for smoking, lipid levels, systolic blood pressure, and family history of CHD. This study suggests, then, that a reasonably modest level of physical fitness can provide a substantial decrease in the risk of dying in women. Additionally, analysis of the relative risk imposed by the presence of a single conventional risk factor for CHD despite high fitness compared to low fitness revealed that fitness levels are more important than high systolic blood pressure (> 140 mmHg), positive family history, and marked obesity in both men and women. In women, low fitness alone also carried a greater risk than elevated blood glucose (42 vs. 0 deaths per 10,000 person-years). Smoking plus high fitness carried a risk roughly equal to that of low fitness alone (22 vs. 25 deaths per 10,000 person-years). Only elevated cholesterol above 6.75 mmol/L carried a greater risk for women than low fitness. In men, fitness was more important than elevated cholesterol, but smoking carried a greater relative risk than low fitness. Although there are several important limitations to this study, such as subject self-selection, middle to high socioeconomic status, and exclusion of individuals with hypertension, diabetes, stroke, or electrocardiographic (ECG) abnormalities, the gender differences in importance of cholesterol, blood glucose, and smoking may be quite meaningful clinically. For example, a woman with low fitness and a high cholesterol level might be expected to do better by reducing her cholesterol level rather than exercising, whereas a man might do better by improving his fitness level. In contrast, a woman with low fitness and an elevated blood glucose level would be well advised to improve her fitness level.

EXERCISE AND PRIMARY PREVENTION OF CARDIOVASCULAR DISEASE

Exercise by Apparently Healthy Women

Millions of women participate regularly in various types of exercise programs. The long-term physiologic consequences to the cardiovascular system are dependent not only on the intensity, duration, and frequency of the exercise but also on whether the exercise is predominantly dynamic or resistive. Dynamic exercise, also termed aerobic or isotonic exercise, can be defined as any exercise in which oxidative phosphorylation is the primary source of energy (19). During dynamic exercise, cardiovascular responses are governed primarily by metabolic demand. Dynamic exercise involves activities such as walking, running, bicycling, swimming, and cross-country skiing, that are rhythmic, alternate contractions of flexor and extensor muscle groups. In contrast, resistive exercise, also called anaerobic, isometric, or static exercise, refers to weight-lifting types of exercise and is fueled primarily by anaerobic glycolysis (20). During resistive exercise, the hemodynamic response is governed primarily by altered autonomic nervous system responses and by mechanical effects, such as increased vascular resistance in vessels compressed in the active muscles and in the thorax (21).

Dynamic Exercise. The cardiovascular responses to single dynamic exercise sessions and to dynamic exercise training are similar in women and men (22). During a single exercise bout, cardiac output increases linearly with oxygen uptake, with the relationship reported to be approximately 6 liters of blood flow per liter of oxygen uptake, with only minor interindividual variations among healthy subjects (23, 24). However, women have been reported to have proportionally higher cardiac outputs than men because of the lower oxygen-carrying capacity of their blood and lower peripheral oxygen extraction (25–27). Increasing heart rates parallel the increased oxygen uptake, with women generally having slightly higher heart rates than men at matched relative exercise intensities (25, 26). At the initiation of upright exercise, stroke volume increases and reaches maximal levels at work rates corresponding to approximately 40% of $\dot{V}O_2$ max in men (25) and 50–60% of $\dot{V}O_2$ max in women (28). Recently, Sullivan et al. (27) reported that increased end-diastolic volumes, decreased end-systolic volumes, and the resultant increased ejection fractions contributed to increased stroke volumes in both men and women. They concluded that the time course and relative magnitude of the ventricular volume changes were not gender dependent. In contrast, earlier reports concluded that approximately 30% of women with angiographically normal coronary arteries failed to increase ejection fraction during exercise (29, 30). During dynamic exercise, muscle and myocardial blood flows are functions of the relative work rate (percent of $\dot{V}O_2$ max) and are not different between genders.

Chronic repetition of these responses through exercise training results in changes in the cardiovascular system that are evident both at rest and during exercise. Although most of the original studies describing the exercise response to dynamic exercise were done with male subjects (19, 23, 31), subsequent studies using women as subjects (4, 31–35) have demonstrated that there are no major gender-related differences in the cardiovascular response to exercise training. Similarly, the response of younger (premenopausal) and older (postmenopausal) women to dynamic exercise training is based on mode, intensity, duration, and frequency of exercise sessions rather than on age or hormonal status.

Resistive Exercise. During resistive exercise, oxygen uptake and heart rate increase but to a smaller extent than during dynamic exercise. Stroke volume is unchanged, as is peripheral resistance. Unlike the situation in dynamic exercise, all blood pressures (systolic, diastolic, and mean) rise. The magnitude of the hemodynamic response to resistive exercise is a function of muscle mass and the percentage of maximal voluntary force production (21, 36).

With repeated resistive exercise training, the cardiovascular system is subjected to a pressure overload. Morganroth et al. (37) reported that resistance-trained male athletes developed an increased ventricular wall thickness with no change in left ventricular volume, a condition analogous to that seen in concentric hypertrophy. Concentric enlargement has not been confirmed by subsequent studies of resistance-trained athletes when data are normalized for body surface area, body mass, lean body mass, or carefully matched control data (38, 39). Fleck (40) has suggested that resistance training increases left ventricular mass only in proportion to the increase in skeletal muscle mass. Since the skeletal muscle hypertrophy response of women to resistance training is considerably less than that of men, less cardiac enlargement would reasonably be expected (41). Cross-sectional studies of female resistance athletes have failed to report concentric myocardial hypertrophy (42, 43). No longitudinal studies of female resistance athletes are available (39).

Effects of Exercise on Cardiovascular Risk Factors

Known CHD risk factors, such as hypertension, obesity, glucose intolerance, and hyperlipidemia, tend to be more prevalent in groups of sedentary women than in regularly exercising women. Although women who are less healthy may choose to be less physically active, dynamic exercise training has been shown to affect each of these risk factors positively.

Blood Pressure. Physical fitness is inversely associated with blood pressure in normotensive women. In a cross-sectional study, Saar et al. (44) reported that lower blood pressures in young women were associated with high levels of fitness. In a large cohort study (45), low-fitness, middle-aged women who were normotensive initially had a 1.52 relative risk of developing hypertension during the next 4 years compared to the highly fit group. The relative risk remained after adjustment for age, initial blood pressure, and initial body mass index (BMI, kg/m^2). Many cross-sectional studies of exercise habits and blood pressure, however, show only weak relationships after correction for BMI (46).

More than 25 years ago, Kral et al. (47) observed postexercise hypotension. Subsequent studies have confirmed that postexercise hypotension is an expected physiologic response that can persist for hours. This response has been noted after both aerobic exercise and resistive exercise (48). The magnitude of the acute postexercise hypotension is similar for normotensive and hypertensive subjects (49). Paulev et al. (50) followed blood pressure recovery for 4 hours after a 20-minute exercise bout by 10 hypertensive women. Blood pressure remained lower than the preexercise level throughout the recovery period. Hagberg et al. (51) followed hemodynamic changes in normotensive older men and women for 1 to 3 hours after a 45-minute exercise bout (50–70% $\dot{V}O_2$ max). During recovery, mean blood pressure and cardiac output were significantly reduced compared to preexercise levels, whereas peripheral resistance was unchanged or slightly increased. Further research is necessary to clarify the mechanisms responsible for postexercise hypotension.

Despite positive associations between physical fitness levels or leisure-time physical activity and blood pressure, exercise training has little effect on resting blood pressure of normotensive individuals. However, there is growing evidence that exercise training may be a useful nonpharmacologic intervention for decreasing blood pressure in hypertensive women (52–54). Urata et al. (54) observed decreases of 15 and 10 mmHg (in systolic and diastolic blood pressures, respectively) following 10 to 20 weeks of moderate exercise by hypertensive men and women. They reported no differences in hemodynamic responses between men and women. In summarizing the information gained from exercise training studies of hypertensive individuals, Seals and Hagberg (55, 56) reported average decreases in both systolic and diastolic blood pressures (11 and 8 mmHg, respectively) following exercise training. They cite methodologic considerations such as type and intensity of exercise or lack of appropriate control groups rather than gender as the factors responsible for inconsistencies among these studies.

Although most adaptations to exercise are proportional to the exercise dose (type, intensity, duration, and frequency), blood pressure responses may not follow this pattern. Hagberg and Seals (56) reported that post-training decreases in blood pressure were unrelated to increases in $\dot{V}O_2$ max. Roman et al. (57) reported blood pressure decreases in 30 hypertensive women subjects following 3 months of aerobic exercise at 70% of maximal heart rate (approximately 50% of $\dot{V}O_2$ max), a level lower than that usually prescribed for cardiovascular conditioning. When exercise was stopped for 3 months, blood pressures returned to preexercise levels. Similar exercise for an additional 12 months again lowered pressures, but increasing exercise intensity did not further lower them. Tipton et al. (58) confirmed this observation in animal studies. Exercise intensities of 40–60% $\dot{V}O_2$ max decreased blood pressures in spontaneously hypertensive rats by 10 to 15 mmHg, whereas intensities of > 75% had no effect on blood pressure. Existing information suggests that the exercise threshold for making positive adjustments in CHD risk factors such as hypertension may be well below that for improved physical fitness. Optimal levels for blood pressure responses may be 40–60% of $\dot{V}O_2$ max rather than the 60–85% of $\dot{V}O_2$ max usually associated with aerobic conditioning for fitness. Perhaps one of the reasons why studies have not universally shown decreases in blood pressure with aerobic training is that the exercise may have been prescribed at too high an intensity. Based on available studies, the blood pressure lowering effect of aerobic training may occur with as little as 3 weeks of training (54) and certainly occurs by 3 months (57).

Resistive exercise has usually been considered contraindicated for hypertensive individuals because weight lifting can elicit high systolic pressures (> 200 mmHg) even in normotensive individuals (59). However, some evidence (albeit preliminary and all in male subjects) exists that resistive training may also maintain lower blood pressures. A small group of adolescent hypertensive boys decreased systolic and diastolic blood pressures by 17 and 6 mmHg, respectively, after a short endurance training program. The decreases were maintained after 20 weeks of resistive training with free weights. Harris and Holly (60) reported no change in systolic blood pressure and a modest reduction in diastolic blood pressure following a 9-week circuit weight-training program in borderline hypertensive male subjects. No investigations of the hypertensive female response to weight-training could be found.

Numerous complex mechanisms have been proposed to explain the exercise-induced chronic reduction in blood pressure. Ultimately, the mechanism(s) must have some effect on either cardiac output or peripheral resistance. A decrease in either heart rate or sympathetic nervous system activity at rest, both of which are frequent consequences of exercise training, would elicit the desired effect on blood pressure. It is not clear whether the training-induced decrease in blood pressure is the result of a change in cardiac output, peripheral resistance, or both (58). In one study (54) using both men and women as subjects, the apparent antihypertensive effect of moderate exercise training may have been mediated by a concurrent decrease in circulating blood volume (3.4 liters/m^2 to 3.0 liters/m^2). Although the usual response to exercise training is an increase in blood volume, the response of subjects with essential hypertension, who perhaps have a hyperkinetic circulation, may be different. Few studies of women have made sufficient hemodynamic measurements to define a mechanism. Exact mechanisms remain unclear and need further study.

Body Weight. Many women exercise, at least in part, to control body weight. Although not a universal finding (61), an inverse relationship between habitual leisure-time exercise and body weight has been observed in large groups of women (62). Leisure-time exercise has also been reported to be a strong predictor of both waist-hip ratios (WHR) and percentage of body fat in women (63, 64). Shangold (65) suggests that inactivity is the most common cause of obesity in women.

Women of normal weight and those who are less than 20% overweight can usually exercise sufficiently to control their weight. The existing evidence points to a a positive effect of aerobic exercise on body weight, percentage of body fat, and fat distribution. Aerobic exercise, such as walking, running, or cycling generally increases lean body mass and decreases body fat in previously sedentary women (66). In normal-weight women, an exercise program of walking done 4 days/week for at least 9 weeks has been shown to result in a decrease in percentage of body fat with no change in total body weight (67). Although a common assumption is that aerobic exercise modes are interchangeable for increasing fitness levels and decreasing body fat, this may not be true. Swimming, a popular exercise for promoting fitness without musculoskeletal stress, may not be appropriate for weight control. Gwinup (68) studied 29 middle-aged nonobese women who exercised in one of three aerobic exercise modes for 1 hour/day for 6 months. The walkers and cyclists lost 11% and 13% of body weight, respectively, but the swimmers had no change in weight. Walking has also been reported to promote loss of abdominal fat more readily than fat at other sites. This response occurs in both men and women (69). Although the effects of resistive exercise training on weight control in women have been inadequately studied, resistive exercise does not have a sufficiently high energy expenditure to be an efficient exercise for weight reduction (66).

Prospective studies have consistently shown that aerobic exercise training has a positive effect on body composition in obese as well as normal-weight women. Franklin et al. (70) reported that although obese and normal-weight women had similar increases in fitness levels, decreases in body fat were larger in the obese women. Epstein and Wing (71) noted that heavy women lose more weight during an exercise program while training at the same intensity as normal-weight women. Despite this, a combination of diet and exercise is necessary for obese women to attain normal body weight and composition (66). Exercise as part of a weight-reduction program may have an additional benefit. Recently, Wood et al. (72) reported that, in a group of premenopausal, obese women, exercise attenuated the decrease in high-density lipoproteins (HDL) usually associated with hypocaloric, low-fat diets.

Exercise may also exert a metabolic effect on obese individuals by lowering insulin levels despite the lack of any change in body composition or glucose tolerance (73). DeFronzo et al. (74) compared seven obese women who exercised for 6 weeks with normal-weight controls of both sexes. Following training, no changes in weight or skinfold thickness were seen, but $\dot{V}O_2$ max increased 17%. Glucose tolerance was normal before training and remained unchanged by the training. Fasting glucose level also did not change and was similar to that of the normal-weight subjects. Fasting insulin, however, decreased by 26% in the obese subjects, demonstrating that hyperinsulinemia associated with obesity can be reduced by exercise training. Although insulin sensitivity increased, it was still less than that of the normal-weight control subjects. Changes in the responses of both peripheral and hepatic tissues are thought to contribute to this response. Krotkiewski and Bjorntorp (75) speculate that the pattern of fat distribution may influence the effect of training on metabolic control. They observed an increase in insulin sensitivity in individuals with android fat distribution (large WHR) but not in those with larger hip dimensions (gynoid pattern).

Glucose Tolerance. Habitual physical activity and level of physical fitness appear to be related to glucose tolerance, insulin sensitivity, and prevalence of diabetes in women as well as in men. Bjorntorp and associates (76) first reported that physically active men had lower fasting and postglucose plasma insulin levels than age- and weight-matched controls. Other cross-sectional studies have reported that athletes have normal or increased glucose tolerance in combination with low basal and low glucose-stimulated insulin levels (77). No evidence is available to suggest a gender difference in this response. Additionally, Frisch et al. (78) reported that the prevalence of diabetes, excluding gestational diabetes, in former female collegiate athletes was significantly less than that in women who had not participated in collegiate athletics. The relative risk of diabetes for nonathletes vs. athletes was 3.4.

As little as a single bout of exercise by an untrained individual may result in increased insulin sensitivity for 12 to 14 hours after exercise (79). This effect has been seen in normal subjects, in insulin-resistant subjects with decreased glucose tolerance, and in individuals with noninsulin-dependent diabetes mellitus (NIDDM) (79, 80). Trained subjects have greater insulin action than untrained subjects for up to 5 days following a single training session.

With exercise training, many studies have confirmed the presence of an improvement or stabilization of both glucose and insulin responses (81). Insulin sensitivity has been shown to increase in humans and in animals. A 30–35% increase in insulin-stimulated glucose utilization has been reported following training (82). In healthy trained subjects of both sexes, insulin sensitivity is increased, and a smaller insulin response to glucose stimulation occurs than in untrained individuals (83, 84). Increased insulin sensitivity following training in women and men 20 to 67 years old was reported to be highly correlated with training-increased $\dot{V}O_2$ max (85). No gender difference was reported. Resistive exercise training has also been reported to improve metabolic control of glucose (86, 87). Van Dam and associates (87) compared the effects of endurance and resistive training on glucose tolerance and insulin sensitivity in postmenopausal women who exercised three times a week for 6 months either on a treadmill (75–85% maximum heart rate) or by lifting weights (maximal effort in each of the major muscle groups). Glucose tolerance and insulin responses were improved in both exercise groups compared to a control group with a greater improvement in the treadmill group (87). The improved metabolic profile, regardless of type of exercise stimulus, is thought to result from improved glucose clearance caused by decreased resistance to insulin at the skeletal muscle (81). Interruption or cessation of training results in decreased glucose tolerance; the training effect is no longer evident after 5 to 7 days of rest (88).

Some controversy exists as to whether endurance training improves glucose tolerance that is already normal (46). Seals et al. (89) reported no change in glucose tolerance that was normal initially in men and women aged 60 to 69 years of age following 1 year of endurance training. However, the insulin response was decreased 8% following 6 months of low-intensity training and further decreased by 23% after an additional 6 months of high-intensity training. Hersey et al. (90) reported significantly improved glucose metabolism as well as decreased insulin after 6 months of endurance training by healthy women aged 70 to 79 years. Shimokata et al. (91) explain the decrease in glucose tolerance that occurs from early adulthood to middle age as a secondary influence of fitness levels and body composition. Holloszy et al. (92) suggest that exercise may be effective in normalizing glucose tolerance in individuals of all ages who are able to secrete insulin and for whom insulin resistance is a problem.

Training appears to improve long-term regulation of hyperglycemia, increase insulin sensitivity, and decrease plasma insulin levels in NIDDM. Studies of physical training in NIDDM have reported no differences in response according to gender. Many of these studies have had predominantly female subjects yet have not addressed the potential effects of hormonal status on the exercise response in NIDDM. Physical activity is also associated with decreased insulin requirements for insulin-dependent diabetes mellitus (81).

Lipid Profile. Although early studies reported only total cholesterol levels, physical activity appears to exert its primary favorable effects on the high-density lipoprotein-2 (HDL_2) subfraction of cholesterol and on triglyceride levels of exercising women. A transient increase in HDL following acute exercise has been reported and is thought to be related to increased lipoprotein lipase (LPL) and clearance of the very low density lipoprotein of triglyceride (93). Although exact mechanisms are unclear, an increase in both adipose and muscle LPL occurs with exercise. Repeated or habitual exercise is frequently associated with high HDL levels (discussed below). However, in some cases, reciprocal changes in subfractions HDL_2 and HDL_3 following exercise may result in no change in total HDL levels (94). In women, HDL concentration appears to be closely associated with training volume, as it is in men (95), but the female response to moderate exercise may be different from the male response (96, 97). However, potential confounders, such as menopausal status, exogenous hormone use (either oral contraceptives or hormone replacement therapy), cigarette smoking, alcohol consumption, dietary composition, or changes in body weight or body composition are numerous and make interpretation of exercise effects difficult. In particular, the effects of body weight and composition are difficult to separate from pure exercise effects. For example, Marti et al. (62) suggest that since leisure-time activity is a strong predictor of waist-hip ratios and percentage of body fat, the effects attributed to activity are not independent but are mediated by body fat content and distribution (WHR).

Nonetheless, many cross-sectional studies have reported that women who engage in endurance exercise have a more favorable lipid profile than inactive women (80, 98–102). For example, high-density lipoproteins have been reported to be higher and triglyceride levels lower in individuals of both genders participating in a range of different activities, including tennis as well as more traditional aerobic exercise training such as running or jogging (103). The relationship to training volume is evident in several studies. One study reported that HDL levels in women (aged 24 to 58 years) were directly related to weekly training distances. HDL in distance runners (50 km/week) was 78mg/dL, in recreational joggers (20 km/week) 70 mg/dL, and in inactive controls, 62 mg/dL (80, 98). The mean ages of these groups were not different, suggesting that menopausal status (pre- or postmenopause) may have been similar. None of the subjects were taking oral contraceptives or hormone replacement therapy. Significant differences among these groups remained after adjustment for dietary intake and body fat content. More recently, Durstine et al. (104) reported similar results with HDL cholesterol levels of 69, 69, 59, and 55 mg/dL for elite women distance runners, good local runners, recreational runners, and sedentary women, respectively. Additionally, the apolipoprotein A-I concentration, which is also inversely related to coronary risk, was higher in the elite and good runners (105). In women who were at least 1 year past the menopause and were not undergoing hormone replacement therapy, Cauley et al. (106) reported that physical activity was related to HDL only when more than 2000 kcal/week were expended in activity.

Physical fitness level, based on treadmill time, has also been reported to be significantly related to HDL concentration in healthy women aged 18 to 65 years old (107). In this study, the association was independent of age and weight. Not all studies, however, have been able to find an independent relationship between fitness or activity level and lipid profile. Haskell et al. (108) found no consistent trends in the association between HDL and exercise tolerance in a large group of women during a treadmill test.

Results of prospective training studies are similar, many demonstrating positive effects (46, 109–111) and others failing to demonstrate significant modifications in the lipid profile (46, 80, 112, 113). The gender difference in response to moderate exercise may account for some of the discrepancy in the results. Ballantyne et al. (112) reported that women who exercised three times/week for 6 months had no increase in HDL, whereas men following the same program increased HDL significantly. Similarly, Brownell et al. (113) reported a 5.1% increase in HDL in men, but a 1% decrease in women, both exercising for 15 to 20 minutes/session at 70% maximum heart rate, three times/week for 10 weeks. HDL has been reported to increase in men following only 1 week of moderate exercise and no change in aerobic capacity (96, 97). The reason for this gender difference is unclear, but it may be related to the generally more favorable lipid profile of premenopausal women and in particular to higher lipoprotein lipase levels in women. Nikkila et al. (114) reported that LPL activity in sedentary premenopausal women was higher than that in male long distance runners.

Exercise volume (intensity, duration, and frequency), as suggested by cross-sectional studies, is critical to the interpretation of prospective studies. For example, Notelovitz (81) found that an exercise program lasting up to 2 years, in which $\dot{V}O_2$ max was increased, had no effect on triglycerides, total cholesterol, or HDL in women aged 40 to 65 years. Notelovitz postulated that the exercise intensity (70% maximum heart rate, < 30 minutes/session three times/week) was not high enough to elicit changes and suggested that 3 to 4 months of fairly strenuous activity (running 10 to 15 miles/week or walking 30 miles/week) is necessary to increase HDL. Rotkis et al. (109) reported that women runners (aged 23 to 37 years) were able to increase HDL levels from 53.5 to 58 mg/dL ($p < .01$) after increasing their average weekly mileage from 13.5 to 44.9 miles over a 4- to 7-month period. The data of Seals et al. (89) suggest an exercise intensity–duration threshold needed to achieve lipid changes in both women and men aged 60 to 69 years old. By walking three times/week for less than 30 minutes/session at 60% maximum heart rate for 6 months (low-intensity training), the older subjects were able to increase $\dot{V}O_2$ max by 12% but did not achieve any changes in lipids, lipoproteins, body weight or skinfold measurements. During the next 6 months, exercise intensity was increased to 80–90% maximum heart rate for 30 to 45 minutes/session. $\dot{V}O_2$ max increased an additional 18%, HDL increased 14%, triglycerides decreased 21%, and both body weight and skinfold measurements also decreased. Total cholesterol and LDL did not change. No gender difference was reported in this older group (88). In a group of older women (61 to 81 years), Whitehurst and Menendez (115) reported decreases in triglycerides and body fat accompanied by increases in HDL in a group of walkers compared to controls after only 8 weeks of walking three times a week but at intensities of 70–80% of predicted maximum heart rate for 40 minutes/session.

Most studies of exercise and lipids have been conducted with endurance exercise as the intervention. The effects of resistive exercise training on lipid profiles of women has been less well studied. In a cross-sectional study, lean women bodybuilders were found to have HDL levels similar to those of a group of lean, aerobically trained women (116). In a prospective study, a group of young women (24 to 30 years old) and men (30 to 36 years old) participated in a weight-lifting program three times a week for 16 weeks (117). Both women and men reduced LDL cholesterol significantly (18% and 16%, respectively). HDL tended to increase but not significantly for either group (women 4.8%; men 15.8%). The women significantly decreased triglyceride levels, but the men did not. Recently, the effects of a resistive exercise program on lipid profiles of obese women were studied (118). The training program resulted in a 58% increase in muscular strength but no change in any of the lipid or lipoprotein levels. The reasons for the difference in LDL and HDL response compared to aerobic exercise is not explained and needs further investigation.

EXERCISE AND SECONDARY PREVENTION OF CARDIOVASCULAR DISEASE

Cardiac Rehabilitation

Cardiac rehabilitation has the potential to improve exercise tolerance by either a change in central hemodynamics, a change in peripheral metabolic response, or both. A survey of cardiac rehabilitation outcomes in multiple studies suggests that exercise training is associated with decreased mortality (119). Two recent reviews of all published randomized trials of cardiac rehabilitation after myocardial infarction (MI) concurred that exercise rehabilitation reduced all-cause mortality by 20–24% and cardiovascular mortality by 23–25% but did not affect the incidence of nonfatal MI (120, 121). O'Connor et al. (120) also found that sudden death was reduced by 37%. Women, however, were included in only 3 of 22 trials and comprised only 143 of 4554 patients studied (3%). These small numbers, plus the limited reporting of outcome by gender in early studies that did include women, make any analysis of the impact of cardiac rehabilitation on the treatment of women impossible. Studies of the effects of exercise training on women heart patients are clearly needed to guide clinical care of women following myocardial infarction.

Patients with congestive heart failure (CHF) represent a unique population in cardiac rehabilitation programs. In patients with CHF, exercise tolerance is limited by fatigue and severe dyspnea. One study (122) reported safe and effective training in 10 patients (one woman) with severely depressed left ventricular function (ejection fraction < 27%). Conversely, Arvan (123) reported that patients with resting ejection fractions of < 40% and ischemia were not able to achieve an adequate training response from a 12-week phase II cardiac rehabilitation program. Although some women were included in this latter study, no comment was made on gender differences, suggesting either that none were observed or the number of women was too small to draw any conclusions. Ellestad (124) cautions that in certain subgroups of patients, such as those with large anterior myocardial infarctions, exercise may have a detrimental effect on left ventricular function and should be avoided.

Although the mechanisms that limit exercise tolerance in CHF are unclear, increased afterload for the right ventricle, increased work of breathing, and decreased oxygen delivery to skeletal muscle all play a part. Sullivan et al. (125) reported an increase in exercise tolerance (23% increase in $\dot{V}O_2$ max) after 4 to 6 months of exercise training in 12 patients (gender not identified) with chronic heart failure (ejection fraction < 24%). The increased $\dot{V}O_2$ max was attributed to an increased maximal cardiac output, increased a-v O_2 difference, increased peak blood flow to active skeletal muscles, and more efficient oxygen and substrate utilization. A 24% (68 second) increase in time to reach the ventilatory anaerobic threshold and a 52% (491 second) increase in submaximal exercise duration following exercise training were reported (126). During submaximal exercise, cardiac output and leg blood flow were unchanged, but blood lactate levels were reduced, suggesting that exercise tolerance was improved by peripheral metabolic or vascular factors. Further studies by Sullivan and Cobb (127) demonstrated that, as in normal subjects, exercise ventilation is closely related to CO_2 production. However, unlike normals, the $\dot{V}E/\dot{V}CO_2$ is increased in CHF. Ventilatory thresholds can be reliably determined, exercise training delays the onset of lactate accumulation, and this delay is associated with improved submaximal exercise tolerance. The evidence, minimal as it is, seems to indicate that exercise training may be helpful in the majority of CHF patients. Far more work is needed on this topic, particularly in terms of the exercise response of women with CHF.

Stroke

The role of exercise training in the secondary prevention of stroke has not been investigated. However, an ample literature on physical therapy demonstrates the usefulness of exercise training in regaining the ability to function independently (128). For this reason alone, physical activity should be included in stroke management.

Peripheral Arterial Disease

Peripheral arterial disease (PAD) affects women with approximately the same frequency as men (129). The major symptomatic manifestation of PAD, intermittent claudication, results in limitation of the ability to walk because of ischemia-induced pain. Although the effect of exercise training on exercise tolerance and the severity of claudication pain has been inadequately studied in women, the evidence from studies of male subjects suggests that exercise training does improve walking ability (130). For example, 19 men were randomly assigned to either a control group or a group that exercised for 1 hour three times/week for 12 weeks. In comparison with the control group, the exercise group increased $\dot{V}O_2$ max by 30% and walk time on a standard treadmill protocol by 123%. Postulated mechanisms associated with improved exercise capacity are improved efficiency of movement, improved peripheral blood flow, decreased blood viscosity, regression of disease or improvement in skeletal muscle metabolism by increased oxygen extraction, and increased oxidative energy production (130). Using an animal model for peripheral arterial insufficiency, Erney and associates (131) reported that better maintained muscle force development, higher peak oxygen uptake, and increased oxygen extraction occurred following 14 to 20 weeks of exercise training. Greater oxygen extraction or redistribution of the limited blood flow to better perfuse the active muscle are the mechanisms postulated to explain the improvements seen in humans. Although studies of exercise training in women with PAD are lacking, adequate information exists to recommend exercise as an important part of treatment in patients with peripheral arterial insufficiency (131, 132).

RISKS ASSOCIATED WITH EXERCISE

Cardiovascular Risks

The cardiovascular risks of exercise are small for the general population but may include cerebrovascular accidents, aortic dissection and rupture, cardiac arrhythmias, myocardial infarction, and sudden death (133, 134). Virtually no information is available on nonfatal cardiovascular complications of exercise in asymptomatic women. Gibbons et al. (135) did, however, calculate a maximal risk estimate (MRE) for the occurrence of a cardiac event during exercise based on 1001 women exercising 110,037 person-hours during a 65-month period. Although there were no cardiac events recorded during that time, MREs consistent with these data within 95% confidence limits were calculated to be between 0.6 and 6.0 events per 10,000 person-hours of exercise for women between 20 and 70 years of age (135). The incidence of sudden exercise-induced death in women is likewise unknown. In men over 30 years old, sudden exercise-related death is usually associated with atherosclerotic coronary artery disease. In general, sudden death in women is less likely to be associated with atherosclerotic heart disease than in men. Whether this is also true for sudden death during exercise is unknown. In younger individuals of both genders, sudden death is usually associated with a variety of cardiac abnormalities, such as hypertrophic cardiomyopathy, aortic stenosis, anomalous coronary arteries, myocarditis, and Marfan's syndrome (136). The relative risk to a young athlete according to gender has not been reported.

The cardiovascular risks during exercise for patients with coronary artery disease are based on data from supervised cardiac rehabilitation programs, in which women participants are few (137). For these reasons, the results may not be applicable to the entire population of heart patients or to women with heart disease. More information on the female response to exercise after heart disease is certainly needed.

Musculoskeletal Injury

Musculoskeletal injuries may occur as an unwanted consequence of exercise participation and are an important deterrent to continuing exercise (138, 139). The incidence of injury has been reported to be between 10 and 50% (140, 141) and is dependent mainly on exercise mode (140, 141) and rate of progression (142). Nonweight-bearing activities, such as stationary cycling or swimming, and low-impact activities such as walking have lower injury rates than high-impact activities such as jogging or aerobic dance. Increasing the intensity or duration of exercise at too fast a rate is a very common cause of injury. A rule of thumb is that exercise should be increased by no more than 10% per week (142). Recently, Pollock et al. (141) investigated the incidence of injury during walk-jog and resistance training programs in older men and women (70 to 79 years old). During a 26-week training program, 2 of 23 (8.6%) in the strength-training group were injured compared to 9 of 21 (42.9%) in the walk-jog group. Eight of the nine injuries in the latter group were associated with increased exercise intensity. In this small sample, two of eight men were injured compared with all six women in the walk-jog group. Further study is necessary to determine whether this is a true gender difference or a reflection of some other factor, such as greater musculoskeletal strength or the more active background characteristic of men. In younger athletic populations, exercise-induced injuries are no more likely in women than in men (143).

SUMMARY

The exercise response in women is in many respects no different from that of men. For example, women improve their fitness levels in the same manner and at the same rate as do men (35). An active lifestyle is associated with decreased incidence and severity of risk factors for cardiovascular disease for both men and women. Neither the mechanisms responsible nor the appropriate exercise dose have been adequately studied in women. The role of exercise in the secondary prevention of cardiovascular disease in women has also been inadequately studied but is potentially quite important. Although much remains to be learned, adequate information is available to justify recommending that exercise be a part of every woman's life.

References

1. Blair SN. Physical activity leads to fitness and pays off. *Physician Sportsmed* 13:145–150, 1985.
2. Harris SS, Caspersen CJ, DeFriese GH, et al. Physical activity counseling for healthy adults as a primary prevention intervention in the clinical setting. *JAMA* 261:3588–3598, 1989.
3. Shvartz E, Reibold RC. Aerobic fitness norms for males and females aged 6 to 75 years: A review. *Aviat Space Environ Med* 61:3–11, 1990.
4. Drinkwater BL. Women and exercise: Physiological aspects. *Exerc Sport Sci Rev* 12:21–51, 1984.
5. Pate RR, Sparling PB, Wilson GE, et al. Cardiorespiratory and metabolic responses to submaximal and maximal exercise in elite women distance runners. *Int J Sports Med* Suppl 8:91–95, 1987.
6. Drinkwater BL, Horvath SM, Wells CL. Aerobic power of females, ages 10 to 68. *J Gerontol* 30:385–394, 1975.
7. Stephens T. Secular trends in adult physical activity: Exercise boom or bust? *Res Q Exerc Sport* 58:94–105, 1987.
8. American College of Sports Medicine. Position statement on the recommended quantity and quality of exercise for developing and maintaining fitness in healthy adults. *Med Sci Sports* 10:vii, 1978.
9. Caspersen CJ, Christenson GM, Pollard RA. Status of the 1990 physical fitness and exercise objectives—Evidence from NHIS 1985. *Public Health Rep* 101:587–592, 1986.
10. Powell KE, PD Thompson, CJ Caspersen, et al. Physical activity and the incidence of coronary heart disease. *Ann Rev Public Health* 8:253–287, 1987.
11. Brunner D, Manelis G, Modan M, et al. Physical activity at work and the incidence of myocardial infarction, angina pectoris and death due to ischemic heart disease. An epidemiological study in Israeli collective settlements (kibbutzim). *J Chron Dis* 27:217–233, 1974.
12. Magnus K, Matroos A, Strackee J. Walking, cycling or gardening, with or without seasonal interruption, in relation to acute coronary events. *Am J Epidemiol* 110:724–733, 1979.
13. Salonen JT, Puska P, Tuomilehto J. Physical activity and risk of myocardial infarction, cerebral stroke and death: A longitudinal study in eastern Finland. *Am J Epidemiol* 115:526–537, 1982.
14. Kannel WB, Sorlie P. Some health benefits of physical activity. The Framingham Study. *Arch Intern Med* 139:857–861, 1979.
15. Lapidus L, Bengtsson C. Socioeconomic factors and physical activity in relation to cardiovascular disease and death: A 12 year follow up of participants in a population study of women in Gothenberg, Sweden. *Br Heart J* 55:295–301, 1986.
16. Marti B, Tuomilehto J, Salonen JT, et al. Relationship between leisure-time physical activity and risk factors for coronary heart disease in middle-aged Finnish women. *Acta Med Scand* 222:223–230, 1987.
17. Salonen JT, Slater JS, Tuomilehto J, et al. Leisure-time and occupational physical activity: Risk of death from ischemic heart disease. *Am J Epidemiol* 127:87–94, 1988.
18. Blair SN, Kohl HW, Paffenbarger RS, et al. Physical fitness and all-cause mortality. A prospective study of healthy men and women. *JAMA* 262(17):2395–2401, 1989.
19. Hammond HK, Froelicher VF. The physiologic sequelae of chronic dynamic exercise. *Med Clin North Am* 69(1):21–39, 1985.
20. O'Toole ML. Gender differences in the cardiovascular response to exercise. In Douglas PS (Ed.), *Heart Disease in Women*. Philadelphia, F.A. Davis, pp. 17–33, 1989.
21. Hill DW, Butler SD. Haemodynamic responses to weightlifting exercise. *Sports Med* 12:1–7, 1991.
22. O'Toole ML, Douglas PS. Fitness: definition and development. In Shangold MM, Mirkin G (Eds.), *Women and Exercise*. Philadelphia, F.A. Davis, pp. 3–19, 1988.
23. Clausen JP. Effect of physical training on cardiovascular adjustments to exercise in man. *Physiol Rev* 57:779–815, 1977.
24. Ekelund LG, Holmgren A. Central hemodynamics

during exercise. *Circ Res* 21 Suppl. 1:1-33–1-43, 1967.
25. Astrand P-O, Cuddy TE, Saltin B, et al. Cardiac output during submaximal and maximal work. *J Appl Physiol* 19:268–274, 1964.
26. Becklake MR, Frank J, Dagenais GR, et al. Influence of age and sex on exercise cardiac output. *J Appl Physiol* 20:938–947, 1965.
27. Sullivan MJ, Cobb FR, Higginbotham MB. Stroke volume increases by similar mechanisms during upright exercise in normal men and women. *Am J Cardiol* 67:1405–1412, 1991.
28. Miles DS, Critz JB, Knowlton RG. Cardiovascular, metabolic, and ventilatory responses of women to equivalent cycle ergometer and treadmill exercise. *Med Sci Sports Exerc* 12:14–19, 1980.
29. Higginbotham MB, Morris KG, Coleman E, et al. Sex-related differences in the normal cardiac response to upright exercise. *Circulation* 70:357–366, 1984.
30. Rodeheffer RJ, Gerstenblith G, Becker LC, et al. Exercise cardiac output is maintained with advancing age in healthy human subjects: Cardiac dilatation and increased stroke volume compensate for a diminished heart rate. *Circulation* 69:703–710, 1984.
31. Blomqvist CG, Saltin B. Cardiovascular adaptations to physical training. *Ann Rev Physiol* 45:169–189, 1983.
32. Kilblom A, Astrand I. Physical training with submaximal intensities in women. II. Effect on cardiac output. *Scand J Clin Lab Invest* 28:163–175, 1971.
33. Flint MM, Drinkwater BL, Horvath SM. Effects of training on women's response to submaximal exercise. *Med Sci Sports Exerc* 6:89–94, 1974.
34. Getchell LH, Moore JC. Physical training: Comparative responses of middle-aged adults. *Arch Phys Med Rehabil* 56:250–254, 1975.
35. Lewis DA, Kamon E, Hodgson JL. Physiological differences between genders: Implications for sports conditioning. *Sports Med* 3:357–369, 1986.
36. Lewis SF, Snell PG, Taylor WF, et al. Role of muscle mass and mode of contraction in circulatory responses to exercise. *J Appl Physiol* 58:146–151, 1985.
37. Morganroth J, Maron BJ, Henry WL, et al. Comparative left ventricular dimensions in trained athletes. *Ann Intern Med* 82:521–524, 1975.
38. Roy A, Doyon M, Dumesnil JG, et al. Endurance vs strength training: Comparison of cardiac structures using predicted normal values. *J Appl Physiol* 64:2552–2557, 1988.
39. George KP, Wolfe LA, Burggraf GW. The "athletic heart syndrome." *Sports Med* 11:300–331, 1991.
40. Fleck SJ. Cardiovascular adaptations to resistance training. *Med Sci Sports Exerc* 20:S146–S151, 1988.
41. Charette SL, McEvoy L, Pyka G, et al. Muscle hypertrophy response to resistance training in older women. *J Appl Physiol* 70:1912–1916, 1991.
42. George KP. Electro- and echocardiographic assessment of female athletes. Master's Thesis, Queen's University, Kingston, Ontario, 1990.
43. Rubal BJ, Al-Muhailani AR, Rosentsweig J. Effects of physical conditioning on the heart size and wall thickness of college women. *Med Sci Sports Exerc* 19:423–429, 1987.
44. Saar E, Chayot R, Meyerstein N. Physical activity and blood pressure in normotensive young women. *Eur J Appl Physiol* 55:64–67, 1986.
45. Blair SN, Goodyear NN, Gibbons LW, et al. Physical fitness and incidence of hypertension in healthy normotensive men and women. *JAMA* 252:487–490, 1984.
46. Marti B. Health effects of recreational running in women. Some epidemiological and preventive aspects. *Sports Med* 11:20–51, 1991.
47. Kral J, Chrastek J, Adamirova J. The hypotensive effect of physical activity. In Raab A (Ed.), *Prevention of Ischemic Heart Disease: Principles and Practice*. Springfield, IL, Charles C Thomas, 1966.
48. Tipton CM. Exercise, training and hypertension: An update. In Holloszy JO (Ed.), *Exercise and Sport Science Reviews*. Baltimore, Williams & Wilkins, 1991, pp 447–505.
49. Kaufman FL, Hughson RL, Schaman JP. Effect of exercise on recovery blood pressure in normotensive and hypertensive subjects. *Med Sci Sports Exerc* 19:17–20, 1987.
50. Paulev P-E, Jordal R, Kristensen O, et al. Therapeutic effect of exercise on hypertension. *Eur J Appl Physiol* 53:180–185, 1984.
51. Hagberg JM, Montain SJ, Martin WH. Blood pressure and hemodynamic responses after exercise in older hypertensives. *J Appl Physiol* 63:270–276, 1987.
52. Jennings G, Nelson L, Nestel P, et al. The effects of changes in physical activity on major cardiovascular risk factors, hemodynamics, sympathetic function, and glucose utilization in man: A controlled study of four levels of activity. *Circulation* 73:30–40, 1986.
53. Nelson L, Jennings GL, Ester MD, et al. Effect of changing levels of physical activity on blood pressure and haemodynamics in essential hypertension. *Lancet* 2:473–476, 1986.
54. Urata H, Tanabe Y, Kiyonaga A, et al. Antihypertensive and volume-depleting effects of mild exercise on essential hypertension. *Hypertension* 9:245–252, 1987.
55. Seals DR, Hagberg JM. The effect of exercise training on human hypertension: A review. *Med Sci Sports Exerc* 16(3):207–215, 1984.
56. Hagberg JM, Seals DR. Exercise training and hypertension. *Acta Med Scand* Suppl 711:131–136, 1986.
57. Roman O, Camuzzi AL, Villalon E, et al. Physical training program in arterial hypertension: A long-term prospective follow-up. *Cardiology* 67:230–241, 1981.
58. Tipton CM, Mathes RD, Marcus KD, et al. Influences of exercise intensity, age and medication on resting systolic blood pressure of SHR populations. *J Appl Physiol* 55:1305–1310, 1983.
59. MacDougal JD, Tuxen D, Sale DG, et al. Arterial blood pressure response to heavy resistance exercise. *J Appl Physiol* 58:785–790, 1985.
60. Harris KA, Holly RG. Physiological responses to circuit weight training in borderline hypertensive subjects. *Med Sci Sports Exerc* 19:246–252, 1987.
61. Blair SN, Jacobs DR, Powell KE. Relationships between exercise or physical activity and other health habits. *Public Health Rep* 100:172–180, 1985.
62. Marti B, Salonen JT, Tuomilehto J, et al. 10-year trends in physical activity in the eastern Finnish adult population: Relationship to socioeconomic and lifestyle characteristics. *Acta Med Scand* 224:195–203, 1988.
63. Marti B, Suter E, Riesen WF, et al. Anthropometric

and lifestyle correlates of serum lipoprotein and apolipoprotein levels among normal non-smoking men and women. *Atherosclerosis* 75:111–122, 1989.
64. Kaye SA, Folsom AR, Prineas RJ, et al. The association of body fat distribution with lifestyle and reproductive factors in a population study of postmenopausal women. *Int J Obesity* 14:583–591, 1990.
65. Shangold MM. Exercise in the menopausal woman. *Obstet Gynecol* Suppl 75(4):53S–58S, 1990.
66. Brownell KD, Rubin CJ, Smoller JW. Exercise and regulation of body weight. In Shangold M, Mirkin G (Eds.), *Women and Exercise*. Philadelphia, F.A. Davis, 1988, pp. 40–54.
67. Cowan MM, Gregory LW. Responses of pre- and post-menopausal females to aerobic conditioning. *Med Sci Sports Exerc* 17:138–143, 1985.
68. Gwinup G. Weight loss without dietary restriction: Efficacy of different forms of aerobic exercise. *Am J Sports Med* 15:275–279, 1987.
69. Despres JP, Tremblay A, Nadeau A, et al. Physical training and changes in regional adipose tissue distribution. *Acta Med Scand* [Suppl] 723:205–212, 1988.
70. Franklin B, Buskirk E, Hodgson J, et al. Effects of physical conditioning on cardiorespiratory function, body composition and serum lipids in relatively normal-weight and obese middle-aged women. *Int J Obesity* 3:97–109, 1979.
71. Epstein LH, Wing RR. Aerobic exercise and weight. *Addictive Behaviors* 5:371–388, 1980.
72. Wood PD, Stefanick ML, Williams PT, et al. The effects on plasma lipoproteins of a prudent weight-reducing diet, with or without exercise, in overweight men and women. *N Engl J Med* 325:461–466, 1991.
73. Bjorntorp P, de Jounge K, Sjostrom L, et al. Physical training in human obesity. II. Effects of plasma insulin in glucose-intolerant subjects without marked hyperinsulinemia. *Scand J Clin Lab Invest* 32:41–45, 1973.
74. DeFronzo RA, Sherwin RS, Kraemer N. Effect of physical training on insulin action in obesity. *Diabetes* 36:1379–1385, 1987.
75. Krotkiewski M, Bjorntorp P. Muscle tissue in obesity with different distribution of adipose tissue: Effects of physical training. *Int J Obesity* 10:331–341, 1986.
76. Bjorntorp P, Fahlen M, Grimby G, et al. Carbohydrate and lipid metabolism in middle-aged, physically well-trained men. *Metabolism* 21:1037–1044, 1972.
77. Lohmann D, Liebold F, Heilmann W, et al. Diminished insulin response in highly trained athletes. *Metabolism* 27:521–542, 1978.
78. Frisch RE, Wyshak G, Albright TE, et al. Lower prevalence of diabetes in female former athletes compared with nonathletes. *Diabetes* 35:1101–1105, 1986.
79. Mikines KJ, Sonne B, Farrell PA, et al. Effect of physical exercise on sensitivity and responsiveness to insulin in humans. *Am J Physiol* 254:E248–E259, 1988.
80. Devlin JT, Hirshman M, Horton ED, et al. Enhanced peripheral and splanchnic insulin sensitivity in NIDDM men after single bout of exercise. *Diabetes* 36:434–439, 1987.
81. Notelovitz M. Exercise and health maintenance in menopausal women. *Ann NY Acad Sci* 592:204–220, 1990.
82. Horton ES. Exercise and physical training: Effects on insulin sensitivity and glucose metabolism. *Diabetes Metab Rev* 2:1–17, 1986.
83. King DS, Dalsky GP, Staten MA, et al. Insulin action and secretion in endurance-trained and untrained humans. *J Appl Physiol* 63:2247–2252, 1987.
84. King DS, Dalsky GP, Clutter WE, et al. Effects of exercise and lack of exercise on insulin sensitivity and responsiveness. *J Appl Physiol* 64:1942–1946, 1988.
85. Rosenthal M, Haskell WL, Solomon R, et al. Demonstration of a relationship between level of physical training and insulin-stimulated glucose utilization in normal humans. *Diabetes* 32:408–411, 1983.
86. Miller WJ, Sherman WM, Ivy JL. Effect of strength training on glucose tolerance and post-glucose insulin response. *Med Sci Sports Exerc* 16:539–543, 1984.
87. Van Dam S, Gillespy M, Notelovitz M, et al. Effect of exercise on glucose metabolism in postmenopausal women. *Am J Obstet Gynecol* 159:82–86, 1988.
88. Burstein R, Polychronakos C, Toews CJ, et al. Acute reversal of the enhanced insulin action in trained athletes: Association with insulin receptor changes. *Diabetes* 34:756–760, 1985.
89. Seals DR, Hagberg JM, Hurley BF, et al. Effects of endurance training on glucose tolerance and plasma lipid levels in older men and women. *JAMA* 252:645–649, 1984.
90. Hersey WC, Hagberg J, Graves J, et al. Effect of exercise training on glucose metabolism in healthy 70–79 year old men and women (Abstract). *Med Sci Sports Exerc* Suppl 21:S45, 1989.
91. Shimokata H, Muller DC, Fleg JL, et al. Age as an independent determinant of glucose tolerance. *Diabetes* 40:44–51, 1991.
92. Holloszy JO, Schultz J, Kusni J, et al. Effects of exercise on glucose tolerance and insulin resistance: Brief review and some preliminary results. *Acta Med Scand* Suppl 711:55–65, 1986.
93. Goodyear LJ, Van Houten, Fronsoe MS, et al. Immediate and delayed effects of marathon running on lipids and lipoproteins in women. *Med Sci Sports Exerc* 22(5):588–592, 1990.
94. Rauramaa R, Salonen JT, Kukkonen-Harjula K, et al. Effects of mild physical exercise on serum lipoproteins and metabolites of arachidonic acid: A controlled randomised trial in middle aged men. *Br Med J* 288:603–606, 1984.
95. Hartung GH, Foreyt JP, Mitchell RE, et al. Relationship of diet to HDL-cholesterol in middle-aged marathon runners, joggers and inactive men. *N Engl J Med* 302:357–361, 1980.
96. Castelli WP. Exercise and high-density lipoproteins (Editorial). *JAMA* 242:2217, 1979.
97. Streja D, Mymin D. Moderate exercise and high-density lipoprotein cholesterol: Observations during a cardiac rehabilitation program. *JAMA* 242:2190–2192, 1979.
98. Moore CE, Hartung GH, Mitchell RE, et al. The relationship of exercise and diet on high-density lipoprotein cholesterol levels in women. *Metabolism* 32(2):189–196, 1983.
99. Vodak PA, Wood PD, Haskell WL, et al. HDL-cholesterol and other plasma lipid and lipoprotein concentrations in middle-aged male and female tennis players. *Metabolism* 29(8):745–752, 1980.
100. Hartung GH, Moore EC, Mitchell R. Relationship of menopausal status and exercise level to HDL cholesterol in women. *Exp Aging* 10:13–18, 1984.

101. Sallis JF, Haskell WL, Wood PD, et al. Vigorous physical activity and cardiovascular risk factors in young adults. *J Chron Dis* 39:115–120, 1986.
102. Wood PD, Haskell WL, Stern S, et al. Plasma lipoprotein distributions in male and female runners. *Ann NY Acad Sci* 301:748–763, 1977.
103. Wood PD, Haskell WL. The effect of exercise on plasma high density lipoproteins. *Lipids* 14(4):417–427, 1979.
104. Durstine JL, Pate RR, Sparling PB, et al. Lipid, lipoprotein, and iron status of elite women distance runners. *Int J Sports Med* (Suppl. 2) 8:119–123, 1987.
105. Durstine JL, Pate RR, Bartoli WP, et al. Apolipoproteins AI and B in elite women runners (abstract). *Med Sci Sports Exerc* 21 (Suppl.):S113, 1989.
106. Cauley JA, Laporte RE, Kuller LH, et al. The epidemiology of high density lipoprotein cholesterol levels in post-menopausal women. *J Gerontol* 37:10–15, 1982.
107. Gibbons LW, Blair SN, Cooper KH, et al. Association between coronary heart disease risk factors and physical fitness in healthy adult women. *Circulation* 67:977–983, 1983.
108. Haskell WL, Taylor HL, Wood PD, et al. Strenuous physical activity, treadmill exercise test performance and plasma high density lipoprotein cholesterol: The Lipid Research Clinics Program Prevalence Study. *Circulation* 62 (Suppl IV):53–61, 1980.
109. Rotkis T, Boyden TW, Pamenter W, et al. High density lipoprotein cholesterol and body composition of female runners. *Metabolism* 30(10):994–995, 1981.
110. Goodyear LJ, Fronsoe MS, Van Houten DR, et al. Increased HDL-cholesterol following eight weeks of progressive endurance training in female runners. *Ann Sports Med* 3:33–38, 1986.
111. Hill JO, Thiel J, Heller PA, et al. Differences in effects of aerobic exercise training on blood lipids in men and women. *Am J Cardiol* 63:254–256, 1989.
112. Ballantyne D, Clark A, Dyker GS, et al. Prescribing exercise for the healthy: assessment of compliance and effects on plasma lipids and lipoproteins. *Health Bull* 32:169–176, 1978.
113. Brownell KD, Bachorik PS, Ayerle RS. Changes in plasma lipid and lipoprotein levels in men and women after a program of moderate exercise. *Circulation* 65:477–483, 1982.
114. Nikkila EA, Taskinen MR, Rehunen S, et al. Lipoprotein lipase activity in adipose tissue and skeletal muscle of runners: Relation to serum lipoproteins. *Metabolism* 27:1661–1667, 1978.
115. Whitehurst M, Menendez E. Endurance training in older women. Lipid and lipoprotein responses. *Physician Sportsmed* 19:95–102, 1991.
116. Elliot DL, Goldberg L, Kuehl KS, et al. Characteristics of anabolic-androgenic steroid-free competitive male and female bodybuilders. *Physician Sportsmed* 15:169–179, 1987.
117. Goldberg L, Elliot DL, Schutz RW, et al. Changes in lipid and lipoprotein levels after weight training. *JAMA* 252(4):504–506, 1984.
118. Manning JM, Dooly-Manning CR, et al. Effects of a resistive training program on lipoprotein-lipid levels in obese women. *Med Sci Sports Exerc* 23:1222–1226, 1991.
119. Dubach P, Froelicher VF. Cardiac rehabilitation for heart failure patients. *Cardiology* 76:368–373, 1989.
120. O'Connor GT, Buring JE, Yusuf S, et al. An overview of randomized trials of rehabilitation with exercise after myocardial infarction. *Circulation* 80:234–244, 1989.
121. May GS, Eberlein KA, Furberg CD, et al. Secondary prevention after myocardial infarction: A review of long term trials. *Prog Cardiovasc Dis* 24:331–352, 1982.
122. Conn EH, Williams RS, Wallace AG. Exercise responses before and after physical conditioning in patients with severely depressed left ventricular function. *Am J Cardiol* 49:296–300, 1982.
123. Arvan S. Exercise performance of the high risk acute myocardial infarction patient after cardiac rehabilitation. *Am J Cardiol* 62:197–201, 1988.
124. Ellestad MH. Is exercise harmful in ischemic heart disease? *Am J Noninvas Cardiol* 1:15–17, 1987.
125. Sullivan MJ, Higginbotham MB, Cobb FR. Exercise training in patients with severe left ventricular dysfunction. Hemodynamic and metabolic effects. *Circulation* 78:506–515, 1988.
126. Sullivan MJ, Higginbotham MB, Cobb FR. Exercise training in patients with chronic heart failure delays ventilatory anaerobic threshold and improves submaximal exercise performance. *Circulation* 79:324–329, 1989.
127. Sullivan MJ, Cobb FR. The anaerobic threshold in chronic heart failure. Relation to blood lactate, ventilatory basis, reproducibility, and response to exercise training. *Circulation* 81(Suppl. II): II-47–II-58, 1990.
128. Sarvner K, Levangie J. *Brunnstrom's Movement Therapy in Hemiplegia*. Philadelphia, J.B. Lippincott, 1992.
129. Criqui MH, Fronek A, Barrett-Connor E, et al. The prevalence of peripheral arterial disease in a defined population. *Circulation* 71:510–515, 1985.
130. Hiatt WR, Regensteiner JG, Hargarten ME, et al. Benefit of exercise conditioning for patients with peripheral arterial disease. *Circulation* 81:602–609, 1990.
131. Erney TP, Mathien GM, Terjung RL. Muscle adaptations in trained rats with peripheral arterial insufficiency. *Am J Physiol* 260 (*Heart Circ Physiol* 29):H445–H452, 1991.
132. Lungren F, Dahllof AG, Lundholm K, et al. Intermittent claudication-surgical reconstruction or physical training? *Ann Surg* 209:346–355, 1989.
133. Thompson PD. Cardiovascular hazards of physical activity. In Terjung R (Ed.), *Exercise and Sport Sciences Reviews* Vol. 10. The Franklin Institute, Philadelphia, 1982, pp. 208–235.
134. Thompson PD. The benefits and risks of exercise training in patients with chronic coronary artery disease. *JAMA* 259:1537–1539, 1988.
135. Gibbons LW, Cooper KH, Meyer BM, et al. The acute cardiac risk of strenuous exercise. *JAMA* 24:1799–1801, 1980.
136. McCaffrey FM, Braden DS, Strong WB. Sudden cardiac death in young athletes. *Am J Dis Child* 145:177–183, 1991.
137. Van Camp SP, Peterson RA. Cardiovascular complications of outpatient cardiac rehabilitation programs. *JAMA* 256:2696–2699, 1986.
138. Dishman RK, Sallis J, Orenstein D. The determinants of physical activity and exercise. *Public Health Rep* 100:158–180, 1985.
139. Pollock ML. Prescribing exercise for fitness and adherence. In Dishman RK (Ed.), *Exercise Adher-*

ence: Its Impact on Public Health. Champaign, IL, Human Kinetics Books, 1988, pp. 259–277.
140. Pollock ML, Gettman LR, Milesis CA, et al. Effects of frequency and duration of training on attrition and incidence of injury. *Med Sci Sports* 9:31–36, 1977.
141. Pollock ML, Carroll JF, Graves JE, et al. Injuries and adherence to walk/jog and resistance training programs in the elderly. *Med Sci Sports Exerc* 23:1194–1200, 1991.
142. O'Neill DB, Micheli LJ. Overuse injuries in the young athlete. *Clin Sports Med* 7(3):591–610, 1988.
143. O'Toole ML, Massimino FA, Hiller WDB, et al. Medical considerations in triathletes: The 1984 Hawaii Ironman Triathlon. *Ann Sports Med* 3:121–123, 1987.

CHAPTER 14

*Psychosocial and Environmental Correlates of Heart Disease**

SUZANNE G. HAYNES, Ph.D.
SUSAN M. CZAJKOWSKI, Ph.D.

During the past 15 years, several reviews have been published on the psychosocial precursors of cardiovascular disease in women (1–6). New observations and insights into this large body of literature will be discussed in this chapter. Controversies in the field will be highlighted, as well as suggestions and needs for future research. This chapter will cover the following topics: the relationship of socioeconomic status, employment status and multiple roles, type A behavior, hostility, depression, and social support to cardiovascular disease (CVD) and cardiovascular risk factors. The lessons learned during the past 15 years from a large body of literature suggest that psychosocial factors, home environment, and work environment are related to the development of cardiovascular disease in women.

SOCIOECONOMIC STATUS

During the last 10 years, scientists have recognized an inverse association between social class and heart disease in women. This research was highlighted by the landmark publication by Feldman el al. (7) showing a marked gradient of death rates from heart disease in women from 1971 to 1984 ranging from 14.0/1000 for women with 0 to 7 years of education to 7.5/1000 for women with 13 or

---
*All material in this chapter is in the public domain, with the exception of any borrowed figures or tables.

more years of education completed. The relative risks (RR) were highest for women aged 45 to 64 (RR = 2.55 for 0 to 7 vs. 12+ years of education), and somewhat lower among women aged 65 to 74 (1.53 for 0 to 7 vs. 12+ years). Even more striking was the fact that the decline in heart disease death rates from 1960 to the period 1971 to 1984 did not bring the rates of the lowest educated women (0 to 7 years of education) in 1971 to 1984 (14.0/1000) to rates comparable to those of the highest educated women (13+ years) in 1960 (12.6/1000). This 25-year gap in rates between the highest and lowest educated women was not explained by the standard coronary risk factors, suggesting other, more serious explanations such as poorer health care, lack of health insurance, sexual discrimination, unfavorable occupational conditions, or increased psychosocial stress as the reasons for higher risk among lower status women.

One of the most intriguing hypotheses as to why women of lower socioeconomic status have higher rates of cardiovascular disease was proposed by Krieger (8), who investigated the effects of discrimination and other forms of subordination and oppression on hypertension. In a study of 101 women aged 20 to 80 years in Alameda County, California, Krieger found that black women who stated that they usually accepted and kept quiet about unfair treatment were 4.4 times more likely to report hypertension than women who said they took action and talked to others (9). This association was not apparent for white women.

In a recent National Heart, Lung, and Blood Institute conference on Women, Behavior and Cardiovascular Disease, Krieger suggested that we need, along with better measures of social class measurement for women, new methodologies that measure and test the objective and subjective components of discrimination and internalized oppression in relation to hypertension as well as other forms of cardiovascular disease (8). It may be that some of the psychosocial variables we will discuss later in this chapter are mere reflections of discriminatory behavior toward the female gender, minority race, or lower socioeconomic groups.

EMPLOYMENT STATUS AND CARDIOVASCULAR DISEASE RISK

One of the most widely discussed and researched topics relating to women during the last decade has been the question "Is working outside the home detrimental to women's health?" The underlying reason for asking this question is curious because the question has rarely been asked about men. Obviously, if working outside the home is a problem for women, then it might also be a problem for men. As will be shown below, the more relevant question is "What occupations or conditions of work are detrimental to women's health?" The answer to this question has significant implications for both women and men and does not imply, as does the previous question, that the female sex is unequivocally affected by the workplace and therefore should refrain from working outside the home.

LaCroix and Haynes (10) reviewed the literature on gender differences in the health effects of workplace roles through 1986 and found that on the basis of nine published studies (11–19), working women appear to be healthier than nonemployed women according to several health indicators (e.g., sick days, limitations in activity, hospital days, incidence of coronary heart disease [CHD], levels of coronary risk factors, and so on). At that time there was limited evidence showing that working women may have a lesser risk of CHD by virtue of more favorable levels of serum cholesterol (10).

Since that review, several additional confirmatory studies have been published. Kritz-Silverstein et al. (20) recently reported data from 242 women aged 40 to 59 years in the Rancho Bernardo Study showing that risk factors favored employed women (20). Employed women smoked fewer cigarettes, drank less alcohol, exercised more, and had significantly lower fasting plasma glucose levels than unemployed women (20). Likewise, recent results from the first Monica Augsburg survey in Germany showed that the mean high-density lipoprotein (HDL) cholesterol level was significantly higher in employed women (64.2 mg/dL) compared with homemakers (62.1 mg/dL), after controlling for a large number of other risk factors including alcohol consumption (21). These studies confirmed the earlier findings by Hazuda et al. (18) in the San Antonio Heart Study, who also found significantly higher HDL levels in employed women compared with homemakers after controlling for a number of other risk factors including alcohol consumption.

Previous studies from the Framingham cohort in the 1960s showed relatively few differences between working women and housewives in the standard coronary risk factors of blood pressure, cigarette smoking, and glucose intolerance (22). In a more contemporary (1987) study of executive women from a professional women's organization, LaRosa (23) found that fewer of these women smoked, but three times as many reported heavy drinking ($\geq$ 25 drinks of alcohol a week) as a matched control from the Centers for Disease Control (CDC) Health Risk Appraisal surveys. However, no statistical testing was reported in that study. In a recent report from the Tecumseh Community Health Study, no significant differences were found in the proportion of women smoking cigarettes at a 1978 to 1979 follow-up for employed women or homemakers (24). However, the proportion of women consuming alcoholic beverages was significantly higher for employed women than for homemakers both at baseline (1959 to 1960) and at follow-up (1978 to 1979). Although these recent studies suggest a higher alcohol consumption in working women, this higher level does not seem to have had a detrimental effect on heart disease and does not seem to explain the higher HDL levels reported above.

These recent and consistent findings of an HDL advantage for working women compared to housewives confirm the preponderance of data showing that employment per se is not detrimental to women's cardiovascular health. In addition, Kotler and Wingard (25) have recently shown in an 18-year follow-up of the Alameda County Study that employed women and housewives did not differ in total mortality risk. Thus, given the consistency of results of studies of employment status, it is probably more appropriate for future research to focus attention on those conditions of work or those selected occupations for which there may be excess cardiovascular risk. This will be discussed in the next section.

OCCUPATIONAL STATUS AND CARDIOVASCULAR DISEASE RISK

In a recent compendium of the latest research on women, work, and health (2), several investigators reported certain conditions of work that pose some cardiovascular risk for women. In a review of eight large epidemiologic studies, Haynes (26) found that most studies of women workers found an elevated prevalence of acute symptoms and chronic health problems (including coronary heart disease) among clerical or sales workers compared with other workers. Cardiovascular mortality rates were elevated in some clerical and sales workers in a Wisconsin study (27), whereas no significant elevations in total mortality were observed in the Tecumseh, Michigan, cohort (28). Since that review, a few additional studies have been published, and again, not all results were consistent. A review of occupational mortality of California women during 1979 to 1981 found high mortality risks among telephone operators; standardized mortality ratios of 156 for ischemic heart disease were found (29). Data from an earlier cohort in Alameda County, California, however, showed no excess risks in all-cause mortality (25). Schlussel et al. (30) reported a significant relationship of clerical occupations to systolic blood pressure in seven New York City work sites. These new studies suggest that clerical work may be associated specifically with death from cardiovascular disease but not with total mortality from all diseases.

The elevations in heart disease mortality observed in telephone operators in California supports research conducted over the last decade on the health effects of video display terminal (VDT) work. In a review of seven cross-sectional studies on the effects of VDTs, Haynes (26) found increased health problems among VDT users compared with nonusers. Although most of the problems were related to fatigue, musculoskeletal pain, anxiety, headaches, and other psychosomatic symptoms, angina pectoris was reported twice as often among VDT workers as in non-VDT workers in a North Carolina study of telephone operators and clerical workers (31). Four studies have reported higher levels of job demands or lower levels of decision making among frequent users of VDTs, indicating one psychosocial mechanism for the reportably higher rates of health problems among clerical workers who use VDTs (26).

One additional occupational group among women that appears to be vulnerable to cardiovascular disease risk is nursing, which is also considered a high-strain (high demand, low control) occupation. The California Mortality Study of women cited previously (29) found that licensed vocational nurses and aides had standardized mortality ratios of 201 (i.e., two times higher than the mortality rates expected). Haynes also reviewed previous studies on nurses, for whom low job control or high workload was associated with poorer job satisfaction, more physiologic symptoms (elevated plasma catecholamines, high systolic blood pressure, and sleep disturbances), or more reports of irritability and stress than were seen in nurses without these work conditions (26). Further studies are needed to confirm whether high-strain conditions in nursing occupations are associated with higher cardiovascular risk.

In conclusion, studies to date suggest that employment per se is not associated with excess risk of coronary heart disease. However, occupations involving clerical work, work using video display terminals, and work that has low control coupled with high demands may be associated with higher morbidity and mortality from heart disease. The work experience of women in the studies noted above may be explained by five important observations made by Hall (32), who studied over 13,000 Swedish working men and women. First, in Sweden as in the United States, women and men are confined to working in jobs that are highly sex segregated. Second, women have fewer occupations and those of a less diverse character from which to choose than men. Third, women have less control over the content and process of their work than men. Fourth, women have less work control than men even in female-segregated jobs. Fifth, white collar workers of both sexes have more control than blue collar workers, but men still have more control regardless of occupation.

These findings support the notion that the source of women's difficulties in certain occupations may be the product of their position within the organization of society as a whole (33). Taking this idea one step further suggests that gender discrimination, as defined by lack of control and decision-making authority for women compared with men in the workplace, may be the key factor explaining the higher rates of heart disease morbidity and mortality in some women's occupations. This intriguing hypothesis should be tested in longitudinal epidemiologic studies.

MULTIPLE ROLES

The risk of women's occupational risk of heart disease has been shown in some previous studies to be heightened by the presence of marital or child-rearing responsibilities (12). For example, in Framingham the 8-year incidence of coronary heart disease increased among women working outside the home as the number of children increased. This effect was particularly marked among clerical workers, for whom the rates were over twice as high in clerical workers with children compared with nonclerical workers with no children (15.4% vs. 6.3%) (12). This effect in clerical workers was not seen in single women or in women without children. Research during the last decade has refined and helped to explain some of these associations. Data from a case-control study of stroke and myocardial infarction in the United Kingdom showed that single women had a significantly lower risk of stroke and myocardial infarction than married women (relative risk 0.49) (34). Although the investigators analyzed parity (0 vs. any) and found no association, they did not stratify the analysis by employment status, nor did they look at parity as a continuous variable (34).

Based on several studies done in the last decade, the excess risks may not be due to the role occupied per se but rather to the quality of the experience within women's social roles (i.e., the balance between rewarding and distressing role attitudes) (33). For example, in a recent study of 202 professional women, career sacrifice and interpersonal sacrifice were significantly associated with self-reported major symptoms of cardiovascular disease (35). Likewise, role integration (i.e., the balance between role stress and role satisfaction for the three roles of employee, spouse, and mother) was significantly associated with perceived health and psychological symptoms in 87 female clerical workers in California (36). Barnett and Marshall (37) recently found in 403 Massachusetts women aged 25 to 55 employed in social work and licensed practical nursing that partner-role quality did not affect the relationship between work overload and psychological distress, nor did having children. However, social work is not generally considered a high-strain occupation, so that the effects noted in this study are unclear. This raises the issue of whether the bearing of multiple children has a psychological as opposed to a physiologic effect on heart disease risk in women.

PSYCHOPHYSIOLOGIC EFFECTS OF MULTIPLE ROLES AND WORK STRESS

Some of the most innovative research in the area of work stress and heart disease has come from studies that have looked at employed women at work, at home, and during sleep for a number of psychophysiologic dimensions. James et al. (38) examined ambulatory blood pressure in 50 normotensive working women employed in technical and clerical jobs. The average blood pressures were 116/78 mmHg at work, 113/74 mmHg at home, and 102/63 mmHg during sleep. A stressful job significantly predicted systolic blood pressure at work, at home, and during sleep in these women. Potential sources of domestic stress were also associated with blood pressure: being married was associated with higher diastolic pressures at work, and having children was significantly associated with higher systolic and diastolic pressures at home (39).

Similar findings have been observed in Sweden by Frankenhaeuser et al. (40), who observed significant norepinephrine excretion after work among female managers at Volvo, although this was not observed among clerical women. Further studies of this genre are needed to help explain the physiologic effects of multiple roles and occupational stress in women.

PERSONALITY AND EMOTIONAL FACTORS

A number of personality, emotional, and behavioral variables have been investigated as possible predictors of CHD in men, and some of these have been linked to CHD incidence and risk in women as well. The main factors considered here are (1) personality traits linked to the type A behavior pattern, such as hostility and related constructs, and (2) negative emotional states, such as depression and anxiety.

Hostility and Related Constructs

As a result of the inconsistent findings, most of them in men, relating the type A behavior pattern to CHD, researchers have focused on identifying components of the type A pattern that are predictive of CHD. The most promising components in this regard include hostility and its related constructs (e.g., the expression of anger), and several lines of research have now confirmed the important role played by hostility in the incidence and mortality of CHD (41–49).

Unfortunately, although hostility and its related constructs have been the subject of increasing efforts to document the aspects of the type A pattern that are most "toxic," these efforts have largely involved studies of men. When women are included, the sample sizes are often too small to permit gender-specific analyses. Thus, only a few studies have explored the relationship of type A components to CHD using sufficient samples of women (see Weidner [50] for a detailed review and critique).

The largest prospective study examining the relationship of type A behavior and its components to CHD in women is the Framingham study (51, 52). In this study, which followed 949 initially healthy women 45 to 77 years of age over an 8- to 10-year period, suppressed hostility (not showing or discussing anger) was found to predict total CHD and angina pectoris in univariate analyses in women under age 65 working outside the home but not in homemakers. However, in multivariate analyses which controlled for standard risk factors as well as for other significant behavioral variables, only the mode of anger expression characterized by not discussing anger remained a significant predictor of CHD and angina pectoris for women working outside the home, but again, not for homemakers. Thus, the Framingham study suggests that a construct that is related to hostility—not discussing anger—is an important factor in CHD incidence at least in one subgroup of women, those working outside the home.

The Life Change Event study followed a representative subsample (372 women and 324 men) of the Tecumseh Community Health study cohort who were 30 to 69 years old at baseline (1971 to 1972). At the 18-year follow-up, suppressed anger (measured by the Harburg Anger expression scale) was found to be a significant predictor of all-cause, CHD, and cancer mortality in women when traditional risk factors were controlled (53).

Another large-scale prospective study of 1462 women aged 38 to 60 years in Gothenburg, Sweden (54), used the Eysenck Personality Inventory and the Cesarec-Marke Personality Schedule to measure a variety of factors related to hostility, including aggression, dominance, and achievement, as well as a number of personality attributes related to neuroticism (passive dependency, neuroticism, and guilt feelings). Other psychosocial factors measured include experience of strain and psychiatric disorders (major and minor depression). Although they did not actually measure hostility and anger expression, the components of the type A behavior pattern most likely to be related to CHD, these investigators did find that low levels of aggression were related to electrocardiographic (ECG) changes indicative of ischemic heart disease. However, none of the other type A–like variables were significantly related to CHD.

Finally, a construct related to hostility—suspiciousness, as measured by Factor L of Cattell's 16PF scale—was found to predict total mortality in a sample of adults (240 women and 260 men) 46 to 71 years of age (55). Unfortunately, this study did not separate cardiovascular-specific deaths, although death due to CHD and other cardiovascular diseases comprised a large proportion of the total mortality figure (45.5% of deaths were due to CHD, and 16% were due to other cardiovascular diseases).

In conclusion, the prospective evidence relating hostility, anger expression, and other similar personality variables to CHD in initially healthy women is mixed. The strongest evidence shows a link between suppression of anger and CHD in women. However, where such evidence exists (51, 53, 55), type A–like components are related either to "softer" end points (e.g., in Framingham, total CHD included angina pectoris), or, as in the study by Barefoot et al. (55), to total mortality rather than CHD-specific mortality. In Julius et al. (53), the suppressed anger variable was related not only to CHD-specific mortality but to cancer and all-cause mortality as well. Further, it must be noted that few prospective studies have been conducted in women, and of those few, standard measures of type A components, such as hostility, were mostly not used (i.e., the Gothenburg study used personality measures that have not typically been used to assess hostility and anger).

In contrast to the few prospective studies of initially healthy women, studies of female coronary artery disease (CAD) patients and those using CHD risk factors as end points suggest that hostility and related affects may play a role in the etiology of CHD in women. For the most part, these studies have used more standard measures of hostility such as the Cook-Medley Hostility scale or structured interview-derived assessments. Several studies have documented a significant relationship between hostility, as measured by the Cook-Medley Hostility Inventory, and CAD severity in male and female angiography patients (56, 57). And in a recent series of studies, Barefoot et al. (58) found that a summary score of subjects' hostile behavior during a structured interview was significantly related to CAD severity in both men and women. The type of hostile behavior most highly related to CAD severity was the indirect challenge, an attempt to challenge the interviewer without direct confrontation. The evidence is not totally consistent in this regard, however. Helmer et al., using a measure derived from the structured interview (59), found a significant inverse relationship between hostility and CAD severity in a sample of 40 women. It is possible that, to some extent, the difference in findings may reflect differences in the scoring of the measures used (e.g., different criteria used for rating the more subtle aspects of hostile behavior, such as the subject's indirect challenge of the interviewer).

Although studies of CAD patients suggest a relationship between hostility and CAD severity in women, these studies are subject to biases inherent in cross-sectional studies using angiography patients (e.g., hostility may be a consequence, not a cause, of CAD; and biases may exist in samples presenting for angiography). However, studies relating hostility, anger, and related constructs to CHD risk factors provide further evidence that these factors may be important predictors of CHD for women. One longitudinal study showed that hostility, as measured by the Cook-Medley scale at age 19, predicted the total cholesterol-to-HDL ratio for men and women at age 42 (60). In addition, several cross-sectional studies have related hostility to lipid levels (61–63). And in a recent study of black and white men and women based on prospective data from the CARDIA study, Knox et al. (64) found a significant linear trend between hostility, as assessed by the Cook-Medley scale, and triglycerides in women. The trend became marginally significant (0.07) after controlling for Body Mass Index and smoking in white women and became nonsignificant after controlling for these factors in black women.

A number of studies have linked hostility to cardiovascular reactivity to stress in women (65–67). These findings are consistent across a variety of measures of hostility, including the Cook-Medley scale (66–67) and Spielberger's State-Trait Anger Scale (STAS) (65). In the latter study, white women showed significant relationships between the STAS-T and systolic and diastolic blood pressures at rest and during the Structured Interview, both of which are laboratory-based assessments. However, black women showed significant associations between the STAS-T and systolic and diastolic blood pressures during the cold pressor test. Furthermore, women, but not men, showed significant positive correlations between all the anger measures used (STAS-T, Framingham Anger Scale, Cognitive Anger, and Somatic Anger subscales of the Cognitive-Somatic Anger Scale) and ambulatory blood pressure at work. In a more recent study, Schechner et al. (68) found significant correlations between casual systolic blood pressure and cognitive anger in white women. And Suarez et al. (66) showed that women with high Cook-Medley Ho scores, in contrast to those with low Ho scores, showed increased cardiovascular reactivity to an interpersonally challenging task. In the only negative finding in this series of studies, Lundberg et al. (62) found significant relationships between Structured Interview–assessed hostility and cardiovascular and neuroendocrine reactivity in men but not in women. It is possible that this finding reflects cultural differences between women in Sweden and those in the United States; further studies of both American and Swedish samples should clarify this issue.

Hostility, as measured by the Cook-Medley scale, has also been related to ambulatory and exercise myocardial ischemia in women (59), and hostile style, as assessed in the type A Structured Interview, was found to be related to the thallium stress test scores of both men and women (69). Finally, research has shown that a relationship between hostility and health behaviors in women exists (58, 64, 70, 71), in that hostility is related to unhealthy behaviors (e.g., smoking initiation and cessation; alcohol intake). In conclusion, the evidence indicating a relationship between hostility and related constructs and CHD risk factors is more consistent than the evidence relating these factors to CHD incidence and mortality in women.

One problem is the fact that the measures of hostility and anger expression used have been developed primarily for use in men and have simply been adopted for use with women. This may be inappropriate, given the fact that women are less likely to self-report hostility (58). This indicates the need for the development of behaviorally based measures that assess the more subtle aspects of hostility that may characterize women's expressions of anger or hostility (e.g., measures which assess indirect as well as direct challenges). In addition, women may respond to different types of situational stressors than men. For example, situations characterized by interpersonal conflict or that mirror the role overload faced daily by many women who have children and work outside the home may evoke greater frustration and anger responses than the stressors often used in studies of men. Future prospective studies should use measures developed specifically to assess hostility and related constructs in women to determine whether hostility is in fact predictive of CHD incidence and mortality in women.

Depression and Anxiety

There now exists a substantial body of evidence linking depression and other negative affects (e.g., anxiety disorders) to CHD in men, and evidence in this regard is accumulating in women as well (72). Unfortunately, as with other psychosocial variables reviewed here, the data are more limited in women. Especially lacking are large-scale prospective studies of initially healthy individuals with sufficient samples of women to establish a causal link of various personality and emotional factors with CHD.

A recent meta-analysis (73) found that depression was strongly and significantly related to CHD in both men and women. Anxiety was also found to be a significant predictor of CHD. Although the number of studies in women are fewer than those in men, several studies of depression and its related negative affects have noted significant relationships between these emotional states and CHD morbidity and mortality. Unfortunately, most of these studies employ case-control, cross-sectional designs, and few prospective studies have been conducted.

One of the few prospective studies available that examined depression as a predictor of CHD in women is the Gothenburg study mentioned previously (54). In this study of 795 initially healthy women who were followed for 12 years, the grade or severity of mental disorder at entry into the study and the severity of major or minor depression at entry were both related to angina pectoris but not to myocardial infarction or CHD death (54). However, only the severity, not the presence of a major depressive disorder, was found to be predictive.

Another prospective study that examined the relationship between negative affects and CHD outcomes is the Framingham study (51, 52). In the Framingham study, housewives with CHD—which included myocardial infarction (MI), sudden cardiac death (SCD), coronary insufficiency syndrome, and angina pectoris—reported greater levels of anxiety and tension than other women (51). In addition, women with more depressive symptoms were more likely to develop CHD than women who reported fewer depressive symptoms. This effect was significant in housewives but was less pronounced and not significant among women who worked outside the home (100). However, the inclusion of angina in the end point raises questions about these findings because anxiety and depression have been associated with noncoronary chest pain in other studies (74).

A number of case-control and retrospective studies have shown a relationship between depression-related affects and both all-cause mortality (75) and sudden cardiac death (76–80) in women. Furthermore, women are more likely to be depressed following MI than are men (81, 82) and are also at greater risk of mortality following MI than are men (83–86). Since a number of studies have linked depression and anxiety with increased risk of morbidity and mortality following an MI for men alone and for combined samples of men and women (87–90), an important research question is whether women's increased risk of mortality following MI is due, at least in part, to their increased anxiety and depression following MI.

In summary, although there are relatively few studies examining the association between depression and CHD incidence and mortality in women, those that do exist suggest a relationship. More research using prospective designs and both healthy and high-risk populations is needed to establish whether negative affects are predictors of cardiovascular disease risk and outcomes in women.

RECENT STUDIES OF TYPE A BEHAVIOR IN WOMEN

In 1986, Haynes reviewed the evidence regarding the relationship between type A behavior and coronary heart disease in women (91). As noted, many investigators have recently focused their research on the examination of type A components, such as hostility. However, new evidence has appeared that supports interest in the overall type A construct. In an 8-year follow-up of the Framingham study offspring (conducted from 1971 to 1975 and from 1979 to 1983), the Framingham type A scale was associated with declines in HDL and increases in the ratio of total cholesterol–HDL among women, albeit at the $p \leq .10$ level (92). However, increases in the latter ratio that reached statistical significance were found in the Framingham trait items in men.

In a case-control study conducted between 1978 and 1981 of myocardial infarction among women under 50 years of age, the Framingham type A scale was significantly associated with MI, with an estimated odds ratio of over twofold (93, 94). A recent case-control study of MI in women aged 20 to 64 years by Palmer et al. (95) found an estimated relative risk of 2.8 when women above the ninetieth percentile were compared with women in the lowest quintile. The relative risks of MI in women studied between 1985 and 1988 were elevated for both working women (2.9) and housewives (2.4) and were higher for professional (5.4) and clerical working women (4.2) compared with blue-collar workers (2.4) (95).

In addition to these studies, the Framingham cohort, for which the original associations between the Framingham type A scale and 8-year CHD incidence were reported (51), has also been followed further for 14 and 20 years (96, 97). At the 14-year follow-up, the Framingham type A scale was still associated with all forms of coronary heart disease in women aged 45 to 64 years; there was a significant relative risk of 1.76 after controlling for standard coronary risk factors (96). The relative risk was significantly reduced to 1.41 (not significant) when patients with angina pectoris were removed. As reported previously by Haynes et al. (51, 52), the risks of type A behavior were strongest when angina pectoris was present. At the 20-year follow-up (97), similar results were observed, and it was further found that among victims of uncomplicated angina, the risk of subsequent coronary morbidity and mortality in women increased by more than fourfold, regardless of behavior type. These later studies have suggested the need to study the meaning of angina pectoris in women (see later discussion). It is of crucial importance to know whether the type A angina patient has some form of cardiovascular disease or whether we are observing a psychologic syndrome that has no cardiovascular consequences.

Finally, in future studies we look forward to the analyses of the relationship of the Framingham type A scale to subsequent heart disease in the Augsburg, Germany, Monica Survey (98), as well as the Framingham Offspring study and other studies in progress.

Type A Behavior, Angina Pectoris, and Neuroticism or Depression

The mystery of the type A behavior–angina pectoris association may be solved by considering the confounding effect of neuroticism or depression on these associations. As mentioned earlier, there is suggestive evidence linking depression to CHD in men and women. In 1987, Booth-Kewley and Friedman (73) reviewed the literature and concluded that subtle depression may be related to cardiac disease. In another study, Swedish women who were depressed were five times as likely to develop angina over a 12-year follow-up period as were nondepressed women (54). In addition, type A behavior has been shown to be associated with neuroticism and depression in previous studies (99), and neuroticism has been shown to be associated with the development of angina pectoris.

To further elucidate this complicated picture, a depression scale was developed and validated in the Framingham study by Fredman (100). The items included becoming easily sad or depressed, getting tired early, having poor concentration, having trouble keeping one's mind on one thing at a time, allowing one's feelings to be easily hurt, crying easily, having a poor appetite, experiencing trouble falling asleep, not feeling calm, being easily upset, feeling depressed when angry, and feeling mixed up or confused when angry. This scale was highly correlated with the Framingham type A scale in women (r = .44). When the association of type A behavior in women aged 45 to 64 with the 8-year incidence of CHD was controlled for high and low depressive symptoms, the risk was only apparent in women with high depressive symptoms, the incidence of CHD being 14.3% in type A and 2.9% in type B. Thus, the association of type A with angina-related CHD was confounded by depressive symptoms.

As Dimsdale has suggested (101), the high rate of depression in women might contribute to the fact that angina is more likely to be the principal manifestation of CHD in women than in men. It is unclear, however, whether depression is a precursor of underlying coronary disease or whether it simply reflects underlying coronary disease per se. The longer term follow-up studies showing an association between depressive symptoms and hard end points suggest that the former explanation cannot be ruled out at this time. The interesting effect of depression on type A women, as suggested by the Framingham analyses, requires further study and replication in other settings.

SOCIAL SUPPORT

A large body of evidence has accumulated during the last 15 years linking social support to total and cardiovascular-specific health (102–104). Many of these studies have included only men; however, in studies that include women, the results are less consistent than those in men (105). These gender differences raise questions about the role of social support in relation to cardiovascular and other diseases in women and whether currently used measures of support are capturing critical aspects of social relationships involving women.

Five prospective studies of social support have included sufficient numbers of women to allow gender comparisons in overall and cardiovascular-specific mortality. In the Alameda County Study (106, 107), a Social Network Index (SNI) based on four items measuring structural support (marital status, number and frequency of contacts with close friends, church group membership, and group affiliation) was found to predict total mortality as well as specific causes of death, including cardiovascular diseases. These results were found for both men and women, although women aged 50 to 59 with a high SNI score were found to have an increased mortality.

In the Tecumseh Community Health Study (108), structure-based support was again found to have a significant inverse relationship to mortality for men, but only one aspect of support, church attendance, was found to be significantly related to mortality for women. A cumulative index of structural support was found to be significantly related to mortality for men but not for women; however, disease-specific analyses found a significant relationship between the cumulative measure of support and ischemic heart disease–related mortality in women. The authors noted that this secondary analysis should be interpreted with caution due to the small sample size involved.

In a study in Evans County, Georgia, Schoenbach et al. (109) found that, for white men and women over age 60, low scores on a cumulative index of structure-based support were related to increased mortality; however, lower support was related to lower mortality for white women under 60. And in a study based on data from the Swedish National Survey of Living Conditions (SNSLC), Orth-Gomer and Johnson (110) found that all-cause mortality rates were highest in the lowest support tertile for both men and women at all ages except the highest age group (65 to 74). Similar findings were reported for cardiovascular-specific mortality as well.

Finally, in a study based in North Karelia, Finland (111), a structure-based measure of support was found to predict total and cardiovascular-specific mortality for men. Although a similar trend was found for women, the relationship was not significant.

In addition to these population-based studies, several studies have examined the relationship of social support to cardiovascular-specific morbidity and mortality in male and female CAD patients referred for angiography. Seeman and Syme (112) found that measures of support that assessed instrumental support and "feeling loved" were negatively related to CAD for the total sample. When gender-specific analyses were performed, these results were replicated for men but not for women. However, the low number of women in this study (40) limits the conclusions that can be drawn from these analyses. Blumenthal et al. (113) found that male and female CAD patients who reported high support and who were classified as type A had a significantly lower incidence of CAD than type A patients with low support. No gender-specific analyses were reported in this study. Williams et al. (114) recently reported that unmarried CAD patients without a confidant had an unadjusted 5-year survival rate of 0.50 compared with 0.82 in patients who were married, had a confidant, or both. In the latter two studies, gender was entered as a variable in the analyses, but there were no significant gender interactions. However, like the Seeman and Syme study, these studies contained very low numbers of women, and thus their ability to detect gender-specific effects is limited. In addition, these studies are subject to confounds inherent in angiographic studies (e.g., selection biases), and so must be interpreted with caution.

Although social support has been consistently linked to total and cardiovascular-specific morbidity and mortality in men, results for women are mixed. The possible reasons for this gender difference have been discussed extensively elsewhere (105, 115). One possibility involves the adequacy of the support measures used—that is, the measures used may not be tapping critical dimensions of support for women, or the meaning of support may be different for men and women. In addition, gender differences exist in the structure and function of support that may affect the relationship of support to health. For example, women have larger and more dense social networks than men (116, 117), are more often the *providers* as well as the *recipients* of support (118), and are more likely to assume caregiving roles, especially with increasing age (118). Thus, women are exposed not only to the positive but also the negative aspects of social interactions to a greater extent than men. Finally, many of the studies discussed above may have had inadequate power to detect gender-specific effects, given either the low numbers of women included in the angiographic studies or the lower incidence of cardiovascular disease in women in the population-based studies.

In summary, research suggests that social support plays a role in women's cardiovascular health, although the relationship is less robust and more complex in women than in men. Further studies are needed, using support measures tailored to women's experiences and with adequate power to test for gender-specific effects, to clarify the nature of the social support–CVD relationship in women.

Conclusions and Future Research

During the past 15 years, a large body of research has accumulated on the relationship between psychosocial and environmental risk factors for cardiovascular disease, as shown below.

- There is a strong inverse association between educational level and heart disease mortality in women.
- Employment outside the home per se is not detrimental to women's cardiovascular health, and working women may have an HDL advantage over housewives.
- Evidence exists to show that occupations involving low control and high demands, such as clerical and nursing jobs, may be associated with cardiovascular disease.
- Suppression of anger has been linked to CHD, although it is not clear whether this includes hard end points.
- Hostility is related to CHD risk factors, cardiovascular reactivity, and unhealthy behaviors.
- Depression is related to the development of angina pectoris in women, with unknown consequences for CHD.
- Type A behavior is associated with angina-related CHD in women but may be confounded by depression.
- Social support is related to cardiovascular health in women, although the relationship is more complex and weaker than that found in men.

As has been noted throughout the text, considerable research is necessary to help elucidate some of the findings reported in this chapter. In particular, longitudinal studies are needed to examine the effect of hostility and anger experience, depression, social support, and high-risk occupations on cardiovascular disease in women. In addition, the medical and psychologic dimensions of angina pectoris in women must be determined in a large-scale epidemiologic study if we are to truly understand the nature of cardiovascular symptoms in women. Finally, the overall societal effect of women's status at the work place and at home should be considered in the design of large-scale studies to further explain the findings reported during the last 15 years of research on the psychologic and environmental correlates of cardiovascular disease.

References

1. Houston BK, Snyder CR (Eds.). *Type A Behavior Pattern: Research, Theory, and Intervention*. New York, Wiley, 1988.
2. Frankenhaeuser M, Lundberg U, Chesney M (Eds.). *Women, Work, and Health: Stress and Opportunities*. New York, Plenum Press, 1991.
3. LaRosa JH. Women, work, and health: Employment as a risk factor for coronary heart disease. *Am J Obstet Gynecol* 158:1597–1602, 1988.
4. Haynes SG, Matthews KA. The association of Type A behavior with cardiovascular disease—Update and critical review. In Houston BK, Snyder CR (Eds.), *Type A Behavior Pattern: Research, Theory, and Intervention*. New York, Wiley, 1988, pp. 51–82.
5. Kringlen E. Psychosocial aspects of coronary heart disease. *Acta Psychiatr Scand* 74:225–237, 1986.
6. Repetti RL, Matthews KA, Waldron I. Employment and women's health. *Am Psychol* 44:1394–1401, 1989.
7. Feldman JJ, Makuc DM, Kleinman JC, et al. National trends in educational differentials in mortality. *Am J Epidemiol* 129:919–933, 1989.
8. Krieger N. Influence of social class, race and gender on the etiology of hypertension among women in the United States. Presented at the Conference on Women, Behavior, and Cardiovascular Disease. Chevy Chase, Maryland, National Heart, Lung, and Blood Institute, September 25–27, 1991.
9. Krieger N. Racial and gender discrimination: Risk factors for high blood pressure. *Soc Sci Med* 30:1273–1281, 1990.
10. LaCroix AZ, Haynes SG. Gender differences in the stressfulness of workplace roles: A focus on work and health. In Barnett RC, Baruch GK, Biener L (Eds.), *Gender and Stress*. New York, Free Press, 1987, pp. 96–121.
11. Hauenstein LS, Kasl S, Harburg E. Work status, work satisfaction and blood pressure among married black and white women. *Psychol Women Q* 1:334–349, 1977.
12. Haynes SG, Feinleib M. Women, work and coronary heart disease: Prospective findings from the Framingham Study. *Am J Public Health* 70:133–141, 1980.
13. Waldron I. Employment and women's health: An analysis of causal relationships. *Int J Health Services* 10:435–454, 1980.
14. Slaby AR. Cardiovascular risk factors in women by their working status. Paper presented at the 22nd Conference on Cardiovascular Disease Epidemiology, San Antonio, Texas, 1982.
15. Verbrugge LM. Multiple roles and physical health of women and men. *J Health Soc Behav* 24:16–30, 1983.
16. Hibbard JH, Pope CT. Employment status, employment characteristics and women's health. *Women Health* 10:59–77, 1985.
17. Verbrugge LM, Madans JH. Social roles and health trends of American women. *Milbank Memorial Fund Quarterly/Health and Society* 63:691–735, 1985.

18. Hazuda HP, Haffner SM, Stern MP, et al. Employment status and women's protection against coronary heart disease: Findings from the San Antonio Heart Study. *Am J Epidemiol* 123:623–640, 1986.
19. House JS, Strecher V, Metzner HL, et al. Occupational stress and health among men and women in the Tecumseh Community Health Study. *J Health Soc Behav*, 27:62–77, 1986.
20. Kritz-Silverstein D, Wingard DL, Barrett-Connor E. Employment status and heart disease risk factors in middle-aged women: The Rancho Bernardo study. *Am J Public Health* 82:215–219, 1992.
21. Haertel U, Heiss G, Filipiak B, et al. Cross-sectional and longitudinal associations between high density lipoprotein cholesterol and women's employment. *Am J Epidemiol* 135:68–78, 1992.
22. Haynes SG, Feinleib M. Clerical work and coronary heart disease in women: Prospective findings from the Framingham Heart Study. In Cohen B G F (Ed.), *Human Aspects in Office Automation*. Amsterdam, Elsevier, 1984, pp. 239–255.
23. LaRosa JH. Executive women and health: Perceptions and practices. *Am J Public Health* 80:1450–1454, 1990.
24. Ebi-Kryston KL, Higgins MW, Keller JD. Health and other characteristics of employed women and homemakers in Tecumseh, 1959–1978. I. Demographic characteristics, smoking habits, alcohol consumption, and pregnancy outcomes and conditions. *Women Health* 16:5–21, 1990.
25. Kotler P, Wingard DL. The effect of occupational, marital, and parental roles on mortality: The Alameda County Study. *Am J Public Health* 79:607–612, 1989.
26. Haynes SG. The effect of job demands, job control, and new technologies on the health of employed women: A review. In Frankenhaeuser M, Lundberg U, Chesney M (Eds.), *Women, Work, and Health: Stress and Opportunities*. New York, Plenum Press, 1991, pp. 157–168.
27. Passannante MR, Nathanson CA. Female labor force participation and female mortality in Wisconsin 1974–1978. *Soc Sci Med* 21:665–668, 1985.
28. House JS, Strecher V, Metznor HL, et al. Occupational stress and health among men and women in the Tecumseh Community Health Study. *J Health Soc Behav* 27:62–77, 1986.
29. Doebbert G, Riedmiller KR, Kizer KE. Occupational mortality of California women, 1979–1981. *West J Med* 149:734–740, 1988.
30. Schlussel YR, Schnall PL, Zimbler M, et al. The effect of work environments and blood pressure. Evidence from seven New York organizations. *J Hypertension* 8:679–685, 1990.
31. Haynes SG. Work stress among women. In Quick JC, Bhayat RS, Dalton JE, et al. (Eds.), *Work Stress and the Role of Health Care Delivery Systems*. New York, Praeger, 1987, pp. 93–110.
32. Hall E. Gender, work control, and stress: A theoretical discussion and an empirical test. *Int J Health Serv* 19:725–745, 1989.
33. Aneshensel CS, Pearlin LI. Structural contexts of differences in stress. In Barnett RC, Baruch GK, Biener L (Eds.), *Gender and Stress*. New York, Free Press, 1987, pp. 75–95.
34. Thompson SG, Greenberg G, Meade TW. Risk factors for stroke and myocardial infarction in women in the United Kingdom as assessed in general practice: A case-control study. *Br Heart J* 61:403–409, 1989.
35. Dixon JP, Dixon JK, Spinner JC. Tensions between career and interpersonal commitments as a risk factor for cardiovascular disease among women. *Women Health* 17:33–57, 1991.
36. Meleis AI, Norbeck JS, Laffrey SG. Role integration and health among female clerical workers. *Res Nurs Health* 12:355–364, 1989.
37. Barnett RC, Marshall NL. The relationship between women's work and family roles and their subjective well-being and psychological distress. In Frankenhaeuser M, Lundberg U, Chesney M (Eds.), *Women, Work, and Health: Stress and Opportunities*. New York, Plenum, 1991, pp. 111–136.
38. James GD, Cates EM, Laragh JH. Parity and perceived job stress elevate blood pressure in young normotensive working women. *Am J Hypertension* 2:637–639, 1989.
39. Pickering TG, James GD, Schnall PL, et al. Occupational stress and blood pressure: Studies in working men and women. In Frankenhaeuser M, Lundberg U, Chesney M (Eds.), *Women, Work and Health: Stress and Opportunities*. New York, Plenum, 1991, pp. 171–186.
40. Frankenhaeuser M, Lundberg U, Fredrikson M, et al. Stress on-off the job as related to sex and occupational status in white-collar workers. *J Org Behav* 10:321–346, 1989.
41. Barefoot JC, Dahlstrom WG, Williams RB Jr. Hostility, CHD incidence and total mortality: A 25-year follow study of 225 physicians. *Psychosom Med* 45:59–63, 1983.
42. Matthews KA, Glass DC, Roseman RH, et al. High drive patterns, and coronary heart disease: A further analysis of some data from the Western Collaborative Group Study. *J Chronic Dis* 30:489–498, 1977.
43. Shekelle RB, Gale M, Ostfeld AM, et al. Hostility, risk of coronary heart disease and mortality. *Psychosom Med* 42:109–114, 1983.
44. Williams RB, Barefoot JC, Shekelle RB. The health consequences of hostility. In Chesley MA, Rosenman RH (Eds.), *Anger and Behavior in Cardiovascular and Behavioral Disorders*. New York, Hemisphere, 1985.
45. Dembroski TM, MacDougall JM, Ta PT, et al. Components of hostility as predictors of sudden death and myocardial infarction in the Multiple Risk Factor Intervention Trial. *Psychosom Med* 51:514–522, 1989.
46. Chesney MA, Ekman P, Triesen WV, et al. Type A behavior: Facial behavior and speech components. *Psychosom Med* 52:307–319, 1990.
47. Hecker MH, Chesney MA, Black GW, et al. Coronary-prone behaviors in the Western Collaborative Group Study. *Psychosom Med* 50:153–164, 1988.
48. Dembroski TM, MacDougall JM, Williams RB, et al. Components of Type A, hostility, anger-in, relationships to angiographic findings. *Psychosom Med* 47:219–233, 1985.
49. MacDougall JM, Dembroski TM, Dimsdale JE, et al. Components of Type A, hostility, anger-in relationships to angiographic findings. *Health Psychol* 4:137–152, 1983.
50. Weidner G. The role of hostility and coronary-prone behaviors in the etiology of cardiovascular disease in women. Presented at Conference on Women, Behavior and Cardiovascular Disease. Chevy Chase,

Maryland, National Heart, Lung, and Blood Institute, September 25–27, 1991.
51. Haynes SG, Feinleib M, Kannel WB. The relationship of psychosocial factors to coronary heart disease in the Framingham study: III. Eight-year incidence of coronary heart disease. *Am J Epidemiol* 111:37–58, 1980.
52. Haynes SG, Feinleib M. Type A behavior and the incidence of coronary heart disease in the Framingham Heart Study. *Adv Cardiol* 29:85–95, 1982.
53. Julius M, Harburg E, Schork MA, et al. Role of marital stress and suppressed anger for women and wives on health risk factors and mortality. Presented at the Conference on Women, Behavior, and Cardiovascular Disease. Chevy Chase, Maryland, National Heart, Lung, and Blood Institute, September 25–27, 1991.
54. Haellstroem T, Lapidus L, Bengtsson C, et al. Psychosocial factors and risk of ischemic heart disease and death in women: A twelve-year follow-up of participants in the population study of women in Gothenburg, Sweden. *Psychosom Res* 30:451–459, 1986.
55. Barefoot JC, Siegler IC, Nowlin JB, et al. Suspiciousness, health, and mortality: A follow-up study of 500 older adults. *Psychosom Med* 49:435–449, 1987.
56. Blumenthal JA, Williams RB, Kong Y, et al. Type A behavior and coronary atherosclerosis. *Circulation* 258:634–639, 1978.
57. Williams RB Jr, Haney TL, Leek L, et al. Type A behavior, hostility and coronary atherosclerosis. *Psychosom Med* 42:539–549, 1980.
58. Barefoot JC, Haney TL, Hershkowitz BD. Hostility and coronary artery disease in women and men. Paper presented at the annual meeting of the Society of Behavioral Medicine, 1991.
59. Helmer DC, Ragland DR, Syme SL. Hostility and coronary artery disease. *Am J Epidemiol* 133:112–122, 1991.
60. Siegler IC, Peterson BL, Barefoot JC, et al. Hostility levels at age 19 predict lipid risk profiles at age 42 (Abstract). *Circulation* (Suppl.) 82:III-228, 1990.
61. Dujovne VF, Houston BK. Hostility-related variables and plasma lipid levels. *J Behav Med* 14:555–565, 1991.
62. Lundberg U, Hedman M, Melin B, et al. Type A behavior in healthy males and females as related to physiological reactivity and blood lipids. *Psychosom Med* 51:113–122, 1989.
63. Weidner G, Sexton G, McLellarn R, et al. The role of Type A behavior and hostility in an elevation of plasma lipids in adult women and men. *Psychosom Med* 48:136–145, 1987.
64. Knox S, Jacobs D, Chesney M, et al. Psychosocial factors and plasma lipids in young adults. Presented at the Society of Behavioral Medicine. New York City, March 25–28, 1992.
65. Durel LA, Carver CS, Spitzer SB, et al. Associations of blood pressure with self-report measures of anger and hostility among black and white men and women. *Health Psychol* 8:557–575, 1989.
66. Suarez EC, Williams RB, Harlan E. Oral contraceptive usage affects cardiovascular responses in low hostile women. *Circulation* (Suppl.) 82:III-577, 1990.
67. Weidner G, Friend R, Ficarrotto TJ. Hostility and cardiovascular reactivity to stress in women and men. *Psychosom Med* 51:36–45, 1989.
68. Schechner RH, Durel LA, Saab PG, et al. Associations of trait measures with blood pressure among black and white men and women. Presented at the Conference on Women, Behavior, and Cardiovascular Disease. Chevy Chase, Maryland, National Heart, Lung, and Blood Institute, September 25–27, 1991.
69. Siegman AW, Johnston GS. Structured interview derived hostility scores and thallium stress test results in men and women. Presented at the Conference on Women, Behavior, and Cardiovascular Disease. Chevy Chase, Maryland, National Heart, Lung, and Blood Institute, September 25–27, 1991.
70. Houston BK, Vavak CR. Cynical hostility: Developmental factors, psychosocial correlates and health behaviors. *Health Psychol* 10:9–17, 1991.
71. Leiker M, Hailey BJ. A link between hostility and disease: Poor health habits. *Behav Med* 14:129–133, 1988.
72. Carney RM, Freedland KE, Smith LJ, et al. Depression and anxiety as risk factors for coronary heart disease in women. Presented at Conference on Women, Behavior and Cardiovascular Disease. Chevy Chase, Maryland, National Heart, Lung, and Blood Institute, September 25–27, 1991.
73. Booth-Kewley S, Friedman HD. Psychological predictors of heart disease: A quantitative review. *Psychol Bull* 101:343–362, 1987.
74. Carney RM, Freedland KE, Ludbrook PA, et al. Major depression, panic disorder and mitral valve prolapse in patients who complain of chest pain. *Am J Med* 89:757–760, 1990.
75. Murphy JM, Monson RR, Olivier DC, et al. Affective disorders and mortality: A general population study. *Arch Gen Psychol* 44:473–480, 1987.
76. Binik YM. Psychosocial predictors of sudden death: A review and critique. *Soc Sci Med* 20:667–680, 1985.
77. Kamarck T, Jennings JR. Biobehavioral factors in sudden cardiac death. *Psychol Bull* 109:42–75, 1991.
78. Talbott E, Kuller LH, Perper J, et al. Sudden unexpected death in women: Biologic and psychosocial origins. *Am J Epidemiol* 114:671–682, 1981.
79. Talbott E, Kuller LH, Detre K, et al. Biologic and psychosocial risk factors for sudden death from coronary disease in white women. *Am J Cardiol* 39:858–864, 1977.
80. Cottington EM, Matthews KA, Talbott E, et al. Environmental events preceding sudden death in women. *Psychosom Med* 42:567–575, 1980.
81. Carney RM, Freedland KE, Jaffe AS. Insomnia and depression prior to myocardial infarction. *Psychosom Med* 52:603–609, 1990.
82. Schleifer SJ, Macari-Hinson MM, Coyle DA. The nature and course of depression following myocardial infarction. *Arch Intern Med* 149:1785–1789, 1989.
83. Wenger NK. Coronary disease in women. *Ann Rev Med* 36:285–294, 1985.
84. Greenland P, Reicher-Reiss H, Goldbourt U, et al. In-hospital and 1-year mortality in 1,524 women after myocardial infarction. *Circulation* 83:484–491, 1991.
85. Welty FK. Gender differences in survival and recovery following cardiovascular disease diagnosis and treatment. Paper presented at Conference on Women, Behavior and Cardiovascular Disease. Chevy Chase, Maryland, National Heart, Lung, and Blood Institute, September 25–27, 1991.
86. Goldberg RJ, Gore JM, Yarzebski J, et al. Sex differences in the incidence and survival rates after

myocardial infarction: A community-based perspective poster presented at the Conference on Women, Behavior and Cardiovascular Disease. Chevy Chase, Maryland, National Heart, Lung, and Blood Institute, September 25–27, 1991.
87. Ahern DK, Gorkin L, Anderson JL, et al. Biobehavioral variables and mortality or cardiac arrest in the Cardiac Arrhythmia Pilot Study (CAPS). *Am J Cardiol* 66:59–62, 1990.
88. Falgar P, Appels A. Psychological risk factors over the life course of myocardial infarction patients. *Adv Cardiol* 29:132–139, 1982.
89. Schleifer SJ, Macari MM, Slater W, et al. Predictors of outcome after myocardial infarction: Role of depression. *Circulation* 74 (Suppl. 2):10, 1986.
90. Stern JJ, Pascale L, Ackerman A. Life adjustment post myocardial infarction: Determining predictive variables. *Arch Intern Med* 137:1680–1685, 1977.
91. Haynes SG. Type A behavior, employment status, and coronary heart disease in women—A review. In Oliver MF, Vedin A, Wilhelmsson C (Eds.), *Myocardial Infarction in Women*. London, Churchill Livingstone, 1986, pp. 66–86.
92. Hubert HB, Eaker ED, Garrison RJ, et al. Lifestyle correlates of risk factor change in young adults: An eight-year study of coronary heart disease risk factors in the Framingham offspring. *Am J Epidemiol* 125:812–831, 1987.
93. Rosenberg L, Miller DR, Kaufman DW, et al. Myocardial infarction in women under 50 years of age. *JAMA* 250:2801–2806, 1983.
94. Rosenberg L. The relation between myocardial infarction and cigarette smoking in women under 50 years of age: Modifying influence of individual risk factors. In Oliver MF, Vedin A, Wilhelmsson C (Eds.), *Myocardial Infarction in Women*. London, Churchill Livingstone, 1986, pp. 150–156.
95. Palmer JR, Rosenberg L, Shapiro S. Type A behavior and myocardial infarction in women. *Am J Epidemiol* 128:892, 1988.
96. Eaker ED, Castelli WP. Type A behavior and coronary heart disease in women: Fourteen-year incidence from the Framingham Heart Study. In Houston BK, Snyder CR (Eds.), *Type A Behavior Pattern: Research, Theory, and Intervention*. New York, Wiley, 1988, pp. 83–97.
97. Eaker ED, Abbott RD, Kannel WB. Frequency of uncomplicated angina pectoris in type A compared with type B persons (the Framingham study). *Am J Cardiol* 3:1042–1045, 1989.
98. Hartel U, Chambless L. Occupational position and Type A behavior: Results from the first Monica Survey, Ausburg F.R.G. *Soc Sci Med* 29:1367–1372, 1989.
99. Smith TW, O'Keeffe JL, Allred KD. Neuroticism, symptom reports, and Type A behavior: Interpretive caution for the Framingham scale. *J Behav Med* 12:1–11, 1989.
100. Fredman L. The demographic and psychosocial correlates of depression among older participants in the Framingham Heart Study. Master thesis, University of North Carolina, School of Public Health, Department of Epidemiology, 1983.
101. Dimsdale JE. Influences of personality and stress-induced biological processes on etiology and treatment of cardiovascular disease in women. In Wenger NK, Speroff L, Packard B (Eds.), *Cardiovascular Health and Disease in Women*. Proceedings of a National Heart, Lung, and Blood Disease Conference, January 22–24, 1992.
102. Broadhead WE, Kaplan BH, James SA, et al. The epidemiologic evidence for a relationship between social support and health. *Am J Epidemiol* 117:521–537, 1983.
103. Cohen S, Syme SL (Eds.). *Social Support and Health*. New York, Academic, 1985.
104. Hazuda HP. A critical evaluation of United States epidemiologic evidence, including a special consideration of ethnic variation. In Shumaker SA, Czajkowski SM (Eds.), *Social Support and Cardiovascular disease*. New York, Plenum (in press, 1992).
105. Shumaker SA, Hill DR. Gender differences in social support and physical health. *Health Psychol* 10:102–111, 1991.
106. Berkman LF. Assessing the physical health effects of social networks and social support. *Ann Rev Pub Health* 5:413–432, 1984.
107. Berkman LF, Syme SL. Social networks, host resistance, and mortality: A nine-year follow-up study of Alameda County residents. *Am J Epidemiol* 109:186–204, 1979.
108. House JS, Robbins C, Metzner HL. The association of social relationships and activities with mortality: Prospective evidence from the Tecumseh Community Health Study. *Am J Epidemiol* 116:123–140, 1982.
109. Schoenbach V, Kaplan BH, Fredman L. Social ties and mortality in Evans County, Georgia. *Am J Epidemiol* 123:577–691, 1986.
110. Orth-Gomer K, Johnson JV. Social network interaction and mortality. *J Chronic Dis* 40:949–957, 1987.
111. Orth-Gomer K. International epidemiological evidence for a relationship between social support and cardiovascular disease. In Shumaker SA, Czajkowski SM (Eds.), *Social Support and Cardiovascular Disease*. New York, Plenum (in press, 1992).
112. Seeman TE, Syme SL. Social networks and coronary artery disease: A comparison of the structure and function of social relations as predictors of disease. *Psychosom Med* 49:341–354, 1987.
113. Blumenthal JA, Burg MM, Barefoot J, et al. Social support, Type A behavior, and coronary artery disease. *Psychosom Med* 49:331–339, 1987.
114. Williams RB, Barefoot JC, Califf RM, et al. Prognostic importance of social and economic resources among medically treated patients with angiographically documented coronary artery disease. *JAMA* 267:520–524, 1991.
115. Berkman LF. Social networks, support, and health: Taking the next step forward. *Am J Epidemiol* 123:559–562, 1986.
116. Antonucci TC, Akiyama H. An examination of sex differences in social support among older men and women. *Sex Roles* 17:737–749, 1987.
117. Vaux A. Variations in social support associated with gender, ethnicity and age. *J Social Issues* 41:89–100, 1985.
118. George LK. Social support and caregiving roles of aging women: Health implications. Paper presented at Seminar Series on Women's Health and Behavior. Bethesda, Maryland, National Institutes of Health, April 3, 1991.

CHAPTER 15

Clinical Implications of Animal Models of Gender Difference in Heart Disease

THOMAS B. CLARKSON, D.V.M.
MICHAEL R. ADAMS, D.V.M.
J. KOUDY WILLIAMS, D.V.M.
JANICE D. WAGNER, D.V.M., Ph.D.

Until relatively recently, animal models have not been used widely to understand gender differences in coronary artery atherosclerosis or pathophysiologic influences on the disease's progression among females. This lack of comparative research resulted primarily from the lack of a suitable animal model. The complexities of coronary atherogenesis in females requires a model with many similarities to women. Consequently, studies in nonprimate animals have not been rewarding.

In 1977 we began to characterize cynomolgus monkeys (*Macaca fascicularis*) for research on "female protection" against coronary artery atherosclerosis. The majority of the data presented in this chapter are based on our research with this model during the past one and a half decades. We review the characteristics of the model, the pathophysiologic basis for female protection, the effect of contraceptive steroids, psychosocial stress, social isolation, pregnancy, central obesity, surgical menopause, and coronary artery vasodilator and vasoconstrictor responses. We have summarized what we believe to be the clinical implications of this research by questions and answers that highlight the observations in monkey models.

ANIMAL MODELS OF GENDER DIFFERENCES AND "FEMALE PROTECTION" IN ATHEROSCLEROSIS RESEARCH

As we have indicated, nonprimate animal models have contributed little to our understanding of gender differences, female protection, or atherogenesis. We have summarized in Table 15–1 criteria for an animal model to be useful in understanding either gender differences in atherogenesis or pathophysiologic mechanisms in female protection.

Pigeons have been widely used in atherosclerosis research (1, 2), although only a single study has focused on estrogen's effect on atherogenesis (3). Chickens have been used more widely to study gender differences and estrogen effects. One of the earliest studies of gender differences in coronary atherosclerosis was the finding that roosters develop more

Table 15–1. CHARACTERISTICS OF A SUITABLE ANIMAL MODEL

- Males develop two to three times more coronary artery atherosclerosis than females
- Ovarian function and menstrual cyclicity are similar to those in women
- Well-established brain (psychosocial) influences on ovarian function exist
- Natural or surgical menopause results in progressing coronary artery atherosclerosis and osteoporosis
- Postmenopausal coronary atherosclerosis and osteoporosis progression are influenced favorably by estrogen replacement

extensive coronary atherosclerosis than do hens (4). Subsequently, estrogen treatment of chickens was found to inhibit progression (5) and promote regression of atherosclerosis (6).

Rabbits are another widely used model for atherosclerosis research. Although significant male-female differences have not been shown, treatment of female rabbits with estrogen has been found to diminish atherosclerosis (7, 8).

Although pigs have been popular animal models in atherosclerosis research (9–11), only a single study has examined the role of gender differences in coronary artery atherosclerosis (12). In that study, coronary artery atherosclerosis was found to be more extensive in female pigs than in male ones.

Cynomolgus monkeys have all of the characteristics delineated in Table 15–1. Males of this species develop main-branch coronary artery atherosclerosis when fed a cholesterol-containing diet (13). Female cynomolgus monkeys share similar reproductive physiologic characteristics with women. These include a 28-day menstrual cycle, qualitatively and quantitatively similar circulating concentrations of gonadotropins and sex steroids, and the natural occurrence of menopause (14). Like premenopausal women, cynomolgus macaque females have significantly higher plasma concentrations of high-density lipoproteins (HDLs) than their male counterparts (15). At necropsy, it was found that females had less coronary artery atherosclerosis than male monkeys. The male-female difference in coronary artery atherosclerosis among monkeys that consumed a moderately atherogenic diet is comparable to the male-female difference in coronary artery lesion extent among New Orleans Caucasians (16).

FACTORS INFLUENCING PROGRESSION OF CORONARY ARTERY ATHEROSCLEROSIS

Contraceptive Steroids

The effects of combination oral contraceptives on coronary heart disease (CHD) risk continue to be controversial (17). However, although these compounds have been in widespread use for 25 years, there is no compelling evidence that there has been a widespread adverse influence on CHD risk. On the contrary, CHD incidence among women in the United States has declined markedly over the same period of time. Also, although there is a well-known increase in CHD risk associated with current oral contraceptive use, present evidence indicates that this increase in risk is largely confined to users of older, high-dose contraceptive formulations who are also cigarette smokers (17–21). In addition, the increase in risk disappears after cessation of oral contraceptive use, suggesting a nonatherogenic mechanism such as thrombosis or vasospasm. Furthermore, some studies actually suggest a decreased risk in past users of oral contraceptives (21), and none provides compelling evidence for an increased CHD risk. Taken together, these epidemiologic findings indicate that oral contraceptives probably do not accelerate, and may in fact inhibit, progression of atherosclerosis. Further evidence to support this conclusion is provided by the work of Engel et al. (22), who studied premenopausal women undergoing coronary angiography for the diagnosis of myocardial infarction. These investigators found that, in contrast to oral contraceptive nonusers, users had little or no angiographic evidence of coronary atherosclerosis.

Because of the great difficulty of studying the pathogenesis of atherosclerosis in human beings, we have used a nonhuman primate model, the cynomolgus macaque with diet-induced atherosclerosis, to study the effects of contraceptive steroids on atherogenesis. In an initial experiment (23), we compared the effects of an oral contraceptive (ethinyl estradiol and norgestrel), an intravaginal ring (17β-estradiol and levonorgestrel), and a placebo vaginal ring (no hormone treatment). Animals consumed the atherogenic diet for 30 months.

None of the contraceptive treatments influenced the prevalence of atherosclerosis. However, treatment did influence the extent of coronary artery atherosclerosis, i.e., plaque size. Treatment with the intravaginal ring resulted in plaques that were larger than those of both control females and oral contraceptive-treated females. This difference in atherosclerosis extent occurred despite the fact that plasma HDL cholesterol concentrations were reduced markedly and to the same extent in both contraceptive-treated groups. The results suggested that the much greater estrogenic influence associated with the ethinyl estradiol–containing oral contraceptive relative to the 17β-estradiol–containing intravaginal ring resulted in inhibition of atherosclerosis despite the pronounced progestin-induced lowering of plasma HDL concentrations. A subsequent study was designed to further clarify these relationships.

In this experiment (24), we compared oral contraceptives that contained equivalent amounts of ethinyl estradiol (50 μg) but structurally and pharmacologically different progestins, norgestrel (500 μg), and ethynodiol diacetate (1 mg). Despite the expected marked influences on plasma lipoproteins (i.e., decreased plasma HDL cholesterol concentrations and changes in HDL subclasses [Fig. 15-1]), the extent of coronary artery atherosclerosis was decreased by both oral contraceptives, and this effect was especially pronounced among females at highest risk due to "atherogenic" plasma lipid profiles (pretreatment total plasma cholesterol–HDL cholesterol ratio > 4.5) (Fig. 15-2).

As estimated by multiple regression analysis, there was a dramatic disparity between observed extent of coronary artery atherosclerosis and the extent of atherosclerosis predicted by theoretically atherogenic effects of the oral contraceptives on plasma lipoprotein patterns (23) (see Fig. 15-3). When all subjects are considered, an approximate doubling of atherosclerosis extent was predicted, whereas a 50–75% reduction in atherosclerosis extent was observed. Among high-risk individuals, the contrast was even more striking. A doubling of atherosclerosis was again predicted, whereas a 75–85% decrease in atherosclerosis extent was observed.

The finding that the oral contraceptive treatment had a large inhibitory influence on the progression of atherosclerosis indicates that, in terms of atherogenicity, steroid-induced changes in plasma lipid concentrations are not the same as changes induced by diet. We have hypothesized that this atherosclerosis-inhibiting effect is due to the ethinyl estradiol component of the oral contraceptives.

These findings are consistent with the data of Haarbo et al. (8) (see Fig. 15-4), who studied the effects of endogenous estrogen and estrogen-progestin combinations on arterial cholesterol accumulation in rabbits fed an atherogenic diet. In these studies, arterial cholesterol accumulation was reduced by two-thirds in rabbits treated with 17β-estradiol given either alone or in combination with the contraceptive progestins norethindrone or levonor-

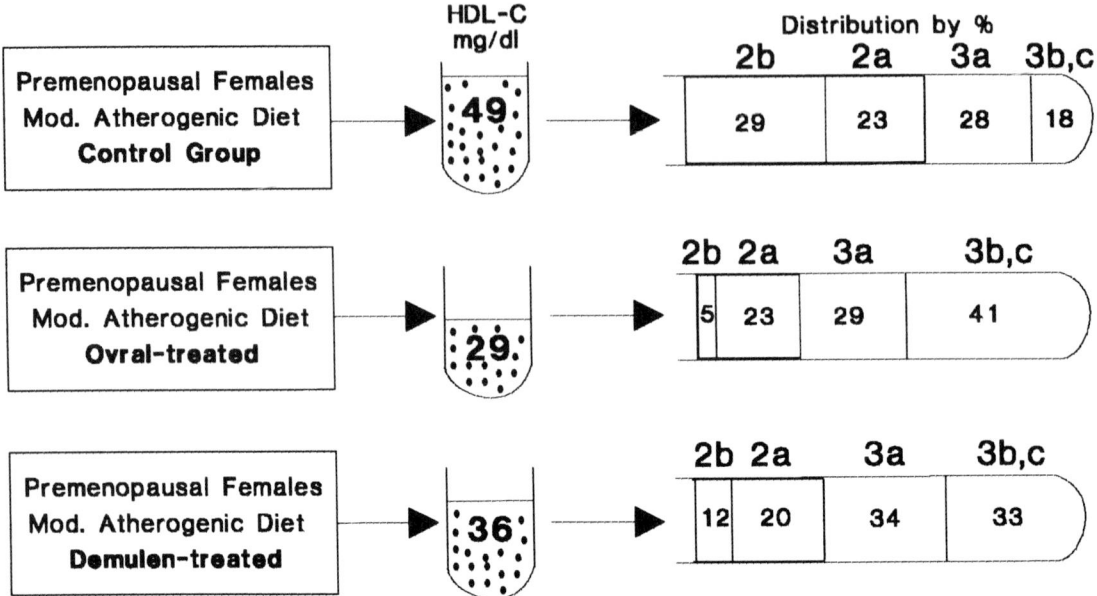

Figure 15–1. Effects of oral contraceptive treatment on plasma high-density lipoprotein cholesterol (HDL-C) concentrations and distribution of HDL subclasses in surgically postmenopausal cynomolgus monkeys. All groups were fed the same moderately atherogenic diet. (Adapted from Clarkson TB, Shively CA, Morgan TM, et al. Oral contraceptives and coronary artery atherosclerosis of cynomolgus macaques. *Obstet Gynecol* 75:217–222, 1990. Reprinted with permission from the American College of Obstetrics and Gynecology.)

gestrel. This effect was not explained by variation in plasma lipoproteins.

In conclusion, it appears that contraceptive progestin-induced lowering of HDL is not atherogenic if a sufficiently potent estrogen is coadministered. The striking difference between the outcome predicted by changes in plasma lipoproteins and the observed outcomes suggests a beneficial effect of estrogen on the artery wall. Mechanisms by which this effect may be mediated will be discussed in a succeeding section of this chapter.

Psychosocial Stress

We have employed the cynomolgus monkey model to study the influence of psychosocial stress on the progression of atherosclerosis. Evidence indicates that males and females respond differently. Studies relevant to psychosocial stress in female monkeys are summarized here.

In study 1 (25), 23 female and 15 male cynomolgus monkeys were fed an atherogenic diet and lived in social groups of five or six.

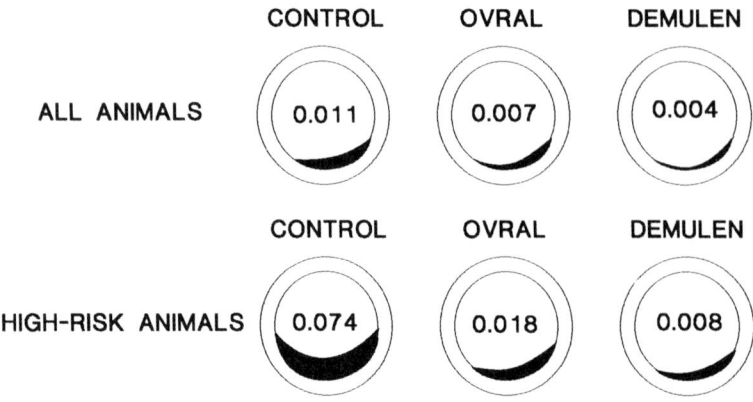

Figure 15–2. Coronary artery plaque area (mm²) in the three experimental groups of monkeys described in Figure 15–1, divided into data from all animals and data from animals considered at high risk for developing atherosclerosis (pretreatment total plasma cholesterol–HDL cholesterol ratio > 4.5). (Adapted from Clarkson TB, Shively CA, Morgan TM, et al. Oral contraceptives and coronary artery atherosclerosis of cynomolgus macaques. *Obstet Gynecol* 75:217–222, 1990. Reprinted with permission from the American College of Obstetrics and Gynecology.)

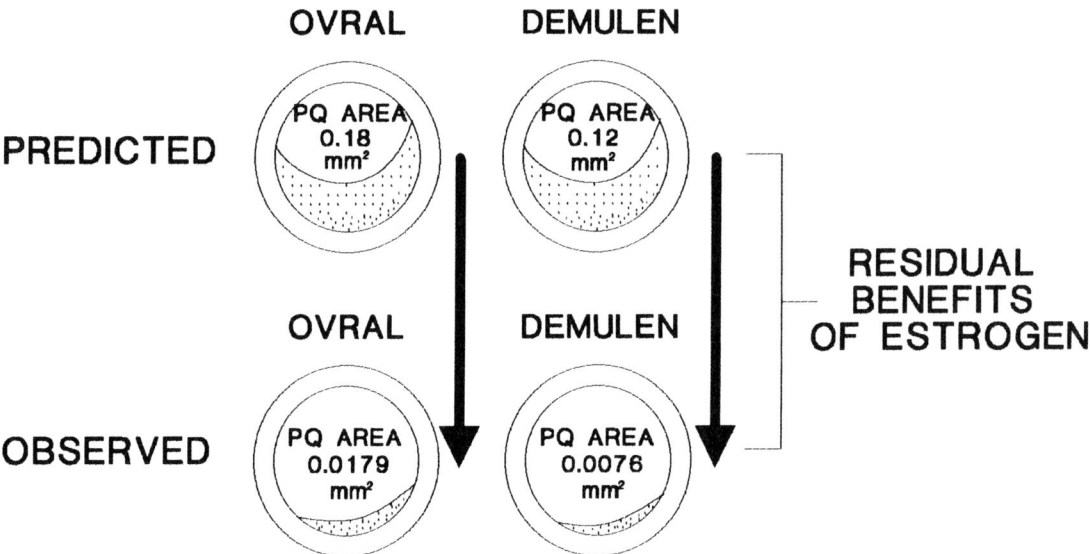

Figure 15–3. Predicted plaque (PQ) area in oral contraceptive–treated cynomolgus monkeys and observed plaque extent. The decrease observed in coronary artery atherosclerosis is thought to result from residual benefits of estrogen replacement. (Adapted from Clarkson TB, Shively CA, Morgan TM, et al. Oral contraceptives and coronary artery atherosclerosis of cynomolgus macaques. *Obstet Gynecol* 75:217–222, 1990. Reprinted with permission from the American College of Obstetrics and Gynecology.)

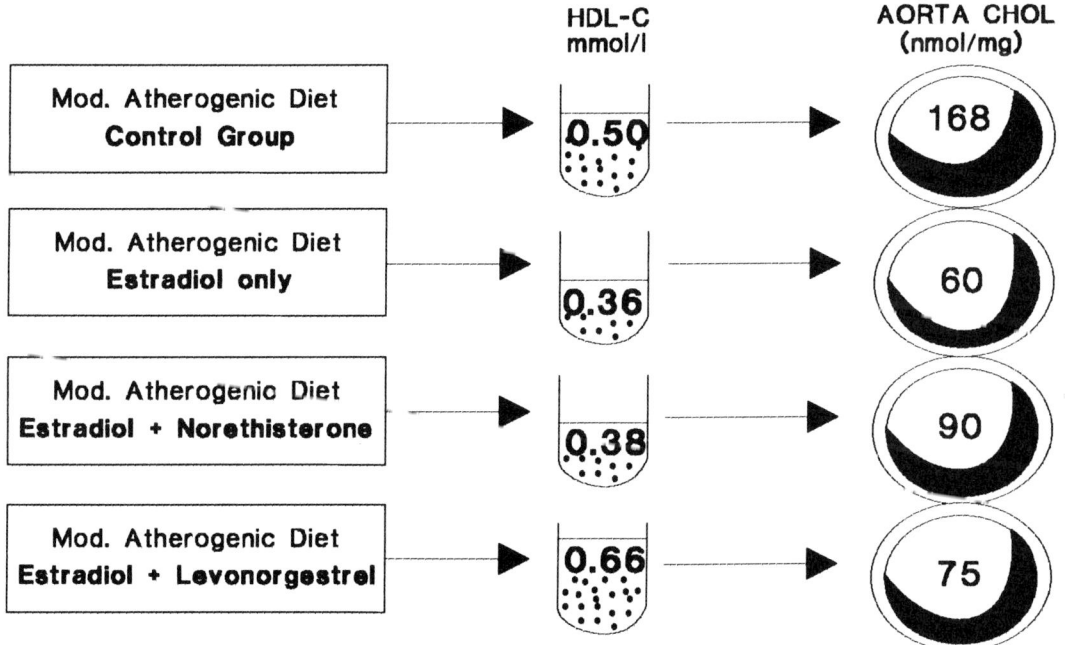

Figure 15–4. Aortic cholesterol accumulation in rabbits treated with estrogen or estrogen-progestin combinations. The reduction in cholesterol accumulation was independent of changes in plasma lipoprotein parameters. (Adapted from Haarbo J, Leth-Espensen P, Stender S, et al. Estrogen monotherapy and combined estrogen-progestogen replacement therapy attenuate aortic accumulation of cholesterol in ovariectomized cholesterol-fed rabbits. *J Clin Invest* 87:1274–1279, 1991; personal communication, Dr. Jens Haarbo.)

The groups of females each contained one vasectomized male (not part of the study). Males lived either in unisexual groups (n = 10), or were the resident male (n = 5) in other groups of females (not part of the study). In addition to the usual physiologic measures (serum lipids, blood pressure, cortisol response to an ACTH challenge), we evaluated ovarian function (daily vaginal swabbing, with blood samples taken for determination of plasma progesterone during the follicular and luteal phases). Finally, the aggressive, submissive, and affiliative responses and relationships of each female were monitored by using focal sampling techniques and an electronic data collection device. The latter data were used to determine dominance ranking within each social group.

The experiment continued for 24 months, after which all animals were evaluated for extent and severity of coronary artery atherosclerosis. Additionally, all females were assigned dominance ranks based on the outcomes of aggressive interactions across the study. Animals that, on average, ranked first or second in their groups were labeled "dominant" for the experiment; all others were considered "subordinate." Although males were somewhat more affected with raised lesions than were females (8 of 15 males, 9 of 23 females), this difference was not significant. However, a pattern of significant differences appeared when the lesion areas of dominant and subordinate females were compared with those of males. Dominant females were significantly less affected than either males or subordinate females, whereas males and subordinate females were equally affected (Fig. 15–5). Thus, female protection in this experiment was defined in part by social status, as only dominant females had less atherosclerosis than males.

In attempting to explain why dominant but not subordinate females were protected from coronary atherosclerosis, we considered serum lipid concentrations, ovarian function, and adrenal-cortical activity. As shown in Table 15–2, subordinate females were characterized by enlarged adrenals and impaired ovarian function relative to dominant animals; serum lipids, however, did not differ among these subgroups. We concluded from this evaluation

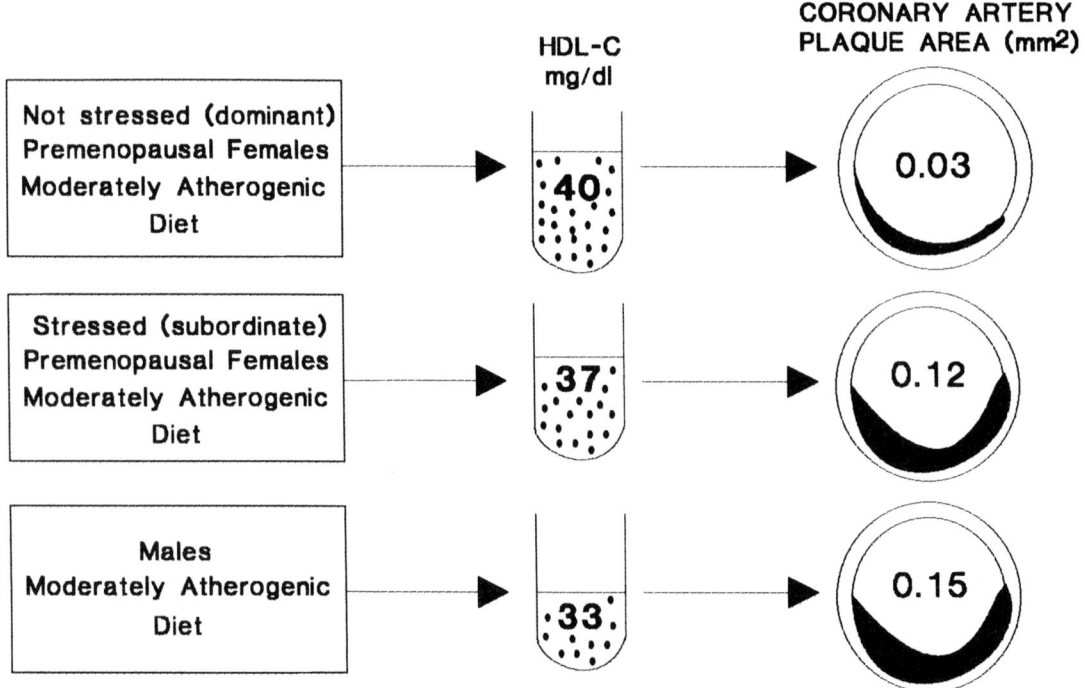

Figure 15–5. HDL cholesterol concentrations and coronary artery plaque (PQ) area in two groups of premenopausal female cynomolgus monkeys (dominant versus subordinate) and in male cynomolgus monkeys. All three groups were fed the same moderately atherogenic diet. Female "protection" from atherosclerosis was found only in the dominant group. (Adapted from Kaplan JR, Adams MR, Clarkson TB, et al. Psychosocial influences on female "protection" among cynomolgus macaques. *Atherosclerosis* 53:283–295, 1984.)

Table 15–2. COMPARISON OF MEDIAN VALUES FOR DOMINANT AND SUBORDINATE FEMALES (Study 1)

Variable	Dominant	Subordinate	P[a]
Aggressive behavior[b]	6.3	3.8	0.02
Submissive behavior[b]	4.7	10.8	0.01
Adrenal weight (mg/kg)	168	201	0.04
Body weight (kg)	3.36	2.86	0.05
High-density lipoprotein cholesterol (mg/dL)	39.8	37.4	>0.10
Total plasma cholesterol: high-density lipoprotein cholesterol	7.74	8.60	>0.10
Peak plasma progesterone (ng/mL)[c]	8.89	3.79	0.01
Percentage anovulatory cycles (%)[d]	3.5	16.5	0.01
Percentage cycles with luteal phase deficiencies (%)[e]	8.9	24.3	0.01

[a]By Mann-Whitney U-test, 2-tailed probabilities.
[b]Behavioral measures expressed in rate of performance/h/monkey.
[c]Peak progesterone determined from luteal phase of 10 randomly chosen cycles from each female.
[d]Anovulatory cycles considered to be those in which peak luteal phase plasma progesterone concentration was <2.0 ng/mL.
[e]Peak luteal progesterone concentrations between 2.0 and 4.0 ng/mL were considered to be indicative of luteal phase deficiencies.
From Kaplan JR, Adams MR, Clarkson TB, et al. Psychosocial influence on female "protection" among cynomolgus macaques. *Atherosclerosis* 53:283–285, 1984.

that female protection could not be explained by the usual risk factors (such as serum lipids); instead, we hypothesized that physiologic factors associated with low social status (e.g., abnormal ovarian or adrenal activity) were probably responsible, at least in part, for the pattern of coronary artery atherosclerosis observed among the females in this experiment (Fig. 15-6). Detailed analyses of both ovarian and adrenal function among these females have been published elsewhere (15, 26); in general, the pattern of impaired ovarian function and elevated adrenal activity observed among subordinates in this experiment is consistent with results observed in other monkeys (27–29).

In a subsequent study (15), we sought to determine whether removal of the ovaries would alter susceptibility to coronary artery atherosclerosis in female cynomolgus monkeys. The results of study 1 indicated that social subordination was associated with increased atherosclerosis of female monkeys. The concurrence of social subordination, impaired ovarian function, and elevated adrenal activity suggested that one or both of these physiologic factors may be capable of exacerbating atherosclerosis. For study 2, we used the females from study 1 as controls. In addition to the 23 control animals, the experiment included 21 ovariectomized females. Like the control animals, the ovariectomized females lived in social groups of five or six, each including a resident male. As in study 1, all relevant physiologic parameters were measured (serum lipid concentrations, blood pressure, cortisol response to ACTH challenge), as were social behavior patterns.

After 24 months, extent of atherosclerosis was measured in the coronary arteries. The results indicated that, overall, ovariectomized animals had more extensive coronary atherosclerosis than did their intact counterparts; however, when partitioned by social status, the data indicated that ovariectomized monkeys were unevenly affected (Fig. 15-7). Subordinate monkeys (ovariectomized or intact) were similar in the extent to which they were affected by atherosclerosis. The significant difference between intact and ovariectomized animals was largely attributable to the markedly worsened extent of atherosclerosis in the dominant females, in which ovariectomy apparently resulted in a relative loss of female protection. Intact subordinate monkeys with ovarian impairment and attendant loss of female protection were apparently not further affected (with respect to atherosclerosis) after complete removal of the ovaries.

Again, the results of this experiment could not be attributed to concomitant variation in serum lipids, which generally did not differ between subordinate and dominant animals or between intact and ovariectomized monkeys. Moreover, the adrenal responses of subordinate animals were greater than those of dominant individuals regardless of ovariectomy (15); it thus seems unlikely that adrenal factors influenced the increased atherosclerosis in the dominant ovariectomized animals.

Overall, the results indicate that ovarian hormones modulate susceptibility to coronary atherosclerosis among female monkeys, suggesting that women may be at increased risk of coronary artery atherosclerosis and hence CHD when ovarian function is impaired. This latter suggestion is supported by the observation that menopause (surgical or natural) is accompanied by an apparently increased risk

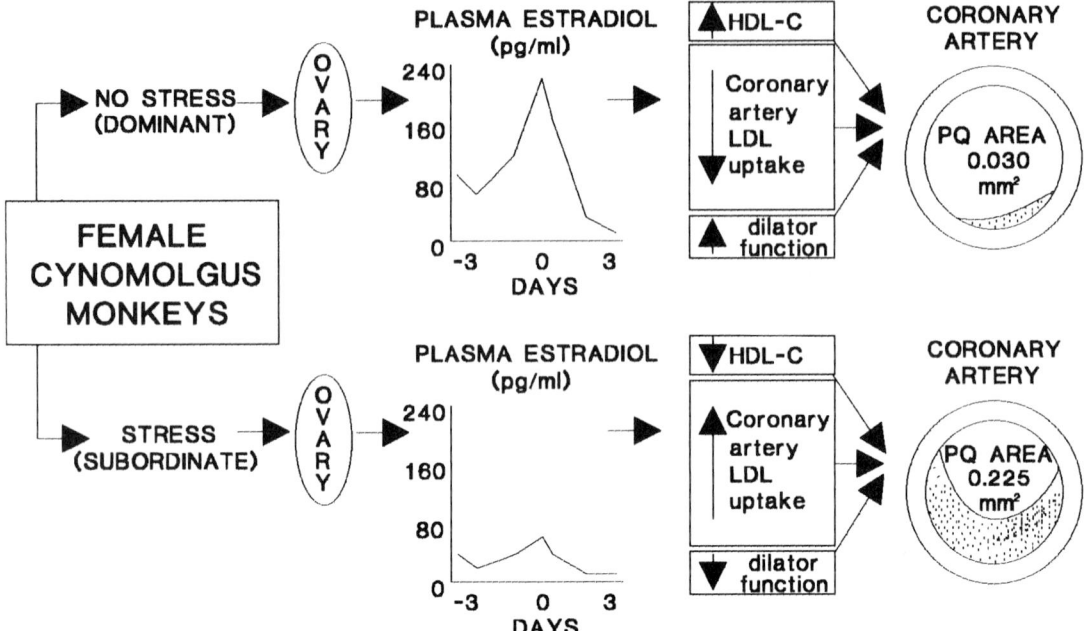

Figure 15–6. Predictors of coronary artery plaque (PQ) area in female cynomolgus monkeys. Effects of ovariectomy, estrogen replacement therapy, changes in lipoprotein parameters, and vasomotion varied in animals of different social status. (Adapted from Kaplan JR, Adams MR, Clarkson TB, et al. Psychosocial influences on female "protection" among cynomolgus macaques. *Atherosclerosis* 53:283–295, 1984.)

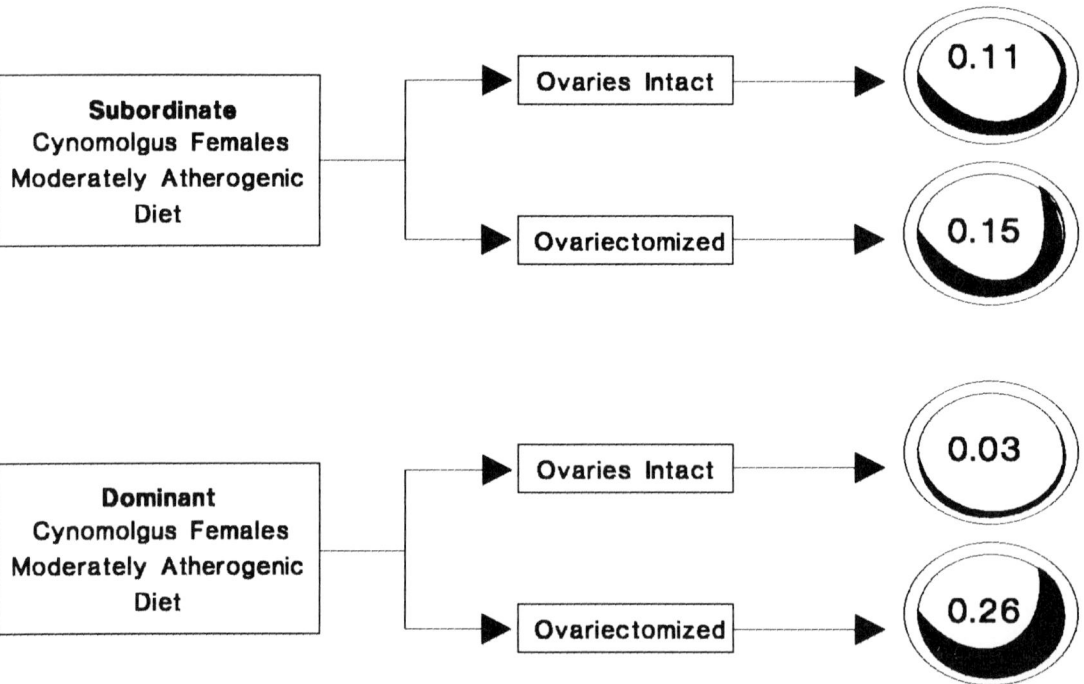

Figure 15–7. Eventual coronary artery plaque area (mm^2) in subordinate versus dominant female cynomolgus monkeys with and without ovariectomy. (Adapted from Kaplan JR, Adams MR, Clarkson TB, et al. Psychosocial influences on female "protection" among cynomolgus macaques. *Atherosclerosis* 53:283–295, 1984.)

of CHD (30–34), and most evidence indicates that estrogen replacement therapy favorably influences coronary risk in postmenopausal women (35). Also, the results of at least one study have linked chronic menstrual irregularity to a significantly increased risk of acute myocardial infarction (36).

As described, spontaneous impairment of ovarian function in cynomolgus monkeys is probably secondary to social subordination. Perturbation of reproductive function associated with stress, particularly the stress of social subordination, is common in mammals and is reminiscent of observations in humans linking emotional distress to ovarian dysfunction. To the extent that impaired ovarian function potentiates atherogenesis, behavioral attributes or responses of individuals that correlate with or contribute to impaired ovarian function may represent, in turn, a behavioral antecedent of coronary disease in women.

Social Isolation

In a third study, we evaluated retrospectively coronary artery atherosclerosis among 77 female monkeys, all of which had been fed the same atherogenic diet. Thirty of the animals had been in an experiment in which all monkeys were housed in single cages, and the other 47 had been maintained in social groups (37) (Fig. 15–8). There were no differences in plasma lipid or lipoprotein concentrations between the two groups. However, females housed in single cages had significantly more coronary artery atherosclerosis than those housed in social groups. As in the other studies, socially subordinate females had more extensive coronary artery atherosclerosis than dominants. Analysis of the data from singly and socially housed females disclosed that single-caged animals had more extensive atherosclerosis than socially dominant females but did not differ from subordinate animals.

The mechanism of coronary artery atherosclerosis among single-caged females is uncertain. It apparently is unrelated to impaired ovarian function. However, we have observed that single-caged male macaques' heart rates are elevated compared with those of group-housed monkeys (38). Elevated heart rate, in turn, is known to potentiate atherogenesis (39). In regard to the causes of elevated heart rates in single-caged animals, we can only speculate that the elements of restraint and social isolation may trigger sympathetic nervous system arousal. The findings reviewed

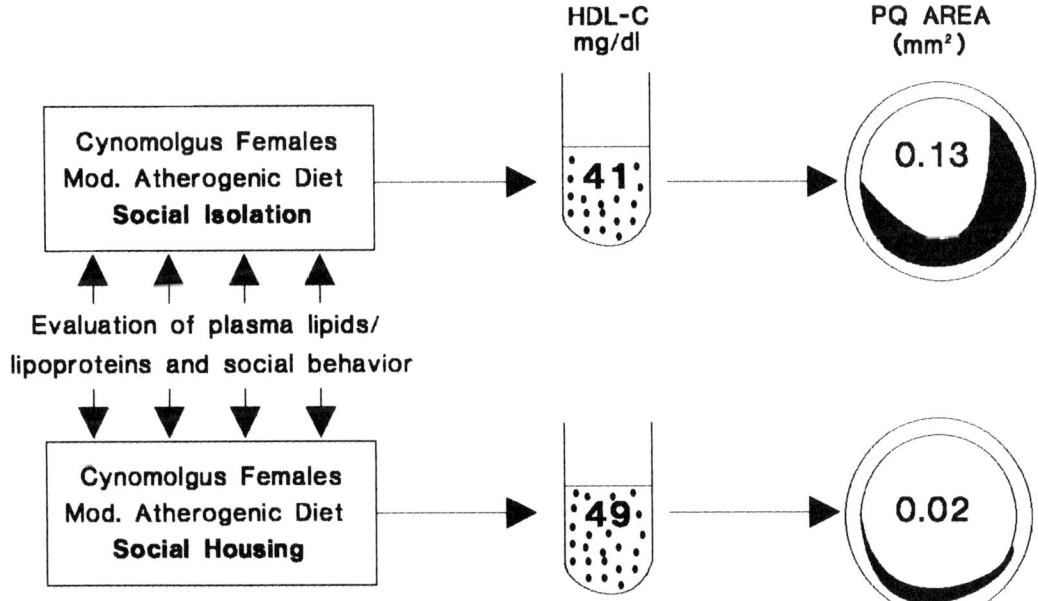

Figure 15–8. Effects of social isolation on coronary artery plaque (PQ) area in premenopausal female cynomolgus monkeys. Plasma lipoprotein concentrations were not significantly different between the two groups. (Adapted from Shively CA, Clarkson TB, Kaplan JR. Social deprivation and coronary artery atherosclerosis in female cynomolgus monkeys. *Atherosclerosis* 77:69–76, 1989.)

here suggest that single caging may represent a significant stress to cynomolgus monkeys and, under some circumstances, may confound experimental outcomes.

Pregnancy

To address further whether endogenous sex hormone concentrations are associated with atherosclerosis progression, we sought to determine whether there was a relationship between pregnancy and atherosclerosis extent in the cynomolgus monkey model (40). In this study, females in one experimental group lived in social groupings with males and were pregnant twice or more, whereas females in a second experimental group lived in social groups with vasectomized males and did not become pregnant during the 30-month study. Females that became pregnant had lower mean total plasma cholesterol concentrations. However, they also had lower plasma HDL cholesterol concentrations and, as a consequence, the ratio of total cholesterol to HDL cholesterol was not different between the two groups.

At necropsy, females that had been pregnant twice or more were found to have less extensive coronary artery atherosclerosis than the females that did not become pregnant (Fig. 15–9). Extent of coronary artery atherosclerosis was inversely related to an index (area under the curve) of the magnitude and duration of pregnancy-related elevations in plasma estradiol concentrations ($r = -0.66$, $p < 0.01$). This estradiol index was the single variable that correlated most strongly with extent of coronary artery atherosclerosis. Total plasma cholesterol and HDL cholesterol were also correlated with extent of atherosclerosis, but less strongly. Plasma progesterone concentration was not correlated with atherosclerosis extent. Thus, pregnancy is relatively protective against coronary artery atherosclerosis in this species, and there is evidence that circulating endogenous estrogen concentrations are associated with a degree of protection.

Central Obesity

Regional obesity is associated with the incidence of CHD and related risk factors in people. Because many premenopausal women are protected, compared with men, against CHD, it is of particular interest to identify characteristics of women who are not protected. These characteristics may give insight into the mechanisms underlying CHD risk. Although prospective epidemiologic studies of body fat distribution have predicted CHD, most of the observed relationships between regional obesity, CHD, and CHD risk factors have been associative rather than causal. At this time, it is not known whether regional obesity is an independent risk factor or whether its relationship to CHD is entirely dependent on other known risk factors, such as plasma lipid concentrations.

The relationships between regional obesity, atherosclerosis, and atherosclerosis risk factors have been studied in female cynomolgus monkeys (41). In a retrospective necropsy study, it was found that females with a relatively high ratio of central to peripheral fat deposition had three times more extensive coronary artery atherosclerosis (Fig. 15–10). In a second experiment, it was found that females with high central fat ratios and females with high levels of whole body obesity were relatively hyperglycemic. Subsequently, it was discovered that females with relatively high whole body obesity and females with relatively central fat deposition had higher blood pressures. Females with relatively central fat deposition had higher total plasma cholesterol and lower HDL cholesterol concentrations as well as exacerbated coronary artery atherosclerosis. Social subordinates were more likely to exhibit a central fat deposition pattern than dominants. These findings suggest that female cynomolgus monkeys may be a potential animal model of the health impact of regional obesity.

Surgical Menopause

Women who have undergone either natural or surgical menopause have rather large increases in the rates of progression of coronary artery atherosclerosis. We have studied surgically postmenopausal cynomolgus monkeys to determine the extent to which they share this pathophysiologic process with women. Figure 15–11 depicts a comparison of plasma HDL cholesterol concentrations and coronary artery atherosclerosis of pre- and postmenopausal cynomolgus monkeys.

Postmenopausal cynomolgus monkeys, like women, have reduced plasma concentrations of HDLs, and we know from other studies that they have increased low-density lipopro-

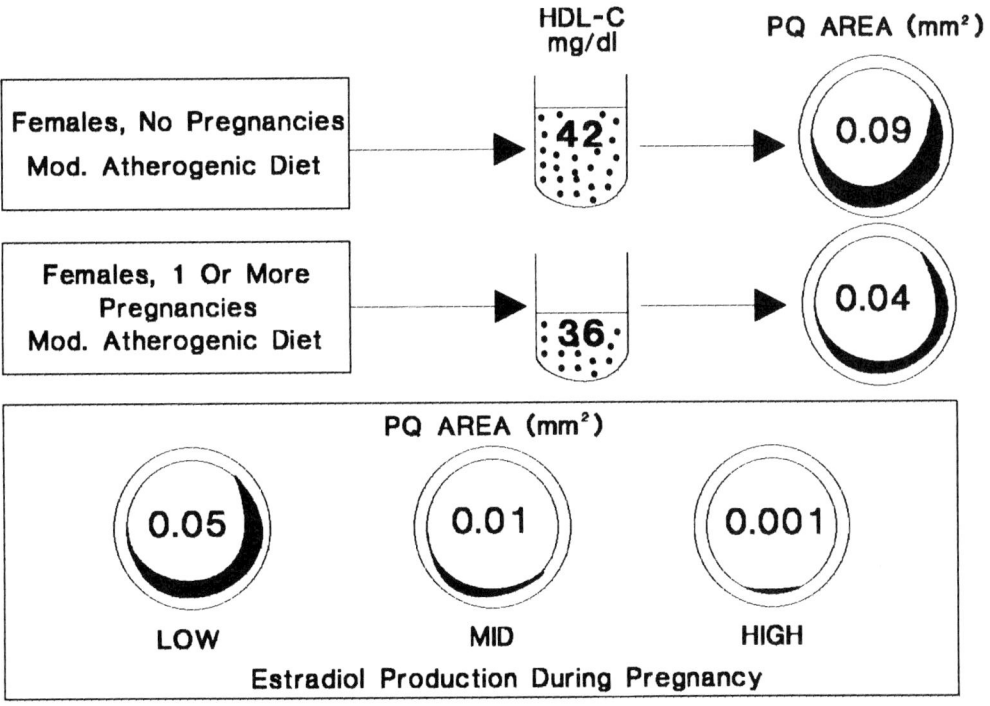

Figure 15–9. Coronary artery plaque (PQ) area was less extensive in female cynomolgus monkeys that had been pregnant at least twice compared with monkeys with no pregnancies. HDL cholesterol concentrations were also lower in the monkeys that had been pregnant at least twice. Extent of plaque area was inversely related to pregnancy-related elevations in plasma estradiol concentrations. (Adapted from Adams MR, Kaplan JR, Koritnik DR, et al. Pregnancy-associated inhibition of coronary artery atherosclerosis in monkeys. Evidence of a relationship with endogenous estrogen. *Arteriosclerosis* 7:378–384, 1987.)

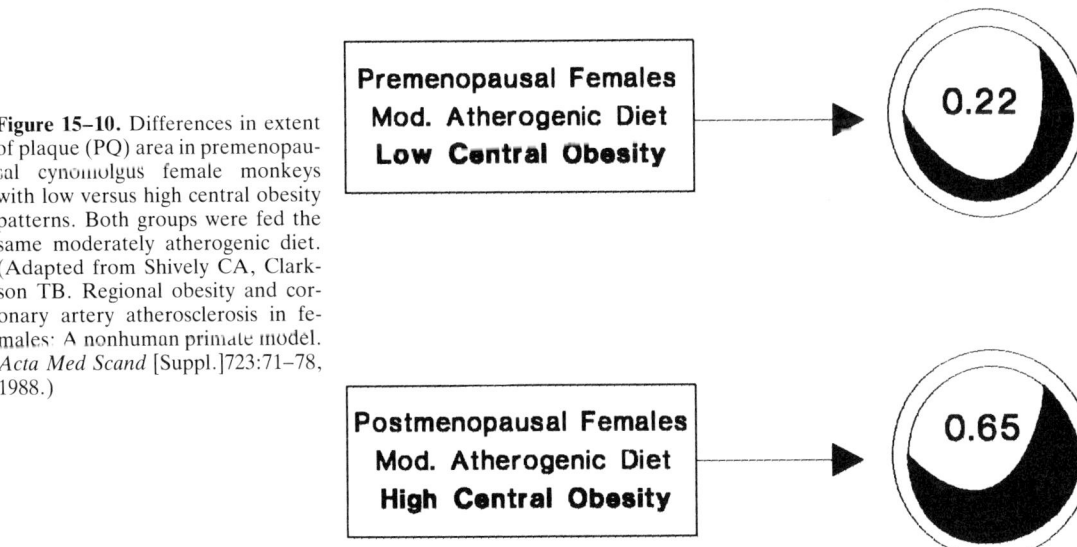

Figure 15–10. Differences in extent of plaque (PQ) area in premenopausal cynomolgus female monkeys with low versus high central obesity patterns. Both groups were fed the same moderately atherogenic diet. (Adapted from Shively CA, Clarkson TB. Regional obesity and coronary artery atherosclerosis in females: A nonhuman primate model. *Acta Med Scand* [Suppl.]723:71–78, 1988.)

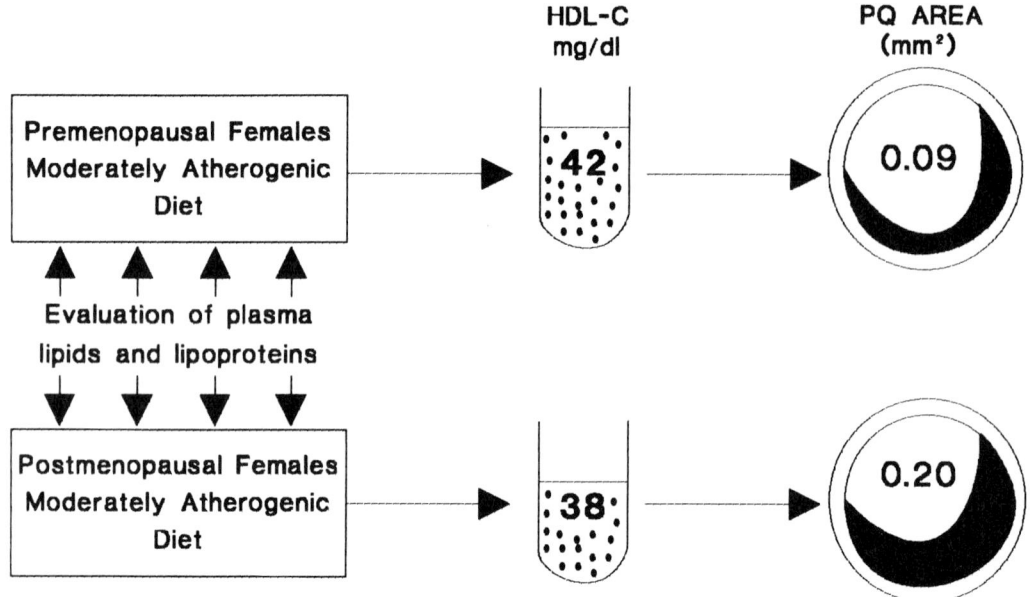

Figure 15–11. Plasma HDL cholesterol (HDL-C) concentrations and coronary artery plaque (PQ) area in premenopausal versus postmenopausal cynomolgus monkeys, both fed the same moderately atherogenic diet. (Adapted from Adams MR, Kaplan JR, Clarkson TB, et al. Effects of psychosocial stress, menopause and pregnancy in coronary artery atherosclerosis. In Eaker ED, Packard B, Wenger NK, et al. [Eds]. *Coronary Heart Disease in Women.* New York, Haymarket Doyma, 1987.)

tein (LDL) accumulation, increased vasoconstrictor responses, and coronary artery atherosclerotic plaques that are much larger than those found in premenopausal monkeys fed the same atherogenic diet for the same length of time.

EFFECTS OF ESTROGEN REPLACEMENT THERAPY

In human populations where CHD is a major public health problem, the incidence of CHD is much lower in premenopausal women than in men of similar age. This gender difference in CHD risk is paralleled by a difference in extent and severity of coronary artery atherosclerosis (42). It is widely believed that ovarian estrogen is responsible for this relative sparing of the coronary arteries; however, it remains uncertain whether CHD risk or atherosclerosis in human beings is influenced by menopause, a state of relative estrogen deficiency (43). Yet there is compelling evidence that estrogen replacement therapy results in a marked reduction in CHD risk in postmenopausal women (44). Mechanisms by which this effect is mediated are poorly understood. Among multiple possibilities are inhibitory effects on atherosclerosis progression, inhibitory effects on coronary thrombosis, and beneficial effects on vasomotor function of coronary arteries. We summarize here the experimental evidence regarding the effects of estrogen deficiency and estrogen replacement therapy on atherosclerosis progression and arterial vasomotor function.

Experimental Evidence: Coronary Artery Atherosclerosis

This discussion emphasizes coronary arteries because (1) the gender difference in atherosclerosis extent is confined to coronary arteries (42); (2) experimental evidence indicates that effects of sex hormones are confined to coronary arteries and perhaps femoral arteries (24, 42, 43); and (3) the effects on coronary arteries are of greatest relevance to CHD, the major clinical sequela of atherosclerosis in human beings. Effects on aortic atherosclerosis, for example, may be of limited relevance and in fact may lead to inappropriate conclusions regarding coronary heart disease.

Among the initial evidence that estrogen inhibits the progression of coronary artery atherosclerosis was a series of studies done in the 1950s at the Michael Reese Research Institute. Ligation of the hen oviduct, which results in a marked elevation in plasma cholesterol concentration, had no effect on the relative resistance of the hen to atherosclerosis, whereas ovariectomy resulted in a marked exacerbation of atherosclerosis (4). In addition, exogenous estradiol in physiologic doses was found to inhibit progression of atherosclerosis and to promote regression of atherosclerosis in this species (6). Subsequent studies using White Carneau pigeons resulted in similar conclusions regarding the inhibitory effects of physiologic doses of estrogen on coronary atherosclerosis (3).

The subject of sex hormones and atherosclerosis received relatively little attention in the 1960s and 1970s. In 1977, McGill and colleagues studied the effects of endogenous estrogens on the extent of atherosclerosis in ovariectomized baboons (45). These studies determined that ovariectomy was not associated with increased extent or severity of diet-induced atherosclerosis. Furthermore, there were no significant effects with either physiologic or pharmacologic estrogen replacement therapy. It is perhaps important to note that, unlike many other primate species, including man, the baboon is relatively resistant to diet-induced hyperlipidemia and atherosclerosis. Furthermore, there is no gender difference in the extent of diet-induced coronary artery atherosclerosis in baboons.

We have employed the cynomolgus monkey model to address the effects of estrogen deficiency and estrogen replacement on atherosclerosis progression. As described elsewhere in this chapter, there is indirect evidence of the effects of endogenous sex hormones on the extent of atherosclerosis. Males and ovariectomized females do not differ in the extent of diet-induced coronary artery atherosclerosis and also have consistently low plasma estradiol concentrations in the range of 20 pg/mL. Atherosclerosis extent is reduced by approximately one-half in intact nonpregnant females, which normally have much higher plasma estradiol concentrations, which range from 60 to 300 pg/mL depending on the time of the menstrual cycle. Atherosclerosis extent is reduced by approximately 25% in pregnant females, which also show sustained dramatic elevations in plasma estradiol concentrations from 300 to 1000 pg/mL.

Direct evidence of an inhibitory effect of physiologic estrogen concentrations on the progression of coronary artery atherosclerosis is provided by the results of a subsequent study (46). In this study, ovariectomized monkeys were assigned randomly to one of three treatment groups: (1) no hormone replacement (n = 17), (2) continually administered 17β-estradiol plus cyclically administered progesterone (n = 20), and (3) continuously administered 17β-estradiol (n = 18). Physiologic patterns of plasma estradiol and progesterone concentrations were maintained by administering the hormones in sustained-release subcutaneous Silastic implants. The experiment lasted 30 months. At necropsy, coronary artery atherosclerosis was inhibited similarly (reduced by approximately half) in animals in both hormone replacement groups (Fig. 15–12). The antiatherogenic effects of hormone replacement were independent of variations in total plasma cholesterol, lipoprotein cholesterol, apoprotein A-1 and B concentrations, average LDL particle size, and HDL subfractional heterogeneity. Similarly, effects of hormone replacement on atherosclerosis could not be accounted for by other risk variables (i.e., blood pressure or carbohydrate tolerance). These findings suggest that an inhibitory influence of estrogen on atherogenesis and CHD must be mediated either through other risk factors not measured in this study or not yet described, or through a direct influence on cellular or biochemical events occurring in the arterial intima.

Estrogen and progesterone receptors have been found in arterial endothelial and smooth muscle cells of several species, including human beings (47–49). Lin et al. reported that estrogen treatment of baboons resulted in a redistribution of arterial intercellular estrogen receptors and increased cellular concentration of progesterone receptors (48). These findings imply a role for sex steroids in the regulation of arterial cell function. Other studies have shown that estrogen treatment results in reductions in lipoprotein-induced arterial smooth muscle cell proliferation (50), inhibition of the myointimal proliferation associated with mechanical endothelial injury (51–53), reduced arterial cholesterol ester influx and hydrolysis (7, 8), inhibition of platelet aggregation (54), decreased collagen and elastin production (55–58), and increased prostacyclin production by arterial smooth muscle cells (59). These studies indicate that estrogen may inhibit atherogenesis by inhibiting foam cell formation, platelet

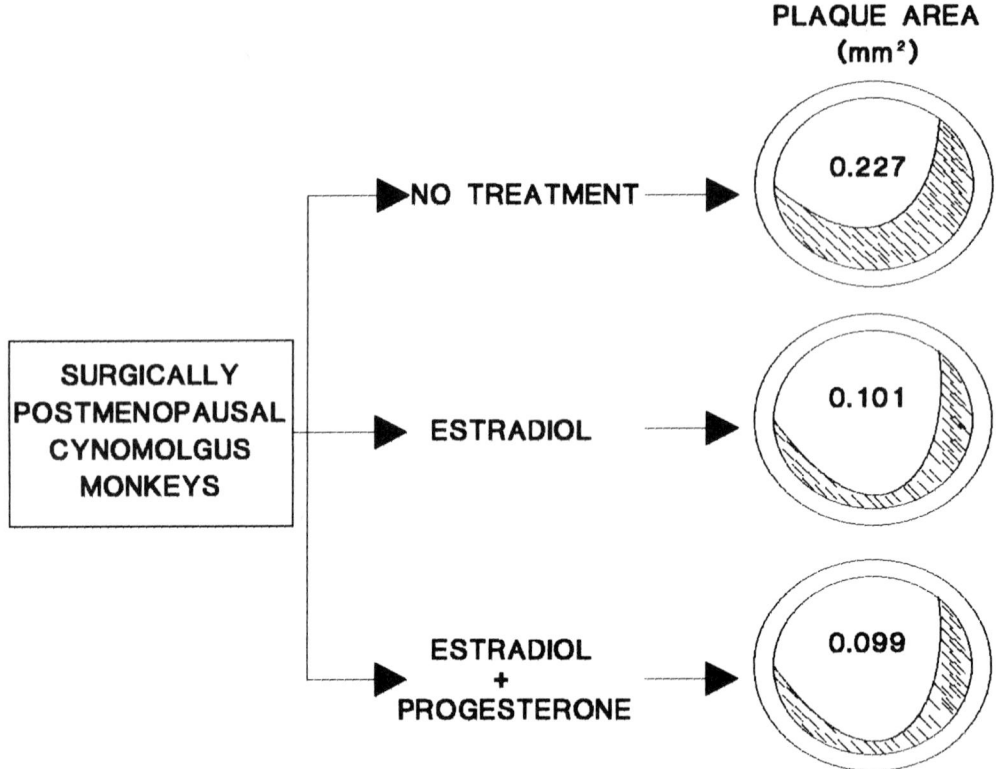

Figure 15–12. Coronary artery plaque area in surgically postmenopausal cynomolgus monkeys was lowest in the group that received continually administered 17β-estradiol and cyclically administered progesterone. Treatment was arranged to mimic the hormonal changes associated with normal ovulation in women. (Adapted from Adams MR, Kaplan JR, Manuck SB, et al. Inhibition of coronary artery atherosclerosis by 17 beta-estradiol in ovariectomized monkeys. Lack of an effect of adding progesterone. *Arteriosclerosis* 10:1051–1057, 1990.)

aggregation, smooth muscle cell proliferation, and the accumulation of collagen and elastin. Subsequent studies in our laboratory have addressed further the effects of sex hormones on arterial lipoprotein metabolism.

ESTROGEN AND PROGESTIN EFFECTS ON ARTERIAL METABOLISM

We have sought to determine the cellular mechanisms for the beneficial effects of estrogens and progestins on atherogenesis. To study the effects of hormone treatment on lipoprotein metabolism, we used LDL coupled to radiolabeled tyramine cellobiose (TC) (60–62). The labeled TC-LDL, originally described by Pittman et al. (63), allows quantification of the accumulation of products of LDL degradation and undegraded LDL in tissue and arterial samples. Furthermore, by using differently labeled LDL (i.e., ^{125}I–TC-LDL and ^{131}I-LDL), it is possible to calculate separately the amount of undegraded and degraded LDL.

Female cynomolgus monkeys were fed an atherogenic diet for short periods of time sufficient to stimulate the early events of atherogenesis but not to develop atherosclerotic plaques. Estrogen and cyclic progesterone were administered to ovariectomized monkeys via Silastic implants in one group (n = 9), resulting in physiologic plasma hormone levels, whereas ovariectomized controls (n = 8) had low to undetectable levels of the hormones. Labeled LDL was injected 24 hours before necropsy, after which the uptake and metabolism of the LDL was determined in various arteries and tissues. Hormone replacement therapy significantly decreased the accumulation of both degradation products of LDL and undegraded LDL in coronary arteries (61) (Fig. 15–13*A*) as well as other arteries (62).

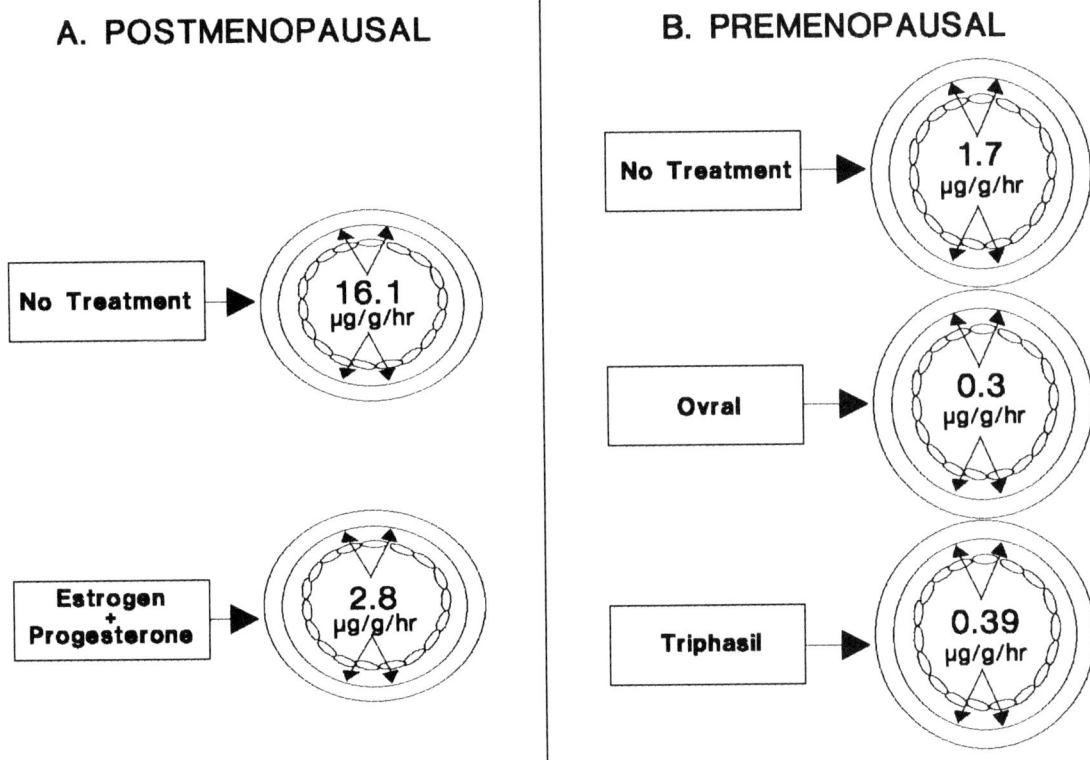

Figure 15–13. *A*, Significantly decreased accumulation of LDL degradation products in the coronary arteries was observed in surgically postmenopausal cynomolgus monkeys receiving hormone replacement therapy. *B*, Oral contraceptive treatment in premenopausal cynomolgus monkeys decreased arterial LDL accumulation despite causing a slightly more atherogenic lipoprotein profile. (Adapted from Wagner JD, Clarkson TB, St. Clair RW, et al. Estrogen and progesterone replacement therapy and coronary artery atherogenesis in surgically menopausal cynomolgus monkeys. *Circulation* 80[Suppl. II]:II-331, 1989 and from Wagner JD, Clarkson TB, St. Clair RW, et al. Estrogen replacement therapy reduces low density lipoprotein accumulation in the coronary arteries of surgically postmenopausal cynomolgus monkeys. *J Clin Invest* 88:1995–2002, 1991.)

Furthermore, with hormone deficiency the coronary arteries had a greater increase in LDL degradation than other arteries, which accurately predicts the increase in coronary artery atherosclerosis in postmenopausal women (62). These changes in arterial LDL metabolism were independent of changes in plasma lipid, lipoprotein, or apoprotein concentrations and occurred without changes in indices of endothelial injury or changes in extra-arterial LDL metabolism (62).

As with estrogen replacement therapy, oral contraceptives also attenuate the accumulation of products of LDL degradation (64). In this study, monkeys were fed an atherogenic diet alone (n = 7) or along with the oral contraceptives Ovral (n = 8) or Triphasil (n = 8) for 16 weeks. Despite causing a slightly more atherogenic lipoprotein profile than diet alone, both contraceptives decreased arterial LDL accumulation (Fig. 15–13*B*). Again, these changes occurred prior to changes in arterial morphology.

The decrease in LDL degradation and accumulation is one mechanism by which we believe that hormone therapy may decrease the incidence of CHD in women. Our findings are consistent with those of Hough and Zilversmit (7), who reported that estrogen treatment (17-estradiol cypionate) in intact female rabbits decreased arterial cholesteryl ester influx and hydrolysis. These decreases occurred independently of plasma cholesterol concentrations and lipoprotein patterns. Thus, in both our studies (61, 62) and in those of Hough and Zilversmit (7), estrogens, with and without progestins, favorably decreased arterial LDL degradation and cholesterol ester hydrolysis independently of lipid and lipoprotein changes.

ESTROGEN AND PROGESTIN EFFECTS ON VASOMOTION

Coronary heart disease develops when blood flow through the coronary arteries is no longer sufficient to meet the metabolic demands of the heart. Development of occlusive atherosclerotic plaque or an occlusive thrombus may reduce blood flow through the coronary arteries, resulting in myocardial ischemia or infarction. However, dynamic changes in vascular smooth muscle tone (resulting in vasospasm) also play an important role in narrowing the lumen of atherosclerotic coronary arteries (65). These factors are not entirely independent, and it is likely that interactions between blood elements, the vascular endothelium, various components of the plaque, and vascular smooth muscle cells are important in the pathogenesis of CHD.

Patients with atherosclerosis are prone to development of coronary vasospasm, particularly at sites of coronary artery stenosis (65, 66). It has become evident that the endothelium is important in modulating vascular smooth muscle cell reactivity (67, 68). Endothelial cells release dilator and constrictor substances that act on the underlying smooth muscle (68, 69). It is thought that atherosclerosis interferes with the normal function of endothelial cells, resulting in impaired release of dilator substances and augmented release of constrictor substances (68, 69). It has been shown experimentally that atherosclerosis impairs dilation and augments constriction to various neurohumoral stimuli, including platelets and white blood cells (70, 71). Thus, a consequence of atherosclerosis is a shift in regulatory responses that promote vasoconstriction and vasospasm.

For the most part, males have been used to examine the effects of atherosclerosis on vasomotion. However, estrogen modulates vascular responses at several arterial sites. Estrogen modulates vascular responses of guinea pig uterine arteries (72) and rabbit arteries in vivo (73, 74). The effect of estrogen on vascular responses in rabbits seems to be site-specific, with estrogen reducing constrictor responses to noradrenalin and the α2-adrenergic antagonist rawuolscine in arteries but not in veins (74). Estrogen augments dilation to both acetylcholine and the calcium ionophore A23187 in the rabbit aorta (but not in the carotid or femoral arteries), suggesting that estrogen may augment release, transport, or viability of endothelium-derived relaxing factors (EDRFs) (74). Preliminary reports by Jiang et al. (75–77) have provided evidence that estradiol promotes endothelium-independent dilation of arteries, has calcium antagonistic properties, and attenuates constriction of rabbit coronary arteries to endothelin-1 (an endothelium-derived constriction factor).

Results of studies in cynomolgus monkeys have indicated that among males, nonatherosclerotic coronary arteries dilate in response to acetylcholine and atherosclerotic coronary arteries constrict (78). Results of a recent study showed that, among surgically postmenopausal female cynomolgus monkeys, atherosclerosis impairs and estrogen replacement (subcutaneous 17β-estradiol) "protects" against impaired dilation of coronary arteries to acetylcholine (Fig. 15–14) (79). In another study, it was determined that estrogen improves endothelium-mediated vascular responses of coronary arteries within 20 minutes of intravenous infusion of pharmacologic doses of ethinyl estradiol (80).

In summary, results of studies with monkeys have suggested that atherosclerosis impairs the vascular responses of coronary arteries in both males and females. Estrogen treatment in postmenopausal females improves the vascular responses of coronary arteries. These findings suggest a mechanism by which estrogen replacement may reduce CHD risk in postmenopausal women.

CLINICAL IMPLICATIONS OF ANIMAL MODEL STUDIES

We have summarized the clinical implications from the cynomolgus monkey studies by questions and answers.

Does contraceptive steroid use hasten coronary atherogenesis?

Monkeys share with women decreases in plasma HDLs when treated with contraceptive steroids; despite this, coronary atherogenesis is diminished (23, 24).

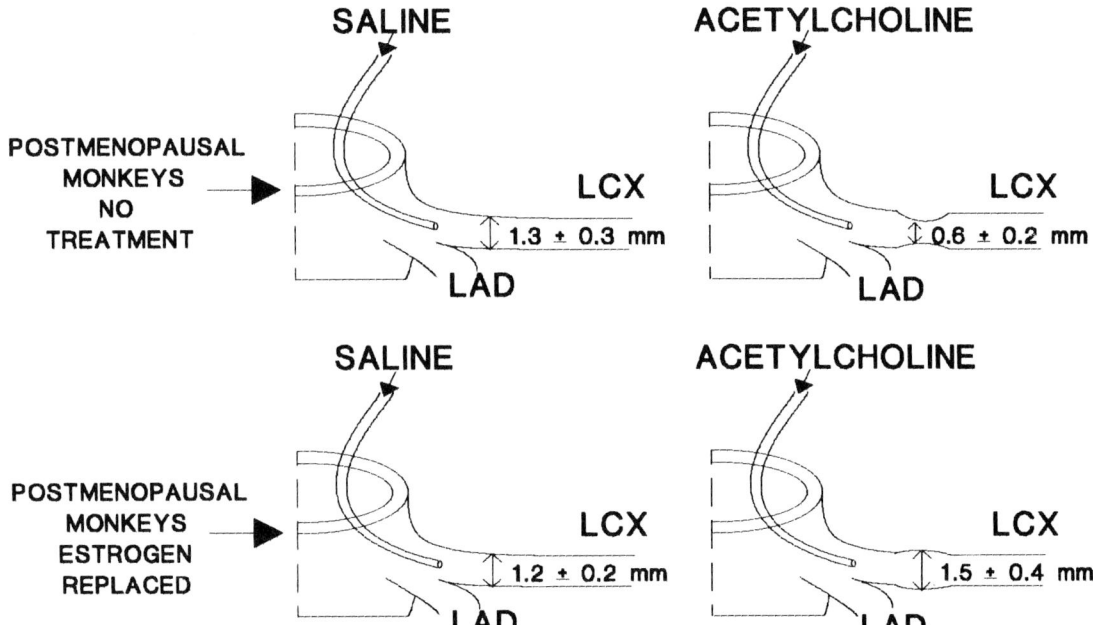

Figure 15-14. Percentage of change in coronary artery diameter in two groups of surgically postmenopausal cynomolgus monkeys in response to intracoronary infusions of saline and 10^{-6}M acetylcholine. Subcutaneous infusion of 17β-estradiol had a protective effect against impaired arterial dilation to acetylcholine. LAD = left anterior descending artery; LCX = left circumflex artery. (Adapted from Williams JK, Adams MR, Klopfenstein HS. Estrogen modulates responses of atherosclerotic coronary arteries. *Circulation* 81:1680–1687, 1990.)

Does psychosocial stress accelerate coronary atherogenesis?

Chronically stressed monkeys have impaired ovarian function, relative estrogen deficiency, early bone loss, and accelerated coronary atherogenesis (15, 25).

Does social isolation affect coronary atherogenesis adversely?

Female monkeys maintained in social isolation have several times more coronary atherosclerosis than their counterparts with social support (37).

Does pregnancy increase or decrease the incidence of coronary atherosclerosis?

Monkeys with multiple pregnancies are protected from coronary artery atherosclerosis and the degree of protection is related to the amount of endogenous estrogen production during pregnancy (40).

Does central obesity increase the progression of coronary atherosclerosis among monkey females?

Increased body mass index of female monkeys is weakly or not associated with coronary atherogenesis, but central (intra-abdominal) obesity is strongly associated with coronary atherogenesis (41).

Does the decreased morbidity and mortality from CHD among postmenopausal women given estrogen replacement therapy result from the decreased extensiveness of coronary atherosclerosis?

Surgically postmenopausal monkeys given physiologic replacement of estrogen show a decrease in the size and extent of coronary artery atherosclerotic plaques of about 50% (see Fig. 15–12) (46).

Is the beneficial effect of postmenopausal estrogen replacement on coronary atherosclerosis modulated by its effect on the plasma lipoproteins?

About 20% of the beneficial effect on coronary artery atherosclerosis in estrogen-replaced postmenopausal monkeys appears to be related to plasma lipoprotein changes (81).

What is the probable mechanism of the beneficial effect of estrogen treatment on coronary atherogenesis?

Studies with both pre- and postmenopausal monkeys suggest that a major mechanism of the coronary atherosclerosis–protective effect of estrogens relates to the markedly decreased uptake of LDL by the coronary arteries (60, 62).

Do estrogen deficiency and estrogen replacement affect the vasodilator and vasoconstrictor responses of coronary arteries?

Nonestrogen-replaced postmenopausal monkeys experience coronary artery vasoconstriction following acetylcholine injection, whereas estrogen-replaced monkeys experience vasodilation when injected with the same amount of acetylcholine (79, 80).

Acknowledgments

Supported in part by Grants P50 HL-45666, R01 HL-38964, and R01 HL-46409, National Institutes of Health, Bethesda, Maryland. The authors wish to thank Ginger Petrick for her expertise in creating the figures and Karen Potvin Klein for her editorial contributions.

References

1. Clarkson TB, Middleton CC, Prichard RW, et al. Naturally occurring atherosclerosis in birds. *Ann NY Acad Sci* 127:685–693, 1965.
2. Adelman SJ, St. Clair RW. Lipoprotein metabolism by macrophages from atherosclerosis-susceptible White Carneau and resistant Show Racer pigeons. *J Lipid Res* 29:643–656, 1988.
3. Prichard RW, Clarkson TB, Lofland HB. Estrogen in pigeon atherosclerosis. Estradiol valerate effects at several dose levels on cholesterol-fed male White Carneau pigeons. *Arch Pathol* 82:15–17, 1966.
4. Stamler J, Pick R, Katz LN. Inhibition of cholesterol-induced coronary atherogenesis in the egg-producing hen. *Circulation* 10:251–254, 1954.
5. Pick R, Stamler J, Rodbard S, et al. The inhibition of coronary atherosclerosis by estrogen in cholesterol-fed chicks. *Circulation* 6:276–280, 1952.
6. Pick R, Stamler J, Rodbard S, et al. Estrogen-induced regression of coronary atherosclerosis in cholesterol-fed chicks. *Circulation* 6:858–861, 1952.
7. Hough JL, Zilversmit DB. Effect of 17-beta estradiol on aortic cholesterol content and metabolism in cholesterol-fed rabbits. *Atherosclerosis* 657–663, 1986.
8. Haarbo J, Leth-Espensen P, Stender SA, et al. Estrogen monotherapy and combined estrogen-progestogen replacement therapy attenuate aortic accumulation of cholesterol in ovariectomized cholesterol-fed rabbits. *J Clin Invest* 87:1274–1279, 1991.
9. Panepinto LM, Phillips RW. The Yucatan miniature pig: Characterization and utilization in biomedical research. *Lab Anim Sci* 36:344–347, 1986.
10. Gal D, Rongione AJ, Slovenkai GA, et al. Atherosclerotic Yucatan microswine: An animal model with high-grade, fibrocalcific, non-fatty lesions suitable for testing catheter-based interventions. *Am Heart J* 119:291–300, 1990.
11. Jacobsson L. Comparison of experimental hypercholesterolemia and atherosclerosis in male and female mini-pigs of the Gottingen strain. *Artery* 16:105–117, 1989.
12. Nichols TC, Bellinger DA, Tate DA, et al. Von Willebrand factor and occlusive arterial thrombosis. A study in normal and von Willebrand's disease pigs with diet-induced hypercholesterolemia and arteriosclerosis. *Arteriosclerosis* 10:449–461, 1990.
13. Strong JP, Eggen DA. Atherosclerosis II. Proceedings of the Second International Symposium on Atherosclerosis 1970, pp. 355–364.
14. Jewett DA, Dukelow WR. Cyclicity and gestational length of *Macaca fascicularis*. *Primates* 13:327–330, 1972.
15. Adams MR, Kaplan JR, Clarkson TB, et al. Ovariectomy, social status, and atherosclerosis in cynomolgus monkeys. *Arteriosclerosis* 5:192–200, 1985.
16. Godsland IF, Wynn V, Crook D, et al. Sex, plasma lipoproteins, and atherosclerosis: Prevailing assumptions and outstanding questions. *Am Heart J* 114:1467–1503, 1987.
17. Mishell DR Jr. Use of oral contraceptives in women of older reproductive age. *Am J Obstet Gynecol* 158:1652–1657, 1988.
18. Realini JP, Goldzieher JW. Oral contraceptives and cardiovascular disease: A critique of the epidemiologic studies. *Am J Obstet Gynecol* 152:792–798, 1985.
19. Thorneycroft IH. Oral contraceptives and myocardial infarction. *Am J Obstet Gynecol* 163:1393–1397, 1990.
20. Thorogood M, Vessey MP. An epidemiologic survey of cardiovascular disease in women taking oral contraceptives. *Am J Obstet Gynecol* 163:274–281, 1990.
21. Stampfer MJ, Willett WC, Colditz GA, et al. Past use of oral contraceptives and cardiovascular disease: A meta-analysis in the context of the Nurses' Health Study. *Am J Obstet Gynecol* 163:285–291, 1990.
22. Engel HJ, Engel E, Lichtlen PR. Coronary atherosclerosis and myocardial infarction in young women—role of oral contraceptives. *Eur Heart J* 4:1–8, 1983.
23. Adams MR, Clarkson TB, Koritnik DR, et al. Contraceptive steroids and coronary artery atherosclerosis in cynomolgus macaques. *Fertil Steril* 47:1010–1018, 1987.
24. Clarkson TB, Shively CA, Morgan TM, et al. Oral contraceptives and coronary artery atherosclerosis of cynomolgus macaques. *Obstet Gynecol* 75:217–222, 1990.
25. Kaplan JR, Adams MR, Clarkson TB, et al. Psychosocial influences on female "protection" among cynomolgus macaques. *Atherosclerosis* 53:283–295, 1984.
26. Kaplan JR, Adams MR, Koritnik DR, et al. Adrenal responsiveness and social status in intact and ovariectomized *Macaca fascicularis*. *Am J Primatol* 11:181–193, 1986.
27. Chamove AS, Bowman RE. Rhesus plasma cortisol response at four dominance positions. *Aggressive Behav* 4:43–55, 1978.
28. Dessi-Fulgheri F, Messeri P, Lupodi PC. A study of testosterone, estradiol, cortisol and prolactin in a socially intact group of Japanese macaques. *Anthropol Contemp* 4:123–127, 1981.

29. Sassenrath EN. Increased adrenal responsiveness related to social stress in rhesus monkeys. *Horm Behav* 1:283–298, 1970.
30. Kannel WB, Hjortland MC, McNamara PM, et al. Menopause and risk of cardiovascular disease. *Ann Intern Med* 85:447–452, 1976.
31. Gordon T, Kannel WB, Hjortland MC, et al. Menopause and coronary heart disease. *Ann Intern Med* 89:157–161, 1978.
32. Talbott E, Kuller LH, Perper J, et al. Sudden unexpected death in women: Biologic and psychosocial origins. *Am J Epidemiol* 114:671–682, 1981.
33. Colditz GA, Willett WC, Stampfer MJ, et al. Menopause and the risk of coronary heart disease in women. *N Engl J Med* 316:1106–1110, 1987.
34. Matthews KA, Meilahn E, Kuller LH, et al. Menopause and risk factors for coronary heart disease. *N Engl J Med* 321:641–646, 1989.
35. Knopp RH. The effects of postmenopausal estrogen therapy on the incidence of arteriosclerotic vascular disease. *Obstet Gynecol* 72:23S–30S, 1988.
36. LaVecchia C, Decarli A, Franceschi S, et al. Menstrual and reproductive factors and the risk of myocardial infarction in women under fifty-five years of age. *Am J Obstet Gynecol* 157:1108–1112, 1987.
37. Shively CA, Clarkson TB, Kaplan JR. Social deprivation and coronary artery atherosclerosis in female cynomolgus monkeys. *Atherosclerosis* 77:69–76, 1989.
38. Adams MR, Kaplan JR, Manuck SB, et al. Persistent sympathetic nervous system arousal associated with tethering in cynomolgus macaques. *Lab Anim Sci* 38:279–281, 1988.
39. Kaplan JR, Manuck SB, Clarkson TB. The influence of heart rate on coronary artery atherosclerosis. *J Cardiovasc Pharmacol* 10 (Suppl 2):S100–S103, 1987.
40. Adams MR, Kaplan JR, Koritnik DR, et al. Pregnancy-associated inhibition of coronary artery atherosclerosis in monkeys. Evidence of a relationship with endogenous estrogen. *Arteriosclerosis* 7:378–384, 1987.
41. Shively CA, Clarkson TB. Regional obesity and coronary artery atherosclerosis in females: A nonhuman primate model. *Acta Med Scand* (Suppl.)723:71–78, 1988.
42. McGill HC Jr, Stern MP. Sex and atherosclerosis. *Atherosclerosis Rev* 4:157–242, 1979.
43. Adams MR, Kaplan JR, Clarkson TB, et al. Effects of psychosocial stress, menopause and pregnancy on coronary artery atherosclerosis. In Eaker ED, Packard B, Wenger NK, et al. (Eds.), *Coronary Heart Disease in Women*. New York, Haymarket Doyma, 1987, pp. 151–157.
44. Bush TL. The epidemiology of cardiovascular disease in postmenopausal women. *Ann NY Acad Sci* 592:263–271, 1990.
45. McGill HC Jr, Axelrod LR, McMahan CA, et al. Estrogens and experimental atherosclerosis in the baboon (*Papio cynocephalus*). *Circulation* 56:657–662, 1977.
46. Adams MR, Kaplan JR, Manuck SB, et al. Inhibition of coronary artery atherosclerosis by 17-beta estradiol in ovariectomized monkeys. Lack of an effect of added progesterone. *Arteriosclerosis* 10:1051–1057, 1990.
47. Lin AL, McGill HC Jr, Shain SA. Hormone receptors of the baboon cardiovascular system. *Circ Res* 50:610–616, 1982.
48. Lin AL, Gonzalez R Jr, Carey KD, et al. Estradiol 17-beta affects estrogen receptor distribution and elevates progesterone receptor content in baboon aorta. *Arteriosclerosis* 6:495–504, 1986.
49. Ingegno MD, Money SR, Thelmo W, et al. Progesterone receptors in the human heart and great vessels. *Lab Invest* 59:353–356, 1988.
50. Fischer-Dzoga K, Wissler RW, Vesselinovitch D. The effect of estradiol on the proliferation of rabbit aortic medial tissue culture cells induced by hyperlipemic serum. *Exp Mol Pathol* 39:355–363, 1983.
51. Rhee CY, Spaet TH, Gaynor E, et al. Suppression of surgically induced vascular intimal hypertrophy by estrogen. *Circulation* 49(Suppl. III):III–92, 1974.
52. Rhee CY, Drouet RO, Spaet TH, et al. Growth inhibition of cultured vascular smooth muscle cells by estradiol. *Fed Proc* 37:474, 1978.
53. Weigensberg BI, Lough H, More MH, et al. Effects of estradiol on myointimal thickening from catheter injury and on organizing white mural nonocclusive thrombi. *Atherosclerosis* 52:252–265, 1984.
54. Johnson M, Ramey E, Ramwell PW. Androgen-mediated sensitivity in platelet aggregation. *Am J Physiol* 232:H381–H385, 1977.
55. Fischer GM. In vivo effects of estradiol on collagen and elastin dynamics in rat aorta. *Endocrinology* 91:1227–1232, 1972.
56. Wolinsky H. Effects of estrogen and progesterone treatment on the response of the aorta of male rats to hypertension. *Circ Res* 30:341–349, 1972.
57. Fischer GM, Swain ML. Effect of sex hormones on blood pressure and vascular connective tissue in castrated and noncastrated male rats. *Am J Physiol* 232:H617–H621, 1977.
58. Beldekas JC, Smith B, Geistenfeld LC. Effects of 17-beta estradiol on the biosynthesis of collagen in cultured bovine aortic smooth muscle cells. *Biochemistry* 20:2161–2167, 1981.
59. Chang W-C, Nakao J, Orimo H, et al. Stimulation of prostacyclin activity by estradiol in rat aorta smooth muscle cell in culture. *Biochim Biophys Acta* 619:107–118, 1980.
60. Wagner JD, Clarkson TB, St. Clair RW, et al. Estrogen replacement therapy and coronary artery atherogenesis in surgically postmenopausal cynomolgus monkeys. *Circulation* 80(Suppl. II):II–331, 1989.
61. Wagner JD, Clarkson TB, St. Clair RW, et al. Estrogen and progesterone replacement therapy reduces low density lipoprotein accumulation in the coronary arteries of surgically postmenopausal cynomolgus monkeys. *J Clin Invest* 88:1995–2002, 1991.
62. Wagner JD, St. Clair RW, Schwenke DC, et al. Regional differences in arterial low density lipoprotein metabolism in surgically postmenopausal cynomolgus monkeys: Effects of estrogen and progesterone replacement therapy. *Arterioscler Thromb* 12:717–726, 1992.
63. Pittman RC, Carew TE, Glass CK, et al. A radioiodinated, intracellularly trapped ligand for determining the sites of plasma protein degradation *in vivo*. *Biochem J* 212:791–800, 1983.
64. Wagner JD, Clarkson TB, Adams MR, et al. The effects of oral contraceptives on coronary artery LDL metabolism in female cynomolgus monkeys. *Circulation* 84(Suppl. II):II–602, 1991.
65. Maseri A, Severi S, De Nes M, et al. "Variant" angina: One aspect of a continuous spectrum of vasospastic myocardial ischemia. Pathogenic mechanisms, estimated incidence and clinical and coronary arterio-

graphic findings in 138 patients. *Am J Cardiol* 42:1019–1035, 1978.
66. Ludmer PL, Selwyn AP, Shook TL, et al. Paradoxical vasoconstriction induced by acetylcholine in atherosclerotic coronary arteries. *N Engl J Med* 315:1046–1051, 1986.
67. Furchgott RF, Zawadski JV. The obligatory role of endothelial cells in the relaxation of arterial smooth muscle by acetylcholine. *Nature* 288:373–376, 1980.
68. Vanhoutte PM. Endothelium and responsiveness of vascular smooth muscle. *J Hypertension* 5(Suppl.):S115–S120, 1987.
69. Vanhoutte PM. Endothelium-dependent contractions in arteries and veins. *Blood Vessels* 24:141–144, 1987.
70. Lopez JAG, Armstrong ML, Piegors DJ, et al. Effects of early and advanced atherosclerosis on vascular responses to serotonin, thromboxane A2, and ADP. *Circulation* 79:698–705, 1989.
71. Lopez JAG, Armstrong ML, Harrison DG, et al. Vascular responses to leukocyte products in atherosclerotic primates. *Circ Res* 65:1078–1086, 1989.
72. Bell C, Coffey C. Factors influencing estrogen-induced sensitization to acetylcholine of guinea-pig uterine artery. *J Reprod Fertil* 66:133–137, 1982.
73. Gisclard V, Miller VM, Vanhoutte PM. Effect of 17 beta-estradiol on endothelium-dependent responses in the rabbit. *J Pharmacol Exp Ther* 244:19–22, 1988.
74. Miller VM, Gisclard V, Vanhoutte PM. Modulation of endothelium-dependent and vascular smooth muscle responses by oestrogens. *Phlebology* 3(Suppl. 1):63–69, 1988.
75. Jiang C, Sarrel PM, Lindsey DC, et al. Endothelium-independent relaxation of rabbit coronary artery by 17 beta-oestradiol in vitro. *Br J Pharmacol* 104:1033–1037, 1991.
76. Jiang C, Sarrel PM, Lindsey DC, et al. 17-beta estradiol has calcium antagonistic properties in the rabbit coronary artery *in vitro*. *Circulation* 84(Suppl. II):II–272, 1991.
77. Jiang C, Sarrel PM, Poole-Wilson PA, et al. Acute effect of 17β estradiol on rabbit coronary artery contractile response to endothelin-1. *Am J Physiol* 263:H271–275, 1992.
78. Williams JK, Vita JA, Manuck SB, et al. Psychosocial factors impair vascular responses of coronary arteries. *Circulation* 84:2146–2153, 1991.
79. Williams JK, Adams MR, Klopfenstein HS. Estrogen modulates responses of atherosclerotic coronary arteries. *Circulation* 81:1680–1687, 1990.
80. Williams JK, Adams MR, Herrington DM, et al. Effects of short-term estrogen treatment on vascular responses of coronary arteries. *J Am Coll Cardiol* 20:452–457, 1992.
81. Clarkson TB, Adams MR, Williams JK, et al. Effects of sex steroids on the monkey cardiovascular system: Relation to changes in serum lipids and lipoproteins? In Christiansen C, Overgaard K (Eds.), Osteoporosis 1990, Proceedings of the Third International Symposium on Osteoporosis and Consensus Development Conference. Copenhagen, Osteopress, 1990, pp. 1798–1805.

# SECTION 4

Pregnancy and the Heart

CHAPTER 16

Cardiovascular Physiology of Pregnancy

PATRICIA LENA COLE, M.D., F.A.C.C.
MARTIN ST. JOHN SUTTON, M.B.B.S., F.A.C.C.

NORMAL PREGNANCY

Symptoms and Signs

A patient who presented to a physician with symptoms of fatigue, dyspnea on exertion, and palpitations would probably undergo a battery of tests designed to evaluate presumed cardiopulmonary disease. A patient presenting with these symptoms who is also pregnant would more than likely be normal (Table 16 1). Pregnancy induces signs and symptoms that often mimic cardiac disease, so an understanding of the normal changes associated with pregnancy is critical in attempting to evaluate the presence of pathology in the pregnant patient.

Pregnancy results in major perturbations in hemodynamics that are outlined later in this chapter. These changes result in hyperventilation and a sensation of breathlessness at rest and dyspnea on exertion (1); as the uterus enlarges, many women develop orthopnealike symptoms. Fatigue is an almost universal symptom, especially during the third trimester. As total body sodium and water increase and the inferior vena cava is compressed by the gravid uterus, peripheral edema results; this finding is present in the vast majority of pregnant women (2, 3). Pressure on the inferior vena cava and the resulting decrease in venous return to the heart also result in lightheadedness or presyncope. Many women complain of palpitations, which usually represent sinus tachycardia, a normal occurrence in pregnancy. Anasarca, paroxysmal nocturnal dyspnea, syncope, hemoptysis, and chest pain are not normal symptoms of pregnancy and warrant investigation.

Table 16–1. SYMPTOMS AND SIGNS IN NORMAL PREGNANCY

Symptoms
Dyspnea
Fatigability
Decreased exercise tolerance
Palpitations
Hyperventilation
Peripheral edema
Signs
Prominent venous pulsations
Basilar rales
Prominent left ventricular impulse
Tachycardia
Third heart sound
Systolic murmur

Clinical signs on general physical examination are altered during pregnancy as a result of the major hemodynamic alterations that occur. The pregnant patient may have full neck veins due to volume overload and the presence of tricuspid regurgitation (4), and prominent precordial pulsations may be present. Basilar atelectasis due to compression of the lower lung fields by the gravid uterus may mimic the pulmonary rales of congestive heart failure. Pedal edema is a common finding, as previously mentioned.

Cardiovascular Examination

The enlarged uterus causes elevation and rotation of the heart, resulting in a leftward displacement of the apical impulse. In addition, the apical impulse is prominent but not sustained. Occasionally, a right ventricular impulse can be palpated just to the left of the sternum.

Heart sounds are altered during pregnancy (5). The first heart sound (closure of the mitral and tricuspid valves) increases in intensity during pregnancy, and the splitting of the two components of the sound (individual valve closure) becomes more exaggerated due to early closure of the mitral valve. It has been suggested that this change may represent hyperkinesis of the left ventricle (6) as well as the increased volume of circulating blood (5). The second heart sound (S_2) remains constant in character until the thirtieth week of pregnancy, when there is a narrowing of the physiologic splitting of the aortic and pulmonic components (5). A third heart sound (S_3) heard just after S_2 is a frequent finding during normal pregnancy, occurring in up to 84% of patients, and does not signify a pathologic condition, as it often does in adults. More than half of all pregnant patients have an audible S_3 before the twentieth week of gestation. A fourth heart sound (S_4) is a common finding in healthy adults but is unusual during pregnancy, occurring in only 4% of patients (5), and is even more rare at delivery (7).

Systolic murmurs are very common during pregnancy (present in 93–96% of patients [5, 8]), and are usually heard in early-to-mid systole. Many of these murmurs represent flow murmurs across the aortic and pulmonic valves due to increased circulating blood volume; in addition, since half of these murmurs are right-sided and vary with respiration, it is likely that a portion of them represent tricuspid regurgitation.

Limacher et al. (9) studied prospectively a cohort of pregnant women beginning at the end of the first trimester, using Doppler echocardiography, and confirmed the presence of tricuspid regurgitation in 43%. Interestingly, in her series, 14 of the patients (17%) showed evidence of minor preexisting but unrecognized cardiovascular abnormalities, including ventricular septal defects and aortic valve disease, that were unmasked by pregnancy.

The concomitant increases in circulating blood volume and cardiac output in pregnancy result in increased intensity of murmurs due to stenotic valvular lesions (6); conversely, the decreased peripheral resistance of pregnancy serves to "unload" the heart, resulting in decreased intensity of regurgitant murmurs (10). Patients who have Barlow's syndrome (click-murmur or mitral valve prolapse) demonstrate similar decreases in the intensity of both the murmur and the systolic click with advancing pregnancy (11, 12).

Diastolic murmurs are infrequent during pregnancy (5) and may represent the after-vibration of a prominent third heart sound (13), increased flow across the tricuspid or mitral valve (14), or dilation of the pulmonary artery (15).

Pericardial "knocks" and systolic ejection clicks do not appear to be common findings in pregnancy, although there are numerous other sounds originating from extra-cardiac sources. Some of these include supraclavicular murmurs originating from the brachiocephalic arteries (6), venous hums originating from the jugular veins (14), and continuous or systolic murmurs heard over the breast (13). Breast murmurs are also referred to as "mammary souffles," and controversy exists about whether they are venous (15) or arterial (16, 17) in origin; there is some speculation that these originate from the junction of the internal mammary and intercostal arteries (18).

Cardiovascular Hemodynamics

Major hemodynamic perturbations occur during normal pregnancy, including changes in measured parameters such as heart rate and blood pressure as well as changes in calculated parameters such as cardiac output and vascular resistance (Table 16–2).

Heart Rate

Mean heart rate during pregnancy is higher than that in the nonpregnant state, averaging 10 to 20 beats/minute faster at term (19–23); the majority of this increase occurs by the eighth week of pregnancy (24, 25). Heart rate has been reported to increase throughout pregnancy (26, 27), but some studies have reported a plateau during the third trimester (21, 24). Multiple pregnancies are associated with a concomitant increase in heart rate above that for singleton pregnancies (28). Maternal posture plays an important role in variations in hemodynamic measurements, with greater heart rate increases occurring in the sitting or standing position and lesser alterations in the left lateral position (29, 30).

The mechanism for the early heart rate increase is not well understood because it occurs earlier in pregnancy than many of the major hemodynamic alterations. Heart rate changes have been postulated to occur in response to hormonal influences (24, 31) and appear to occur prior to the hemodynamic demands made by the fetoplacental unit (32).

Blood Pressure

Although a few studies have reported no alterations in blood pressure during pregnancy (26, 33, 34), most suggest that blood pressure alterations do occur. The magnitude of these alterations is a function of age, parity, and gestation and also appears to be profoundly affected by maternal position at the time the measurements are taken.

Christianson (35) studied a group of 6662 white women of varying age and parity and analyzed the changes in blood pressure that occurred throughout pregnancy. For any given level of parity, both mean systolic and mean diastolic pressures increased throughout pregnancy as a function of advancing age ($>$ 35 years). The effects of parity were opposite—i.e., the mean systolic blood pressure within each age group decreased as parity increased (Fig. 16–1). When these data were analyzed after excluding hypertensive disorders of pregnancy, the observed pattern persisted. Gestational changes included an early decrease (by the seventh or eighth week) in both systolic and diastolic blood pressures (23, 31), which continued through the middle trimester with a gradual rise in pressure as term approached.

Table 16–2. CARDIOCIRCULATORY CHANGES DURING NORMAL PREGNANCY

Parameter	1st Trimester	2nd Trimester	3rd Trimester
Blood volume	↑	↑ ↑	↑ ↑ ↑
Cardiac output	↑	↑ ↑ ↑	↑ ↑
Stroke volume	↑	↑ ↑ ↑	↔ or ↓
Heart rate	↑	↑ ↑	↑ ↑ ↑
Systolic blood pressure	↔	↓	↔
Diastolic blood pressure	↓	↓ ↓	↔
Pulse pressure	↑	↑ ↑	↔
Systemic vascular resistance	↓	↓ ↓ ↓	↓ ↓
Oxygen consumption	↔ or ↑	↑ ↑	↑ ↑ ↑
Left ventricular volume	↔	↑	↑
Left ventricular systolic function	↔	↔	↔

↔, no change compared to nonpregnant level; ↑, small increase; ↑ ↑, moderate increase; ↑ ↑ ↑, large increase; ↓, small decrease; ↓ ↓, moderate decrease; ↓ ↓ ↓, large decrease.
From Elkayam U, Gleicher N. Hemodynamics and cardiac function during normal pregnancy and the puerperium. In Elkayam U, Gleicher N (Eds.), *Cardiac Problems in Pregnancy*. New York, Alan R Liss, 1990, pp. 5–24.

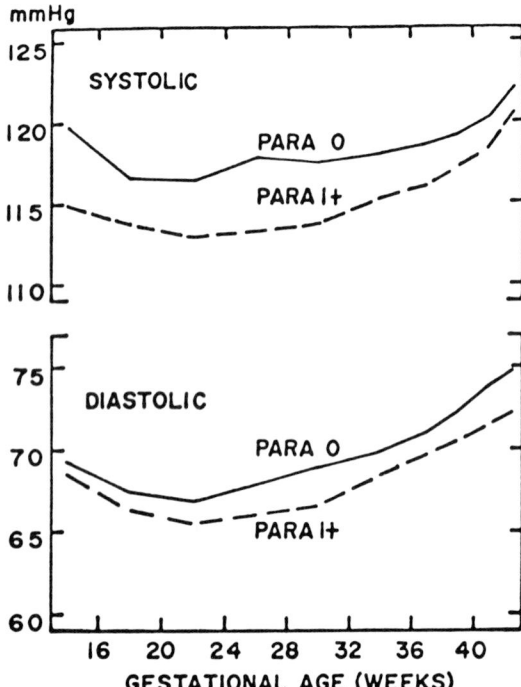

Figure 16–1. Mean blood pressure by gestational age and parity for white gravidas 25 to 34 years of age who delivered single, live, term babies. (From Christianson R. Studies on blood pressure during pregnancy. Influence of parity and age. *Am J Obstet Gynecol* 125:509–513, 1976.)

The pregnancy-induced fall in blood pressure during midpregnancy with a rise toward term has been described in other studies (27, 36, 37), and the magnitude of the changes appears to be a function of maternal position, the lowest blood pressure measurements occurring in the left lateral position (37, 38). The presence of twins does not alter blood pressure response to pregnancy.

Blood (Plasma–Red Blood Cell) Volume

Pregnancy results in profound changes in maternal blood volume, with increases in both the plasma component and red blood cell mass. A wide variety of techniques have been used to study pregnancy-induced changes in blood volume, including the carbon monoxide method (39), radioactive tracer techniques (40, 41), and Evans' blue dye (42–44). Recently, position emission tomography has been used to determine maternal blood volume in the placenta (45).

Although there is general agreement that plasma volume increases in pregnancy, the magnitude and timing of this increase varies among different studies. Plasma volume begins to increase as early as 6 weeks of pregnancy (31, 46), and volume expansion continues throughout the second trimester (21, 46). Thereafter, to term, there are reports of continued increases in plasma volume (29), as well as decreases (21, 44) and lack of change (47). The reason for the discrepancies among studies is unresolved but may be related to the maternal position in which the measurements were made (48). In addition, some studies have reported that blood volume is indexed to body weight, but if the "tracer" does not equilibrate in all body compartments (for example, blue dye), the values calculated will be spuriously low, and the differences will become more pronounced toward term (43). Reported increases in plasma volume during pregnancy range from 22–65% (40, 43), with most studies showing a mean increase of 50% (39, 41, 46, 97). There is a wide range of individual variation with reports of increases of up to 121% in individual patients (19). Red blood cell (RBC) mass increases progressively throughout pregnancy, with mean increases of 30–40% (49). Although increases in RBC mass parallel increases in plasma volume, the volume changes are of greater magnitude and result in a relative decrease in the ratio of RBC mass to plasma volume (19) (Fig. 16–2). The latter was described in the 1800s as "serous plethora" by Kiwisch (50) but is now referred to as the "physiologic anemia of pregnancy."

Blood volume consists of RBC mass and plasma volume, and, as expected, the blood volume increases seen during pregnancy parallel the increases of these two components. Alterations in blood volume correlate directly with the number of fetuses in multiple pregnancies (47, 51), age, parity (43), placental weight (47), and fetal weight (41, 52). Maternal size has been variably reported to correlate (41) and not to correlate (52) with increases in blood volume during pregnancy.

The causes of blood volume changes during pregnancy are multifactorial and poorly understood (53–55). Pregnancy is associated with elevated renin and aldosterone levels, both of which serve to accentuate salt and water retention. Renin-angiotensin activity has been shown to be affected during oral contraceptive (OC) use (56), and this effect is believed to be

Figure 16–2. Percentage changes in blood volume, plasma volume, and red blood cell (RBC) mass during pregnancy. (From Scott DE. Anemia in pregnancy. *Obstet Gynecol Annu* 1:219, 1972.)

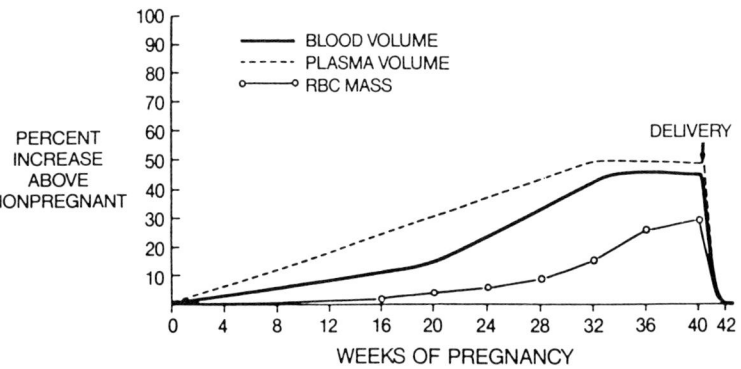

due to the estrogen component of contraceptives. Thus, it has been postulated that alterations in the renin-angiotensin cycle during pregnancy may be hormonally mediated. Estrogen administration has been shown to result in plasma volume expansion (57, 58). In addition, both estrogen and progesterone affect aldosterone levels, leading to salt retention and increased total body volume. Additionally, progesterone causes relaxation in smooth muscle in the walls of veins (59).

Longo (32) has suggested additional mechanisms that may be responsible for the increase in blood volume occurring during pregnancy, including (1) hormonal stimulation of erythropoiesis by prolactin, progesterone, and chorionic somatomammotropin, and (2) the development of a low-resistance vascular circuit (the placenta), which acts like an arteriovenous shunt.

Although the actual mechanism of the pregnancy-induced increase in blood volume is not clear, its development appears to be an important component of a healthy pregnancy. A decrease in the expected augmentation of blood volume during pregnancy has been associated with various complications of pregnancy such as prematurity, intrauterine growth retardation, oligohydramnios, maternal diabetes, toxemia, and hypertension (32, 42).

Regional Blood Flow

Marked alterations in blood flow to various organs occur during pregnancy. The most marked alteration involves the uterus. First trimester uterine blood flow has been estimated to be 50 mL/minute, increasing to 500 mL/minute at term (60, 61). With refinement of the measurements made using Doppler techniques, unilateral ascending arterial uterine blood flow has been shown to increase from 94.5 mL/minute in the nonpregnant state to nearly 350 mL/minute near term (62, 63) (Fig. 16–3). The diameter of the ascending uterine artery progressively increases from approximately 1.5 mm in the nonpregnant state to almost 4 mm at term (62) (Fig. 16–4). Resistance, assessed as the peak systolic-to-end-diastolic flow ratio, declined throughout pregnancy (62) (Fig. 16–4). The marked alterations in uterine blood flow are thought to result from local hormonal effects in addition to central hemodynamic alterations (64, 65) and, as with all other hemodynamic measurements made during pregnancy, vary with maternal position (66).

Other organs also receive an augmented blood supply during pregnancy, specifically the skin, kidneys, mammary glands, and extremities. Blood flow to the skin, measured by photoelectric flow sensors, is significantly increased by 16 weeks of gestation and remains elevated throughout gestation (67). Similar increases were noted for blood flow to the mucous membranes (68). Hormonal changes result in structural alterations in the calyces, pelvis, and ureters of the kidney and are accompanied by flow alterations of up to 50% above nonpregnant values, including increases in glomerular filtration rate and renal plasma flow (69). Mammary blood flow throughout pregnancy and lactation has been studied using Doppler techniques (63). Blood flow increases up to 24 weeks' gestation and then remains elevated until term. Lactation is accompanied by a 50% increase in blood flow velocity over prepartum levels, but these velocities return to prepartum levels during the maintenance phase of lactation. Blood flow to the extremities also increases during pregnancy, with more marked alterations to the hands than to the lower extremities (70, 71); blood flow to the

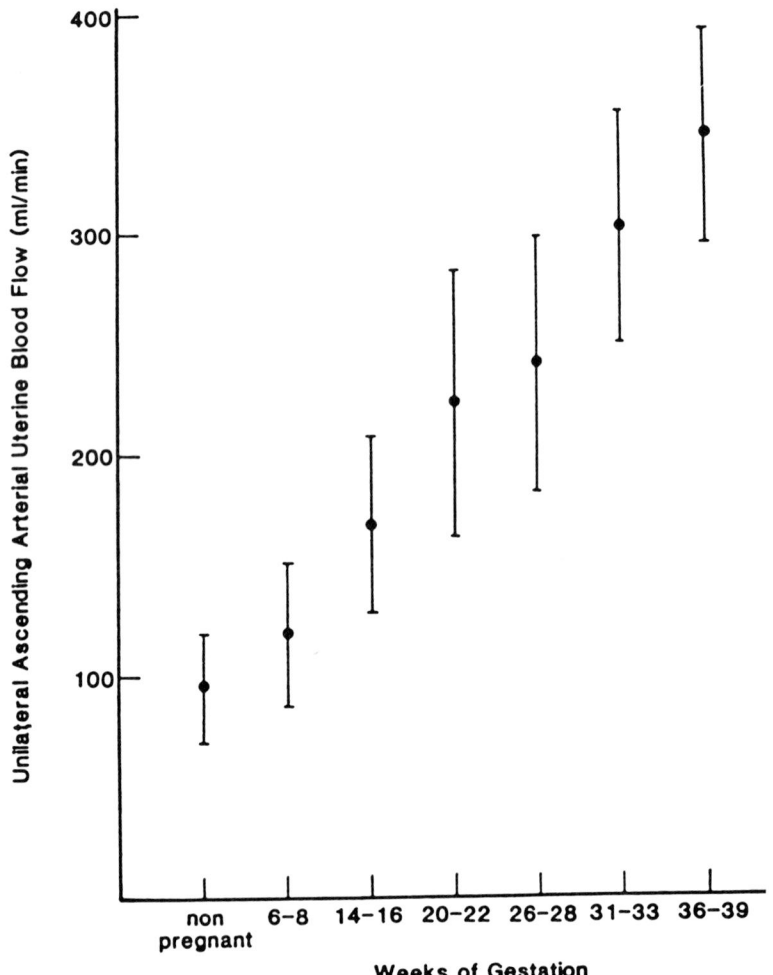

Figure 16–3. Changes in uterine blood flow during pregnancy. (From Thaler I, Manor D, Itskovitz J, et al. Changes in uterine blood flow during human pregnancy. *Am J Obstet Gynecol* 162:121–125, 1990.)

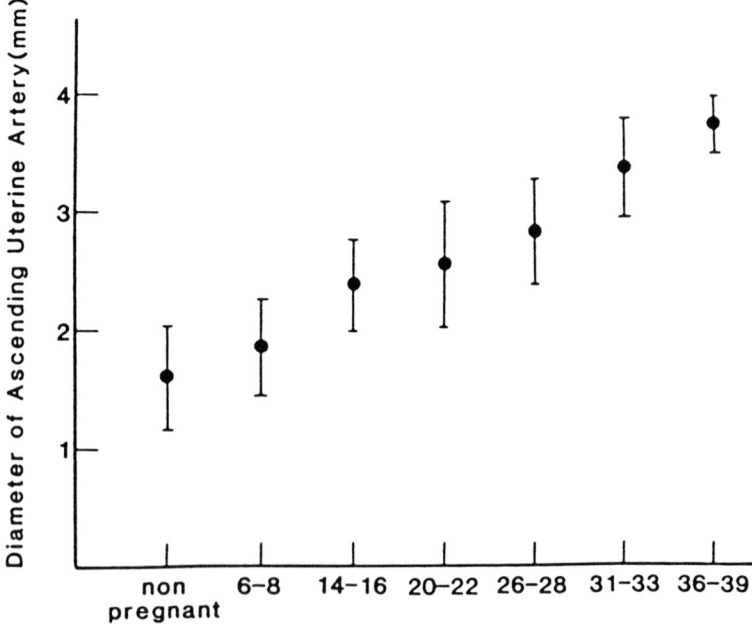

Figure 16–4. Diameter of ascending uterine artery at different gestational ages. (From Thaler I, Manor D, Itskovitz J, et al. Changes in uterine blood flow during human pregnancy. *Am J Obstet Gynecol* 162:121–125, 1990.)

lower extremities declines as term approaches, possibly owing to compression of the vena cava (72).

In contrast to the organs mentioned above, blood flow to the liver and brain does not appear to change during pregnancy.

Central Blood Pressures

In 1949 Hamilton measured hemodynamics in 68 pregnant patients and 32 nonpregnant controls by means of right heart catheterization (73). He described no change in right atrial pressure during pregnancy. Several years later, Bader et al. used a similar technique in 46 pregnant women of varying gestational ages to measure central blood pressures (34). In this study, right ventricular and pulmonary artery systolic pressures were normal, as were pulmonary capillary wedge pressures. Right ventricular end-diastolic pressures increased during the third trimester but returned toward normal just prior to delivery. These authors postulated that elevated right ventricular end-diastolic pressure was consistent with increased intrapleural pressure owing to elevation of the diaphragm from the gravid uterus. Similar findings of elevated right ventricular end-diastolic pressure were also reported by Rose et al. (74).

Other authors suggest that both right- and left-sided filling pressures remain normal during pregnancy and that the only hemodynamic changes are increases in output measurements and decreases in resistance measurements (75, 76) (Table 16–3).

CALCULATED HEMODYNAMICS

Cardiac Output

The magnitude of increase in cardiac output during pregnancy was initially described in the early 1900s (77), and since that time numerous techniques have been employed to determine cardiac output alterations, including dye dilution, Fick calculation using oxygen saturation, thermodilution, impedance cardiography, and Doppler ultrasound.

Table 16–3. NORMAL HEMODYNAMIC VALUES

Place and Kind of Measurement	Units	Nonpregnant	Late Pregnancy[a]
Right atrium			
Pressure (mean)	mm Hg	<7	<7
O_2 saturation	%	65–75	60–70
Right ventricle			
Pressure (systolic-diastolic)	mm Hg	<25/7	<25/7
O_2 saturation	%	65–75	60–70
Pulmonary artery			
Pressure (systolic-diastolic)	mm Hg	<25/12	<25/12
Pressure (mean)	mm Hg	<16	<16
O_2 saturation	%	65–75	60–70
Pulmonary capillary wedge			
Pressure (mean)	mm Hg	<13	<13
O_2 saturation	%	>90	>90
Left atrium			
Pressure (mean)	mm Hg	<13	<13
O_2 saturation	%	>90	>90
Left ventricle			
Pressure (systolic)	mm Hg	<130	<120[b]
Pressure (end-diastolic)	mm Hg	<13	<13
O_2 saturation	%	>90	>90
Cardiac index	L/min/M²	2.5–4.0	3.5–5.0
Stroke volume	mL/beat	60–70	70–100
Heart rate	beats/min	60–80	70–105
Systemic vascular resistance	dynes·sec·cm⁸	1200–1600	600–800
Pulmonary vascular resistance	dynes·sec·cm⁸	120–200	60–100

[a]Lateral recumbency.
[b]Body surface area should be calculated from prepregnant weight.
From Metcalfe J, McAnulty J, Ueland K (Eds.). *Heart Disease and Pregnancy.* Boston, Little, Brown, 1986, pp. 55–82.

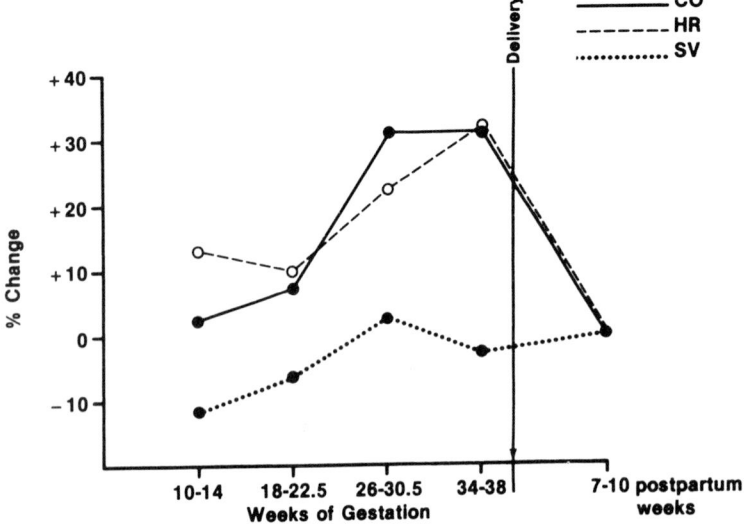

Figure 16–5. Percent changes in cardiac output (CO), heart rate (HR), and stroke volume (SV) during gestation with the postpartum period used as a control. (From Mashini I, Albazzaz S, Fadel H, et al. Serial non-invasive evaluation of cardiovascular hemodynamics during pregnancy. Am J Obstet Gynecol 156:1208–1213, 1987.)

Most reports have documented increases in cardiac output of 30–50% during pregnancy (19, 29, 33), but there is lack of agreement on the timing of these increases. Recent studies have suggested that changes in cardiac output occur early (23, 25), with a 22% rise in cardiac output by the eighth week of gestation and peak cardiac output occurring by the beginning of the third trimester (21, 78) (Fig. 16–5). Early reports of a decline in cardiac output near term were challenged because the maternal position confounded the results. It is well known that in the supine position the gravid uterus obstructs both inferior vena caval flow (79) and abdominal aortic flow (80). Serial studies suggest that changes in position from the supine to the left lateral position are associated with increases in cardiac output (20, 26, 37, 81). Some subsequent reports have demonstrated a decline in cardiac output toward term regardless of maternal position (29, 82) (Fig. 16–6), whereas others have failed to demonstrate this decline toward term (83, 84). Increases in cardiac output are higher in twin than in single pregnancies (Fig. 16–7).

Studies of cardiac output in the past have utilized measurement techniques that are either not reliable, such as the nitrous oxide technique used by early investigators (19), or require invasive assessment such as the Fick method (which requires arterial and venous blood samples) or the thermodilution method (which requires placement of a pulmonary artery catheter). Basal measurements may be affected by sympathetic nervous system stimulation during invasive techniques. Thus, there has been great interest recently in the use of noninvasive methods of assessing cardiac output such as M-mode and cross-sectional echocardiography, impedance cardiography, and Doppler techniques.

Cardiac output (CO) derived from M-mode echocardiography is calculated from stroke volume (SV) (CO = SV × heart rate [HR]), which is defined as the systolic change in the cube of left ventricular internal dimensions, a technique that makes many assumptions about ventricular shape (85).

Impedance cardiography is a noninvasive technique that measures changes in transtho-

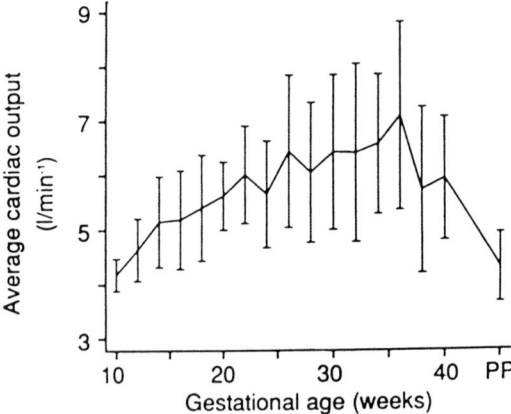

Figure 16–6. Serial changes in cardiac output throughout pregnancy and postpartum using Doppler echocardiography. (From Vered Z, Poler M, Gibson P, et al. Noninvasive detection of morphologic and hemodynamic changes during normal pregnancy. Clin Cardiol 14:327–334, 1991.)

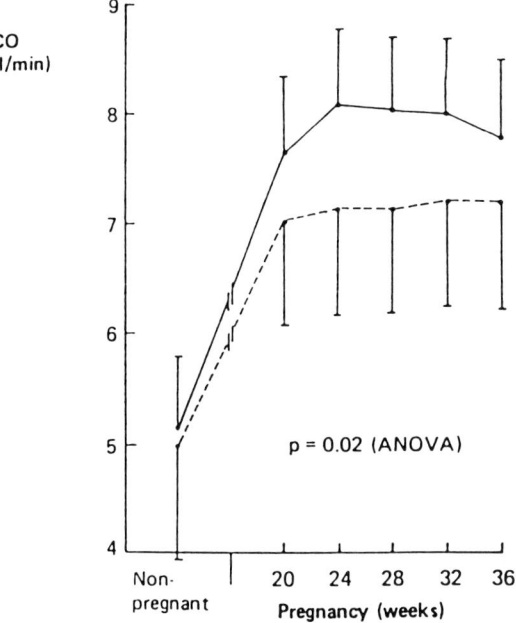

Figure 16–7. Serial measurements of cardiac output during singleton (*dotted line*) and twin (*solid line*) pregnancies. Figures shown represent mean and 95% confidence interval. (From Robson SC, Hunter S, Boys R, et al. Hemodynamic changes during twin pregnancy. A Doppler and M-mode echocardiogram study. *Am J Obstet Gynecol* 161:1273–1278, 1989.)

racic electrical resistance associated with ejection of blood into the pulmonary circulation. Studies using early bioimpedance technology to measure cardiac output correlated poorly with thermodilution techniques (86), but newer bioimpedance technology has resulted in measurements that correlate better with accepted techniques such as thermodilution (87, 88). In one study (88), measurements of cardiac output following anesthesia had a poor correlation with thermodilution, suggesting that the technique was not useful following pharmacologic administration. In addition, although this technique may be useful for measuring relative changes during pregnancy, it appears to be less useful for measurements of absolute values (89).

Doppler echocardiographic techniques have now been used extensively to measure cardiac output changes during pregnancy, and these techniques appear to yield results that are reproducible and correlate closely with other reliable methods (85, 90–94). Some authors suggest that, due to inherent variability in the Doppler technique, this test is more useful for determining changes that occur longitudinally in the same patient rather than for describing alterations across patient groups (95). Serial cardiac output determinations using Doppler techniques (96, 97) have correlated with previous invasive testing in showing that cardiac output increases begin early in gestation, peak by the beginning of the third trimester, and decline toward term. Thus, Doppler echocardiography is a safe and accurate alternative for measuring cardiac output in pregnancy.

Systemic Vascular Resistance and Pulmonary Vascular Resistance

Systemic vascular resistance (SVR) declines during pregnancy (23, 27, 31, 33, 34), the majority of the decline occurring by the eighth week of gestation (23, 31). These alterations in SVR during pregnancy appear to parallel blood pressure changes, showing a gradual rise in levels from the second trimester to term (33). The mechanism for this finding is not clear, but it has been postulated that the decline in SVR is hormonally mediated (65). In addition, the development of a low-resistance uteroplacental circuit is thought to play an important role in the decline in SVR (37).

Little information exists concerning alterations in pulmonary vascular resistance (PVR) during pregnancy, but available data suggest that unlike SVR, PVR remains constant during pregnancy (75). Since cardiac output increases and mean pulmonary capillary wedge pressure (PCWP) remains unchanged (33), the absence of a change in PVR requires a concomitant increase in mean pulmonary artery ($\overline{PA}$) pressures $\left([PVR = \dfrac{\overline{PA} - \overline{PCWP}}{CO}] \right)$. However, in one study in which central pressures during pregnancy were measured directly (34), no significant changes in pulmonary artery pressure were documented except in response to exercise. The maternal position during this catheterization study was not specified, and thus position could be the explanation for the difference between studies.

Cardiac Size and Function

Echocardiography has been a useful noninvasive tool for serial determinations of left ventricular size and function during pregnancy; measurements thus generated have advanced the understanding of cardiovascular adaptive responses to pregnancy.

In one of the earliest studies, Rubler et al. evaluated pregnant women in different gestational stages by measuring indices of function (stroke volume, cardiac output) as well as size (left ventricular end-diastolic volume) using M-mode echocardiography (26). She reported a pregnancy-induced increase in cardiac size as well as contractility. Using a similar technique, Katz et al. (37) studied a group of pregnant women serially throughout pregnancy and described increases in both end-diastolic diameter and volume of the ventricular chambers but found no alteration in indices of cardiac function such as percentage of fractional shortening or ejection fraction. Similar preservation of heart function during pregnancy despite increasing ventricular size has subsequently been described (20, 98). In a study of twin pregnancies, Veille et al. (28) demonstrated that despite increases in contractility in twin compared to singleton pregnancies, left ventricular dimensions were not different; the authors concluded that this represented reduced cardiovascular reserve. Capeless and Clapp (23) studied a group of women prior to conception and followed serial M-mode measurements throughout pregnancy. Significant increases were seen in end-diastolic volume, the majority of which occurred by 8 weeks of gestation; ejection fraction did not change. In this study, the women were used as their own prepregnant controls, whereas other studies have used 6-week postpartum measurements as controls. Evidence is accumulating that some cardiac measurements (e.g., aortic diameters) do not revert to prepregnant values (99), and thus the postpartum state may not be an appropriate control for hemodynamic comparison. Vered and colleagues (82) studied a group of pregnant patients from the first trimester throughout pregnancy and postpartum using M-mode and two-dimensional echocardiography. In contrast to previous studies, this group found no significant changes in either ejection fraction or left ventricular dimensions throughout pregnancy. The authors postulated that the lack of change in ventricular size may have been due to limitations in measurement techniques.

Cole et al. used two-dimensional echocardiography to study a group of pregnant volunteers during the last trimester of pregnancy and made serial measurements to 14 weeks postpartum (98). Left ventricular volumes (systolic and diastolic) and mass were all significantly higher during pregnancy, but no change in ejection fraction was demonstrated. During pregnancy-induced left ventricular remodeling, changes in volume and mass appeared to occur concurrently, so that end-systolic stress and ejection fraction, both determinants of left ventricular function, remained unchanged. Thus, major changes in the geometry of the left ventricle occur throughout pregnancy, yet this adaptive remodeling does not affect left ventricular function, whereas in pathologic states alterations in left ventricular size and shape have a profound impact on function (100–103).

EXERCISE DURING PREGNANCY

Concerns About Exercise in Pregnancy

During the past decade a large proportion of women of reproductive age have begun to engage in regular exercise programs to maintain their cardiovascular health. Recommendations concerning the level and duration of exercise for pregnant women have been difficult to formulate owing to the relative lack of definitive data on the risks and benefits of exercise for both mother and fetus. In addition to an improved sense of well-being, the benefits of exercise during pregnancy may include control of weight gain (104), a decreased likelihood of caesarean section (105), increase in work capacity (106), and a reduction in the incidence of depression (Table 16–4). Exercise exacerbates the increased hemodynamic demands imposed by pregnancy, and concern for fetal well-being has generated interest in the development of guidelines for the safety of exercise during pregnancy.

Pregnancy causes musculoskeletal alterations such as relaxation of ligaments and joints

Table 16–4. POTENTIAL BENEFITS OF EXERCISE DURING PREGNANCY

Control of weight gain
Sense of well-being
Decreased likelihood of cesarean section
Increase in work capacity
Reduced incidence of depression

that may result in decreased stability and an increased susceptibility to sprain injury. These changes lead to the wide-based gait characteristic of pregnancy and may result in discomfort during exercise. Furthermore, the gravid uterus alters the center of balance, producing strain on the back muscles and ligaments and leading to lordosis. The weight gain of pregnancy increases the cardiac work load at any level of exercise (Table 16–5).

Apart from maternal alterations induced by exercise during pregnancy, there are concerns about the effects of exercise on the fetus. Fetal hypoxia may result from shunting of blood away from the uteroplacental vessels toward the exercising muscle. During exercise, maternal hyperthermia is postulated to have an adverse effect on the fetus. It is not clear what effect, if any, is produced by maternally generated metabolic acids on the fetus. Finally, the repetitive mechanical displacement of the fetus during vigorous exercise may play a role in inducing premature delivery, decreased fetal weight, or placental abruption.

Guidelines for an appropriate exercise program during pregnancy should be based on a careful analysis of the available data on maternal and fetal responses to exercise as well as on evaluation of the individual patient, her prior level of conditioning, and the current state of the pregnancy (see later section, Guidelines for Exercise During Pregnancy).

Effects of Exercise

Maternal Cardiovascular Effects

During the past several decades there has been an increasing awareness of the health benefits of cardiovascular fitness, which includes a low-fat, low-cholesterol dietary intake and a regular exercise program. Cardiovascular changes induced by pregnancy are well known, but the effects of exercise during pregnancy on maternal and fetal well-being are less well understood. The perceived benefits of exercise during pregnancy include better control of weight gain, shorter labor, and faster return to baseline after delivery. However, until recently little information has been available on the potential adverse effects on the fetus such as miscarriage or prematurity, smaller fetal weight, and increased incidence of fetal abnormalities.

The hemodynamic changes induced by pregnancy are described elsewhere in this chapter; exercise results in additional demands on the cardiovascular system. Studies of exercise in pregnant animals have generally measured exercise response during maximal exercise, and thus they are not useful in predicting exercise response in humans due to the potential fetal risks of exercising to exhaustion.

Studies of exercise during pregnancy have demonstrated that heart rate increases with exercise (107). However, at low or moderate work loads, data on heart rate response vary, with some reports showing augmentation of heart rate during exercise in pregnant patients (108) and other reports suggesting that pregnancy dampens heart rate augmentation (109). This variability is due in part to the type of exercise utilized (110). Heart rate at maximal exercise (exercise to exhaustion) appears to be the same in pregnant and nonpregnant subjects (111).

Sady et al. found that pregnancy did not alter the blood pressure response to rest and exercise (111), although this finding contrasts with findings in other studies, which showed a drop in systolic and diastolic resting blood pressures with pregnancy (35).

Measurements of cardiac output during exercise in pregnancy have yielded conflicting results, some studies showing no change in exercise cardiac output compared to nonpregnant controls (34, 112), and other studies showing increases in cardiac output in pregnant patients compared with controls regardless of the length of gestation (109, 110, 113, 114). The reason for the discrepancies among these studies is not clear, but it may reflect the methods used to calculate cardiac output (Fick versus nitrous rebreathing versus dye dilution techniques). One of the few studies that has systematically examined the hemodynamic responses to submaximal and maximal exercise, both antepartum and postpartum (111), demonstrated an increase in oxygen consumption

Table 16–5. POTENTIAL ADVERSE EFFECTS OF EXERCISE DURING PREGNANCY

Increased susceptibility to injury
Discomfort from exercise
Shunting of blood from fetus to exercising muscle
Adverse fetal effects
Decreased fetal weight
Premature delivery
Maternal hyperthermia
Hypoxia secondary to shunting

and cardiac output at rest during pregnancy compared with postpartum but showed a lower systemic (a-v) O_2 difference. The increase in cardiac output and decrease in (a-v) O_2 difference in the pregnant versus the nonpregnant state persisted during all work loads of exercise, but the differences in oxygen consumption in the antepartum and postpartum periods disappeared with both submaximal and maximal exercise. The authors concluded that the coupling of the pregnancy-induced increase in cardiac output with increased systemic oxygen demand is unaffected by pregnancy, and that the pregnancy-induced increased cardiac output and lower (a-v) O_2 difference were consistent with increased blood flow to nonexercising tissue (e.g., the gravid uterus). The lack of difference in oxygen consumption during exercise in the antepartum and postpartum states demonstrated in this study has not been consistently found in other studies (109, 115). At least one study suggested that these differences may be due to the basic level of conditioning of the participants (116) because well-conditioned women were able to exercise at a more "efficient" level in terms of oxygen requirements.

Metabolic alterations resulting from exercise are normal during pregnancy, with significant increases shown in norepinephrine, epinephrine, and glucagon during light exercise (107, 108). Most studies have demonstrated that hemodynamic changes return to baseline within 30 minutes following exercise.

Uterine Placental Blood Flow

A major concern in regard to exercise during pregnancy is that blood may be shunted away from the uterus to exercising skeletal muscle, resulting in deleterious effects on the fetus. There has been little systematic investigation of this topic due in part to the technical difficulty of measuring uterine blood flow during exercise. Available studies suggest that uterine blood flow is preserved and no change in uteroplacental resistance occurs immediately following moderate exercise in healthy (117–120) but not in hypertensive women (121). Morrow (122) demonstrated an increase in uterine vascular resistance but unaltered umbilical circulation during exercise in healthy pregnant women. However, the maternal position during exercise was not specified, and there is evidence that uterine flow may be compromised during exercise in the supine position (123).

Fetal Hemodynamic Effects

Ultimately, interpretation of the adverse effects of exercise during pregnancy must take into account the actual effects on the fetus because the uteroplacental unit has extensive compensatory mechanisms that may reduce the impact of exercise-induced alterations on the fetus. One method of assessing fetal effects is heart rate measurement. Fetal heart rate is characterized by beat-to-beat variability, and intrauterine fetal distress is commonly manifested by fetal bradycardia or loss of heart rate variability.

Studies have demonstrated increases, decreases, and no change in fetal heart rate after maternal exercise (118, 122, 124–127). It is assumed that fetal tachycardia represents an appropriate response, but it is unclear whether this represents a compensatory response induced by hypoxia, a result of increased circulating catecholamines, or fetal well-being. Although the results of one study (128) suggested that fetal heart rate response during cycle exercise testing may be of value in screening pregnant women for uteroplacental insufficiency, there has been no study correlating exercise-induced alterations in fetal heart rate with adverse outcome.

Effects of Exercise on Pregnancy Outcome

Few studies designed to evaluate maternal and fetal hemodynamic alterations in response to exercise have correlated the findings with the outcome of pregnancy. Adverse pregnancy outcomes include spontaneous abortion, decreased fetal weight, decreased Apgar scores, prematurity, birth complications, and congenital malformations. In a study designed to assess pregnancy outcome, Clapp (129) evaluated 119 physically active women throughout pregnancy, using exercise protocols designed to allow a 50–80% maximum intensity of exercise. The author concluded that exercise at this level during pregnancy did not adversely affect pregnancy outcome. The same author prospectively studied 336 women who continued jogging during pregnancy. Although birth weights were greater in women who stopped exercising in the third trimester, overall there was no increased incidence of adverse pregnancy outcomes. There is also evidence that continuing moderate exercise during pregnancy may have beneficial effects on such outcome measurements as length of hospital stay, incidence of cesarean section, length of labor, and Apgar scores (105, 106). Many of the available studies are small but show no consistent effect of exercise on fetal growth, length of gestation, or fetal outcome (106, 130, 131).

Thus, although there is concern that the uteroplacental effects of maternal exercise may have deleterious effects on fetal well-being, there is no evidence that continuing moderate exercise during pregnancy results in an adverse outcome.

Guidelines for Exercise During Pregnancy

Because of the recent interest in the health benefits of exercise, especially in young women of reproductive age, as well as concerns about the potential fetal risks of maternal exercise, guidelines have been established concerning exercise during pregnancy. In 1985 the American College of Obstetricians and Gynecologists (ACOG) reviewed the available data and made recommendations about the intensity and duration of exercise during pregnancy (132) (Table 16–6). These guidelines suggest limiting exercise to 15-minute periods performed on a regular basis (three times a week) and avoiding exercise that involves jerky or bouncy movements. Care should be taken to avoid maternal tachycardia (rates > 140 beats/minute) and hyperthermia (core body temperature > 38°C). These guidelines were designed to be safe for the general pregnant population; however, in women with preexisting cardiovascular disease or problems that develop during pregnancy, the guidelines should be modified appropriately. These guidelines may appear conservative for women who are well-conditioned and who have exercised regularly and vigorously prior to becoming pregnant. The ACOG recommendations should be viewed as a framework for exercise guidelines that can be used by the physician based on careful assessment of the individual patient.

Various authors have made recommendations about specific forms of exercise (133–

Table 16–6. AMERICAN COLLEGE OF OBSTETRICIANS AND GYNECOLOGISTS GUIDELINES FOR EXERCISE DURING PREGNANCY AND POSTPARTUM

Pregnancy and Postpartum
1. Regular exercise (at least three times per week) is preferable to intermittent activity. Competitive activities should be discouraged.
2. Vigorous exercise should not be performed in hot, humid weather or during a period of febrile illness.
3. Ballistic movements (jerky, bouncy motions) should be avoided. Exercise should be done on a wooden floor or a tightly carpeted surface to reduce shock and provide sure footing.
4. Deep flexion or extension of joints should be avoided because of connective tissue laxity. Activities that require jumping, jarring motions or rapid changes in direction should be avoided because of joint instability.
5. Vigorous exercise should be preceded by a five-minute period of muscle warm-up. This can be accomplished by slow walking or stationary cycling with low resistance.
6. Vigorous exercise should be followed by a period of gradually declining activity that includes gentle stationary stretching. Because connective tissue laxity increases the risk of joint injury, stretches should not be taken to the point of maximum resistance.
7. Heart rate should be measured at times of peak activity. Target heart rates established in consultation with the physician should not be exceeded.
8. Care should be taken to gradually rise from the floor to avoid orthostatic hypotension. Some form of activity involving the legs should be continued for a brief period.
9. Liquids should be taken liberally before and after exercise to prevent dehydration. If necessary, activity should be interrupted to replenish fluids.
10. Women who have led sedentary lifestyles should begin with physical activity of very low intensity and advance activity levels very gradually.
11. Activity should be stopped and the physician consulted if any unusual symptoms appear.

Pregnancy Only
1. Maternal heart rate should not exceed 140 beats per minute.
2. Strenuous activities should not exceed 15 minutes in duration.
3. No exercise should be performed in the supine position after the fourth month of gestation is completed.
4. Exercises that employ the Valsalva maneuver should be avoided.
5. Caloric intake should be adequate to meet not only the extra needs of pregnancy, but also of the exercise performed.
6. Maternal core temperature should not exceed 38°C (100.4°F).

From American College of Obstetricians and Gynecologists. *Exercise During Pregnancy and the Postnatal Period. Home Exercise Programs.* Washington, D.C., American College of Obstetricians and Gynecologists, 1985, p. 4.

135). In general, nonweight-bearing activities (cycling) are preferred to weight-bearing activities (jogging) because they lessen the risk of developing musculoskeletal problems. Any exercise should be avoided when the environmental temperature is high. The intensity and duration of any activity that involves large muscle groups (tennis, jogging) should be decreased during pregnancy. Exercise in the supine position should be avoided, especially in the last trimester, because of the hemodynamic consequences of the gravid uterus in this position. Scuba diving, contact sports, ice skating, and waterskiing should be avoided or modified during pregnancy; in addition, other high-risk activities (sky diving, mountain climbing, downhill skiing) should be avoided altogether. Racquet sports (tennis, squash, racquetball) are acceptable in moderation, as are walking, cycling, swimming, and low-impact aerobics. Weight-lifting, which can cause muscle or joint injury to the back, should be modified to prevent such musculoskeletal injuries, and caution has been urged regarding activities that result in the Valsalva maneuver.

In conclusion, decisions about exercise during pregnancy should be individualized, taking into account the general physical status of the patient and any pregnancy-induced physical ailments; the ACOG recommendations should be used as a guideline.

LABOR, DELIVERY, AND POSTPARTUM PERIOD

Labor and Delivery

Hemodynamic Changes

Profound hemodynamic changes take place during labor and delivery, and the magnitude of these changes appears to be directly related to the levels of pain and anxiety; thus analgesia plays an important role in attenuating these changes.

Several studies have demonstrated an augmentation in heart rate during uterine contractions of nearly 20% over the augmented baseline heart rate of pregnancy (136, 137), whereas other studies have suggested that no important change in heart rate occurs (138, 139). Systolic and diastolic blood pressures and mean arterial pressure rise during labor with each uterine contraction (136, 137, 139, 140), and there is evidence that pulmonary pressures rise as well (141). Uterine contractions result in a transient autotransfusion of up to 500 mL of blood into the central venous system (65); this increased venous return to the heart results in augmentation of stroke volume and, consequently, cardiac output. Cardiac output increases markedly during uterine contractions regardless of the method used to measure it (136, 137, 142). It has been postulated that all of these hemodynamic alterations are augmented by an increase in circulating catecholamine levels, which are known to be increased during labor and delivery (143). Like resting hemodynamic parameters, these measurements are affected by the maternal position, with different measurements in the left lateral decubitus and the supine positions.

Blood loss during delivery also affects hemodynamics because of the change in volume as well as the compensatory responses it evokes such as tachycardia. Blood volume lost during delivery has been estimated to be 500 mL for a vaginal delivery, 900 mL for a vaginal twin delivery, and more than 900 mL for a singleton cesarean section (40, 144, 145). Primiparas appear to have greater blood loss than multiparas, and an episiotomy results in an additional blood loss of 150 mL (144).

Hemodynamics during labor and delivery are markedly affected by a wide range of variables, including the level of pain and analgesia and the mode of delivery (vaginal or cesarean section).

Effect of Anesthesia

Ueland and Hansen and colleagues (139, 146–148) described markedly different hemodynamic responses to several forms of anesthesia; more pronounced alterations occurred in women who received local anesthetics than in those who received caudal anesthesia. Spinal and epidural (plus epinephrine) anesthesia resulted in a decrease in both blood pressure and cardiac output, whereas the smallest hemodynamic alteration was seen with epidural (without epinephrine) anesthesia. Intubation results in transient alterations in hemodynamics in addition to changes resulting from pharmacologic agents alone (147). For any given type of anesthesia, vaginal deliveries appear to result in less hemodynamic perturbation than cesarean sections.

Administration of nonanesthetic medications also affects central hemodynamics during labor and delivery. Pitocin is commonly used to initiate labor as well as to decrease postdelivery blood loss. Use of this agent results in hypotension and an increased cardiac output (30). Obstetric practice employs prostaglandins to induce labor as well as to induce therapeutic abortion. Uterine smooth muscle is profoundly affected by these compounds, but even in large doses they have relatively few effects on cardiovascular hemodynamics (149).

Postpartum Involution of Changes

Immediately after delivery there is a marked increase in intravascular volume (43, 150), most likely due to the sudden release of inferior vena caval obstruction; this, in combination with pain-induced tachycardia, results in major increases in cardiac output (21, 34, 142), which then rapidly returns to baseline (136, 150, 151). Heart rate also changes rapidly immediately after delivery, decreasing by up to 17 beats/minute (37, 137, 139). Despite marked changes in these parameters, blood pressures do not alter markedly after delivery (43, 142).

The hemodynamic changes that occur during pregnancy rapidly return to baseline after delivery. By the fifth postpartum week, heart rate, blood volume, cardiac output, and left ventricular diameter and thickness are all significantly lower than at term (34, 43, 82, 98, 152, 153).

Many studies have used postpartum measurements as the baseline when women are used as their own controls on the assumption that hemodynamic parameters return to normal postpartum. However, evidence is mounting that some anatomic and hemodynamic changes of pregnancy may not be transient. Aortic size and compliance appear to remain elevated postpartum, and multiparous women have larger and more compliant aortas than primiparous women (99). Blood flow to the hand remains significantly elevated past the sixth postpartum week (70). Breast feeding, with its attendant effects on plasma volume (154), may alter the time course of involution of pregnancy-induced changes.

MATERNAL CARDIAC DIAGNOSTIC TESTING IN PREGNANCY

Although women of reproductive age are generally healthy and require little in the way of cardiac diagnostic or therapeutic intervention, problems do occasionally arise that require assessment or therapy. These problems may be due to preexisting cardiovascular conditions that are exacerbated by pregnancy, or they may be due to difficulties that first become manifest during pregnancy. The risks to the fetus from cardiac diagnostic testing are almost all attributable to exposure of the fetus to ionizing radiation. In the absence of radiation there is virtually no cause for concern.

Tests Not Involving Ionizing Radiation

Electrocardiography

Interpretation of abnormalities on electrocardiography (ECG) must take into account the normal changes that occur as a function of pregnancy itself (Table 16–7). Heart rate during pregnancy is faster (24), which results in small changes in the P–R and Q–T intervals but no alteration in P-, QRS, or T-wave amplitude (155). Both leftward and rightward shifts in the QRS axis occur during pregnancy (156, 157) owing to rotation of the heart due to the enlargement of the gravid uterus. No important shifts occur in the P- or T-wave axis. ST segments are generally stable during pregnancy (158, 159), so the presence of ST segment elevation or depression should be interpreted as abnormal.

Premature atrial and ventricular beats are common, but with the exception of rare episodes of Wenckebach (160), conduction abnormalities are not normally found during pregnancy. Rhythm disturbances during pregnancy are uncommon (161–163). Upshaw (164) examined ECG data obtained during labor and delivery in 13 women and docu-

Table 16–7. ELECTROCARDIOGRAPHIC CHANGES IN PREGNANCY

Increased heart rate
Decreased P–R and QRS intervals
QRS axis shifts
Premature atrial and ventricular beats

mented a wide variety of rhythm disturbances including premature atrial, ventricular, and nodal contractions, sinoatrial arrest, wandering atrial pacemaker, paroxysmal supraventricular tachycardia, and sinus tachycardia. Although the group studied was small, all of the subjects demonstrated some departure from normal sinus rhythm. None of the patients in this study developed bundle branch block or atrioventricular block. Of interest, 3 of the 13 patients developed "ischemic" 1-mm ST segment depression, but tachycardia (HR = 140 bpm) was present in all three cases, which may therefore have represented a rate-related change.

Echocardiography (M-Mode, Two-Dimensional, Doppler, Color Flow)

Echocardiography is an extremely valuable noninvasive cardiovascular diagnostic tool that involves the use of sound waves. Echocardiography has great utility in evaluating the anatomy and function of cardiac chambers, the appearance of the valvular structures, the pericardium, proximal aorta, and origin of the coronary arteries. The addition of Doppler and color flow technology to echocardiography has enhanced its ability to quantify stenotic and regurgitant valvular lesions and intracardiac shunts and to provide information about pulmonary artery pressures and systolic and diastolic cardiac function. Doppler techniques are also valuable in assessing the uteroplacental circulation (165) in patients with complications of pregnancy or fetal abnormalities (166–168).

Echocardiography is an extremely important diagnostic tool because it provides information that was previously available only by cardiac catheterization or radionuclide technology (both of which involve ionizing radiation). There is no information to suggest that echocardiographic sound waves are harmful to the fetus (169).

Systolic Time Intervals

This diagnostic tool utilizes information obtained from simultaneous recording of the phonocardiogram, carotid pulse tracing, and electrocardiogram to describe sequential phases of left ventricular systole. Although early descriptions of left ventricular chamber function were made using this technique, the advent of high-quality echocardiography has rendered this technique obsolete.

Stress Testing

Although exercise to the point of exhaustion is not recommended during pregnancy, exercise stress testing at low or moderate levels of activity may be valuable in the pregnant patient for obtaining information about functional capacity or evidence of ischemia. There is virtually no information about the use of thallium perfusion scanning as an adjunct to stress testing during pregnancy. Thallium is a radioactive tracer that is injected intravenously. Because of its albumin binding it is assumed that little crosses the placenta, although theoretically leaks can occur. The risks to the fetus are not well described. In addition, there are few data on the use of adenosine or dipyridamole as alternatives to exercise. (Both adenosine and dipyridamole require thallium scanning or two-dimensional echocardiography for assessment of ischemia.) In the absence of resting abnormalities on the electrocardiogram, stress testing without thallium normally provides adequate information about ischemia. Thus, it is prudent to avoid thallium scans during pregnancy unless the information is critical to patient management and cannot be obtained by other means such as echocardiography.

Magnetic Resonance Imaging

Nuclear magnetic resonance imaging (NMR or MRI) is a diagnostic imaging tool that involves exposure to high magnetic fields. Mechanisms by which MRI may be harmful include (1) orientation changes in molecules leading to changes in membrane permeability, (2) potential changes in enzyme kinetics, (3) reduction in nerve conduction velocity, (4) superposition of low potentials on natural biopotentials (170). Although it is known that MRI induces changes in electrocardiograms (170), there is currently no demonstration of harmful effects in humans, or evidence of reproducible genetic biochemical or cellular effects at field strengths of less than 20,000 gauss. Currently, there is no evidence that this diagnostic technique results in unusual hazards to the fetus (170, 171), although avoidance of MRI scanning has been recommended in the first trimester of pregnancy (172).

Cardiac Diagnostic Tests Utilizing Ionizing Radiation

Chest X-ray

Although chest x-rays involve radiation exposure, the dose is small, amounting to less than 0.5 mrad to the fetus (173). There is no need for routine chest x-rays during pregnancy. When cardiac disease is suspected, echocardiography is more accurate and poses no radiation risk. In patients with pulmonary disease, especially pulmonary hypertension, in whom a chest x-ray evaluation is of diagnostic importance, the radiation risk is low and can be further reduced by shielding the uterus with a lead shield.

Pregnancy results in normal changes to the cardiopulmonary silhouette on chest x-ray (174). The gravid uterus results in an elevation of the diaphragm, which causes a rotation of the heart to a more horizontal plane and an increased cardiothoracic ratio and increased lung markings. There is a straightening of the left upper cardiac border and a pseudo-enlargement of the left atrium due to the lordosis of pregnancy (64, 175). Small pleural (176) and pericardial (177) effusions may be normal findings in pregnancy and in the postpartum period.

Radionuclide Ventriculography

Radionuclide ventriculography (RVG) utilizes a radioactive tracer that is administered intravenously; a scintillation angiogram is then produced by detection of radiation by a gamma camera during phases of the cardiac cycle. This diagnostic test is useful to assess overall cardiac function and regional wall motion abnormalities and to detect intracardiac shunts. Maternal and fetal radiation exposure is different from that for external beam radiation such as a chest x-ray because the radioactive material is carried directly to the target organs by the circulatory system. The maternal whole-body radiation dose from an RVG is 290 mrad (178), but the effective radiation dose to the fetus is unclear. Various models have been used to estimate fetal radiation exposure from radiopharmaceutical agents (179, 180). Exposure depends on total dose, target organ, and volume of distribution. One commonly used tracer is technetium-99m, which is bound to albumin and therefore is theoretically less likely to cross the placental barrier. However, radionuclide techniques should be avoided whenever possible during pregnancy, and much of the information available from an RVG can now be obtained accurately and with less risk using Doppler echocardiography techniques.

Cardiac Perfusion Scanning

Perfusion scanning utilizes a radioactive tracer, usually thallium or technetium, which is injected intravenously to obtain information about myocardial perfusion. Both thallium and technetium are albumin bound, and thus do not easily cross the placenta; the effective fetal radiation dose is probably less than the estimated maternal dose of 360 mrem (thallium) or 200 mrem (technetium).

Since many radionuclide isotopes are excreted through the bladder, and local concentration of radiation in the bladder is in close proximity to the fetus, the pregnant woman should be cautioned to empty her bladder frequently following such a test. As with other tests involving radiation exposure, perfusion scanning should be avoided unless the information to be obtained is crucial for patient management and cannot be obtained by other tests that do not involve the use of radiation.

Cardiac Catheterization

Right Heart Catheterization. Placement of a pulmonary artery balloon wedge (Swan-Ganz) catheter can provide extremely useful information for the diagnosis and management of the pregnant patient who has preexisting heart disease or has developed problems during pregnancy. Often these balloon flotation catheters can be positioned without the use of fluoroscopy, especially from the right internal jugular vein. If high pulmonary artery pressures or the presence of tricuspid regurgitation makes placement difficult, brief use of fluoroscopy may aid in placing the catheter. The radiation dose to the fetus can be minimized by appropriate shielding. The radiation exposure to both mother and fetus is a function of the length of time fluoroscopy is used; an estimate of fetal radiation dose during fluoroscopy to the pelvis is approximately 1.25 rad/minute (181), and some authors estimate even less (182). Fluoroscopy of the chest with appropriate lead shielding of the pelvis further reduces fetal exposure.

Left Heart Catheterization. Certain suspected emergencies such as acute myocardial infarction or aortic dissection may necessitate the use of left heart catheterization during pregnancy. This test should be avoided if the necessary diagnostic information can be generated by any other test. Cardiac catheterization delivers a radiation dose that varies widely and is estimated to range from 500 mrad up to 47 rad (183–185) to the chest with lesser amounts directed at the abdomen. Only a portion of the dose delivered to the maternal abdomen is actually delivered to the fetus, and the actual fetal dose is not known, although it has been estimated to be 1650 mrad (184). Fetal exposure can be reduced by using the brachial instead of the femoral approach, by shielding the abdomen appropriately with a lead shield, and by using the absolute minimum fluoroscopic and ciné time.

Computed Tomographic Scans

There are a limited number of cardiovascular diagnoses that are made optimally by computed tomographic (CT) scans in pregnant women; even the diagnosis of aortic dissection may be made by alternative means such as transesophageal echocardiography. Estimates in the literature suggest that the radiation dose from a maternal chest CT scan is on the order of 2 to 10 mrad (186), but that 1 meter away the dose is reduced to 1 to 2 mrad. Fetal dose depends on technical factors such as the type of equipment used and the dose necessary for resolution as well as the location of CT. The fetal dose will be higher if the abdominal aorta is being visualized than if the thoracic aorta is the region of interest. Ultra-fast ciné CT is a new imaging tool that is likely to occupy an important place in cardiovascular assessment. There is virtually no information about the use of this diagnostic tool and radiation risks to the fetus.

Positron Emission Tomography

Positron emission tomography (PET) is a noninvasive imaging technique that is useful for studying the regional kinetics of positron-emitting radiotracers. Radioactive tracers that are commonly used include carbon-11 and nitrogen-14.

Although PET scanning has been used to study pharmacokinetics in the fetomaternal unit (187), there is little information about its safety, which is directly related to exposure of the fetus to the radioactive tracer.

EFFECTS OF RADIATION DURING PREGNANCY

Occasionally signs or symptoms arise during pregnancy that necessitate the use of cardiac diagnostic tests. In addition, patients with preexisting cardiovascular abnormalities require close evaluation and, rarely, cardiovascular intervention during pregnancy. Although recent advances in technology have resulted in accurate noninvasive cardiovascular tests that do not involve ionizing radiation, occasionally testing requires exposure of both mother and fetus to radiation. Knowledge of the hazards and effects of the total radiation dose and the timing of the exposure help to minimize fetal risk (Table 16–8).

Table 16–8. FETAL RADIATION DOSE IN MATERNAL CARDIOVASCULAR DIAGNOSTIC TESTING USING IONIZING RADIATION

Test	Estimated Maternal Dose	Estimated Fetal Dose
Chest radiograph		0.5 mrad
Radionuclide ventriculogram	290 mrem	
Thallium perfusion scan	360 mrem	
Technetium scan	200 mrem	0.48 mrem/mCi maternal dose
Cardiac catheterization		1.25 rad/minute of fluoroscopy
Computed tomogram	2 to 10 rad	

The effects of radiation on the fetus depend on the gestational age at which exposure occurs and can be divided into three main phases. During the preimplantation period (0 to 2 weeks) the effects appear to be "all or none" (188). Radiation either induces spontaneous resorption of the fertilized egg, or the pregnancy progresses in the normal fashion, possibly due to the inherent "plasticity" of development of this early embryo. During the period of organogenesis (2 to 9 weeks) exposure to radiation results in congenital malformations (188); large doses of radiation (50 rad) have been shown to cause skeletal and central nervous system abnormalities in addition to uterine growth retardation (189). Fetal development occurs along a strict timetable, so the type of abnormality induced is a function of the exact time of the radiation exposure from conception. During the second and third trimesters, the major risk of fetal radiation exposure is the development of childhood leukemia (190) and other malignancies (191). Although the development of most organs is complete by 9 to 12 weeks, the brain continues to grow and thus remains sensitive to the effects of radiation throughout pregnancy. Numerous reports have correlated radiation exposure to mental retardation and microcephaly (188, 192). More subtle forms of neurologic deficit such as behavior disorders are suspected to be a result of low levels of ionizing radiation, but there are virtually no data to support this speculation. Radiation exposure to the fetal gonads may result in chromosomal abnormalities that become manifest in the following generation.

In addition to the timing of the radiation exposure during gestation, the radiation dose is critical in assessing fetal risk. The incidence of spontaneous embryo resorption during the first 2 weeks of gestation is approximately 25–50%, and a dose of 10 rad is estimated to increase that number by 0.1%. During the period of organogenesis (from implantation to 8 or 9 weeks), a dose of 200 rad will produce a 100% incidence of congenital abnormalities, whereas a dose of 10 rad results in a 1% increase in malformations over a baseline of 5–10%. A fetal dose of 1 rad is estimated to increase the existing genetic mutation rate by 0.1%. A dose of 1 to 2 rad during weeks 8 to 15 is estimated to double the rate of severe mental retardation (192). Second and third trimester risks are primarily related to the development of childhood cancer. Data are scarce, but it has been estimated that a dose of 1 rad increases the risk of childhood malignancy by two cases per 100,000 births to a total of six cases in 100,000 live births (193), or by 0.9% (194).

The maximum acceptable fetal radiation dose has been set at 500 mrem (195), although some authors have suggested that a 10-rad exposure is "safe" (i.e., no recommendation would be made to terminate the pregnancy). If the fetal dose is in excess of 25 rad, elective pregnancy termination should be recommended because the risk of adverse outcome is high.

Although convincing data about low levels of radiation (fetal dose < 500 mrem) do not exist, it is assumed that because exposure occurs on a continuum, subtle changes in behavior or cancer risk may still exist. Thus, prudent management of the pregnant patient dictates avoidance of all radiation exposure unless the benefits of the information generated by such tests outweigh the risks to the fetus. If the use of ionizing radiation is imperative, such as cardiac catheterization in a pregnant patient with an acute myocardial infarction or aortic dissection, attempts should be made to minimize radiation exposure by any means possible.

References

1. Milne J, Howie A, Pack A. Dyspnoea during normal pregnancy. *Br J Obstet Gynecol* 85:260–263, 1978.
2. Hytten E, Thomson A, Taggart N. Total body water in normal pregnancy. *J Obstet Gynecol Br Commonw* 73:553–561, 1966.
3. Robertson E. The natural history of oedema during pregnancy. *J Obstet Gynecol Br Commonw* 78:520–529, 1971.
4. Cole P, St John-Sutton M. Normal cardiopulmonary adjustments to pregnancy. *Cardiovasc Clin* 19:37–56, 1989.
5. Cutforth R, MacDonald C. Heart sounds and murmurs in pregnancy. *Am Heart J* 71:741–747, 1966.
6. Perloff J. Pregnancy and cardiovascular disease. In Braunwald E (Ed.), *Heart Disease*. Philadelphia, W.B. Saunders, 1984, pp. 1763–1781.
7. O'Rourke R, Ewy G, Marcus F, et al. Cardiac auscultation in pregnancy. *Med Ann D C* 39:92–94, 1970.
8. Goldberg L, Uhland H. Heart murmurs in pregnancy: A phonocardiographic study of their development, progression and regression. *Dis Chest* 52:381–386, 1967.
9. Limacher M, Ware J, O'Meara M, et al. Tricuspid regurgitation during pregnancy: two-dimensional and pulsed doppler echocardiographic observations. *Am J Cardiol* 55:1059–1062, 1985.
10. Marcus F, Ewy G, O'Rourke R, et al. The effect of pregnancy on the murmurs of mitral and aortic regurgitation. *Circulation* 41:795–805, 1970.

11. Haas J. The effects of pregnancy on the midsystolic click and murmur of the prolapsing posterior leaflet of the mitral valve. *Am Heart J* 92:407–408, 1976.
12. Devereux R, Perloff J, Reicheck N, et al. Mitral valve prolapse. *Circulation* 54:3–14, 1976.
13. Harvey W. Alterations of the cardiac physical examination in normal pregnancy. *Clin Obstet Gynaecol* 18:51–63, 1975.
14. Elkayam U, Gleicher N. Changes in cardiac findings during normal pregnancy. In Elkayam U, Gleicher N (Eds.), *Cardiac Problems in Pregnancy*. New York, Alan R Liss, 1990, pp. 31–38.
15. Hurst J, Staton J, Hubbard D. Precordial murmurs during pregnancy and lactation. *N Eng J Med* 259:515–517, 1958.
16. Grant R. A precordial systolic murmur of extracardiac origin during pregnancy. *Am Heart J* 52:944–946, 1956.
17. Scott J, Murphy J. Mammary souffle: Report of two cases simulating patent ductus arteriosus. *Circulation* 18:1038–1043, 1958.
18. Tabatznik B, Randall T W, Hersch C. The mammary souffle of pregnancy and lactation. *Circulation* 22:1069–1073, 1960.
19. Walters W, Lim Y. Changes in the maternal cardiovascular system during human pregnancy. *Surg Gynecol Obstet* 131:765–784, 1970.
20. Laird-Meeter K, Van de Ley G, Bom T, et al. Cardiovasculatory adjustments during pregnancy—An echocardiographic study. *Clin Cardiol* 2:328–332, 1979.
21. Roy S, Malkani P, Virik R, et al. Circulatory effects of pregnancy. *Am J Obstet Gynecol* 96:221–225, 1966.
22. Airaksinen K, Salmela P, Ikaheimo M, et al. Effect of pregnancy on autonomic nervous function and heart rate in diabetic and nondiabetic women. *Diabetes Care* 10:748–751, 1987.
23. Capeless E, Clapp J. Cardiovascular changes in early phase of pregnancy. *Am J Obstet Gynecol* 161:1449–1453, 1989.
24. Clapp J. Maternal heart rate in pregnancy. *Am J Obstet Gynecol* 152:659–660, 1985.
25. Robson S, Hunter S, Boys R, et al. Serial study of factors influencing changes in cardiac output during human pregnancy. *Am J Physiol* 256:H1060–1065, 1989.
26. Rubler S, Damani P, Pinto E. Cardiac size and performance during pregnancy estimated with echocardiography. *Am J Cardiol* 40:534–540, 1977.
27. Atkins A, Watt J, Milan P, et al. A longitudinal study of cardiovascular dynamic changes throughout pregnancy. *Eur J Obstet Gynecol Reprod Biol* 12:215–224, 1981.
28. Veille J, Morton M, Burry K. Maternal cardiovascular adaptations to twin pregnancy. *Am J Obstet Gynecol* 153:261–263, 1985.
29. Ueland K, Novy M, Peterson E, et al. Maternal cardiovascular dynamics. IV. The influence of gestational age on the maternal cardiovascular response to posture and exercise. *Am J Obstet Gynecol* 104:856–863, 1969.
30. Ueland K, Metcalfe J. Circulatory changes in pregnancy. *Clin Obstet Gynecol* 18:41–50, 1975.
31. Clapp J, Seaward B, Sleamaker R, et al. Maternal physiologic adaptations to early human pregnancy. *Am J Obstet Gynecol* 159:1456–1460, 1988.
32. Longo L. Maternal blood volume and cardiac output during pregnancy: A hypothesis of endocrinologic control. *Am J Physiol* 245:R720–R729, 1983.
33. Mashini I, Albazzaz S, Fadel H, et al. Serial noninvasive evaluation of cardiovascular hemodynamics during pregnancy. *Am J Obstet Gynecol* 156:1208–1213, 1987.
34. Bader R, Bader M, Rose D, et al.: Hemodynamics at rest and during exercise in normal pregnancy as studied by cardiac catheterization. *J Clin Invest* 34:1524–1536, 1955.
35. Christianson R. Studies on blood pressure during pregnancy. Influence of parity and age. *Am J Obstet Gynecol* 125:509–513, 1976.
36. Gallery E, Hunyor S, Ross M, et al. Predicting the development of pregnancy-associated hypertension: The place of standardized blood pressure measurement. *Lancet* 1:1273–1275, 1977.
37. Katz R, Karliner J, Resnik R. Effects of a natural volume overload state (pregnancy) on left ventricular performance in normal human subjects. *Circulation* 58:434–441, 1978.
38. Kinsella S, Spencer J. Blood pressure measurement in the lateral position. *Brit J Obstet Gynecol* 96:1110–1112, 1989.
39. Chesley L. Plasma and red cell volumes during pregnancy. *Am J Obstet Gynecol* 112:440–450, 1972.
40. Pritchard J. Changes in the blood volume during pregnancy and delivery. *Anaesthesiology* 26:393–399, 1965.
41. Ueland K. Maternal cardiovascular dynamics. VII. Intrapartum blood volume changes. *Am J Obstet Gynecol* 126:671–677, 1976.
42. Goodlin R, Dobry C, Anderson J, et al. Clinical signs of normal plasma volume expansion during pregnancy. *Am J Obstet Gynecol* 145:1001–1007, 1983.
43. Adams J. Cardiovascular physiology in normal pregnancy: Studies with the dye dilution technique. *Am J Obstet Gynecol* 67:741–759, 1954.
44. Thomson K, Hirsheimer A, Gibson J, et al. Studies on the circulation in pregnancy. III. Blood volume changes in normal pregnant women. *Am J Obstet Gynecol* 36:48–59, 1938.
45. Berglund L, Lilja A, Andersson J, et al. Maternal blood volume in placenta of the rhesus monkey measured in vivo by positron emission tomography. *Gynecol Obstet Invest* 31:1–7, 1991.
46. Lund C, Donovan J. Blood volume during pregnancy. *Am J Obstet Gynecol* 98:393–403, 1967.
47. Rovinsky J, Jaffin H. Cardiovascular hemodynamics in pregnancy. I. Blood and plasma volumes in multiple pregnancy. *Am J Obstet Gynecol* 93:1–15, 1965.
48. Chesley L, Duffus G. Posture and apparent plasma volume in late pregnancy. *J Obstet Gynecol Br Commonw* 78:406–412, 1971.
49. Pritchard J. Hematologic aspects of pregnancy. *Clin Obstet Gynecol* 3:378–385, 1960.
50. Miller J, Keith N, Rowntree L. Plasma and blood volume in pregnancy. *JAMA* 65:779–782, 1915.
51. Fullerton W, Hytten F, Klopper A, et al. A case of quadruplet pregnancy. *J Obstet Gynecol Br Commonw* 72:791–796, 1965.
52. Hytten F, Paintin D. Increase in plasma volume during normal pregnancy. *J Obstet Gynecol Br Commonw* 70:402–407, 1963.
53. Schrier R, Durr J. Pregnancy: An overfill or underfill state. *Am J Kidney Dis* 9:284–289, 1987.
54. Davison J, Lindheimer M. Volume homeostasis and

osmoregulation in human pregnancy. *Bailliére's Clin Endocrin Metab* 3:451–472, 1989.
55. Gallery E, Brown M. Volume homeostasis in normal and hypertensive human pregnancy. *Bailliére's Clin Obstet Gynecol* 1:835–851, 1987.
56. Tapia H, Johnson C, Strong C. Effect of oral contraceptive therapy on the renin-angiotensin system in normotensive and hypertensive women. *J Obstet Gynecol* 41:643–649, 1973.
57. Ueda S, Fortune V, Bull B, et al. Estrogen effects on plasma volume, arterial blood pressures, interstitial space, plasma proteins and blood viscosity in sheep. *Am J Obstet Gynecol* 155:195–201, 1986.
58. Hart M, Hosenpud I, Hohimer A, et al. Hemodynamics during pregnancy and sex steroid administration in guinea pigs. *Am J Physiol* 249:R179–R185, 1985.
59. McCausland A, Hyman C, Winsor T, et al. Venous distensibility during pregnancy. *Am J Obstet Gynecol* 81:472–479, 1961.
60. Assali N, Rauramo L, Pertonen T. Measurement of uterine blood flow and uterine metabolism. VIII. Uterine and fetal blood flow and oxygen requirement in early human pregnancy. *Am J Obstet Gynecol* 79:86–98, 1960.
61. Metcalfe J, Romney S, Ramsey L, et al. Estimation of uterine blood flow in normal human pregnancy at term. *J Clin Invest* 34:1632–1638, 1955.
62. Thaler I, Manor D, Itskovitz J, et al. Changes in uterine blood flow during human pregnancy. *Am J Obstet Gynecol* 162:121–125, 1990.
63. Thoresen M, Wesche J. Doppler measurements of changes in human mammary and uterine blood flow during pregnancy and lactation. *Acta Obstet Gynecol Scand* 67:741–745, 1988.
64 Metcalfe J, McAnulty J, Ueland K (Eds.). *Burwell and Metcalfe's Heart Disease and Pregnancy: Physiology and Management*. Boston, Little, Brown, 1986.
65. Elkayam U, Gleicher N. Hemodynamics and cardiac function during normal pregnancy and the puerperium. In Elkayam U, Gleicher N (Eds.), *Cardiac Problems in Pregnancy*. New York, Alan R Liss, 1990, pp. 5–24.
66. Lunell N, Nylund L, Lewander R, et al. Uteroplacental blood flow in pre-eclampsia measurements with indium-113m and a computer-linked gamma camera. *Clin Exp Hypertens* B1:105–117, 1982.
67 Katz M, Sokal M. Skin perfusion in pregnancy. *Am J Obstet Gynecol* 137:30–33, 1980.
68. Fabricant N. Sexual functions and the nose. *Am J Med Sci* 239:498–502, 1960.
69. Lindheimer M, Katz A. The kidney in pregnancy. *N Engl J Med* 283:1095–1097, 1970.
70. Ginsberg J, Duncan S. Peripheral blood flow in normal pregnancy. *Cardiovasc Res* 1:132–137, 1967.
71. Abramson D, Flachs K, Fierst S. Peripheral blood flow during gestation. *Am J Obstet Gynecol* 45:666–671, 1943.
72. Herbert C, Banner E, Wakim K. Variations in the peripheral circulation during pregnancy. *Am J Obstet Gynecol* 76:742–745, 1958.
73. Hamilton H. The cardiac output in normal pregnancy. *J Obstet Gynecol Br Emp* 56:548–552, 1949.
74. Rose D, Bader M, Bader R, et al. Catheterization studies of cardiac hemodynamics in normal pregnant women with reference to left ventricular work. *Am J Obstet Gynecol* 72:233–244, 1956.
75. Yeomans E, Hankins G. Cardiovascular physiology and invasive cardiac monitoring. *Clin Obstet Gynecol* 32:2–12, 1989.
76. Evaluation of health. In Metcalfe J, McAnulty J, Ueland K (Eds.), *Heart Disease and Pregnancy*. Boston, Little, Brown, 1986, pp. 55–82.
77. Elkayam U, Gleicher N. Cardiovascular physiology of pregnancy. In Elkayam U, Gleicher N (Eds.), *Cardiac Problems in Pregnancy: Diagnosis and Management of Maternal and Fetal Disease*. New York, Alan R Liss, 1982, pp. 5–26.
78. Rovinsky J, Jaffin H. Cardiovascular hemodynamics in pregnancy. II. Cardiac output and left ventricular work in multiple pregnancy. *Am J Obstet Gynecol* 95:781–794, 1966.
79. Kerr M. The mechanical effects of the gravid uterus in late pregnancy. *J Obstet Gynecol Br Commonw* 72:513–529, 1965.
80. Bieniarz J, Crottogini J, Curuchet E, et al. Aortocaval compression by the uterus in late human pregnancy. II. An arteriographic study. *Am J Obstet Gynecol* 100:203–217, 1968.
81. Vorys N, Ullery J, Hanusek G. The cardiac output changes in various positions in pregnancy. *Am J Obstet Gynecol* 82:1312, 1961.
82. Vered Z, Poler S, Gibson P, et al. Noninvasive detection of the morphologic and hemodynamic changes during normal pregnancy. *Clin Cardiol* 14:327–334, 1991.
83. Lees M, Taylor S, Scott D, et al. A study of cardiac output at rest throughout pregnancy. *J Obstet Gynecol Br Commonw* 74:319, 1967.
84. Walters W, Mac Gregor W, Hills M. Cardiac output at rest during pregnancy and the puerperium. *Clin Sci* 30:1–11, 1966.
85. Robson S, Dunlop W, Moore M, et al. Combined doppler and echocardiographic measurement of cardiac output: Theory and application in pregnancy. *Br J Obstet Gynecol* 94:1014–1027, 1987.
86. Milsom I, Forssman L, Sivertsson R, et al. Measurement of cardiac stroke volume by impedance cardiography in the last trimester of pregnancy. *Acta Obstet Gynecol Scand* 62:473–479, 1983.
87. Masaki D, Greenspoon J, Ouzounian J. Measurement of cardiac output in pregnancy by thoracic electrical bioimpedance and thermodilution. *Am J Obstet Gynecol* 161:680–684, 1989.
88. Secher N, Arusbo P, Andersen L, et al. Measurements of cardiac stroke volume in various body positions in pregnancy and during caesarean section: A comparison between thermodilution and impedance cardiography. *Scand J Clin Lab Invest* 39:569–576, 1979.
89. Myhrman P, Granerus G, Karlsson K, et al. Cardiac output in normal pregnancy measured by impedance cardiography. *Scand J Clin Lab Invest* 42:513–520, 1982.
90. Easterling T, Watts H, Schmucker B, et al. Measurement of cardiac output during pregnancy: Validation of Doppler technique and clinical observations in pre-eclampsia. *Obstet Gynecol* 69:845–850, 1987.
91. Easterling T, Carlson K, Schmucker B, et al. Measurement of cardiac output in pregnancy by Doppler technique. *Am J Perinatology* 7:220–222, 1990.
92. Lee W, Rokey R, Cotton D. Noninvasive maternal stroke volume and cardiac output determinations by pulsed Doppler echocardiography. *Am J Obstet Gynecol* 158:505–510, 1988.

93. Nishimura R, Callahan M. Noninvasive measurement of cardiac output by continuous wave Doppler echocardiography: Initial experience and review of the literature. *Mayo Clin Proc* 59:484–489, 1984.
94. Robson S, Murray A, Peart I, et al. Reproducibility of cardiac output measurements by cross-sectional and Doppler echocardiography. *Br Heart J* 59:680–684, 1988.
95. Robson S, Boys R, Hunter S. Doppler echocardiographic estimation of cardiac output: Analysis of temporal variability. *Eur Heart J* 9:313–318, 1988.
96. McLennan E, Haites N, Rawles J. Stroke and minute distance in pregnancy: a longitudinal study using Doppler ultrasound. *Br J Obstet Gynecol* 94:499–506, 1987.
97. James C, Banner T, Levelle J, et al. Noninvasive determination of cardiac output throughout pregnancy. *Anesthesiology* 63:A434, 1985.
98. Cole P L, Plappert T, Saltzman D, et al. Changes in left ventricular architecture, load and function during pregnancy. *J Am Coll Cardiol* 9:43A, 1987.
99. Hart M, Morton M, Hosenpud J, et al. Aortic function during normal human pregnancy. *Am J Obstet Gynecol* 154:887–891, 1986.
100. Carabello B, Nolan S, McGuire L. Assessment of preoperative left ventricular function in patients with mitral regurgitation: Value of end-diastolic wall stress—end-systolic volume ratio. *Circulation* 64:1212–1217, 1981.
101. Grossman W, Braunwald E, Mann T, et al. Contractile state of the left ventricle in man as evaluated from end-systolic pressure-volume relations. *Circulation* 56:845–852, 1977.
102. Reichek N, Wilson J, St. John-Sutton M, et al. Noninvasive determination of left ventricular end-systolic stress: Validation of the method and initial application. *Circulation* 65:99–108, 1982.
103. Gunther S, Grossman W. Determinants of ventricular function pressure-overload hypertrophy in man. *Circulation* 59:679–688, 1979.
104. Clapp J, Dickstein S. Endurance exercise and pregnancy outcome. *Med Sci Sports Exerc* 16:556–562, 1984.
105. Hall D, Kaufmann D. Effects of aerobic and strength conditioning on pregnancy outcomes. *Am J Obstet Gynecol* 157:1199–1203, 1987.
106. Kulpa P, White B, Visscher R. Aerobic exercise in pregnancy. *Am J Obstet Gynecol* 156:1395–1403, 1987.
107. Artal R, Platt L, Sperling M, et al. Exercise in pregnancy. I. Maternal cardiovascular and metabolic response in normal pregnancy. *Am J Obstet Gynecol* 140:123–127, 1981.
108. Cooper K, Hunyor S, Boyce E, et al. Fetal heart rate and maternal cardiovascular and catecholamine responses to dynamic exercise. *Aust NZ J Obstet Gynecol* 27:220–223, 1987.
109. Pivarnik J, Lee W, Clark S, et al. Cardiac output responses of primigravid women during exercise determined by the direct Fick technique. *Obstet Gynecol* 75:954–959, 1990.
110. McMurray R, Katz V, Berry M, et al. Cardiovascular responses of pregnant women during aerobic exercise in water: A longitudinal study. *Int J Sports Med* 9:443–447, 1988.
111. Sady S, Carpenter M, Thompson P, et al. Cardiovascular response to cycle exercise during and after pregnancy. *J Appl Physiol* 66:336–341, 1989.
112. Knuttgen H, Emerson K. Physiological response to pregnancy at rest and during exercise. *J Appl Physiol* 36:549–553, 1974.
113. Ueland K, Novy M, Metcalfe J. Cardiorespiratory response to pregnancy and exercise in normal women and patients with heart disease. *Am J Obstet Gynecol* 115:4–10, 1973.
114. Guzman C, Caplan R. Cardiorespiratory responses to exercise during pregnancy. *Am J Obstet Gynecol* 108:600–605, 1970.
115. Pernoll M, Metcalfe J, Scheenker T, et al. Oxygen consumption at rest and during exercise in pregnancy. *Respir Physiol* 25:285–293, 1975.
116. Clapp J. Oxygen consumption during treadmill exercise before, during and after pregnancy. *Am J Obstet Gynecol* 161:1458–1464, 1989.
117. Baumann H, Huch A, Huch R. Doppler sonographic evaluation of exercise-induced blood flow velocity and waveform changes in fetal, uteroplacental and large maternal blood vessels in pregnant women. *J Perinatal Med* 17:279–287, 1989.
118. Steegers E, Buunk G, Binkhorst R, et al. The influence of maternal exercise on the uteroplacental vascular bed resistance and the fetal heart rate during normal pregnancy. *Eur J Obstet Gynecol Reprod Biol* 27:21–26, 1988.
119. Moore D, Jarrett J, Bendick P. Exercise induced changes in uterine artery blood flow as measured by Doppler ultrasound, in pregnant subjects. *Am J Perinatol* 5:94–97, 1988.
120. Rauramo I, Forss M. Effect of exercise on maternal hemodynamics and placental blood flow in healthy women. *Acta Obstet Gynecol Scand* 67:21–25, 1988.
121. Rauramo I, Forss M. Effect of exercise on placental blood flow in pregnancies complicated by hypertension, diabetes or intrahepatic cholestasis. *Acta Obstet Gynecol Scand* 67:15–20, 1988.
122. Morrow R, Ritchie J, Bull S. Fetal and hemodynamic responses to exercise in pregnancy assessed by Doppler ultrasonography. *Am J Obstet Gynecol* 160:138–140, 1989.
123. Morris N, Osborn S, Wright H. Effective uterine blood flow during exercise in normal and pre-eclamptic pregnancies. *Lancet* 2:481–484, 1956.
124. Clapp J. Fetal heart rate response to running in midpregnancy and late pregnancy. *Am J Obstet Gynecol* 153:251–252, 1985.
125. Dressendorfer R. Fetal heart rate response to maternal exercise testing. *Physician Sports Med* 8:90–100, 1980.
126. Artal R, Paul R, Romem Y, et al. Fetal bradycardia induced by maternal exercise. *Lancet* 2:258–260, 1984.
127. Golomer E, Arfi J, Sud R, et al. Exercise and pregnancy. Study of the changes in heart rate in pregnancy when performing standardized moderate exercise. *J Gynecol Obstet Biol Reprod* 18:295–302, 1989.
128. Pomerance J, Gluck L, Lynch V. Maternal exercise as a screening test for uteroplacental insufficiency. *Obstet Gynecol* 44:383–387, 1979.
129. Clapp J. The effects of maternal exercise on early pregnancy outcome. *Am J Obstet Gynecol* 161:1453–1457, 1989.
130. Pomerance J, Gluck L, Lynch V. Physical fitness in pregnancy: Its effect on pregnancy outcome. *Am J Obstet Gynecol* 119:867–876, 1974.
131. Collings C, Curet L, Mullin J. Maternal and fetal

responses to a maternal aerobic exercise program. *Am J Obstet Gynecol* 145:702–707, 1983.
132. American College of Obstetricians and Gynecologists. *Home Exercise Programs.* Washington D.C., American College of Obstetricians and Gynecologists, 1985, p. 4.
133. Paisley J, Mellion M. Exercise during pregnancy. *Am Fam Physician* 38:143–150, 1988.
134. Mullinax K, Dale E. Some considerations of exercise in pregnancy. *Clin Sports Med* 5:559–570, 1986.
135. Fishbein E, Phillips M. How safe is exercise during pregnancy. *J Obstet Gynecol Neonatal Nursing* 19:45–49, 1990.
136. Robson S, Dunlop W, Boys R, et al. Cardiac output during labor. *Br Med J* 295:1169–1172, 1987.
137. Adams J, Alexander A. Alterations in cardiovascular physiology during labor. *Am J Obstet Gynecol* 12:542–549, 1958.
138. Ueland K, Hansen J. Maternal cardiovascular dynamics: II. Posture and uterine contractions. *Am J Obstet Gynecol* 103:1–7, 1969.
139. Ueland K, Hansen J. Maternal cardiovascular dynamics III. Labor and delivery under local and caudal anaesthesia. *Am J Obstet Gynecol* 103:8–18, 1969.
140. Winner W, Romney S. Cardiovascular responses to labor and delivery. *Am J Obstet Gynecol* 95:1104–1114, 1966.
141. Metcalfe J, Ueland K. Maternal cardiovascular adjustments to pregnancy. *Prog Cardiovasc Dis* 16:363–374, 1974.
142. Hendricks C, Quilligan E. Cardiac output during labor. *Am J Obstet Gynecol* 71:953–972, 1956.
143. Jones C, Greiss F. The effect of labor on maternal and fetal circulating catecholamines. *Am J Obstet Gynecol* 144:149–153, 1982.
144. Newton M, Mosey L, Egli G, et al. Blood loss during and immediately after delivery. *Obstet Gynecol* 17:9–18, 1961.
145. Wilcox C, Hunt A, Owen C. The measurement of blood lost during cesarean section. *Am J Obstet Gynecol* 77:772–779, 1959.
146. Ueland K, Gills R, Hansen J. Maternal cardiovascular dynamics I. Cesarean section under subarachnoid block anaesthesia. *Am J Obstet Gynecol* 100:42–54, 1968.
147. Ueland K, Hansen J, Eng M, et al. Maternal cardiovascular dynamics V. Cesarean section under thiopental nitrous oxide and succinylcholine anaesthesia. *Am J Obstet Gynecol* 108:615–622, 1970.
148. Ueland K, Akamatsu T, Eng M, et al. Maternal cardiovascular dynamics VI. Cesarean section under epidural anaesthesia without epinephrine. *Am J Obstet Gynecol* 114:775–780, 1972.
149. Karim S, Hillier K, Sommers K, et al. The effects of prostaglandin E$_2$ and F$_2$ administered by different routes on uterine activity and the cardiovascular system in pregnant and non-pregnant women. *J Obstet Gynecol Br Commonw* 78:172–179, 1971.
150. Brown E, Sampson J, Wheeler E, et al. Physiologic changes in the circulation during and after obstetric labor. *Am Heart J* 34:311–333, 1947.
151. Robson S, Boys R, Hunter S, et al. Maternal hemodynamics after normal delivery complicated by postpartum hemorrhage. *Obstet Gynecol* 74:234–239, 1989.
152. Robson S, Hunter S, Moore M, et al. Hemodynamic changes during the puerperium: a doppler and M-Mode echocardiographic study. *Br J Obstet Gynecol* 94:1028–1039, 1987.
153. Robson S, Dunlop W, Hunter S. Hemodynamic changes during the early puerperium. *Br Med J* 294:1065, 1987.
154. Bond C. Blood volume changes in the lactating rat. *Endocrinology* 63:285–289, 1958.
155. Carruth J, Mirvis S, Brogan D, et al. The electrocardiogram in normal pregnancy. *Am Heart J* 102:1075–1078, 1981.
156. Schwartz D, Schamroth L. The effect of pregnancy on the frontal plane QRS axis. *J Electrocardiol* 12:279–281, 1979.
157. Wenger N, Hurst J, Strozier V. Electrocardiographic changes in pregnancy. *Am J Cardiol* 13:774–778, 1964.
158. Boyle D, Lloyd-Jones R. The electrocardiographic ST segment in pregnancy. *J Obstet Gynecol Br Commonw* 73:986–987, 1966.
159. Oram S, Holt M. Innocent depression of the ST segment and flattening of the T wave during pregnancy. *J Obstet Gynecol Br Commonw* 68:765–770, 1961.
160. Copeland G, Stern T. Wenckebach periods in pregnancy and puerperium. *Am Heart J* 56:291–298, 1958.
161. Feldman L, Hill H. The electrocardiogram of the normal heart in pregnancy. *Am Heart J* 10:110–117, 1934.
162. Brodsky M, Sato D, Oster P, et al. Paroxysmal ventricular tachycardia with syncope during pregnancy. *Am J Cardiol* 58:563–564, 1986.
163. McMillan T, Bellet S. Ventricular paroxysmal tachycardia: report of case in a pregnant girl of 16 years with apparently normal heart. *Am Heart J* 7:70–78, 1931.
164. Upshaw C. A study of maternal electrocardiograms recorded during labor and delivery. *Am J Obstet Gynecol* 107:17–27, 1970.
165. Watson P, Young W, Hegge F. Doppler measurements of maternal and fetal blood flow. *Clin Obstet Gynecol* 30:948–955, 1987.
166. Al-Ghazali W, Chapman M, Allan L. Doppler assessment of cardiac and uteroplacental circulations in normal and complicated pregnancies. *Br J Obstet Gynecol* 95:575–580, 1988.
167. Kurjak A, Alfirevic Z, Miljan M. Conventional and color doppler in the assessment of fetal and maternal circulation. *Ultrasound Med Biol* 14:337–354, 1988.
168. McPartland P, Pearce J. Doppler blood flow in pregnancy. *Placenta* 9:427–450, 1988.
169. Bioeffects considerations for the safety of diagnostic ultrasound. American Institute of Ultrasound in Medicine. Bioeffects Committee. *J Ultrasound Med* 7(9 Suppl):S1–S38, 1988.
170. Budinger TF. Nuclear magnetic resonance (NMR) in vivo studies: known thresholds for health effects. *J Comput Assist Tomogr* 5:800–811, 1981.
171. Thomas A, Morris P. The effects of NMR exposure in living organisms. I: a microbial assay. *Br J Radiol* 54:615–621, 1981.
172. Underwood R, Firmin D. *An Introduction to Magnetic Resonance of the Cardiovascular System.* London, Current Medical Literature, 1988.
173. Baker D. Radiology, is there an occupational hazard? *Am Ind Hyg Assoc J* 49:17–20, 1988.
174. Turner A. The chest radiograph in pregnancy. *Clin Obstet Gynecol* 18:65–74, 1975.

175. Szekely P, Snaith L. *Heart Disease and Pregnancy*. Edinburgh, Churchill Livingstone, 1974.
176. Hughson W, Friedman P, Feigin D, et al. Postpartum pleural effusion: A common radiologic finding. *Ann Intern Med* 97:856–858, 1982.
177. Enein M, Zina A, Kassem M, et al. Echocardiography of the pericardium in pregnancy. *Obstet Gynecol* 69:851–853, 1987.
178. Bakal C, Strauss H. Radionuclide imaging. In Morganroth J, Parisi AF, Pohost GM (Eds.), *Noninvasive Cardiac Imaging*. Chicago, Year Book, 1983, pp. 22–52.
179. Smith E, Warner G. Estimates of radiation dose to the embryo from nuclear medicine procedures. *J Nucl Med* 17:836–839, 1976.
180. Husak V, Wiedermann M. Radiation absorbed dose estimates to the embryo from some nuclear medicine procedures. *Int J Nucl Med* 5:205–207, 1980.
181. Syed I, Samols E. Medical xray exposure of the human embryo and fetus. *Health Physics* 42:61–64, 1982.
182. Baker M, Vandergrift J, Dalrymple G. Fetal exposure in diagnostic radiology. *Health Physics* 37:237–239, 1979.
183. Wagner L, Lester R, Saldana L. *Exposure of the Pregnant Patient to Diagnostic Radiation*. Philadelphia, J.B. Lippincott, 1985.
184. Metcalfe J, McAnulty J, Ueland K (Eds.). *Burwell and Metcalfe's Heart Disease and Pregnancy: Evaluation of Health*. Boston, Little, Brown, 1986.
185. Elkayam U, Gleicher N. Diagnostic approaches to maternal heart disease during pregnancy. In Elkayam U, Gleicher N (Eds.), *Cardiac Problems in Pregnancy*. New York, Alan R Liss, 1990, pp. 41–45.
186. McCullough E, Payne J. Patient dosage in computed tomography. *Radiology* 129:457–463, 1978.
187. Lindberg B, Hartvig P, Lilja A, et al. Positron-emission tomography: A new approach to feto-maternal pharmacokinetics. *Gynecol Obstet Invest* 31:1–7, 1991.
188. Jankowski C. Radiation and pregnancy: Putting the risks in proportion. *Am J Nursing* 86:260–265, 1986.
189. Brent RL. Radiation teratogenesis. *Teratology* 21:281–298, 1980.
190. Graham S, Levin M, Lilienfeld A, et al. Preconception, intrauterine and postnatal irradiation as related to leukemia. *National Cancer Institute Monograph* 19:347–371, 1966.
191. Stewart A, Webb J, Giles D, et al. Malignant disease in childhood and diagnostic irradiation in utero. *Lancet* 2:447, 1956.
192. Miller R. Intrauterine radiation exposure and mental retardation. *Health Physics* 55:295–298, 1988.
193. Bushong S. Policies for managing the pregnant employee. *Radiol Management* 6:2–5, 1984.
194. Wagner L, Haymon L. Pregnancy and women radiologists. *Radiology* 145:559–562, 1982.
195. Deluca S, Castronovo F. Radiation exposure in diagnostic studies. *Am Fam Physician* 36:101–103, 1987.

CHAPTER 17

Pregnancy with Preexisting Heart Disease

JOHN D. RUTHERFORD, M.B.Ch.B., F.R.A.C.P., F.A.C.C.
MARK E. HANDS, M.B., B.S., F.R.A.C.P.

GENERAL MANAGEMENT STRATEGIES

Some cardiac conditions associated with pregnancy are "well tolerated" and can withstand the known increases in cardiac output and profound fall in systemic vascular resistance associated with normal pregnancy, whereas others are "poorly tolerated" and are likely to be aggravated by these cardiovascular changes (Table 17–1). The likelihood of a successful outcome of pregnancy can usually be assessed with confidence if careful attention is paid to the symptomatic status of patients and to accurate noninvasive cardiac diagnosis and monitoring. Two-dimensional echocardiography has obviated the need for cardiac catheterization in most patients (1, 2), although this is often required in the occasional patients with acute ischemic syndromes. Even in patients with mild symptoms and well-tolerated cardiac disease daily periods of rest are recommended during pregnancy. Additionally, attention to diet with mild to moderate sodium restriction (if appropriate) and prompt diagnosis and treatment of intercurrent infections are important. Pathologic anemia should be promptly treated. Last, as term is approached, joint consultations with the attending obstetrician, cardiologist, and subsequently, anesthesiologists are important requirements of clear, careful, coordinated planning.

Myocardial Infarction

Acute myocardial infarction is rare during pregnancy, but the greatest maternal mortality occurs in patients who sustain the myocardial

Table 17-1. PROGNOSIS OF CARDIAC CONDITIONS DURING PREGNANCY

Well Tolerated During Pregnancy	Poorly Tolerated During Pregnancy
1. Asymptomatic, i.e., *NYHA*[a] *Class I*	1. Breathless at rest, i.e., *NYHA Class IV*
2. Mild to moderate *valvular regurgitation:* AR, MR If sinus rhythm is maintained the normal fall in systemic vascular resistance during pregnancy should reduce regurgitation	2. Moderate to severe *valvular stenosis:* MS, AS In patients with mitral stenosis the increased cardiac output and relatively shortened diastolic filling period (associated with increased heart rate) tend to elevate left atrial pressure
3. *Left-to-right shunt* without pulmonary hypertension (atrial septal defect, ventricular septal defect, patent ductus arteriosus) The normal fall in systemic vascular resistance during pregnancy should reduce left-to-right shunting	3. *Right-to-left shunt:* Eisenmenger's syndrome In patients with a fixed, elevated pulmonary vascular resistance the normal fall in systemic vascular resistance during pregnancy will increase right-to-left shunting
4. Mild to moderate *pulmonary valve stenosis*	4. *Primary pulmonary hypertension*
5. Mild to moderate *idiopathic hypertrophic subaortic stenosis* The increase in left ventricular volume occurring with pregnancy usually diminishes outflow obstruction	5. *Marfan's syndrome* Especially with aortic root dilation or moderate to severe valvular regurgitation
	6. *Myocardial infarction* Especially with moderate to severe ventricular dysfunction

AR = aortic regurgitation, MR = mitral regurgitation, MS = mitral stenosis, AS = aortic stenosis.
[a]New York Heart Association.

infarction late in pregnancy. Most maternal deaths occur either at the time of the infarction (usually resulting in an undelivered child) or within the next few weeks, usually in relation to the onset of labor and delivery (3). Postpartum myocardial infarction may also be associated with a high mortality (4). Approximately 90 cases have been reported in the English literature (5), and coronary morphology has been defined in about one-third of all reported cases, either by angiography or autopsy. Most of the cases have been reported in women over 35 years of age, and significant coronary atherosclerosis has been found in nearly 40% of patients. Coronary thrombosis has been involved in 10–30% of patients (angiographic evidence of total occlusion of the coronary vessel with otherwise normal vessels), and coronary aneurysm or dissection has been involved in 10% (6). With the trend towards increased maternal age the usual risk factors for coronary artery disease are important (high cholesterol, cigarette smoking, hypertension, diabetes mellitus, and a family history), but in younger patients estrogen use and cigarette smoking assume great importance (7). Last, cocaine abuse is also associated with acute myocardial infarction in this age group and should always be suspected.

The care of the pregnant patient with an acute myocardial infarction follows the same general principles as are used for the care of any patient with an acute infarction. Thrombolytic therapy is contraindicated, and percutaneous transluminal coronary angioplasty can be considered in a patient with ongoing myocardial infarction and continuing pain, especially if there is hemodynamic compromise (5). If anticoagulation is necessary, heparin is the drug of choice (Table 17-2). Obviously, if any invasive procedure is performed requiring fluoroscopic guidance, then the fetus must be adequately protected from excessive radiation. In the event of sudden maternal demise, careful planning must have occurred to achieve prompt rescue of a potentially viable fetus. The method of delivery needs to be individualized, and if a trial of labor and a vaginal delivery are contemplated, the limits to the duration of labor must be clearly defined and the team should be prepared to perform a cesarean section if necessary. Data on maternal and fetal outcomes of pregnancy in patients who have previously had a myocardial infarc-

Table 17-2. CARDIOVASCULAR DRUGS IN PREGNANCY

Drug	Placental Transfer	Adverse Fetal or Neonatal Effects	Teratogenic	FDA Class	Breast Feed
Amiodarone	Yes	Hypothyroidism, premature birth, hypotonia, large fontanelle		C	No
Atenolol	Yes	Low birth weight		B	Yes
Captopril	Yes	Second, third trimester use associated with skull hypoplasia, hypotension, anuria, oligohydramnios, death		C, 1st trimester D, trimesters 2 and 3	Yes
Digitalis	Yes	Low birth weight		A	Yes
Furosemide	Yes	Decreased Na$^+$, K$^+$, glucose		C	Yes
Heparin	No	Abortion		C	Yes
Hydralazine		Thrombocytopenia, acute distress		B	Yes
Isoproterenol	?	Tachycardia No adequate human studies		C	No data
Labetalol	Yes	No adequate human studies		C	Yes
Lidocaine	Yes	Bradycardia and CNS toxicity (keep maternal blood levels < 4 μg/mL)		B	No data
Mexilitine	Yes	Bradycardia, small infants, low APGAR, hypoglycemia		C	Yes
Phenytoin	Yes	Mental or growth retardation	Yes	X	No
Procainamide	Yes	None		B	Yes
Propranolol	Yes	Growth retardation, prematurity, hypoglycemia, bradycardia, respiratory depression		D	Yes (Observe infants carefully)
Quinidine	Yes	Thrombocytopenia		C	Yes
Sodium nitroprusside	Yes	Potentially toxic No adequate human studies		C	No
Thiazides	Yes	Decreased Na$^+$, K$^+$, glucose		D	+/− Can suppress lactation
Verapamil	Yes	No adequate human studies		C	Yes
Warfarin	Yes	Abortion, hemorrhage	Yes	X	Yes

tion are limited. As with other patients surviving acute myocardial infarction, the ultimate prognosis depends on the cumulative amount of myocardial damage sustained. Patients with poor left ventricular function have a poor prognosis, whereas those sustaining minimal left ventricular damage without evidence of residual ischemia may be expected to do reasonably well with a subsequent pregnancy. Among the few reported cases of pregnancy in patients with prior myocardial infarction there have been no maternal deaths. These data should be interpreted cautiously because of the small number of patients involved (13).

Cardiac Arrhythmias

The principles of antiarrhythmic therapy during pregnancy have been carefully documented (8). The most common arrhythmias during pregnancy include premature atrial or ventricular beats, reentrant supraventricular tachyarrhythmias, and occasionally tachyarrhythmias associated with the Wolff-Parkinson-White syndrome. If myocardial contractile function is thought to be normal, there is usually no need to treat asymptomatic or mildly symptomatic patients with ventricular or supraventricular premature beats. A history of caffeine use, alcohol use, or other precipitants of arrhythmias (e.g., sympathomimetic amine inhalers for asthma) are sought. There are a number of reports of paroxysmal supraventricular tachyarrhythmias that occur only during pregnancy (9). They are usually well tolerated and require active therapy only if they are very frequent or are associated with uncomfortable symptomatology or hemodynamic compromise. Vagal maneuvers are always taught to the patient and should be attempted initially in patients with such arrhythmias. If vagal maneuvers are ineffective, patients should be treated with digitalis, beta-blocking drugs, adenosine, or intravenous verapamil. Occasionally, cardioversion with or without quinidine therapy may be needed to achieve sinus rhythm.

Ventricular tachycardia can occur in pregnant patients and has been reported in the absence of detectable organic heart disease (8, 10, 11). Therapy with lidocaine is used acutely, and subsequent recurrence is prevented either with beta-blocking drugs, procainamide, or quinidine.

In the event of cardiopulmonary resuscitation during pregnancy the main objective is to resuscitate the mother before the onset of fetal viability (approximately the twenty-fourth week of gestation). After this stage of pregnancy, consideration has to be given to delivery of the fetus, which is usually expedited by emergency cesarean section if 15 minutes or more of cardiopulmonary resuscitation is unsuccessful or even earlier if it is not adequate (12).

Marfan's Syndrome

Because Marfan's syndrome has autosomal dominant inheritance, 50% of patients with this syndrome will have affected children. The syndrome does not skip generations. In patients with the classic syndrome and cardiac involvement, life expectancy is reduced to one-half, and most individuals die of a complication such as aortic rupture or dissection, heart failure secondary to valvular regurgitation, or infective endocarditis (13).

In patients with Marfan's syndrome, if cardiovascular involvement is minimal, the pregnancy may be tolerated without serious problems (14). Women with mild aortic dilation and no evidence of aortic regurgitation have a small risk of dissection, and monitoring with six to eight weekly echocardiograms is appropriate (15). Women who have moderate or severe cardiovascular dysfunction may be at considerable risk during pregnancy. The highest incidence of aortic dissection in women occurs during the third trimester and first postpartum month, and most dissections have occurred in women with aortic regurgitation or evidence of marked aortic root enlargement (15). It is recommended that women with Marfan's syndrome who are considering pregnancy should be assessed clinically, and echocardiography should be performed to look for aortic root dilation or valvular dysfunction. There is a relatively small risk of aortic dissection during pregnancy provided the patient is asymptomatic, the aortic root diameter is less than 40 mm, and there is no significant valvular dysfunction (14). Nevertheless, patients should be followed at a "high-risk" clinic. A normal noninduced vaginal delivery should be aimed for, and sudden increases in blood pressure or contractility should be treated or avoided. Beta-blockers are given to virtually all patients with Marfan's syndrome, even during pregnancy, because they have been shown to reduce the rate of aortic dilation and risk of complications (16). It is felt that the maternal advantages of beta-blockers far outweigh their potential adverse effects for the fetus. Even in patients with a normal aortic root and no evidence of valvular dysfunction, the presence of Marfan's syndrome alone can predispose the patient to a poor outcome with morbid or fatal events (17).

Valvular Heart Disease

Acute rheumatic fever with carditis is rare during pregnancy but is associated with increased fetal and maternal mortality (18). Patients with mild or moderate degrees of mitral and aortic regurgitation usually tolerate pregnancy well because systemic vascular resistance falls markedly during pregnancy and "afterloads" the heart. Either cardiac rhythm changes or the increase in cardiac output during pregnancy can lead to hemodynamic compromise in patients with severe degrees of valvular regurgitation. Both the increased heart rate and cardiac output associated with pregnancy compromise patients with severe aortic and mitral valvular stenoses.

Mitral valve stenosis is the most common, most important cardiac valvular problem during pregnancy. The symptoms of breathlessness on exertion, orthopnea, nocturnal dyspnea, or nocturnal cough may occur for the first time during pregnancy, usually in the middle trimester. Atrial fibrillation aggravated either by altered hemodynamics or concurrent infection in such patients may be associated with the onset of acute pulmonary edema. Two-dimensional echocardiography should be performed and will usually provide an accurate assessment of the severity of mitral stenosis. Patients with significant mitral stenosis who are symptomatic early in pregnancy despite treatment with diuretics are unlikely to tolerate the hemodynamic stress of labor and delivery. They are also at risk of developing pulmonary edema with tachyarrhythmias or with concurrent infection. Other patients with mitral stenosis who are either asymptomatic or have minor symptoms on a moderate medical regimen tolerate pregnancy remarkably well. Treatment modalities that can help individual patients include bed rest, appropriate diuretic therapy, restriction of sodium, prompt treatment of intercurrent infections, and home help to care for other children in the family. The new onset of tachyarrhythmias such as atrial fibrillation or supraventricular tachycardia can precipitate a medical emergency in patients with significant mitral stenosis. Acute pulmonary edema often ensues if the ventricular rate is not controlled rapidly or if normal sinus rhythm is not regained. Too often, ineffective attempts at heart rate control over a period of hours are accompanied by a deterioration in maternal or fetal status. Therefore, for rapid atrial fibrillation associated with symptoms or evidence of pulmonary edema, we prefer prompt cardioversion. The efficacy and safety of such an approach have been demonstrated (19), and rapid restoration of the hemodynamic status of the mother will improve the outlook for the fetus.

With severe mitral stenosis there is a pregnancy-related mortality, the times of greatest risk being labor, delivery, and the immediate postpartum period (20). Uterine contractions can elevate left atrial pressure by ~ 7 mm Hg transiently (21) and in patients with New York Heart Association (NYHA) class III or class IV symptoms a mean postpartum rise in pulmonary capillary wedge pressure of approximately 10 mm Hg may be anticipated (22). It has been recommended that in such patients there should be oxygen administration, labor in the lateral recumbent position, a Swan-Ganz catheter placed in the pulmonary artery to monitor hemodynamics, and a therapeutic reduction of the pulmonary capillary wedge pressure to approximately 14 mm as a desired goal (22). The same authors recommend epidural anesthesia in the active phase of labor, careful monitoring in the puerperium and reservation of cesarean section for obstetric reasons only.

In patients with significant mitral stenosis and more than class II symptomatology early in pregnancy, consideration should be given to either mitral balloon valvuloplasty (for significant mitral stenosis) or surgical intervention. Percutaneous balloon valvuloplasty of patients with severe mitral stenosis has been successfully performed during pregnancy (23), and mitral valvotomy or replacement with cardiopulmonary bypass can be successful for mother and fetus (24). Pregnancy does not influence the maternal surgical results, but there is a fetal mortality of approximately 10%, and surgery early in pregnancy may be associated with abortion and later in pregnancy with premature labor (25). Normothermic perfusion at high pressure and flow during cardiopulmonary bypass is probably safest for the fetus.

ANTICOAGULATION DURING PREGNANCY

The clinical situations in which anticoagulants are required during pregnancy include patients with heart valve prostheses, patients with acute dysrhythmia and mitral valve disease and associated paroxysmal or chronic atrial fibrillation, and patients who need prophylaxis against recurrent pulmonary thromboembolism.

Oral Anticoagulants—Warfarin and Related Drugs

Warfarin crosses the placental barrier and is teratogenic. There is a 5–15% risk of "warfarin embryopathy" (central nervous system abnormalities including microcephaly, optic atrophy, and hydrocephalus [26]) when warfarin is used in the first trimester of pregnancy. Later maternal hemorrhagic complications and fetal death can occur, and both intracerebral and retroplacental hemorrhages have been described. Warfarin requirements do not usually change during pregnancy, and the concentration of warfarin in breast milk is low, so that patients taking full-dose warfarin therapy can breast feed without affecting the clotting mechanisms of their infants (27, 28).

Heparin

Heparin is not teratogenic and does not cross the placenta, although its use is associated with maternal and fetal hemorrhage and possibly with premature labor (29). The complications of heparin therapy during pregnancy include hemorrhage, thrombocytopenia, osteopenia, and hypoaldosteronism. Transient heparin-induced thrombocytopenia may occur in up to 10% of patients (30). Antiplatelet immunoglobulin antibodies have been demonstrated in up to 10% of patients on heparin therapy and may also be associated with heparin-associated thrombocytopenia–thrombosis, which more frequently occurs with beef lung heparin. This latter major complication can be associated with significant mortality and may be heightened if the patient has been treated previously with heparin. Clinically important thrombocytopenia, with or without associated thrombosis, is unusual. Heparin is not detectable in breast milk.

Heparin is the anticoagulant of choice during pregnancy, and its administration on an ambulatory basis is feasible (31). High-dose subcutaneous heparin is regulated by obtaining a trough level (the lowest partial thromboplastin time [PTT] level before the next dose), which should be a few seconds above normal. A level drawn midway between doses should give a PTT of approximately one and a half times the control PTT. Outpatients can monitor high-dose subcutaneous heparin injections with a finger-stick PTT machine. Apart from intermittent subcutaneous administration, other routes include long-term ambulatory subcutaneous infusion (32) and permanent venous access via a Hickman catheter (33). At the onset of labor heparin injections are discontinued and are usually resumed 12 hours after normal vaginal delivery. Warfarin can be started on the first postpartum day, and both heparin and warfarin are overlapped for 3 to 5 days when full-dose anticoagulation is required. With the onset of labor, if a patient is fully anticoagulated with warfarin, fresh frozen plasma is usually administered.

Prosthetic Heart Valves

Increasing numbers of patients with prosthetic heart valves are contemplating pregnancy. The mother is exposed to the risks of infective endocarditis and thromboembolism, and anticoagulation increases the risk for mother and fetus. Clearly, antiplatelet agents (aspirin, dipyridamole) do not protect the mother sufficiently from thromboembolism to make their use advisable in pregnant women with prosthetic heart valves (34). Low-dose heparin does not protect against prosthetic heart valve thrombosis; however, long-term high-dose subcutaneous heparin sufficient to anticoagulate the mother fully may be given during pregnancy and may be self-administered by the patient two or three times daily at home (35). Warfarin derivatives provide effective protection against maternal thromboembolism but are teratogenic early in pregnancy. Warfarin use is also associated with significant fetal wastage (36). We prefer to manage patients with high-dose, self-administered subcutaneous heparin throughout pregnancy rather than using a regimen of heparin in the first and third trimesters and warfarin in the middle of pregnancy.

Cardiac Shunts

Patients who have undergone a successful repair of an atrial or ventricular septal defect or patent ductus arteriosus and who are asymptomatic and have normal hemodynamics have a maternal risk during pregnancy that is similar to that of a normal population (37). However, patients with persistent cyanotic heart disease or significant pulmonary hypertension are at significant risk for morbid or fatal events during pregnancy.

Left-to-Right Cardiac Shunts. The most common abnormalities encountered in women of childbearing age are atrial or ventricular septal defects. In the absence of significant cardiac symptomatology or pulmonary hypertension, the outcome of pregnancy is usually normal and uncomplicated because the degree of left-to-right shunting tends to diminish with the normal fall in systemic vascular resistance during pregnancy. Maternal and fetal problems can occur during pregnancy in patients with shunts associated with cardiac dysrhythmias, pulmonary hypertension, or right heart failure.

Right-to-Left Shunts, Eisenmenger's Syndrome. The term Eisenmenger's syndrome usually applies to patients with large intracardiac defects that allow free communication between the systemic and pulmonary circulations at the aortic, ventricular, or atrial level. Such patients have predominantly right-to-left shunting secondary to *fixed* and *markedly* elevated pulmonary vascular resistance (38). The term Eisenmenger's complex is used to describe the condition of a large ventricular septal defect associated with a marked, fixed, and elevated pulmonary vascular resistance resulting in a predominantly right-to-left shunt. With pregnancy and the usual maternal hemodynamic alterations (including an increased cardiac output and a fall in systemic vascular resistance), patients with Eisenmenger's syndrome will develop more right-to-left shunting. As a consequence, they may experience deeper cyanosis, a reduced systemic arterial oxygen saturation, and a rise in hematocrit. Such patients with Eisenmenger's syndrome and severe pulmonary hypertension should be counseled not to become pregnant. This is one of the few cardiac conditions for which sterilization is usually recommended because pregnancy is rarely tolerated (39). Maternal mortality approaches 30–50%, and the majority of deaths occur during or within the first week following delivery. There is a perinatal mortality of approximately 30%. If feasible, therapeutic abortion is indicated because cesarean sections and other operations are all associated with increased maternal risk. If interruption of pregnancy is not feasible or is declined, supportive measures include avoidance of operative procedures and avoidance of hypotension, hypovolemia, and thromboembolic phenomena. Gleicher and colleagues (39) recommend hospitalization and prolonged bed rest plus anticoagulation of patients from midpregnancy, noninduced labor, administration of high concentrations of oxygen during labor, epidural anesthesia, and vaginal delivery (noninduced) with elective low forceps delivery used to shorten the second stage of labor. Despite these active measures, maternal mortality still remains substantial in the first week following delivery.

References

1. Raymond R, Underwood DA, Mooide DS. Cardiovascular problems in pregnancy. *Cleve Clin J Med* 54:95, 1987.
2. Elkayam U. Pregnancy and cardiovascular disease. In Braunwald E (Ed.), *Heart Disease: A Textbook of Cardiovascular Medicine*. Philadelphia, W.B. Saunders, 1992, pp. 1790–1809.
3. Hankins GDV, Wendall GD, Leveno KJ, et al. Myocardial infarction during pregnancy. *Obstet Gynecol* 65:139, 1985.
4. Beary JF, Summer WR, Bulkley BH. Postpartum acute myocardial infarction: A rare occurrence of uncertain etiology. *Am J Cardiol* 43:158, 1979.
5. Hands ME, Johnson MD, Saltzman DH, et al. The cardiac, obstetric and anesthetic management of pregnancy complicated by acute myocardial infarction. *J Clin Anesth* 2:258, 1990.
6. Movsesian MA, Wray RB. Postpartum myocardial infarction. *Br Heart J* 62:154, 1989.
7. Croft P, Hannaford PC. Risk factors for acute myocardial infarction in women: Evidence from the Royal College of General Practitioners Oral Contraception Study. *Br Med J* 298:165, 1989.
8. Rotmensch HH, Elkayam U, Irishman W. Antiarrhythmic drug therapy during pregnancy. *Ann Intern Med* 98:487, 1983.
9. Szekely P, Snaith L. Paroxysmal tachycardia in pregnancy. *Br Heart J* 15:195, 1953.
10. Braverman AC, Bromley BS, Rutherford JD. New onset ventricular tachycardia during pregnancy. *Int J Cardiol* 33:409, 1991.
11. Brodsky MA, Sato DA, Oster PD, et al. Paroxysmal

ventricular tachycardia with syncope during pregnancy. *Am J Cardiol* 58:563, 1986.
12. Lee RV, Rodgers BD, White LM, et al. Cardiopulmonary resuscitation of pregnant women. *Am J Med* 81:311, 1986.
13. Murdock JL, Walker BA, Halpern BL, et al. Life expectancy and causes of death in the Marfan syndrome. *N Engl J Med* 286:804, 1972.
14. Pyeritz RE. Maternal and fetal complications of pregnancy in the Marfan syndrome. *Am J Med* 71:784, 1981.
15. Pyeritz RE. The Marfan syndrome. *Am Fam Physician* 34:83, 1986.
16. Pyeritz RE. Propranolol retards aortic root dilatation in the Marfan syndrome. *Circulation* 68 (Suppl III):365, 1983.
17. Rosenblum NG, Grossman AR, Mennuti MT, et al. Failure of serial echocardiographic studies to predict aortic dissection in the pregnant patient with Marfan's syndrome. *Am J Obstet Gynecol* 146:470, 1983.
18. Sullivan JM, Ramanathan KB. Management of medical problems in pregnancy—severe cardiac disease. *N Engl J Med* 313:304, 1985.
19. Metcalfe J, McAnulty JH, Ueland K. *Burwell and Metcalfe's Heart Disease and Pregnancy: Physiology and Management.* Boston, Little, Brown, 1986.
20. Ueland K. Intrapartum management of the cardiac patient. *Clin Perinatol* 8:155, 1981.
21. Jakobi P, Adler Z, Zimmer EZ, et al. Effect of uterine contractions on left atrial pressure in a pregnant woman with mitral stenosis. *Br Med J* 298:27, 1989.
22. Clark SL, Phelan JP, Greenspoon J, et al. Labor and delivery in the presence of mitral stenosis: Central hemodynamic observations. *Am J Obstet Gynecol* 152:984, 1985.
23. Safian RD, Berman AD, Sachs B, et al. Percutaneous balloon mitral valvuloplasty in a pregnant woman with mitral stenosis. *Cathet Cardiovasc Diagn* 15:103, 1988.
24. Becker RM. Intracardiac surgery in pregnant women. *Ann Thorac Surg* 36:453, 1983.
25. Bernal JM, Miralles PJ. Cardiac surgery with cardiopulmonary bypass during pregnancy (review). *Obstet Gynecol Surv* 41:1, 1986.
26. Pettifor JM, Benson R. Congenital malformations associated with administration of oral anticoagulants during pregnancy. *J Pediatr* 86:459, 1975.
27. Orme M L'E, Lewis PJ, de Swiet M, et al. May mothers given warfarin breast feed their infants? *Br Med J* 1:1564, 1977.
28. McKenna R, Cole ER, Vasan U, et al. Is warfarin sodium contraindicated in the lactating mother? Clinical and laboratory observation. *J Pediatr* 103:325, 1983.
29. Howell R, Fidler J, Letsky E, et al. The risks of antenatal subcutaneous heparin prophylaxis: A controlled trial. *Br J Obstet Gynaecol* 90:1124, 1983.
30. Calhoun BC, Hesser JW. Heparin associated antibody with pregnancy. Discussion of two cases. *Am J Obstet Gynecol* 156:964, 1987.
31. Henny CP, Ten Cate MT, Buller HR, et al. Ambulatory heparin treatment. *Lancet* 1:615, 1982.
32. Rabinovici J, Mani A, Barkai G, et al. Long-term ambulatory anticoagulation by constant subcutaneous infusion in pregnancy. *Br J Obstet Gynaecol* 94:89, 1987.
33. Nelson DM, Stempel LE, Fabri PJ, et al. Hickman catheter use in a pregnant patient requiring therapeutic heparin anticoagulation. *Am J Obstet Gynecol* 149:461, 1984.
34. Salazar E, Zajarias A, Gutierrez N, et al. The problem of cardiac valve prosthesis, anticoagulants and pregnancy. *Circulation* 70 (Suppl. I):1–169, 1984.
35. Iturbe-Alessio I, Fonseca M, Mutchinik O, et al. Risks of anticoagulant therapy in pregnant women with artificial heart valves. *N Engl J Med* 315:1390, 1986.
36. Sareli P, England MJ, Berk MR, et al. Maternal and fetal sequelae of anticoagulation during pregnancy in patients with mechanical heart valve prostheses. *Am J Cardiol* 63:1462, 1989.
37. Perloff JK. Congenital heart disease and pregnancy. In Gleicher N (Ed.), *Principles of Medical Therapy in Pregnancy*. New York, Plenum Medical Books, pp. 665–671.
38. Graham TP. The Eisenmenger syndrome in adult congenital heart disease. In Roberts WD (Ed.), *Adult Congenital Disease*. Philadelphia, F.A. Davis, 1987, pp. 567–581.
39. Gleicher N, Midwall J, Hochberger D, et al. Eisenmenger's syndrome and pregnancy. *Obstet Gynecol Surv* 34:721, 1979.

CHAPTER 18

Heart Disease Arising During Pregnancy

KAREN B. JAMES, M.D.

The state of pregnancy in some women can precipitate cardiovascular disorders not previously present in seemingly well individuals. These cardiovascular disease states arising during pregnancy often occur unexpectedly and pose risks to both mother and fetus. Cardiovascular disorders that may present for the first time during pregnancy include (1) toxemia, (2) systemic hypertension, (3) peripartum cardiomyopathy, (4) aortic dissection, and (5) pulmonary hypertension. The first two disorders are the most common and the most amenable to treatment. The other disorders—peripartum cardiomyopathy, aortic dissection, and pulmonary hypertension—can be disastrous and sudden in presentation but fortunately are rare.

TOXEMIA

Toxemia, previously known as preeclampsia, is a systemic disease unique to pregnancy in which proteinuria, central nervous system irritability, and renal, hematologic, and hepatic abnormalities occur. In fulminant toxemia or eclampsia, convulsions and consumptive coagulopathy may ensue. Hypertensive disorders may also occur during pregnancy without the features of toxemia; these are discussed later in this chapter.

The American Obstetrical Committee has defined a blood pressure of 130/80 mm Hg as the upper limit of normal for pregnant women. Rises of 30 mm Hg systolic or 15 mm Hg diastolic between monthly visits or above prepregnancy levels are considered abnormal regardless of the absolute levels. These recommendations are based on data that blood pressures above 125/75 mm Hg prior to the thirty-sixth week of gestation are associated with increased fetal risk, with fetal mortality rising in direct linear relation to maternal diastolic blood pressure elevations above 90 mm Hg (1).

The incidence of toxemia in the United States is 7% of all pregnancies; there is a bimodal distribution with peaks in young primigravidas and older multiparas (2). Toxemia, along with hemorrhage, infection, and cardiac disease, was the leading cause of maternal mortality in the mid-1950s, according to data collected by the Committee on Maternal Welfare of the Massachusetts Medical Society (3). In contrast, the same study found that in the 1980s, the leading causes of maternal death were trauma (homicides, suicides, motor vehicle accidents) and pulmonary emboli. With specific regard to toxemia, the maternal mortality rate fell from 5/100,000 live births in 1954–1957 to 1/100,000 subsequently (1958–1985), representing an 82% decline. The decrease in toxemia-associated maternal mortality is due to a reduction in intracranial hemorrhage, which is believed by the Committee to have been related to poor blood pressure control. They noted that improved medical care including aggressive management of hypertension in toxemia has clearly played an important role in decreasing maternal mortality from this disease (3).

Clinical Features

Weight gain with edema is often the first sign of toxemia, although edema is often present in normal pregnancy. The edema in toxemia may be more generalized, however, involving the upper body (face and hands) as well as the feet and ankles. In toxemia, a rise in blood pressure and proteinuria follow shortly, with onset usually after the thirty-second week of gestation. Hypertension occurring during the first trimester is usually due to chronic hypertension or, rarely, to toxemia resulting from a hydatidiform mole (4). Furthermore, hypertension that persists past delivery rarely is due to persistent toxemia; it usually represents persistent essential hypertension (4). The cardiac examination, aside from hypertension, is usually normal unless frank left ventricular failure or pulmonary edema occurs secondary to severe hypertension.

Headache, epigastric pain, visual disturbances, and apprehension may occur in toxemia. In advanced cases, central nervous system irritability, hyperreflexia, seizures, and even cerebral hemorrhage or edema may occur. Retinal edema, hemorrhages, and exudates may sometimes occur in the optic fundus as well.

Pathophysiology

Renin-Angiotensin and Prostaglandin Physiology in Toxemia

There is a 30–50% rise in cardiac output and a 50% increase in plasma volume during pregnancy (5). Although cardiac output rises in normal pregnancy, the blood pressure falls owing to a marked decrease in peripheral vascular resistance (4). In toxemia the vascular resistance increases instead, leading to the hypertension.

Renin secretion, which is markedly elevated during normal pregnancy, leads to elevated angiotensin levels (4, 6, 7). Angiotensin contributes to hypertension in two ways: it is a potent vasoconstrictor, and it leads to volume expansion by stimulating aldosterone secretion. Plasma renin levels are increased by up to eightfold in normal pregnancy, and yet in normal pregnancy the blood pressure falls. How is this paradox explained?

It is postulated that normal pregnancy represents a state of angiotensin insensitivity that begins in the first trimester and lasts throughout pregnancy. This insensitivity to angiotensin is inferred by the fact that a vasodilated state persists in the pregnant woman despite a marked increase in plasma renin and angiotensin levels (6, 7). Furthermore, despite a markedly expanded volume status, aldosterone may not be suppressed in response to increased sodium intake in normal pregnancy (7).

If angiotensin insensitivity does indeed prove ultimately to be a major explanation of why hypertension occurs in toxemia, the mechanism might be related to modulation of angiotensin II receptors on smooth muscle. Animal studies with rats, for example, have shown that vascular sensitivity to angiotensin can be modified by renal artery clipping or sodium loading, which leads to increased vascular receptor affinity for angiotensin (8).

Toxemic women display loss of angiotensin insensitivity as early as the eighteenth week of pregnancy. Postulated modulators of angiotensin sensitivity include altered levels of angiotensinase (4), angiotensin-converting enzyme (4), and prostaglandins (9). Prostaglandins are most likely an important modulator of angiotensin sensitivity in normal and toxemic pregnancies.

Prostacyclin (PGI_2) is a vasodilatory prostaglandin that antagonizes angiotensin. Prostacyclin is primarily synthesized by endothelium, but it has also been shown to be produced by the myometrium, placenta, umbilical vascular tissue, and kidney. Prostaglandin synthesis is enhanced during pregnancy, as evidenced by elevated urinary and plasma concentrations of metabolites of PGI_2 synthesis.

Evidence of altered prostaglandin modulation in toxemia is based on the finding that administration of prostaglandin inhibitors to normotensive women in the third trimester causes increased sensitivity to angiotensin (9). Further evidence that toxemia is a "prostacyclin deficiency state" arises from the fact that production of 6-keto-PGF_1, a stable metabolite of PGI_2, is decreased in toxemic pregnancies (10, 11). Placental production of PGI_2 and urinary concentrations of PGI_2 are also decreased in toxemia (12, 13).

An alternative explanation to lack of angiotensin insensitivity in toxemia is the possible presence of a pressor substance (14–17). Previous studies have shown that transfusion of sera, plasma, or whole blood from toxemic women into normal volunteers, animals, or back into the same patient postpartum results in hypertension (18, 19). However, the results of these studies have been inconsistent (20, 21). Perfusion of blood vessels in vitro with sera from toxemic women has also been shown to cause vasoconstriction, supporting the theory of a pressor substance contributing to toxemia (22, 23). Isolation of such a substance would provide yet another clue to the understanding of this most intriguing disease.

Last, other peptides may be altered in toxemia, but their role as cause or effect is currently unknown. For example, atrial natriuretic peptide (ANP), a vasodilatory hormone first described in atrial myocytes, has been shown to have specific receptors on the normal human placenta (24). Other investigators have observed that peripheral ANP concentrations may increase significantly in toxemic patients (25). A decreased affinity of placental ANP receptors in toxemic women has been shown, suggesting a down-regulation of these receptors in this entity. The functional significance of ANP and other peptides is unknown, but it represents a stimulating area for further investigation (26).

The Placenta in Toxemia

Placental growth in normal pregnancy is associated with a tenfold increase in blood flow (27, 28). The spiral arteries supplying the placenta undergo marked morphologic alterations in pregnancy, mediated by trophoblast invasion into the media of these vessels (29–31). In the first trimester, degeneration of the internal elastic lamina of the spiral arteries occurs with denudement of the smooth muscle and elastin (32–34). In the second trimester, endovascular trophoblastic invasion extends into the myometrial segments of the spiral arteries (32–34). These changes of normal placentation allow for maximal fetal blood flow at low resistance.

In toxemia, the trophoblast-induced physiologic changes are restricted to the decidual segments of the spiral arteries of the placental bed. The endovascular trophoblastic invasion does not extend to the myometrial segments, thus leaving these segments of spiral arteries to retain their musculoelastic architecture and their vasoconstrictive capabilities (35, 36). The basal and myometrial portions of the spiral arteries in toxemic patients have been shown subsequently to undergo "acute atherosis" (37). This pathologic lesion includes extensive lipid necrosis (35, 36), myointimal cell hyperplasia (38), platelet deposition, mural thrombosis, and fibrinoid necrosis (35, 36). The hyperplastic vascular smooth muscle proliferation promotes vasospasm. The net result is reduced fetal blood flow and increased responsiveness to vasoconstrictors such as angiotensin and thromboxane.

Vasculopathy in Toxemia

Toxemia is a multisystem disorder characterized by fibrin deposition in the microcirculation of various organs. Renal involvement in toxemia correlates well with the level of proteinuria, which can range from minimal to frank nephrosis. Renal biopsies vary from patient to patient depending on the degree of renal involvement, but the typical renal biopsy in toxemia reveals swollen endothelial and mesangial cells. The endothelial cells usually contain large vacuoles with fibrinlike deposition. (39)

In normal pregnancies, the glomerular filtration rate and renal blood flow increase; normal creatinine levels average 0.45 ± 0.06 mg/dl compared with 0.67 ± 0.17 mg/dl in nonpregnant women (39). Uric acid clearance increases concomitantly in normal pregnancy. The opposite occurs in toxemia owing to the renal glomerular insult, and there is a decrease in uric acid clearance. In fact, hyperuricemia correlates well with the clinical severity of toxemia, with the histologic lesion seen on renal biopsy, and with decreased survival of the fetus (39).

Hepatic dysfunction with elevation of lactate dehydrogenase and transaminase levels may occur in toxemia. Percutaneous liver biopsies in toxemic women have shown fibrin deposits in this organ also with patchy areas of necrosis (40). Another hepatic lesion seen in toxemic women is the acute fatty liver of pregnancy. One review reported the presence of toxemia in 22% of 49 patients who had fatty liver of pregnancy (41). The specific organ systems involved in toxemia may vary from patient to patient, and numerous syndromes have been described. One such example is the HELLP syndrome, which describes toxemic patients with hemolysis, elevated liver enzymes, and low platelet count (42).

The central nervous system may be involved in toxemia. The most common cause of death in toxemia is cerebral hemorrhage. Convulsions are an ominous sign in this disease. Microscopically, fibrin deposits have been reported in the brains of patients dying of eclampsia. Grossly, petechial, thrombotic, and hemorrhagic lesions have been described. Both uncontrolled hypertension and coagulopathy contribute to these lesions. Other central nervous system lesions in toxemia include central venous thrombosis and cerebral edema. Newer brain imaging modalities, including computed tomographic and magnetic resonance scanning, have provided further insight into the changes in the brain that occur in toxemia. Cerebral edema has been a predominant finding and has been reported to improve with clinical improvement (43, 44). Cerebral vasospasm has been implicated as a cause of cerebral edema based on angiographic evidence (45).

Pathologically, the heart is not a major target organ in toxemia. One postmortem study, however, did disclose contraction band necrosis in 12 of 34 hearts of eclamptic patients. These findings suggest that coronary vasospasm may have occurred (46).

Other organs involved in toxemia include the pancreas, with acute pancreatitis being thought to be due to an ischemic process (47). Microthrombi in the lungs can cause ventilation-perfusion defects in toxemia (48). Adult respiratory distress syndrome has also been described in toxemia (49).

Coagulopathy in Toxemia

Although normal pregnancy represents a physiologic hypercoagulable state with increases in factors VII, VIII, and X and a decline in plasminogen activator, toxemia represents a state of marked aberration in the coagulation system. In toxemic women, antithrombin III (50), plasminogen (51), α_2-plasmin inhibitor (51), and factor XIII (51) are further decreased, and fibrinopeptide A (50), bradykinin (51), and D-dimer fibrin degradation products (52) are increased. Although fibrin degradation products are frequently elevated in toxemia, frank disseminated intravascular coagulation (DIC) is usually absent. However, in some toxemic patients chronic DIC should be considered responsible for the coagulation profile. Repeated infusions of tissue thromboplastin have been shown to lead to chronic DIC in experimental animals (53, 54).

The platelet component of the hemostatic system also undergoes changes and activation in toxemia. Platelet counts may decrease during or even before overt toxemia appears (55). Platelet size may be increased, indicating increased turnover (56). Concentrations of platelet factor 4, serotonin, and β-thromboglobulin may be increased, indicating in vivo platelet aggregation (57, 58). Lastly, platelets may exhibit altered responsiveness in toxemic patients, indicating aggregation-disaggregation abnormalities. Increased circulating von Willebrand factor (vWF) concentrations may be noted in toxemia, which may contribute to platelet aggregation (59). In fact, thrombotic thrombocytopenic purpura is sometimes indistinguishable from toxemia (60).

Just as prostaglandins are thought to play a pivotal role in the hypertension of toxemia through increased angiotensin sensitivity, imbalances in prostaglandin synthesis are thought to contribute to the coagulopathy of toxemia. Specifically, a relative deficiency of prostacyclin might tip the balance between thromboxane, a potent vasoconstrictor that promotes platelet aggregation, and prostacyclin, to favor thrombosis. Walsh reported that the placenta in toxemic patients produces seven times more thromboxane than prostacyclin, whereas in a normal pregnancy the placenta produces equal quantities of these prostaglandins (61). Another study reported that renal prostacyclin synthesis is decreased by 50% and thromboxane A_2 is normal in women with toxemia and in their infants (62). Hence, an aberration in prostaglandin synthesis may help to explain, at least in part, both the hypertensive and the thrombotic manifestations of toxemia. The thrombotic tendencies are manifested by the multiorgan fibrin deposition described previously. Recently, plasma from toxemic patients has been found to contain a substance that is cytotoxic to endothelial cells in monolayer culture (63, 64). Characterization of this substance may promote further understanding of the effect of toxemia on blood vessels and on coagulation.

Integrated View of Toxemia

Multiple aspects of toxemia have been discussed, including the vasoconstrictive and hematologic aspects and their links to prostacyclin deficiency. Pathologic placentation is the earliest anatomic aberration in toxemia, and this too is linked to prostaglandins. In the pathologic placentation of toxemia, failure of trophoblastic migration occurs, as discussed earlier. Trophoblasts are capable of PGI_2 synthesis, and this PGI_2 production has two important functions: (1) it promotes trophoblastic invasion, and (2) it prevents clotting in the low-pressure intervillous space (65). If there is a pathologic shift in the PGI_2-thromboxane ratio in the toxemic placenta, this shift favors fibrin deposition.

Further evidence indicates that toxemia may be a primary trophoblast-related disorder involving fibrin deposition in the placenta and placental vasoconstriction with uteroplacental ischemia. Elegant studies using dogs have demonstrated that the placenta is the source of the signal for maternal hypertension (66, 67). If a clamp is placed on the aorta below the renal arteries in a nonpregnant dog, hypertension does not occur. However, if a clamp is placed on the aorta below the renal arteries of a *pregnant* dog, hypertension occurs. If the pregnant uterus is then removed, it is impossible to induce hypertension. It is the placenta, not the uterus, that leads to the hypertension, because women with abdominal pregnancies can also develop toxemia (68). Likewise, the placenta and not the fetus is the source because toxemia has been reported in patients with hydatidiform moles (4).

Treatment

Primary prevention is the first step in treating toxemia of pregnancy. Close monitoring of blood pressure, weight gain, and renal function is important. Close attention should be paid to patients at risk, including those with a family history of toxemia, a prior occurrence of the disease, the very young, and older women. Nonmedical therapies include restriction of activity and salt intake. Generally, in the presence of toxemia, hospitalization is indicated.

For specific antihypertensive treatment in patients with either toxemia or hypertension of pregnancy, concern previously existed that reducing arterial blood pressure with drugs would compromise uteroplacental blood flow. This concern has been found to be without scientific foundation; measurements of uterine blood flow in toxemic women have demonstrated an increase in flow with antihypertensive treatment (69). Excellent clinical studies have shown that treatment of hypertension decreases risk to the fetus (70, 71). However, there is no specific firm consensus on a standard antihypertensive approach to hypertension in pregnancy. Proposed pharmacologic treatments include antiplatelet agents as well as more conventional antihypertensive agents. The pros and cons of aspirin and of each class of antihypertensive drug will therefore be reviewed here.

The role of antiplatelet agents in toxemia is controversial. On the negative side, it was earlier stated that administration of prostaglandin inhibitors to normotensive pregnant women in their last trimester increased their sensitivity to angiotensin (9). On the other hand, it is possible that antiplatelet agents may prevent platelet thrombosis and progressive maternal-placental endothelial damage when used in the appropriate dosage. Use of aspirin in doses above 80 mg inhibits both thromboxane and prostacyclin. In contrast, aspirin in low doses reduces thromboxane synthesis without impairing prostacyclin production (72).

A randomized, placebo-controlled, double-blind trial of low-dose aspirin in primigravida women who were found to have an increased pressor response to infused angiotensin at 28 weeks gestation was performed by Wallenberg et al (73). Forty-six women with abnormal responses to angiotensin were randomized to groups that received either aspirin (60 mg/day) or placebo. All subsequent cases of preeclampsia occurred in the placebo group. There were no premature deliveries in the treated group. The incidence of small-for-gestational-age infants was 19% versus 39% in the treated and placebo groups, respectively. No maternal hemorrhagic complications occurred. The authors concluded that low-dose aspirin begun at 28 weeks may prevent toxemia in primigravida patients who are predisposed to it.

Concerns about aspirin administration during pregnancy include potential risks for congenital anomalies, neonatal bleeding, and ductal closure. Several studies have suggested that aspirin use may be associated with an increased occurrence of coarctation of the aorta (74), conotruncal anomalies (74), aortic stenosis (75), and hypoplastic left heart syndrome (75). However, the net overall increase in risk for congenital heart disease rises from only 0.2 to 0.4%. This risk can be avoided simply by deferring aspirin use until after organogenesis is completed.

There have been several reports of instances of neonatal cerebral hemorrhage, petechiae, hematuria, and subconjunctival hemorrhage in infants of mothers ingesting aspirin (76). However, there have not been sufficient randomized trials to establish whether these risks are significantly increased with maternal aspirin use. This issue merits further study.

Concern about aspirin use causing ductal closure has been expressed in isolated case reports (77). Several animal studies have shown that administration of cyclooxygenase inhibitors in late pregnancy causes ductal constriction (77–79). A study utilizing fetal echocardiography in humans demonstrated that use of indomethacin was associated with transient ductal constriction (80). However, in several controlled trials utilizing antiprostaglandin agents for preterm labor management, ductal closure was not a problem clinically (81–83).

Dietary manipulation that includes increases in the intake of eicosapentaenoic acid has been proposed. This group of fatty acids competes with arachidonic acid as a substrate for the cyclooxygenase enzyme, leading to a different set of products. One of these is PGI_3, which has platelet antiaggregatory activity that adds to the effect of PGI_2. As might be expected, the incidence of toxemia is extremely low in Greenland Eskimos, less than 1% (82). Therefore, dietary supplementation with cod liver oil might be a reasonable, though not highly palatable, alternative to aspirin (83).

It was previously felt that diuretics could potentially exacerbate volume depletion in toxemia. However, a review of nine randomized trials involving 11,000 women concluded that diuretics decreased the incidence of toxemia (87). Furthermore, the incidence of stillbirth was reduced by one-third in the diuretic-treated women compared with controls, and there was no increase in perinatal mortality. Thiazides reduced blood pressure by mechanisms other than pure natriuresis. Both thiazides and furosemide have been shown to increase PGI_2 synthesis.

Beta-adrenergic blocking drugs have been shown to be effective in treating hypertension and toxemia during pregnancy. Prior concerns that these drugs might induce premature labor by stimulating uterine β_2-receptors have proved groundless (86). A study using oxprenolol showed that fetal growth and development were superior with oxprenolol compared with methyldopa (88). Labetalol, a combined α- and β-blocker with an α-to-β antagonism ratio of 1:4, is considered by some to be the drug of choice for acute treatment of hypertension in toxemia (89). The usual dose for severe hypertension is 20 mg intravenously given over 2 minutes, followed, if necessary, by 40- or 80-mg doses at 10-minute intervals up to a total dose of 300 mg. Alternatively, a continuous infusion of labetalol can be administered, giving a total of 50 to 300 mg at a rate of 2 mg/minute.

Methyldopa is a central adrenergic antagonist that has been commonly used during pregnancy. Late follow-up studies of children born of mothers who used methyldopa during pregnancy have revealed normal physical and mental development (90). The relatively slow 4- to 6-hour onset of intravenous methyldopa as well as the somnolence it causes and its relative ineffectiveness have caused methyldopa to be replaced often by the β-adrenergic blockers.

Clonidine is another central adrenergic antagonist that activates central presynaptic α_2-receptors. Clonidine has been used in pregnancy both in women with toxemia and in those with essential hypertension. It is effective and well tolerated but is generally recommended only for more severe cases of hypertension. The drug has not been reported to compromise maternal or fetal well-being. The most common side effects are sedation and rebound hypertension if the drug is suddenly discontinued (91).

The major vasodilators that have been used in pregnancy include hydralazine, diazoxide, nitroprusside, and magnesium sulfate. Magnesium sulfate and hydralazine increase PGI_2 synthesis. Although magnesium sulfate has been used extensively in treatment of toxemia in the past, it has only transient, mild antihypertensive effects achieved by causing smooth muscle relaxation and inhibiting acetylcholine release from the sympathetic ganglia. Magnesium sulfate can cause myocardial and myometrial depression and has a narrow toxic-therapeutic window. There are more potent, safer vasodilators currently available for use in hypertension in pregnancy with or without toxemia.

Hydralazine is a vasodilator that acts directly on vascular smooth muscle, reducing peripheral vascular resistance and leading to a compensatory increase in heart rate. Side effects include tachycardia, tremor, headache, flushing, and nausea. Occasionally a lupuslike syndrome is seen with higher doses (200 to 300 mg/day), but occurrence of this syndrome during pregnancy is reportedly rare (92). Hydralazine has been widely used in hypertensive pregnancies, orally or parenterally. Often concomitant β-blockers are helpful in treating the reflex tachycardia that occurs with hydralazine use. Hydralazine crosses the placenta and also is excreted in breast milk in small amounts (93). The usual oral dose of hydralazine is 10 mg four times a day for 2 to 4 days, followed by titration upward if needed to 25 mg four times a day for 1 week, followed by 50 mg four times a day thereafter if the blood pressure still remains elevated. Serum levels are higher in patients with a slow acetylation rate; these patients therefore require lower doses of hydralazine.

Prazosin is a peripherally acting selective α_1-antagonist vasodilator. This drug reduces both arterial and venous vascular resistance. As a result, venous pooling with postural hypotension is a potential side effect that has a peculiar effect of occasional syncope following the first dose. This drug has been shown to be useful in gestational hypertension (94), but it must be used with caution owing to the hypotensive effect. The alpha blockade can possibly affect uterine labor. Another side effect of this drug is tachyphylaxis. In general, there are other effective vasodilators, discussed earlier, that merit use during pregnancy.

Nitroprusside, a potent vasodilator that acts on smooth muscle, is often used in hypertensive emergencies in *nonpregnant* patients. However, studies in pregnant ewes have demonstrated accumulation of cyanide in the fetus (95). This threat has limited the use of nitroprusside in patients with hypertension in pregnancy. Diazoxide is a potent intravenous arteriolar vasodilator that can be used effectively in 30- to 50-mg boluses over 5 to 15 minutes or until blood pressure falls to a safe range in pregnant women with severe hypertension. This drug may cause cessation of labor in 50% of cases owing to smooth muscle relaxation. Oxytocic agents can be used if needed to reinitiate labor when appropriate.

Calcium channel blockers are another class of antihypertensive agents. These drugs inhibit calcium ion influx, leading to decreased contractility, vasodilation, and slowing of atrioventricular nodal conduction. Nifedipine is an effective antihypertensive agent, but it has been shown to be teratogenic in rats when given in doses 30 times the maximum recommended human dose. There are no controlled studies of its use in human pregnancy. However, in the treatment of acute hypertension in patients with toxemia, it has reportedly been effective (96). Calcium channel blockers have been reported to improve placental and renal perfusion (96). They also have been shown to decrease levels of thromboxane and to reverse the thrombocytopenia of preeclampsia, portending useful roles in the treatment of toxemia (96, 97). Like vasodilators, calcium channel blockers may cause cessation of labor.

The last class of antihypertensives to be mentioned is the angiotensin converting-enzyme inhibitors. Although no teratogenic effects have been reported in animal studies, these drugs do lower uterine blood flow and reduce fetal survival in gravid rabbits, probably due to decreased uterine prostacyclin synthesis (98). In reports of the use of these drugs in pregnancy, there are isolated instances of miscarriage, stillbirth, patent ductus arteriosus, and acute fetal renal failure (99). Because angiotensin sensitivity is a suspected mechanism in toxemia, it is theoretically likely that angiotensin converting-enzyme inhibitors would be effective antihypertensive agents in this setting. However, the aforementioned side effects have precluded their extensive study and use in toxemic women. Therefore, at this time, because other classes of antihypertensive drugs are available, this class should be avoided in the treatment of hypertension and toxemia during pregnancy.

Despite all of these therapies for toxemia and hypertension, the definitive cure for toxemia of pregnancy is delivery of the fetus. Advances in neonatology in recent years may allow this option to be used earlier in cases of complex or fulminant toxemia. The rapidity with which toxemia resolves upon delivery supports the earlier described direct link to the placenta or fetus and gravid reproductive organs.

SYSTEMIC HYPERTENSION DURING PREGNANCY

Other hypertensive disorders during pregnancy besides toxemia also pose significant risks to the mother and fetus. Specific risks to the fetus caused by hypertension include intrauterine death, intrauterine growth retardation, placental insufficiency or abruption, and premature delivery (100). Risks to the hypertensive pregnant woman herself include left ventricular failure, cerebral hemorrhage, and predisposition to toxemia.

There is a lack of uniformity in the classification of types of hypertensive disorders during pregnancy. However, one useful classification is as follows: (1) chronic hypertension of any cause (blood pressure above 140/90 mm Hg in the first trimester), (2) pregnancy-induced hypertension (an increase in systolic blood pressure by 30 mm Hg above either prepregnancy level or first trimester values and a diastolic increase of 15 mm Hg), (3) preeclampsia, (4) eclampsia (both of which were discussed earlier in the section on toxemia), (5) chronic hypertension with superimposed toxemia, and (6) late or "transient" hypertension (101). Preciseness of classification is often difficult. Sometimes a patient may have chronic hypertension that was not detected previously if she had had no regular physician visits prior to pregnancy. The normal physiologic changes in peripheral vascular resistance that occur during pregnancy may confuse the picture further. The physiologic decrease in vascular resistance and blood pressure that occurs during the first half of pregnancy may mask previous chronic hypertension. When the blood pressure rises later in pregnancy to its previous levels, the patient may be misdiagnosed as having toxemia rather than chronic hypertension, especially if there is edema, which occurs commonly even in normal pregnancy in up to 80% of women.

Pathophysiology

It is possible that some types of "nontoxemic" hypertension that arise during pregnancy only, in the absence of preexisting or chronic hypertension, may overlap in etiology with full-blown toxemia. These types of hypertension arising only during pregnancy may possibly represent milder manifestations of the pathophysiology induced by the previously discussed alterations in angiotensin and prostaglandin balance seen in toxemia.

With regard to chronic or preexisting hypertension, few renal functional studies of essential hypertension have been performed in human pregnancy. However, there have been elegant animal studies in this area. Baylis and Reckelhoff investigated the renal hemodynamics associated with pregnancy in spontaneously hypertensive rats using micropuncture single-nephron studies (102). Their work showed that in normotensive pregnant rats, glomerular filtration rate (GFR) rises owing to increases in plasma flow, whereas glomerular capillary blood pressure remains unchanged owing to parallel reductions in preglomerular and efferent arteriolar resistance. Surprisingly, in spontaneously hypertensive rats that have undergone repeated pregnancies, no renal impairment is found. Pregnancy was felt to have an antihypertensive effect in most rat models of hypertension for reasons that are not clear.

Studies on the renal hemodynamic response in pregnant women with essential hypertension are scanty and contradictory. Lindheimer et al. reported high inulin clearances in seven pregnant women with essential hypertension, suggesting a gestational increase in GFR (103). In contrast, Sarles et al. reported low GFR and renal plasma flow in pregnant women with essential hypertension (104). It is clear that more studies on hypertension in pregnancy are needed.

Nisell et al. studied β_2-adrenoreceptors on lymphocytes of healthy nonpregnant women, healthy pregnant women, and women with hypertension during pregnancy (105). The healthy pregnant women had significantly fewer β_2-receptor–binding sites than the pregnant women (47.1 ± 5.6 vs. 73.6 ± 10.5 fentamoles × mg^{-1} protein), and the hypertensive pregnant women displayed intermediate values. Adrenaline-induced rises in plasma cyclic AMP also tended to be lower in normal pregnancy. The authors concluded that a reduction of β_2-receptor function occurs during normal pregnancy but is less pronounced in hypertensive pregnant women. They also noted an altered relationship between β_2-vasodilator responses and densities of β_2-receptors on lymphocytes during pregnancy. How these data fit into the puzzle of hypertension during pregnancy merits further investigation; the results may have therapeutic implications in terms of the specific role of beta antagonists in the treatment of hypertension during pregnancy.

Treatment

The cornerstones of treatment of hypertension during pregnancy include salt restriction, close follow-up by an obstetrician and an internist, and pharmacologic treatment if the above measures alone fail to normalize blood pressure. The aims of antihypertensive therapy in hypertension during pregnancy are twofold: to attain normotension in the mother to avoid morbidity and to protect the second patient, the fetus, from the effects of maternal hypertension as well as from the potential side effects of the antihypertensive drug therapy. The use of antihypertensive agents during pregnancy was previously discussed in the section on toxemia and does not differ in uncomplicated hypertension.

For women whose hypertension is "pregnancy-induced," delivery of the fetus will provide the cure. For women with preexisting chronic hypertension that is sometimes first discovered during pregnancy, regular long-term medical follow-up and treatment are warranted long beyond pregnancy to avoid the later complications of hypertension, namely, atherosclerotic cardiovascular disease.

PERIPARTUM CARDIOMYOPATHY

Peripartum cardiomyopathy (PPCM) is a dilated cardiomyopathy that occurs in the last month of pregnancy or within the first 5 months after delivery in the absence of any other preexisting heart disease. This rare disorder represents less than 1% of all cardiac problems associated with pregnancy in the United States and has a frequency of 1/1300 to 1/4000 deliveries in this country (106). Peripartum cardiomyopathy has been observed with increased frequency in older women, in twin pregnancies, in toxemia, and with multiparity (107). In some forms of familial dilated cardiomyopathy, patients present first with heart failure in the peripartum period (108).

Clinical Features

The symptoms of peripartum cardiomyopathy are those of congestive heart failure. A literature survey by Veille of 329 cases of peripartum cardiomyopathy found that dyspnea was the most common symptom in 91%, cough in 80%, and orthopnea in 65%; palpitations, hemoptysis, chest pain, and abdominal pain also occurred in decreasing order of frequency (107). Veille reported that the most frequent physical signs in PPCM were cardiomegaly (95%), tachycardia (84%), and pulmonary rales (72%), with hypertension and dysrhythmias occurring less frequently. Emboli, either pulmonary or systemic, can complicate PPCM. Walsh et al. reported that thromboembolic phenomena can occur in up to 53% of PPCM cases (109, 110).

The electrocardiogram is often abnormal in this condition, with findings including atrial enlargement or ventricular hypertrophy, ST-T segment alterations, bundle branch block, arrhythmias, and other nonspecific changes. On catheterization, right and left filling pressures are elevated, although severe pulmonary hypertension is unusual. The cardiac output is generally depressed. Coronary arteriography is typically normal. Echocardiography reveals diminished left ventricular function, usually global, although occasionally regional asynergy is seen. Mural thrombi and regurgitant atrioventricular valves secondary to annular dilatation may also be seen on echocardiography.

Pathologically, the features of PPCM are the same as those seen in idiopathic dilated cardiomyopathy. Grossly, there is four-chamber dilatation and often mural thrombi, but the coronary arteries are usually normal. Microscopically, the findings are nonspecific and can include myocyte hypertrophy, degeneration, fibrosis, or necrosis. Sometimes inflammation or frank myocarditis is found, the potential significance of which is discussed below (106, 111–113).

Pathophysiology

Peripartum cardiomyopathy is diagnosed only after all forms of preexisting heart disease have been excluded. In a review of 28 women diagnosed with peripartum cardiomyopathy at Parkland Memorial Hospital between 1973 and 1984, 21 were eventually found to have other underlying cardiovascular abnormalities that explained their congestive heart failure (114). Silent mitral stenosis was found in four women by echocardiography or autopsy; aortic stenosis was also found in one. Fourteen women had congestive heart failure explicable on the basis of the increased physiologic demands of pregnancy in concert with a complication of pregnancy (e.g., toxemia), with underlying heart disease, such as hypertensive heart disease. Ultimately, only 7 of 28 (25%) of the women in this study were found to have peripartum cardiomyopathy without other underlying causes of heart failure. Although controversy exists about whether PPCM is a distinct entity, it does have some unique features—specifically, the temporal relationship to late pregnancy as well as the tendency to recur with future pregnancies.

There is an unusual form of peripartum cardiomyopathy found in Nigeria that is probably unrelated to PPCM in the United States. The Nigerian form of PPCM is probably secondary to social rituals practiced there. In Nigeria it is customary for pregnant women to lie for many hours on a baked-mud bed over a fire and eat large quantities of a dried salt known as kanwa (106, 111). As expected, this custom can lead to volume overload and ventricular dilatation without any actual decrease in ventricular contractility. This is different from the peripartum cardiomyopathy seen in the United States, where significant left ventricular impairment is generally seen. It is interesting to note that a subset of women with PPCM has also been described in Brazil, where some women with PPCM have high-output failure with elevated cardiac indices (115). In this report, there were no obvious cultural or medical reasons such as hyperthyroidism, anemia, or thiamine deficiency that could explain the high-output failure in this subset.

A number of explanations for PPCM have been postulated previously, all without a proven basis. These have included nutritional factors, small vessel intramural arterial heart disease, hormonal changes, fetal antigens, and drug hypersensitivity (106, 111, 114).

The most intriguing explanation of the genesis of PPCM centers upon myocarditis, either viral or immune. A study from Johns Hopkins Hospital described endomyocardial biopsy findings in 18 consecutive women with peripartum cardiomyopathy. Fourteen of the eighteen patients (78%) had myocarditis on biopsy (116). Biopsies were performed 6 to 195 days after delivery, with a mean biopsy time of 69 days postpartum. Melvin et al. had previously described three consecutive women with PPCM, all of whom revealed myocarditis on biopsy (117). Sanderson reported "healing myocarditis" on endomyocardial biopsy in 5 of 11 women with PPCM in Africa (111). O'Connell reported an incidence of myocarditis of 29% on endomyocardial biopsy in 14 women with PPCM (112).

These differences in the reported incidence of myocarditis in PPCM may stem either from differences in myocardial biopsy interpretation or from the timing of the biopsy. Biopsy interpretation in the Johns Hopkins study, for example, utilized the Dallas criteria, whereby active myocarditis is diagnosed when there is mononuclear cell infiltration associated with myocyte necrosis or degeneration without evidence of marked fibrosis or cellular hypertrophy (116, 118). Borderline myocarditis using the Dallas criteria is classified as the presence of a significant mononuclear cell infiltrate without clear-cut myocyte necrosis. However, in many instances, lymphocytic infiltration of the myocardium with or without myocyte degeneration can be a nonspecific finding associated with catecholamine release, coronary reperfusion, and use of certain medications (119–121).

Timing of an endomyocardial biopsy in relation to the onset of congestive heart failure may also account for variations in the diagnosis of myocarditis or in the intensity of inflammatory response. It is likely that myocarditis behaves like other human inflammatory responses in that the mononuclear cell infiltrate gradually resolves over time and the amount of fibrosis that subsequently ensues varies (118). The extent to which the inflammation resolves and the rate at which this occurs spontaneously are extremely variable. O'Connell and Melvin described a high incidence of myocarditis on biopsy in patients with PPCM when the biopsy was performed within 1 week of the onset of heart failure (112, 117). This suggests that the earlier the myocardial biopsy is performed, the higher the likelihood of diagnosing myocarditis, leading to the finding of a higher frequency of this diagnosis. Midei et al. found that myocarditis may be present on biopsy in patients with PPCM on average 1 month after the onset of symptoms, and occasionally as long as 195 days postpartum (116).

The two leading suspected causes of myocarditis in PPCM are viral and immune factors. Immunologic studies in humans have shown that suppressor cell activity during pregnancy is enhanced, which might increase the susceptibility to viral infections. Studies utilizing mice have suggested that susceptibility to myocarditis is enhanced in pregnant mice exposed to certain viruses, including coxsackie viruses. It has been shown that pregnant mice infected with encephalomyocarditis virus exhibit greater natural killer cell activity and myocardial damage than do nonpregnant infected mice (122). It has further been demonstrated that in the presence of an increased cardiac workload, virus-induced lesions in the heart multiply (123, 124). Subsequently it has been theorized that PPCM results from the increased susceptibility to the stresses of pregnancy in some women, leading to the development of viral myocarditis. Stamler et al. described several cases of PPCM in which they thought that increased cardiac stresses during pregnancy—namely, sepsis, coagulopathy, anemia, or strenuous overexertion—acted synergistically with the stress of pregnancy to precipitate PPCM in susceptible women (125). In the murine animal model, sustained strenuous exercise combined with coxsackie virus infection has been shown to depress immune function and lead to increased titers of myocardial virus and increased mortality (126). Despite the suspicions that viruses may play a role in predisposing to PPCM, they have not been isolated in the myocardium in this disease. Likewise, plasma viral titers for viruses such as coxsackie virus and echo virus have not been found in increased frequency in women with PPCM compared with healthy breast-feeding women (127).

Therefore, viruses may play an indirect rather than a direct role in PPCM. Postviral myocarditis is probably autoimmune in origin (128). Hormonal alterations in pregnancy due to progesterone acting on T-cell expression may predispose certain pregnant women to myocarditis. Additional insight into the immunology of PPCM was provided by Sanderson, who reported an increased proportion of helper to inducer T-cells ($T_4:T_8$) by monoclonal antibody techniques in patients with dilated cardiomyopathy. Two of the patients in this group had peripartum cardiomyopathy (111). Some investigators have reported enhanced maternal suppressor cell activity in human pregnancy (123). Others have suggested that the passage of fetal suppressor cells to the mother during the third trimester results in a rebound phenomenon 2 to 6 months postpartum, a common time of occurrence of peripartum cardiomyopathy (129).

The above data support a possible role of immune, cell-mediated factors in myocarditis, especially with regard to peripartum cardiomyopathy. On the other hand, the humoral aspect of immunity has not been shown to play a major role. Levels of serum immunoglobulins and heart muscle autoantibodies were not found to be significantly different in women with peripartum cardiomyopathy and healthy breast-feeding controls (130).

Treatment

In the United States, the mortality associated with peripartum cardiomyopathy is high, ranging from 25–50% (106). In one study, the mortality rate was highest in the first year at 11% and declined therafter (131). In this study, 52% of the women with PPCM improved without further recurrences of heart failure. Heart failure recurred after subsequent pregnancies in 27%, and 13% had recurrent heart failure unrelated to pregnancy (131). Progression to dilated cardiomyopathy in this cohort occurred in 9%. Cardiac deaths were most common in those with recurrent or progressive heart failure (131). Causes of death included refractory heart failure, arrhythmias, and thromboembolic phenomena. Normalization of cardiac size within a year is one of the most favorable predictors of long-term outcome. The prognosis is poor in patients with PPCM when significant cardiomegaly persists longer than 6 months and in patients with low left ventricular ejection fractions (112, 132). In one study, patients with PPCM who had a poor outcome (death, need for transplantation, or persistent functional class III or class IV) had significantly greater left ventricular end-diastolic diameters compared with women who had a good outcome (69 ± 6 mm vs. 58 ± 7 mm, p < .005) (133).

When the heart remains dilated, the prognosis is therefore poor. Subsequent pregnancies are strongly discouraged in this group of patients. However, in those whose ventricular function returns to normal, it has been reported that further pregnancy can be undertaken cautiously with anticipation of a normal fetal outcome and a low risk of recurrent left ventricular dysfunction (134). It is possible, however, that even in women whose heart size becomes normal, subclinical ventricular impairment may persist. Hadjimiltiades et al. reported a woman who "recovered" from peripartum heart failure but at 10 months postpartum still exhibited a decrease in ventricular functional reserve during bicycle radionuclide stress ventriculography (135).

The medical management of heart failure associated with PPCM is the same as that for heart failure in general, including salt restriction, diuretics, digoxin, vasodilators, and antiarrhythmics when appropriate. The judicious use of diuretics is reasonable in the face of volume overload. As discussed earlier, diuretics are no longer viewed as deleterious in pregnancy when they are clinically indicated.

Digitalis is an inotrope commonly used in patients with heart failure and is safe to use in pregnant patients in therapeutic range. The "final" word on the efficacy of digitalis in heart failure, in general, remains unanswered and is the aim of an ongoing multicenter collaborative trial being conducted by the National Institutes of Health. Digitalis is useful for controlling ventricular rate in women with PPCM with atrial fibrillation.

Afterload reduction can be accomplished in these patients with hydralazine, a vasodilator. Its main side effect is reflex tachycardia, which unfortunately can increase myocardial oxygen consumption. Captopril, an angiotensin converting-enzyme inhibitor, is an effective afterload-reducing agent. However, it has been associated with reduced fetal survival in pregnant rabbits and ewes (98, 99). Therefore, this is not a first-line drug of choice in pregnancy.

Bed rest has been advocated in the past, but no controlled studies have proved its efficacy (136). If anticoagulation is needed for those at highest risk of embolization, such as those with mural thrombi, there may be some increased risk to the fetus. However, heparin is the preferred anticoagulant in the third trimester because it does not cross the placenta and has a short half-life.

Women with peripartum cardiomyopathy should undergo serial echocardiographic evaluation throughout the antepartum and postpartum periods to monitor left ventricular function. Intrapartum, cardiac function should be monitored, if indicated, with a pulmonary arterial catheter in any high-risk patient to optimize hemodynamics during the increased stress of delivery. Optimal care throughout delivery requires a multidisciplinary approach involving an obstetrician, cardiologist, anesthesiologist, and pediatrician. Often vaginal delivery is possible with careful medical management.

In some patients with PPCM, decompensation may occur despite the above measures, requiring more intense therapy with parenteral inotropes. Dopamine causes predominantly β_1 effects on the heart when used at 2 to 10 µg/kg/minute, producing improvement in myocardial contractility, stroke volume, and cardiac output. Another effective inotrope with a lesser tendency toward tachycardia is dobutamine. This direct-acting myocardial β_1 stimulant increases cardiac output in dosages ranging from 2 to 10 µg/kg/minute, and occasionally it is used in doses of up to 20 µg/kg/minute.

Aside from the pharmacologic management of heart failure in PPCM, a word must be said about treatment of the possible underlying cause of cardiomyopathy. As discussed earlier, exciting data are accumulating that myocarditis is prominent in women with PPCM and may be causative. In the Johns Hopkins prospective study myocarditis was found by endomyocardial biopsy in 14 of 18 (78%) women with PPCM (116). Of those 14, 10 were treated with immunosuppressive therapy consisting of oral prednisone (1 mg/kg/day) and azathioprine (1.5 mg/kg/day) for 6 to 8 weeks. Nine of the ten treated women with myocarditis showed subjective and objective improvement on echocardiography and nuclear ventriculography. There was resolution or substantial improvement of myocarditis on follow-up endomyocardial biopsies in the ten treated women. Of note, four patients with myocarditis not treated with immunosuppressives also improved. However, this study does suggest that immunosuppressive treatment in patients with myocarditis and persistent left ventricular dysfunction may improve left ventricular function and, therefore, the prognosis. Others have reported similar results in the past in small series; Melvin et al. reported a 100% response rate to immunosuppressive treatment in three patients with PPCM (117). There were no serious complications with immunosuppression in the Johns Hopkins study, nor was there any apparent rebound deterioration of left ventricular function following discontinuation of immunosuppression. Preliminary evidence therefore supports early endomyocardial biopsy in patients with PPCM as well as consideration of immunosuppressive treatment in those whose left ventricular function fails to normalize after 1 week. Further study of the role played by myocarditis in peripartum cardiomyopathy as well as in idiopathic dilated cardiomyopathy remains a most intriguing area. A prospective double-blind national cooperative trial of myocarditis and its treatment in patients with peripartum cardiomyopathy is warranted.

For the unfortunate woman with peripartum cardiomyopathy who continues to have refractory heart failure despite aggressive medical management, orthotopic cardiac transplantation remains an option in qualified patients. Current 1-year survival rates after heart transplantation are 80+%, with 5-year survivals of 70%. An ongoing problem in transplantation is the limited number of donors, but technology sometimes allows "bridging" of the critical patient with devices such as ventricular assist devices or artificial hearts until a donor is available. Hovsepian et al. reported successful use of a left ventricular assist device for 48 hours until a donor heart became available for a 20-year-old woman with PPCM who had cardiogenic shock (137). Another newer procedure available to patients with refractory symptoms of congestive cardiomyopathy is the latissimus dorsi cardiomyoplasty procedure, in which the left latissimus dorsi muscle is wrapped around the failing heart and then paced, gradually training the skeletal muscle to function as cardiac muscle and eventually augmenting cardiac performance after several months (138). This novel and still investigational procedure may become an option for women with severe refractory heart failure secondary to peripartum cardiomyopathy.

There are burgeoning areas of ongoing research in the treatment of heart failure, including the role of myocarditis and its treatment in peripartum cardiomyopathy and the growing number of options available to those with severe end-stage heart failure, including the sickest victims of PPCM. Answers to the many questions raised will help to brighten the outlook not only for the pregnant woman with peripartum cardiomyopathy but for all patients with heart failure as well.

PULMONARY HYPERTENSION IN PREGNANCY

Pulmonary hypertension during pregnancy may be due to preexisting heart disease such as congenital heart disease, to mitral stenosis, or to recurrent pulmonary emboli. Pulmonary hypertension may also exist without any underlying cause; in these instances, the disease is diagnosed as primary pulmonary hypertension. Primary pulmonary hypertension occurs most frequently in women (60–90%) of childbearing age, and therefore it is sometimes diagnosed first during pregnancy, which generally worsens the condition.

In general, pulmonary hypertension occurring during pregnancy carries a poor prognosis. In pulmonary hypertension secondary to congenital heart disease, Rosenberg et al. reported a 66% mortality in women with Eisenmenger's syndrome undergoing cesarean section (139). Others have reported a 30.3% maternal and a 28.3% perinatal mortality rate in pregnancies complicated by pulmonary hypertension secondary to Eisenmenger's syndrome (140). In a review of the literature on primary pulmonary hypertension in pregnancy, McCaffrey and Dunn noted a maternal mortality of nearly 40% in women with primary pulmonary hypertension in pregnancy, even when they were asymptomatic or only mildly symptomatic (141). For these reasons, pregnancy in women with pulmonary hypertension is strongly discouraged, and therapeutic abortion should be considered in those who are already pregnant.

Primary pulmonary hypertension has an average survival of 2 to 3 years, but some patients have survived more than 10 years (142). Adverse prognostic indicators include right ventricular failure, low cardiac index (<2 to 2.5 liters/minute/m^2), high right atrial pressure (>10 mm Hg), and elevated pulmonary vascular resistance (>1000 to 1500 dyne·second·cm^{-5}). Absolute pulmonary artery pressure is a poor prognostic indicator (143, 144).

Clinical Features

In primary pulmonary hypertension as well as in pulmonary hypertension due to a specific cause, onset is often insidious. Exertional dyspnea may be an early symptom that may over time progress to dyspnea at rest. As the disease advances, syncope occurs and is thought to be due to acute right heart decompensation with a fall in cardiac output. Later, symptoms of right heart failure ensue.

Physical examination may disclose findings of right heart failure. A parasternal heave, augmented pulmonic second heart sound, right ventricular gallop, and murmurs of tricuspid and pulmonic insufficiency may be noted on cardiac examination. Hepatomegaly, liver pulsation, neck vein distention, and peripheral edema may be seen (145).

Right heart catheterization reveals pulmonary artery pressures that are two to four times above normal, often equalling or exceeding the systemic blood pressure, and there is a concomitant increase in pulmonary vascular resistance. The pulmonary capillary wedge pressure is normal in primary pulmonary hypertension, and cardiac output may be decreased owing either to diminished blood flow to the left ventricle due to right ventricular failure, or to bulging of the septum due to a dilated right ventricle with compromise of left ventricular cavity filling (146).

Pathophysiology

The pathophysiology of primary pulmonary hypertension involves a progression from increased right ventricular afterload to right ventricular hypertrophy and dilatation, and finally to right ventricular failure. The right ventricle hypertrophies in response to increased pulmonary vascular resistance to continue to generate adequate pressure for flow. Dilatation occurs, which augments preload and maintains cardiac output through the Frank-Starling mechanism (142, 147). Systemic hypotension or arrhythmias can compromise the demand-availability curve and precipitate possible frank ischemia (147, 148).

Cardiac output rises by 40% in pregnancy. During labor and delivery, large volume shifts occur that may be hazardous in patients with pulmonary hypertension. Labor, especially if painful, may increase the demands on cardiac output by a further 50–60%. Oxygen consumption rises by 20% during pregnancy and increases markedly with painful contractions by up to 63% (149, 150). During the first 3 to 4 days postpartum, cardiac output and pulmonary blood volume remain high. The noncompliant pulmonary vessels and reduced vascular bed are unable to accommodate this increased volume. In addition, in a woman with pulmonary hypertension the increased cardiovascular demands occurring during labor and delivery may increase pulmonary pressure sufficiently to precipitate acute right ventricular failure with severely diminished cardiac output and sudden death. In the review by McCaffrey and Dunn, seven of nine maternal deaths were sudden and involved hemodynamic collapse (141).

In primary pulmonary hypertension, the heart reveals right ventricular hypertrophy on postmortem examination with patent coronary arteries and atheroma of the large pulmonary arteries. The medium-sized pulmonary arteries exhibit intimal proliferation and medial hypertrophy. In the pulmonary arterioles, extensive and often obliterative intimal proliferation with "plexiform lesions" is seen; these are dilated endothelium-lined channels in arterioles that communicate with the adjacent venules (151). Thrombi are often present, possibly due to sluggish flow or recurrent emboli. The etiology of the pulmonary vascular disease in primary pulmonary hypertension is unknown. Anderson et al. have postulated that a primary abnormality may be a hyperactive, proliferating endothelium capable of synthesizing vasoactive substances, which in turn initiate spasm associated with pulmonary hypertension (151). Other investigators have theorized that in many cases, recurrent silent miliary pulmonary emboli are the initial events that lead secondarily to the vascular structural changes.

Why pulmonary hypertension during pregnancy has such a dismal prognosis is unknown. The high mortality suggests a deleterious effect of pregnancy. Even when factors that worsen pulmonary vascular resistance during the peripartum period (hypoxia, acidosis, increased intrathoracic pressure, hypothermia, increased catecholamines, and certain anesthetics) are minimized, there are still unexplained increases in pulmonary vascular resistance (152–154).

Amniotic fluid embolism has been suggested as a risk factor during delivery in women with pulmonary hypertension. However, histologic examination has failed to show features that could be interpreted as residue of amniotic embolism (155). Pulmonary arterial blood samples have also failed to reveal evidence suggestive of amniotic fluid embolism (156).

The most intriguing explanation for why pulmonary hypertension becomes worse with pregnancy is possible widespread thrombosis of the small vessels in the pulmonary arterial system in the postpartum period (153, 155). Conditions favoring this occurrence in pregnant women with pulmonary hypertension include a greatly reduced pulmonary vascular bed, diminished production of tissue plasminogen activator by pulmonary endothelium, and high levels of pregnancy-related plasminogen activator inhibitor at delivery. Newer and more sensitive radionuclide imaging modalities and hematologic assays may allow further investigation of the possible thrombotic etiology of pulmonary hypertension exacerbation in pregnancy. This could have major therapeutic implications in justifying a more aggressive antithrombotic approach in these extremely sick women.

Treatment

Women with primary pulmonary hypertension or pulmonary hypertension secondary to other causes should avoid pregnancy owing to the high mortality and apparent deleterious effect of pregnancy on the disease. Despite this recommendation, some women still undertake pregnancy of their own will owing to failed contraception or to unawareness of the underlying pulmonary hypertension.

The initial step in management of the pregnant woman with pulmonary hypertension is assessment of the severity of the pulmonary hypertension. Right ventricular failure is an ominous finding and mandates treatment as best possible once diagnosed (141). Serial echocardiography provides an estimate of pulmonary arterial pressure derived from Doppler-estimated right ventricular systolic pressure. Right atrial and ventricular size and function can also be followed by echocardiography (142). Pulmonary arterial catheterization provides measurements of right ventricular preload (right atrial pressure), cardiac output, and right ventricular afterload (pulmonary vascular resistance). There are some risks associated with right heart catheterization in this setting, with data indicating a 4% mortality (141, 144). Atropine, epinephrine, and a transvenous pacemaker should be available if needed for severe bradycardia during right heart catheter insertion. Insertion of the catheter may be hindered by tricuspid insufficiency, a large right ventricle, or low cardiac output. These difficulties of pulmonary artery catheterization, however, are outweighed by the value of the information gained.

According to the literature, the best maternal survival occurs with vaginal delivery, although there may be a selection bias because those undergoing cesarean section are possibly sicker. Cesarean section imposes increased risks of anesthesia, hemorrhage, uterine manipulation, potential for embolism, and sepsis (156, 157). If vaginal delivery is undertaken, however, facilities for cesarean section must be available if needed.

In terms of medical management during the antepartum period, consideration should be given to hospitalization around the twenty-eighth to thirtieth week of gestation to minimize cardiovascular demands. If right ventricular failure is present, activity restriction, digoxin, oxygen, and diuretics may be needed (142).

Use of oral calcium channel blockers in primary pulmonary hypertension has shown some encouraging results, although the responsiveness of the pulmonary vasculature of any given patient is variable. Nifedipine has been shown to cause selective pulmonary vasodilation in some patients, with a mean reduction in pulmonary artery pressure of 6 ± 5 mm Hg in those who respond to the drug (158). As previously discussed, the effect of calcium channel blockers in human pregnancy needs further investigation, but in the case of a pregnant woman with pulmonary hypertension, the potential benefit to the mother must be weighed against the potential risk to the fetus.

The use of anticoagulants is controversial, but it seems reasonable to give low dose heparin prophylaxis to women with low cardiac output at bed rest (142, 144). If future research strongly supports the theory of a thrombotic etiology for pregnancy-induced worsening of pulmonary hypertension, perhaps anticoagulation use should be more aggressive in these patients. Anticoagulants do carry an increased risk to the fetus, as discussed previously, and can also compromise anesthetic use by spinal or epidural blockade, necessitating their discontinuation far enough in advance of delivery to allow normalization of coagulation parameters.

During delivery, blood loss must be monitored and hypovolemia avoided because any decrease in venous return may cause a precipitous drop in cardiac output in the presence of a dilated, impaired right ventricle. Hemodynamic monitoring is essential during labor and delivery. Systemic hypotension should likewise be aggressively treated. Aortocaval compression and the Valsalva maneuver, which also compromise venous return, should be avoided.

Worsening of pulmonary vascular resistance or cardiac output during parturition and in the postpartum period may be improved by pulmonary vasodilators, inotropes, or cautious volume augmentation. Oxygen is the most potent pulmonary vasodilator and should always be utilized. Of the medications available, pulmonary vasodilators are the preferred option, but unfortunately not all women will be responsive. Because there is no currently available specific pulmonary pharmacologic vasodilator, systemic hypotension remains a limitation. Specific parenteral vasodilators include sodium nitroprusside, glyceryl trinitrate, and prostaglandins. Nitroprusside has been used successfully in this setting, but its limitations include systemic vasodilation and cyanide toxicity in the mother and fetus (143, 159). Glyceryl trinitrate is an effective pulmonary vasodilator that has lesser systemic effects as well as minimal effects on the fetus and uterine activity (160). For these reasons, it is the vasodilator of choice. Prostaglandins, PGE_1, and prostacyclin have been used in patients with primary pulmonary hypertension. However, in the pregnant woman, PGI_1 may cause increased uterine tone and fetal distress (161). Prostacyclin may cause systemic hypotension and also has mild uterine relaxant properties (162).

Inotropic support may improve right ventricular function in some instances, but the parenteral inotropes are not without limitations (163). Dopamine, at doses of less than 10 μg/kg/minute, causes some pulmonary vasoconstriction and has detrimental effects on uterine blood flow (150). Noradrenaline has been shown to be effective in animal studies in improving cardiac output during acute rises in pulmonary vascular resistance (163). Dobutamine and isoproterenol can potentially cause myocardial ischemia by producing systemic vasodilation with hypotension and increased myocardial oxygen consumption (142).

However, they produce pulmonary vasodilation and have minimal effects on the uterine vasculature (142).

In labor, natural onset is the preferred mode. Oxytocin has previously been reported to cause acute circulatory deterioration. It may cause systemic vasodilation, an acute rise in pulmonary vascular resistance, and a fall in cardiac output (164). Ergometrine and prostaglandin F_2 are similarly to be avoided owing to their pulmonary vasoconstrictive effects.

For anesthetic management, adequate analgesia is important because unrelieved pain leads to increased cardiopulmonary demands. Parenteral opioids are to be avoided owing to the risk of respiratory depression with resultant respiratory acidosis and pulmonary vasoconstriction. Epidural local anesthetics attenuate the pain response, but the risk of extensive sympathetic blockade with venodilation and hypotension resulting from decreased systemic vascular resistance exists (165, 166). Use of epidural combined fentanyl-bupivacaine has been reported during delivery in patients with pulmonary hypertension with hemodynamic stability (152). Successful use of intrathecal morphine in the first stage of labor has also been reported (167). Slow anesthetic induction has been advised to minimize the risk of tachycardia and hypertension. Fentanyl has been recommended as the sole anesthetic agent in patients with poor right ventricular function and relative hemodynamic stability because it has minimal effects on myocardial contractility and pulmonary vascular resistance (168). Pancuronium has been recommended as the relaxant of first choice because it avoids bradycardia and excessive hypotension (168). Isoflurane is the volatile agent of choice because it causes the least myocardial depression and has pulmonary vasodilatory properties (169).

In the rare woman with pulmonary hypertension who survives pregnancy and the postpartum period, the prognosis remains poor, with an average survival of 2 to 3 years (142). Future pregnancies are strongly discouraged, and sterilization should be considered. Single lung transplantation for primary pulmonary hypertension in some centers has yielded promising results. Interestingly, Cooper et al. have shown that the replacement of just *one* of the diseased lungs in patients with primary pulmonary hypertension leads to an immediate, marked improvement in pulmonary artery pressures and cardiac output. In their series, the mean pulmonary artery pressures in seven patients undergoing single lung transplantation for pulmonary hypertension fell from 92 ± 7 mm Hg preoperatively to 29 ± 6 mm Hg at 13 weeks postoperatively (170). Further animal and human research and technical improvements in single lung transplantation are needed, however, to circumvent its difficulties, namely, rejection, infection, and reperfusion injury. Nonetheless, these exciting results lend some hope to the desperately ill woman with pulmonary hypertension who is fortunate enough to survive pregnancy.

AORTIC DISSECTION IN PREGNANCY

Although aortic dissection is uncommon in women less than 40 years of age, pregnancy significantly increases the risk of this occurrence. In one study, 50% of all aortic dissections in women of childbearing age occurred with pregnancy (171). Pregnancy is a risk factor, therefore, for aortic dissection. Other risk factors associated with pregnancy-related dissection include advanced age, hypertension, multiparity, Marfan's syndrome, trauma, coarctation of the aorta, and bicuspid aortic valves (172). Aortic dissection during pregnancy has been described, not surprisingly, in Ehlers-Danlos type IV syndrome (173). However, in 63% of dissections during pregnancy, none of these predisposing factors were found (172). Arterial dissection in sites other than the aorta also occur more frequently in pregnancy. Coronary artery dissection leading to myocardial infarction or sudden death has been described in the peripartum period (174).

Clinical Features

Aortic dissection during pregnancy occurs most commonly in the third trimester, when cardiac output and blood volume are maximal, although dissection can occur in any stage of pregnancy or in the postpartum period. One of the most common symptoms of aortic dissection is chest and back pain, often described as "tearing" pain in the interscapular region. Acute heart failure or shock may ensue if the dissection involves the aortic root and leads to acute aortic insufficiency or tamponade. Associated symptoms depend on which arterial trees are involved in the dissection. Stroke, myocardial infarction, paralysis, limb ischemia, and visceral ischemia are all potential complications, depending on the extent of the dissection. The associated physical findings depend on the organs compromised by the dissection. Pulse asymmetry and an aortic insufficiency murmur (if the aortic root is involved) are among the more common findings with aortic dissection. The chest roentgenogram may reveal widening of the superior mediastinum. Echocardiography, CT scanning, or magnetic resonance imaging often reveals an intimal flap with a false lumen. Transesophageal echocardiography has proved extremely useful in recent years in diagnosing aortic dissection.

Pathophysiology

The cause of aortic dissection in pregnancy is unclear. The most attractive theories involve the hemodynamic and hormonal changes of pregnancy as inciting causes. During pregnancy, stroke volume and cardiac output increase. Compression of the inferior vena cava by the gravid uterus causes further changes in hemodynamics. Hypertension, if it accompanies the pregnancy, is a known risk factor for dissection. The mechanism by which hypertension predisposes to dissection is unknown because the process has been difficult to reproduce in the animal model. It is theorized that increased arterial pressure may lead to tears in weakened areas of the media. Hypertension is also felt to accelerate the age-related degenerative process in arteries.

Although Marfan's syndrome is a risk factor for aortic dissection in pregnancy, in 63% of dissections no Marfan's syndrome or other predisposing causes are found (172). However, with specific regard to Marfan's syndrome in pregnancy, Pyeritz reported that 20 of 32 pregnant women with Marfan's syndrome either died or had aortic dissection in the peripartum period (175). The author noted that aortic disease that was present prior to pregnancy in women with Marfan's syndrome was a major risk factor for maternal mortality. He observed that aortic root diameters of less than 4 cm on echocardiography carried a lower risk of dissection. Careful echocardiographic assessment of the aortic root is therefore merited in women with Marfan's syndrome who anticipate pregnancy (176). Avoidance of pregnancy in these women should be considered owing to the dire consequences of potential dissection.

The pathologic diagnosis of cystic medial necrosis has frequently been reported in patients with aortic dissection. However, the pathologic criteria for this diagnosis are variable. Generally, the media is the site of major disruption in the vessel, in which separation of the outer third of the arterial wall occurs; this is associated with intramural hemorrhage and fibrin deposition. The elastic fibers may also be fragmented.

Biochemical alterations are thought to occur in connective tissue during pregnancy owing to alterations in hormonal levels, especially elevated estrogen concentrations. When norethynodrel plus mestranol (Enovid) was administered to pregnant rabbits, changes in the animals' vasculature were observed (177). Specifically, degenerative changes in the aorta occurred, with fragmentation of the reticulum, reduction in collagen, decrease in acid mucopolysaccharides, and loss of resilience in the elastic fibers of the aorta. These histologic changes appear to be hormonally related and may be responsible in part for why pregnancy predisposes to aortic dissection. In other settings involving aortic dissection or rupture, other hormones have been implicated. For example, in patients with preexisting abdominal aortic aneurysm undergoing cardiac surgery, an increased risk of abdominal aortic aneurysm rupture has been noted; this has been thought to be due to increased amounts of elastin induced by other surgical procedures. Perhaps this hormone and others are intertwined with the alterations in reproductive hormones that occur during pregnancy. Further investigation of these hormonal modulators may provide important insights into the etiology of aortic dissection both in pregnancy and in arterial catastrophes in both genders.

Treatment

The earliest step in treatment of aortic dissection is recognizing the diagnosis in the pregnant patient. When dissection in pregnancy is discovered, immediate delivery by cesarean section is generally indicated if the fetus will survive. If the fetus is too premature for delivery, surgical repair may be attempted. In general, however, the fetus has a poor tolerance of cardiopulmonary bypass and has a high mortality, particularly during surgeries requiring a longer time on bypass (178).

Management of aortic dissection during pregnancy is otherwise similar to its management in the nonpregnant patient. The blood pressure must be lowered. The usual antihypertensive agents used have been sodium nitroprusside combined with a β-adrenergic blocking drug. As noted previously, nitroprusside does carry with it the risk of cyanide toxicity. Labetalol, a combined α- and β-adrenergic blocker, has been a useful antihypertensive agent in the setting of aortic dissection in pregnancy. Particularly if dissection is proximal, emergency surgery is indicated. If the aortic root is involved, concomitant aortic valve replacement is usually indicated. When possible it is preferable to wait up to 48 hours after delivery of the infant to avoid excessive bleeding from the placental site during anticoagulation for cardiopulmonary bypass.

The cardiovascular diseases that arise during pregnancy represent a unique and often unexpected challenge in management and are often best tackled by a multidisciplinary approach. Successful treatment of these diseases is most gratifying, in that two young lives, that of the mother and the infant, may be preserved in fortunate cases. Hope is available now even to those afflicted with possibly the two most dismal disorders of pregnancy, peripartum cardiomyopathy and pulmonary hypertension, due to continuing improvements in cardiac and lung transplantation. The exciting ongoing research in these disorders can lead only to continued improvement in the outlook for future generations of pregnant women stricken with these devastating diseases.

References

1. Chesley LC. *Hypertensive Disorders in Pregnancy*. New York, Appleton-Century-Crofts, 1978.
2. Chesley LC. The remote prognosis of eclamptic women. *Am Heart J* 93:407, 1977.
3. Sachs BP, Brown DA, Driscoll SG, et al. Hemorrhage, infection, toxemia, and cardiac disease, 1954–85: causes for their declining role in maternal mortality. *Am J Public Health* 78:671, 1988.
4. Ferris TF. Toxemia and hypertension. In Burrow GN, Ferris TF (Eds.), *Medical Complications During Pregnancy* (2nd ed.). Philadelphia, W. B. Saunders, 1982.
5. Burwell CS, et al. Circulation during pregnancy. *Arch Intern Med* 62:979, 1938.
6. Ferris TF, Stein JH, Kauffman J. Uterine blood flow and uterine renin secretion. *J Clin Invest* S1:2827, 1972.

7. Weir RJ, Brown JJ, Fraser R, et al. Plasma renin, renin substrate, angiotensin II, and aldosterone in hypertensive disease of pregnancy. *Lancet* 1:291, 1973.
8. Brunner HR, Chanes P, Wallach R, et al. Angiotensin II vascular receptors: Their avidity in relationship to sodium balance, the autonomic nervous system and hypertension. *J Clin Invest* S1:58, 1972.
9. Everett RB, Worley RJ, MacDonald RG, et al. Effect of prostaglandin synthetase inhibition on pressor response to angiotensin II in human pregnancy. *J Clin Endocrinol Metab* 46:1007, 1978.
10. Remuzzi G, Marchesi D, Mecca G, et al. Reduction of fetal vascular prostacyclin activity in pre-eclampsia. *Lancet* 2:310, 1980.
11. Makila UM, Wiinikka L, Ylikorkala O. Evidence that prostacyclin deficiency is a specific feature in pre-eclampsia. *Am J Obstet Gynecol* 148:772, 1984.
12. Goodman RP, Killam P, Brash AR, et al. Prostacyclin production during pregnancy: Comparison of production during normal pregnancy and pregnancy complicated by hypertension. *Am J Obstet Gynecol* 142:817, 1982.
13. Walsh WS, Behr MJ, Allen NH. Placental prostacyclin production in normal and toxemic pregnancies. *Am J Obstet Gynecol* 151:110, 1985.
14. Raab W, Schroeder G, Wagner R, et al. Vascular reactivity and electrolytes in normal and toxemic pregnancy. *J Clin Endocrinol* 16:1196, 1956.
15. Abdul-Karim R, Assali NS. Pressor response to angiotensin in pregnant and nonpregnant women. *Am J Obstet Gynecol* 82:246, 1961.
16. Talledo DE, Chesley LC, Zuspan FP. Renin-angiotensin system in normal and toxemic pregnancies. III. Differential sensitivity to angiotensin II and norepinephrine in toxemia of pregnancy. *Am J Obstet Gynecol* 100:218, 1968.
17. Gant NF, Daley GL, Chard S, et al. A study of angiotensin II pressor response throughout primigravid pregnancy. *J Clin Invest* 52:2682, 1973.
18. Tatum HJ, Mule JG. The hypertensive action of blood from patients with preeclampsia. *Am J Obstet Gynecol* 83:1028, 1962.
19. Pirani BB, MacGillivray I. The effect of plasma retransfusion on the blood pressure in the puerperium. *Am J Obstet Gynecol* 121:221, 1975.
20. Host HF. Experimental investigations of hypertonia. *Acta Med Scand* 77:28, 1931.
21. Page EW. The effect of eclamptic blood upon the urinary output and blood pressure of human recipients. *J Clin Invest* 17:207, 1938.
22. Puffer HW, Cheek SE, Oakes GK, et al. Vasoactive effect of sera from preeclamptic patients. *Am J Obstet Gynecol* 142:468, 1982.
23. Puffer HW, Warner NE, Martin CB Jr. Preliminary observations of the effect of serum from patients with toxemia of pregnancy. *Bibl Anat* 12:13, 173.
24. Hatjis CG, Grogan D. Atrial natriuretic peptide receptors (ANP) in normal human placentas. *Am J Obstet Gynecol* 159:587, 1988.
25. Thomsen JK, Storm TL, Thamsburg G, et al. Atrial natriuretic peptide concentrations in pre-eclampsia. *Br Med J* 294:1508, 1987.
26. Hatjis CG, Grogan DM. Changes in placental atrial natriuretic peptide receptors associated with severe toxemia of pregnancy. *Placenta* 10:153, 1989.
27. Rosenfield CR, Morris AM Jr, Makowski EL, et al. Circulatory changes in reproductive tissues of ewes during pregnancy. *J Gynecol Invest* 5:252, 1974.
28. Edman CD, Devereux WP, Parker CR, et al. Placental clearance of maternal androgens: A protective mechanism against fetal virilization. *Proc Soc Gynecol Invest* Abstract No. 67, 1979.
29. Robertson WB, Khong TY, Brosens I, et al. The placental bed biopsy: Review from three European centers. *Am J Obstet Gynecol* 155:401, 1986.
30. Pijnenborg R, Dixon G, Robertson WB, et al. Trophoblastic invasion of the human decidua from 8 to 18 weeks of pregnancy. *Placenta* 10:3, 1989.
31. Orsini MW. Trophoblastic giant cell and endovascular cells associated with pregnancy in the hamster (*Cricetus anuratus*). *Am J Anat* 94:273, 1954.
32. DeWolf F, DeWolf-Peeters C, Brosens I. Ultrastructure of the spiral arteries in the human placental bed at the end of normal pregnancy. *Am J Obstet Gynecol* 117:833, 1973.
33. Brosens I, Robertson WB, Dixon HG. The physiological response of the vessels of the placental bed to normal pregnancy. *J Pathol Bacteriol* 93:569, 1967.
34. Pijnenborg R, Robertson WB, Brosens I, et al. Reveiw article: Trophoblast invasion and the establishment of haemochorial placentation in man and laboratory animals. *Placenta* 2:71, 1981.
35. DeWolf F, Robertson WB, Brosens I. The ultrastructure of acute atherosis in hypertensive pregnancy. *Am J Obstet Gynecol* 123:164, 1975.
36. Robertson WB, Brosens I, Dixon HG. The pathological response of the vessels of the placental bed to hypertensive pregnancy. *J Pathol Bacteriol* 93:581, 1967.
37. Hertig AT. Vascular pathology in the hypertensive albuminuric toxaemias of pregnancy. *Clinics* 4:602, 1945.
38. Levin M, Stroobant P, Walters M, et al. Platelet-derived growth factors as possible mediators of vascular proliferation in the sporadic hemolytic uraemic syndrome. *Lancet* 2:830, 1986.
39. Ferris TF. Pregnancy complicated by hypertension and renal disease. *Adv Intern Med* 35:269, 1990.
40. Arias F, Mancilla-Jiminez R. Hepatic fibrinogen deposits in preeclampsia. *N Engl J Med* 295:578, 1976.
41. Hatfield AK, Stein JH, Greenberger NJ, et al. Idiopathic acute fatty liver of pregnancy. Death from extrahepatic manifestation. *Am J Digest Dis* 17:167, 1972.
42. Duffy BL. HELLP syndrome and the anaesthetist. *Anaesthesia* 43:223, 1988.
43. Kolawole TM, Patel PJ, Yagub B, et al. Computed tomographic changes of the brain in toxemia of pregnancy. *Curr J Radiol* 11:46, 1990.
44. Raroque HG, Orrison WW, Rosenberg GA. Neurologic involvement of toxemia of pregnancy: Reversible MRI lesions. *Neurology* 40:167, 1990.
45. Lewis LK, Hinshaw DB, Will AD, et al. CT and angiographic correlation of severe neurological disease in toxemia of pregnancy. *Neuroradiology* 30:59, 1988.
46. Bauer TW, Moore GW, Hutchins GM. Morphologic evidence for coronary artery spasm in eclampsia. *Circulation* 65:255, 1982.
47. Vardi J, Fields GA. Microangiopathic hemolytic anemia in severe pre-eclampsia. *Am J Obstet Gynecol* 119:617, 1974.
48. Starkie CM, Harding LK, Fletcher DJ, et al. Intra-

vascular coagulation and abnormal lung-scans in preeclampsia and eclampsia. *Lancet* 2:889, 1971.
49. Anderson HF, Lynch JP, Johnson TRB. Adult respiratory distress syndrome in obstetrics and gynecology. *Obstet Gynecol* 55:291, 1980.
50. Weiner C, Keller S. Preeclampsia is not associated with excess fetal clotting. *Obstet Gynecol* 68:871, 1986.
51. Hayakawa M, Maki M. Coagulation-fibrinolytic and kinin-forming systems in toxemia of pregnancy. *Gynecol Obstet Invest* 26:181, 1988.
52. Terao T, Maki M, Ikenove T, et al. The relationship between clinical signs and hypercoagulable state in toxemia of pregnancy. *Gynecol Obstet Invest* 31:74, 1991.
53. Schneider CL. The active principle of placental toxin: Thromboplastin; its inactivator in blood: Antithromboplastin. *Am J Physiol* 149:123, 1947.
54. Schneider CL. Complications of late pregnancy in rabbits induced by experimental placenta trauma. *Surg Gynecol Obstet* 90:613, 1950.
55. Clark SJ, Phelan JR, Allen SH, et al. Antepartum reversal of hematologic abnormalities associated with the HELLP syndrome: A report of three cases. *J Reprod Med* 31:70, 1986.
56. Stubbs TM, Lazarchick J, Van Dorsen JP. Evidence of accelerated platelet production and consumption in nonthrombocytopenic preeclampsia. *Am J Obstet Gynecol* 155:263, 1986.
57. Douglas J, Shah M, Lowe GDO, et al. Fibrinopeptide A and beta-thromboglobulin levels in preeclampsia and hypertensive pregnancy (abstract No. 0007). *Thromb Haemostas* 46:8, 1981.
58. Kaplan KL, Owen J. Plasma levels of beta-thromboglobulin and platelet factor 4 as indices of platelet activation in vivo. *Blood* 57:199, 1981.
59. Thornton CA, Bonhar J. Factor VIII-related antigen and factor VIII coagulant activity in normal and preeclamptic pregnancy. *Br J Obstet Gynaecol* 84:919, 1977.
60. Byrnes JJ, Moake JL. Thrombotic thrombocytopenic purpura and the hemolytic-uremic syndrome: Evolving concepts of pathogenesis and therapy. *Clin Haematol* 15:413, 1986.
61. Walsh SW. Preeclampsia: An imbalance in placental prostacyclin and thromboxane production. *Am J Obstet Gynecol* 152:335, 1985.
62. Ylikorkala O, Pekonen F, Viinikka L. Renal prostacyclin and thromboxane in normotensive and preeclamptic pregnant women and their infants. *J Clin Endocrinol Metab* 63:1307, 1986.
63. Rodgers GM, Taylor RN, Roberts JM. Serum from preeclamptic women contains a factor which damages human endothelial cells (abstract No. 12). Presented at the 35th Annual Meeting of the Society of Gynecologic Investigation, Baltimore, March 17–20, 1988.
64. Rappaport V, Hirata G, Yap HK, et al. Anti-endothelial cell antibodies in severe preeclampsia (abstract No. 84). Presented at the 35th Annual meeting of the Society for Gynecologic Investigation, Baltimore, March 17–20, 1988.
65. Rakoczi I, Tihanyi K, Falkay G, et al. Prostacyclin production in trophoblast. In Lewis PJ, Moncada S, O'Grady J (Eds.), *Prostacyclin in Pregnancy*. New York, Raven Press, 1983, pp. 15–23.
66. Ogden E, Hildebrand GJ, Page EW. Rise of blood pressure during ischemia of the gravid uterus. *Proc Soc Exp Biol Med* 43:49, 1940.
67. Gyongyossy A, Kelentey B. An experimental study of the effect of ischaemia of the pregnant uterus on the blood pressure. *J Obstet Gynaecol Br Commonw* 65:617, 1958.
68. Benjamin F, Craig CJT. Uterine distension and preeclamptic toxemia. *J Obstet Gynaecol Br Commonw* 68:827, 1961.
69. Masotti G, Galanti G, Poggesi L, et al. Differential inhibition of prostacyclin production and platelet aggregation by aspirin. *Lancet* 2:1213, 1979.
70. Wallenburg HCS, Dekker GA, Makovitz JW, et al. Low-dose aspirin prevents pregnancy-induced hypertension and pre-eclampsia in angiotensin-sensitive primigravidae. *Lancet* 1:1, 1986.
71. Slone D, Heinonem OP, Kaufman DW, et al. Aspirin and congenital malformations. *Lancet* 1:1373, 1976.
72. Zierler S, Rothman KJ. Congenital heart disease in relation to maternal use of bendectin and other drugs in early pregnancy. *N Engl J Med* 313:347, 1985.
73. Stuart MJ, Gross SJ, Elrad H, et al. Effects of acetylsalicylic-acid ingestion on maternal and neonatal hemostasis. *N Engl J Med* 307:909, 1982.
74. Arcilla RA, Thilenius DG, Ranniger K. Congestive heart failure from unsuspected ductal closure in utero. *J Pediatr* 75:74, 1969.
75. Sharpe GL, Larsson KS, Thalme BE. Studies on closure of the ductus arteriosus. XII. In utero effect of indomethacin and sodium salicylate in rats and rabbits. *Prostaglandins* 9:585, 1975.
76. Powell JG, Cochrane RL. The effects of the administration of fenoprofen or indomethacin to rat dams during late pregnancy with special reference to the ductus arteriosus of the fetuses and neonates. *Toxicol Appl Pharmacol* 45:783, 1978.
77. Olley PM, Bodach E, Heaton J, et al. Further evidence implicating E-type prostaglandins in the patency of the lamb ductus arteriosus. *Eur J Pharmacol* 34:247, 1975.
78. Moise KJ Jr, Huhta JC, Sharif DS, et al. Indomethacin in the treatment of premature labor: Effects in the fetal ductus arteriosus. *N Engl J Med* 319:327, 1988.
79. Niebyl JR, Blake DA, White RD, et al. The inhibition of premature labor with indomethacin. *Am J Obstet Gynecol* 136:1014, 1980.
80. Dudley DKL, Hardie MS. Fetal and neonatal effects of indomethacin used as a tocolytic agent. *Am J Obstet Gynecol* 151:181, 1985.
81. Tyler HM, Saxton CAPD, Parry MJ. Administration to man of UK 37, 248-01, a selective inhibitor of thromboxane synthetase. *Lancet* 1:629, 1981.
82. Dyerberg J, Bang HO. Preeclampsia and prostaglandins (letter to the editor). *Lancet* 1:1267, 1985.
83. Tobin A. Fish oil supplementation (letter to the editor). *Lancet* 1:1046, 1988.
84. Lunell NO, Nylund L, Lewander R, et al. Uteroplacental blood flow in pregnancy hypertension after the administration of a beta-adrenoreceptor blocker, pindolol. *Gynecol Obstet Invest* 18:269, 1984.
85. Horvath JS, Korda A, Child A, et al. Hypertension in pregnancy: A study of 142 women presenting before 32 weeks gestation. *Med J Aust* 143:19, 1985.
86. Rubin PC, Butters L, Clark DM, et al. Placebo-controlled trial of atenolol in treatment of pregnancy associated hypertension. *Lancet* 1:431, 1983.
87. Collins R, Yusuf S, Peto R. Overview of randomized

trials of diuretics in pregnancy. *Br Med J* 290:17, 1985.
88. Gallery EDM, Saunders DM, Hunyor SN, et al. Randomized comparison of methyldopa and oxprenolol for treatment of hypertension in pregnancy. *Br Med J* 1:1591, 1979.
89. Lunell NO, Persson B, Aragon G, et al. Circulatory and metabolic effects of acute beta 1-blockage in severe pre-eclampsia. *Acta Obstet Gynecol Scand* 58:443, 1979.
90. Ounsted M, Cockburn J, Moar VA, et al. Maternal hypertension with superimposed pre-eclampsia: Effects on child development at 7½ years. *Br J Obstet Gynecol* 90:644, 1983.
91. Horvath JS, Phippard A, Korda A, et al. Clonidine hydrochloride—a safe and effective antihypertensive agent in pregnancy. *Obstet Gynecol* 66:634, 1985.
92. Drayer JI, Zegarelli EC. Hypertension and pregnancy. In Douglas PS, Brest AN (Eds.), *Heart Disease in Women*. Philadelphia, F.A. Davis, 1989, pp. 97–111.
93. Liedholm H, Melander A. Drug selection in the treatment of pregnancy hypertension. *Acta Obstet Gynecol Scand* (Suppl.) 118:49, 1984.
94. Rubin PC, Butters L, Low RA, et al. Clinical pharmacological studies with prazosin during pregnancy complicated by hypertension. *Br J Clin Pharmacol* 16:543, 1983.
95. Shoemaker CT, Meyers M. Sodium nitroprusside for control of severe hypertensive disease of pregnancy: A case report and discussion of potential toxicity. *Am J Obstet Gynecol* 149:171, 1984.
96. Erbel R, Brand G, Meyers J, et al. Emergency treatment of hypertensive crisis with sublingual nifedipine. *Postgrad Med J* 59 (Suppl. 3):134, 1983.
97. Rubin PC, Butters L, McCabe R. Nifedipine and platelets in pre-eclampsia. *Am J Hypertens* 1:175, 1988.
98. Ferris TF, Weir EK. The effect of captopril on uterine blood flow and prostaglandin synthesis in the rabbit. *J Clin Invest* 71:80, 1983.
99. Kreft C, Plouin PF, Tchobioutschy C, et al. Angiotensin and converting enzyme inhibitors during pregnancy: A summary of 22 patients given captopril and 9 given enalapril. *Br J Obstet Gynaecol* 95:42, 1988.
100. Rubin PC. Treatment of hypertension in pregnancy. *Clin Obstet Gynaecol* 13:307, 1986.
101. Sullivan JM. *Hypertension and Pregnancy*. Chicago, Year Book, 1987.
102. Baylis C, Reckelhoff JF. Renal hemodynamics in normal and hypertensive pregnancy: Lessons from micropuncture. *Am J Kidney Dis* 17(2):98, 1991.
103. Lindheimer MD, Katz AI. Effects of hypotonic expansion on sodium and water excretion in hypertensive non-preeclamptic primigravidas. *Am J Obstet Gynecol* 111:1053, 1971.
104. Sarles HE, Hill SS, LeBlanc AL, et al. Sodium excretion patterns during and following intravenous sodium chloride loads in normal and hypertensive pregnancies. *Am J Obstet Gynecol* 102:1, 1968.
105. Nisell H, Mortinsson A, Hjemdahl P. Reduced B_2-adrenoreceptor sensitivity in normal pregnancy but not in pregnancy-induced hypertension. *Gynecol Obstet Invest* 25:262, 1988.
106. Homans DC. Peripartum cardiomyopathy. *N Engl J Med* 312:1432, 1985.
107. Veille JC. Peripartum cardiomyopathies: A review. *Am J Obstet Gynecol* 148:805, 1984.
108. Michels VV, Moll PP, Miller FA, et al. The frequency of familial dilated cardiomyopathy in a series of patients with idiopathic dilated cardiomyopathy. *N Engl J Med* 326:77, 1992.
109. Walsh JJ, Burch GE. Post partum heart disease. *Arch Intern Med* 108:817, 1961.
110. Walsh JJ, Burch GE, Black WC, et al. Idiopathic myocardiopathy of puerperium (post-partal heart disease). *Circulation* 32:19, 1965.
111. Sanderson JE, Olsen EGJ, Gatei D. Peripartum heart disease: An endomyocardial biopsy study. *Br Heart J* S6:285, 1986.
112. O'Connell JB, Costanzo-Nardin MR, Subramanian R, et al. Peripartum cardiomyopathy: Clinical, hemodynamic, histologic and prognostic characteristics. *J Am Coll Cardiol* 8:52, 1986.
113. James KB, Healy BP. Heart disease arising during or secondary to pregnancy. In Douglas PS, Brest AN (Eds.), *Heart Disease in Women*. Philadelphia, F.A. Davis, 1989, pp. 81–96.
114. Cunningham G, Pritchard JA, Heinkins GDV, et al. Peripartum heart failure: Idiopathic cardiomyopathy or compounding cardiovascular events? *Obstet Gynecol* 67:157, 1986.
115. Marin-Neto JA, Maciel BC, Urbanetz LLT, et al. High output failure in patients with peripartum cardiomyopathy: A comparative study with dilated cardiomyopathy. *Am Heart J* 121:134, 1990.
116. Midei MG, DeMent SH, Feldman AM, et al. Peripartum myocarditis and cardiomyopathy. *Circulation* 81:922, 1990.
117. Melvin KR, Richardson PJ, Olsen EGJ, et al. Peripartum cardiomyopathy due to myocarditis. *N Engl J Med* 307:731, 1982.
118. Edwards WD, Holmes DR, Reeder GS. Diagnosis of active lymphocytic myocarditis by endomyocardial biopsy—Quantitative criteria for light microscopy. *Mayo Clin Proc* 57:419, 1982.
119. Gavras H, Kremer D, Brown JJ, et al. Angiotensin- and norepinephrine-induced myocardial lesions: Experimental and clinical studies in rabbits and man. *Am Heart J* 89:321, 1975.
120. Hutchins GM, Bulkley BH. Correlation of myocardial contraction band necrosis and vascular patency. *Lab Invest* 36:642, 1977.
121. Fenoglio JJ, McAllister HA, Mullieh FG. Drug related myocarditis: I. Hypersensitivity myocarditis. *Hum Pathol* 12:900, 1981.
122. Yokoyama S, Kanda T, Suzuki T, et al. Response of NK cell activity in postpartum myocarditis due to experimental viral infection. *Circulation* Suppl 84(4):II-634, 1991.
123. Korithavongs T, Dossetor JB. Suppressor cells in human pregnancy. *Transplant Proc* 10:911, 1978.
124. Virus, immunology and the heart (editorial). *Lancet* 2:1111, 1979.
125. Stamler J, Horowitz SF, Goldman ME, et al. Peripartum cardiomyopathy—A role for cardiac stress determinants other than pregnancy? *Mt Sinai J Med* 56(4):285, 1989.
126. Lerner AM. Coxsackie virus cardiomyopathy. *J Infect Dis* 120:496, 1969.
127. Cenac A, Gaultier Y, Devillechabrolle A, et al. Enterovirus infection in peripartum cardiomyopathy. *Lancet* 2:968, 1988.
128. Rose NR, Herskowitz A, Neumann DA, et al. Autoimmune myocarditis: A paradigm of post-infec-

tion autoimmune disease. *Immunol Today* 9:117, 1988.
129. Froelich CJ, Goodwin JS, Bankhurst AD, et al. Pregnancy, a temporal fetal graft of suppressor cells in autoimmune disease? *Am J Med* 69:329, 1980.
130. Cenac A, Beaufils H, Soumara I, et al. Absence of humoral autoimmunity in peripartum cardiomyopathy. A comparative study in Nigeria. *Intern J Cardiol* 26:49, 1990.
131. Adesanya CO, Angorin FI, Adeoshun IO, et al. Peripartum cardiac failure. A ten year follow-up study. *Trop Geogr Med* 41:190, 1989.
132. Demakis JG, Rahimtoola SH, Sutton GG, et al. Natural course of peripartum cardiomyopathy. *Circulation* 44:1053, 1971.
133. Carvalho A, Brandao A, Martinez EE, et al. Prognosis in peripartum cardiomyopathy. *Am J Cardiol* 64:540, 1989.
134. Sutton MSJ, Cole P, Plappert M, et al. Effects of subsequent pregnancy on left ventricular function in peripartum cardiomyopathy. *Am Heart J* 121:1776, 1991.
135. Hadjimiltiades S, Panidis IP, Segal BL. Recovery of left ventricular function in peripartum cardiomyopathy. *Am Heart J* 112:1097, 1986.
136. Burch GE, McDonald CD, Walsh JJ. The effect of prolonged bed rest on postpartal cardiomyopathy. *Am Heart J* 81:186, 1971.
137. Hovsepian PG, Ganzel B, Sohi GS, et al. Peripartum cardiomyopathy treated with a left ventricular assist device as a bridge to cardiac transplantation. *S Med J* 82(4):527, 1989.
138. Moreira LFP, Seferian P, Bocchi E, et al. Survival improvement with dynamic cardiomyoplasty in patients with dilated cardiomyopathy. *Circulation* 84 (Suppl III):III-296, 1991.
139. Rosenberg B, Suisan K, Peretz BA, et al. Eisenmenger syndrome and Schwangerschaft. *Reg Anaesth* 7:131, 1984.
140. Gliecher N, Midwall J, Hochberger D, et al. Eisenmenger's syndrome and pregnancy. *Obstet Gynecol Surv* 34:721, 1979.
141. McCaffrey RM, Dunn LJ. Primary pulmonary hypertension in pregnancy. *Obstet Gynecol Surv* 19:567, 1964.
142. Rich S. Primary pulmonary hypertension. *Prog Cardiovasc Dis* 31:205, 1988.
143. Rich S, Levy P. Characteristics of surviving and nonsurviving patients with primary pulmonary hypertension. *Am J Med* 76:573, 1984.
144. Kanemoto N. Natural history of pulmonary hemodynamics in primary pulmonary hypertension. *Am Heart J* 114:407, 1981.
145. Braunwald E (Ed.). *Heart Disease. A Textbook of Cardiovascular Medicine* (3rd ed.). Philadelphia, W.B. Saunders, 1988, pp. 793–814.
146. Weber KJ, Janicki JS, Schroff SG, et al. The right ventricle: Physiological and pathophysiological considerations. *Crit Care Med* 11:323, 1983.
147. Burrows FA, Klinck JR, Rabinovitch M, et al. Primary pulmonary hypertension in children: Perioperative management. *Can Anaesth Soc* 33:606, 1986.
148. D'Alonzo GE, Bianott LA, Pohil RL, et al. Comparison of progressive exercise performance of normal subjects and patients with primary pulmonary hypertension. *Chest* 92:57, 1987.
149. Cheek TG, Gutsche BB. Maternal physiological alterations during pregnancy. In Shnider S, Levinson G (Eds.), *Anaesthesia for Obstetrics* (2nd ed.). Baltimore, Williams & Wilkins, 1987, pp. 3–13.
150. Mangano D. Anaesthesia for the pregnancy cardiac patient. In Shnider SM, Levinson G (Eds.), *Anaesthesia for Obstetrics* (2nd ed.). Baltimore, Williams & Wilkins, 1987, pp. 345–351.
151. Anderson EG, Simon G, Reid L. Primary and thrombo-embolic pulmonary hypertension: A quantitative pathological study. *J Pathol* 110:273, 1973.
152. Robinson DE, Leicht CH. Epidural anaesthesia with low dose bupivacaine and fentanyl for labour and delivery in a parturient with severe pulmonary hypertension. *Anesthesiology* 68:285, 1988.
153. Slomka F, Salmerson S, Zetlaoui P, et al. Primary pulmonary hypertension and pregnancy: Anaesthetic management for delivery. *Anesthesiology* 69:959, 1988.
154. Nelson DM, Main E, Crafford W, et al. Peripartum heart failure due to primary pulmonary hypertension. *Obstet Gynecol* 62(5):58, 1983.
155. Weir EK. Diagnosis and management of primary pulmonary hypertension. In Weir EK, Reeves JT (Eds.), *Pulmonary Hypertension*. New York, Futura, 1984, pp. 142–143.
156. Pritchard JA, MacDonald PC, Gant NF. Caesarean section and caesarean hysterectomy. In Williams JW (Ed.), *Obstetrics* (17th ed.). Norwalk, Conn, Appleton-Century-Crofts, 1985, pp. 867–886.
157. Feijen HWH, Hein PR, Lakwikj-Vondrovilova EL, et al. Primary hypertension and pregnancy. *Eur J Obstet Gynecol Reprod Biol* 15:159–164, 1983.
158. Rich S, Brundage BH, Levy PS. The effect of vasodilator therapy on the clinical outcome of patient with primary pulmonary hypertension. *Circulation* 71(6):1191, 1985.
159. Roberts NV, Keast PJ. Pulmonary hypertension and pregnancy—a lethal combination. *Anaesth Intens Care* 18:366, 1990.
160. Pearl RG, Rosenthal MH, Schroeder JS, et al. Acute hemodynamic effects of nitroglycerin in pulmonary hypertension. *Ann Intern Med* 99:9, 1983.
161. Bygdeman M, Kivon S, Mukhorjee T, et al. Effect of intravenous infusion of prostaglandin E1 and E2 on motility of the pregnant uterus. *Am J Obstet Gynecol* 102:317, 1968.
162. Swahn ML, Lundstrom V. The effect of intravenous and intrauterine administration of prostacyclin on non-pregnant uterine contractility in vivo. *Acta Obstet Gynecol Scand* Suppl. 113:47, 1983.
163. Prewitt RM, Glugone M. Treatment of right ventricular dysfunction in acute respiratory failure. *Crit Care Med* 11:346, 1983.
164. Rall RT, Sclufer LS. Drugs and uterine motility. In Gilman A, Goodman LS, Rall T, et al. (Eds.), *The Pharmacological Basis of Therapeutics* (7th ed.). New York, Macmillan 1985, pp. 926–945.
165. Brownridge P, Cohen SE. Neural blockade for obstetrics and gynecologic surgery. In Cousins MJ, Bridenbaugh PO (Eds.), *Neural Blockade* (2nd ed.). Philadelphia, J.B. Lippincott, 1988, pp. 593–634.
166. Cousins MJ, Bromage PR. Epidural neural blockade. In Cousins MJ, Bridenbaugh PO (Eds.), *Neural Blockade* (2nd ed.). Philadelphia, J.B. Lippincott, 1988, pp. 253–360.
167. Abboud TK, Raya J, Noveihed R, et al. Intrathecal morphine for the relief of labour pain in a parturient

with severe pulmonary hypertension. *Anesthesiology* 59:477, 1983.
168. Gravlec GP, Ramsay FM, Roy RC, et al. Rapid administration of a narcotic and neuromuscular blocker. A hemodynamic comparison of fentanyl, sufentanil, pancuronium and vecuronium. *Anesth Anal* 67:39, 1988.
169. Cheng DCH, Edelest G. Isoflurane and primary pulmonary hypertension. *Anaesthesia* 43:22, 1988.
170. Pasque MK, Trulock EP, Kaiser LR, et al. Single-lung transplantation for pulmonary hypertension. *Circulation* 84:275, 1991.
171. Pumphrey CW, Fay T, Weir I. Aortic dissection during pregnancy. *Br Heart J* 55:106, 1986.
172. Konishi IY, Tatsuta N, Kumada K, et al. Dissecting aneurysm during pregnancy and the puerperium. *Jpn Circ J* 44:726, 1980.
173. Williams GB, Gott VL, Brawley RK, et al. Aortic disease associated with pregnancy. *J Vasc Surg* 8:470, 1988.
174. Bulkley BH, Roberts WC. Isolated coronary arterial dissection: A complication of cardiac operations. *J Thorac Cardiovasc Surg* 67:148, 1974.
175. Pyeritz RE. Maternal and fetal complications of pregnancy in the Marfan syndrome. *Am J Med* 71:784, 1981.
176. Come PC, Bulkley BH, McKusick VA, et al. Echocardiographic recognition of silent aortic root dilatation in Marfan's syndrome. *Chest* 72:789, 1977.
177. Danforth DN, Manalo-Estrella P, Buckingham JC. The effect of pregnancy and of Enovid on the rabbit vasculature. *Am J Obstet Gynecol* 88:952, 1964.
178. Becker RM. Intracardiac surgery in pregnant women. *Ann Thorac Surg* 36:453, 1983.

Index

Note: Page numbers in *italics* refer to illustrations; page numbers followed by t refer to tables.

Abortion, fetal radiation hazard and, 323
  spontaneous, autoimmune disorders and, 243
    thrombocythemia and, 244
ACE (angiotensin-converting enzyme) inhibitors, fetal injury from, 95, 343–344
  postinfarction, 55
Activin, 154, *154*
Aerobic capacity, 253–254
Age, angina and, 27
  at menopause, 156
  blood pressure and, 63–66, *65*
  CHD and, 26, 27
  lipoproteins and, *181*
  mitral valve prolapse and, 119
  restriction of care based on, 34
  smoking and, 218–219, 218t
  thrombolytic therapy and, 53, 54
Aggression, 274
Alcohol drinking, employment status and, 270–271
  restriction of, in hypertension, 90
Amenorrhea, hormonal replacement therapy and, 171
Amiodarone, in pregnancy, 331t
AMIS (Aspirin in Myocardial Infarction Study), 55
Amniotic fluid embolism, pulmonary hypertension and, 350–351
Amputation, in peripheral arterial disease, 146
Anagrelide, 244
Androgen(s), cardiac effects of, 72, 107–108
  estradiol production and, 155–156
  hypertension and, 73–77, *74*, *76*
  menopause and, 157, *157*
  menstrual cycle and, 156
  smoking and, 222
Androgenicity, of progestins, 160
Androstenedione, menopause and, 157, *157*
  menstrual cycle and, 156
  smoking and, 222
Anesthesia, during labor, 318–319

Anesthesia *(Continued)*
  in patient with pulmonary hypertension, 352
Anger, 273–274
Angina, clinical manifestations of, 26t, 27–28, 28t, 45
  drug therapy for, 45
  nonspecific chest pain and, 27–28, 28t
  perception of, 11–12
  smoking and, 219–220
  Type A behavior and, 277
  unstable, 33
  variant, 28
Angiography, postinfarction, 56
Angioplasty, in peripheral arterial disease, 146
  percutaneous transluminal coronary. See *Percutaneous transluminal coronary angioplasty (PTCA)*.
Angiotensin II, 71–72
  toxemia and, 338–339
Angiotensin-converting enzyme (ACE) inhibitors, fetal injury from, 95, 343–344
  postinfarction, 55
Animal models, 283–302
  gender differences and, 283–284, 284t
  of arterial metabolism, 296–298, *297*
  of central obesity, 292, *293*, 299
  of hormonal replacement therapy, 294–296, *296*, 299
  of hypertension, 69, 73–77, *74*, *76*
    in pregnancy, 344
  of lipoprotein metabolism, 296–298, *297*, 299
  of menopause, 292, *293*, 294
  of oral contraceptive effects, 284–286, *286*, *287*, 298
  of peripartum cardiomyopathy, 347
  of pregnancy, 292, *293*, 299
  of psychosocial stress, 286, 288–289, *288*, 289t, *290*, *291*, 299
  of social isolation, 291–292, *291*
  of vasomotion, 298, *299*, 300
Anticardiolipins, 243
Anticoagulation therapy, 247

361

Anticoagulation therapy *(Continued)*
  in pregnancy, 239, 240, 331t, 333–334, 348
  in pulmonary hypertension of pregnancy, 351–352
Antihypertensive agents, 92
  clinical trials of, 83–88, 84t
    Australian, 85–86
    Elderly Patients in Primary Care, 86
    Hypertension Detection and Follow-up Program, 83–85
    Medical Research Council, 86–87
    pooled results of, 88
    Swedish Trial in Old Patients with Hypertension, 87
    Systolic Hypertension in the Elderly Program, 87
    U.S. Public Health Service, 83
  in pregnancy, 94–95
  in pregnancy complicated by aortic dissection, 354
  in toxemia of pregnancy, 94, 341–342
  other cardiovascular risk factors and, 95
  quality of life and, 95–96
Antiphospholipid syndrome, 242–244, 243t
Antithrombin III deficiency, 240
Anular calcification, mitral valve, 127
Anuloaortic ectasia, 128, *129*
Anxiety, 275–276
  mitral valve prolapse syndrome and, 120t, 122t
Aortic dissection, in pregnancy, 353–354
  Marfan's syndrome and, 130–131, 332, 353
  repair of, 131
Aortic root dilatation, 128, *129*, 332–333
Aortic valve, anuloaortic ectasia and, 128, *129*
  bicuspid, 127–128
  regurgitation from, 126–127
  stenosis of, 128
Apoproteins, 175–176, 177t, 178–179
  genetic disorders of, 179
Arrhythmias, in pregnancy, 319–320, 332
  ventricular, postinfarction, 31
Arterial disease. See *Coronary heart disease (CHD)*; *Peripheral vascular disease.*
Arteriography, coronary, 34–35
  recommendations for, 38
Aspirin in Myocardial Infarction Study (AMIS), 55
Aspirin therapy, for stroke prevention, 141
  in myeloproliferative syndromes, 244
  in pregnancy, 243, 244
  in toxemia of pregnancy, 94, 341–342
  postinfarction, 55
  research on, 10, 44, 55, 245–246
  vs. ticlopidine, 246
Atenolol, in pregnancy, 331t
Atherectomy, 48
Atherosclerosis, animal models of, 283–284, 284t. See also *Animal models.*
  diabetes and, 208–210, 208t
  hormonal replacement therapy and, 167–168, *168*, *169*
  lipoproteins and, 180, 182, 241–242
  obesity and, 201–203
  oral contraceptives and, 161–162
  regression of, 51
Atrial fibrillation, in pregnancy, 333
  stroke and, 141, 142
Atrial natriuretic peptide, toxemia and, 339
Australian Therapeutic Trial in Mild Hypertension, 84t, 85–86
Autoimmune disorders, peripartum cardiomyopathy and, 347
  thrombosis and, 242–244, 243t
Autonomic nervous system, hypertension and, 70

Azathioprine, in peripartum cardiomyopathy, 348

Baboons, research using, 295
Becker's muscular dystrophy, 113
Behavior modification techniques, for smokers, 224
  in hypertension, 91
Beta blocking agents, 45
  in pregnancy, 95, 332–333
  in toxemia of pregnancy, 342
  postinfarction, 54–55
Bias. See *Gender bias.*
Biopsy, endomyocardial, in peripartum cardiomyopathy, 346–347, 348–349
Blacks, diabetes among, 206, 206t
  female, CHD mortality among, 5, 6t
    postinfarction, 32
  hypertension among, 63–66
    body weight and, 199
    CHD and, 80
  obesity among, 198, *198*
Bleeding, thrombolytic therapy and, 54
Bleeding time, 232
Blood circulation, in pregnancy, 309, *310*, 311
Blood loss, during childbirth, 318
Blood pressure, 63–67. See also *Hypertension.*
  age and, 63–66, *65*
  body weight and, 199
  classification of, 64t
  during labor, 318
  estrogen and, 76, 77, 164, *165*
  exercise and, 256–257
  in mitral valve prolapse syndrome, 121
  in pregnancy, 93, 307–308, *308*, 311, 311t, 337
    with exercise, 315
  measurement of, 88–89
  menopause and, 65
  trends in, 66–67
Blood volume, in pregnancy, 308–309, *309*
  postpartum, 319
Body fat distribution, animal studies of, 292, *293*, 299
  cardiovascular risk and, 197–198, *198*
  diabetes and, 207
  hyperinsulinemia and, 200–201, *200*
  hypertension and, 199
  lipoprotein levels and, 183, 200
Body mass index, 197, 197t
Body weight, 197, 197t. See also *Obesity.*
  exercise and, 257–258
  in mitral valve prolapse syndrome, 121
  reduction of, 205
    in hypertension, 90
    in obesity, 204
    lipoprotein levels and, 183
  smoking and, 198–199, 223–224
Bone loss, menopause and, 156
Breast cancer chemotherapy, thromboembolic complications of, 245
Breast feeding, blood flow and, 309
  cardiovascular drugs and, 331t
Breast tissue, scintigraphy and, 36
Bruit, carotid, stroke and, 139–140
Bypass surgery. See *Coronary artery bypass graft (CABG) surgery.*

CABG. See *Coronary artery bypass graft (CABG) surgery.*
Caffeine, hypertension and, 91
Calcification, coronary artery, fluoroscopy in, 37–38
　mitral valve, 125–126
　　anular, 127
Calcium channel blockers, 45
　in pregnancy, 343
　in pulmonary hypertension of pregnancy, 351
Calcium supplementation, in hypertension, 91
　in pregnancy, 94
Cancer, chemotherapy for, thromboembolic complications of, 244–245
　coagulation abnormalities and, 244–245
　perceived risk of, 11
Captopril, in pregnancy, 331t
　in pregnancy complicated by cardiomyopathy, 348
　sexual function and, 96
Carbohydrates, intolerance to, estrogens and, 164–165
　oral contraceptives and, 161
　metabolism of, 191–193, *192*, 192t, 193t
　　pregnancy and, 193
Cardiac. See also *Heart* entries.
Cardiac catheterization, in pregnancy, 321–322
　postinfarction, 45, 56
　pulmonary hypertension of pregnancy, 351
　referral after, 45, 56
Cardiac hypertrophy, concentric, exercise and, 255–256
　gender differences in, 110–113, *111*
　hypertension and, 72, 110–111, *111*
Cardiac output, during labor, 318
　exercise and, 255
　hypertension and, 70–71
　in pregnancy, 311–313, *312*, *313*
　　with exercise, 315–316
　obesity and, 204
　postpartum, 319
Cardiac rehabilitation, 261. See also *Exercise therapy.*
　after CABG surgery, 52
　after myocardial infarction, 56
　after PTCA, 51–52
Cardiac rupture, 31, 112
Cardiac shunts, in pregnancy, 330t, 335
Cardiography, impedance, cardiac output measurement by, 312–313
Cardiomyopathy, diabetic, 210–211
　peripartum, 345–349
　　clinical features of, 345–346
　　pathophysiology of, 346–347
　　treatment of, 347–349
　X-linked, 113
Cardiopulmonary resuscitation, in pregnancy, 332
Cardiovascular disease. See also *Coronary heart disease (CHD)* and specific disorders.
　diabetes and, 208–210, 208t
　employment and, 270–273
　estrogens and, 157–158
　exercise and, 254
　　risks from, 262
　gender differences in, 3–4
　hematologic risk factors for, 240–241
　hormonal replacement therapy and, 167–171, *168–170*, 168t
　obesity and, *202*
　oral contraceptives and, 161–162
　perception of, 11–13
　prevention levels in, 17t, 18t
　progestins and, 170–171

Cardiovascular disease *(Continued)*
　psychoemotional factors and, 273–277
　smoking and, 119–222
　social support and, 277–279
　socioeconomic status and, 269–270
Cardiovascular examination, in pregnancy, 306–307, 311t
Cardioversion, in atrial fibrillation, in pregnancy, 333
Carotid bruit, stroke and, 139–140
Carotid endarterectomy, 140, 141–142
CASS. See *Coronary Artery Surgery Study (CASS).*
Catecholamines, carbohydrate metabolism and, 192–193, 193t
Catheterization. See *Cardiac catheterization.*
Central nervous system, in toxemia, 340
Cerebrovascular disease. See also *Stroke.*
　in toxemia, 340
Charleston Heart Study, on hypertension among blacks, 80
CHD. See *Coronary heart disease (CHD).*
CHEC (Community Hypertension Evaluation Clinic) program, 64
Chemotherapy, thromboembolic complications of, 244–245
Chest pain. See also *Angina.*
　mitral valve prolapse syndrome and, 120t, 122t
　nonspecific, 27–28, 28t, 35–36
　syndrome X and, 28, 46
Chest x-ray, in pregnancy, 321
Chewing gum, nicotine, 224–225
Chickens, research using, 284, 295
Childbirth, anesthesia at, 318–319
　aortic dissection and, 354
　hemodynamic changes during, 318
　heparin and, 334
　mitral stenosis and, 333
　peripartum cardiomyopathy and, 348
　pulmonary hypertension and, 351
Children, multiple role stress and, 272, 273
Cholesterol, 175, *176*, 178–179. See also *Lipoprotein(s).*
　age and, *181*
　diabetes and, 207–208
　estrogens and, 166–167, *166*, *167*, 168, 237
　lowering of, 185–187, 186t
　menopause and, 158
　normal levels of, 186t
　obesity and, 200
　oral contraceptives and, 162, *162*
　　animal studies of, 285–286, *286*, 287
　progestins and, 170–171
　stroke and, 140–141
Chronic myelogenous leukemia, 244
Chylomicrons, 175, *176*, *176*, 178
Cigarettes, low-yield, nicotine and carbon monoxide levels in, 220–221
Circulation, blood, in pregnancy, 309, *310*, 311
Claudication, intermittent, 143–144, 144t
　exercise in, 262
　hypertension and, 82–83
Clerical workers, risks among, 271
Clonidine, in pregnancy, 342–343
Clotting factors. See *Coagulation factors.*
Coagulation, 232–233, *232*
　abnormalities of, 8, 241–245
　　autoimmune, 242–244, 243t
　　inherited, 239–240, 240t
　　malignancy and, 244–245
　disseminated intravascular, in pregnancy, 239, 240
　estrogen and, 165, *166*

Coagulation *(Continued)*
   hormonal replacement therapy and, 237
   oral contraceptives and, 236, 236t
   vascular surface and, 234–235, *234*, 234t
Coagulation factors, 232–235, *232*, 241
   activated endothelium and, 234, 234t
   deficiencies of, 239–240, 240t
   hormonal replacement therapy and, 237
   in complicated pregnancy, 238–239, 240, 340
   in uncomplicated pregnancy, 235
   oral contraceptives and, 236, 236t
Cocaine abuse, myocardial infarction and, 330
Colestipol, 51
Collagen, hormones and, 108
Communication, patient-physician, 14–15, 15t
Community Hypertension Evaluation Clinic (CHEC) program, 64
Compliance, barriers to, 18t
   with risk-reduction regimes, 17–18
Computed tomography (CT), in pregnancy, 322
Congestive heart failure, diabetes and, 210–211
   exercise in, 261
   gender differences in, 110–111
   hypertension and, 78–79
   peripartum cardiomyopathy and, 345–346
Conjugated equine estrogens, 163
Coronary arteriography, 34–35
   recommendations for, 38
Coronary artery(ies), calcification of, fluoroscopy in, 37–38
   size of, PTCA results and, 48
Coronary artery bypass graft (CABG) surgery, 49–51
   diabetes and, 209, 210
   gender differences and, 33–35, 45, 49
   graft patency after, 50
   long-term survival after, 50–51, 51t
   obesity and, 205
   operative mortality from, 49–50, 49t
   postinfarction, 56
   rehabilitation after, 52
   results of, 32, 34, 50–51, 51t
   symptom relief after, 50
Coronary Artery Surgery Study (CASS), on angina, 27
   on CABG mortality, 32
   on congestive heart failure, 111
   on diabetes, 210
   on referral for surgery, 45
Coronary heart disease (CHD). See also *Cardiovascular disease* and specific disease.
   age and, 26, 27
   death rates for, 5–6, *5*, 6t, 25t, *184*
   diabetes and, 183–185, *184*, 208–210, 208t
   employment and, 270–273
   exercise and, 254
      risks from, 262
   gender differences in, 3–4, 7, 25–27, 26t
   hormonal replacement therapy and, 167–169, *168–170*, 168t
   hyperinsulinemia and, 201
   hypertension and, 79–81
   obesity and, 201–205, *202–204*
   oral contraceptives and, 161–162, 161t
   perception of, 11–13
   psychoemotional factors and, 273–277
   smoking and, 219–222
   social support and, 277–279
   socioeconomic status and, 269–270
   CT (computed tomography), in pregnancy, 322

Cynomolgus monkey, 283–284. See also *Animal models*.
Cystathionine synthase deficiency, 242
Cystic medial necrosis, aortic dissection and, 354
Cytochrome C oxidase, 107
Cytokines, activated endothelium and, 234

Death rates, 5–6, *5*, 6t, 25t, *184*
   by disease, *4*
   diabetes and, *184*, 209–210
   educational level and, 269–270
   exercise and, 254
   for deep venous thrombosis, 142
   for peripartum cardiomyopathy, 347
   for peripheral arterial disease, 145, 145t
   for pulmonary hypertension in pregnancy, 349
   for stroke, 137–138
   hormonal replacement therapy and, 167–168, 168t
   hypertension and, 78, *78*, 84–85
   maternal, 338
   myocardial infarction and, 29–30, 52
   operative, after CABG surgery, 49–50, 49t
   oral contraceptives and, *162*
   thrombolytic therapy and, 53–54, 53t, 54t
Deep venous thrombosis, 142–143, *143*. See also *Thrombosis*.
   in pregnancy, 238–239
      factor deficiencies and, 240
   oral contraceptives and, 160–161
Dehydroepiandrosterone, menopause and, 157, *157*
Delivery, anesthesia at, 318–319
   aortic dissection and, 354
   hemodynamic changes during, 318
   heparin and, 334
   mitral stenosis and, 333
   peripartum cardiomyopathy and, 348
   pulmonary hypertension and, 351
Depression, 275–276
   angina and, 277
Diabetes mellitus, 191–216
   atherosclerosis and, 208–210, 208t
   cardiac effects of, 210–211
   CHD and, *184*, 208–210, 208t
   congestive heart failure and, 210–211
   diagnostic criteria for, 194t
   epidemiology of, 205–206, 206t
   estrogens and, 164–165
   exercise and, 207, 211, 258–259
   genetic factors in, 206–207
   gestational, 194–195, 194t
   hypertension and, 208
   impaired glucose tolerance and, 194, 194t
   insulin resistance in, 193–194
   insulin-dependent, 195, 206
   lipoprotein levels and, 183–185, 207–208
   noninsulin-dependent, 195, *196*, 206
      prevention and treatment of, 211
   normal carbohydrate metabolism vs., 191–193, *192*, 192t, 193t
   obesity and, 195, 197–198, 207
   oral contraceptives and, 161
   postinfarction ventricular function in, 31
   revascularization procedures in, 209–210
   secondary, 195
Diagnostic testing, 33–39
Dialysis, hypertension and, 79
Diazoxide, in pregnancy, 343

Diet, in hypertension, 90–91
  in toxemia, 342
  lipoprotein levels and, 182–183
  obesity and, 199
Digitalis, in peripartum cardiomyopathy, 348
  in pregnancy, 331t
Dipyridamole, aspirin with, 246
  CABG surgery and, 50
Disability, from stroke, 141
Discrimination, 270
  occupation and, 272
Dissection, aortic. See *Aortic dissection*.
  arterial, in pregnancy, 353
Disseminated intravascular coagulation, in pregnancy, 239, 240
Diuretics, in toxemia, 342
Dobutamine, in peripartum cardiomyopathy, 348
  in pulmonary hypertension of pregnancy, 352
Doctor-patient relationship. See *Physician-patient relationship*.
Dopamine, in peripartum cardiomyopathy, 348
  in pulmonary hypertension of pregnancy, 352
Doppler echocardiography, cardiac output measurement by, 313
  in pregnancy, 320
Doppler ultrasonography, in carotid disease, 140
Drugs. See specific agents or classes.
Duchenne's muscular dystrophy, 113
Dyslipoproteinemias, 179–180, 180t
  diabetes and, 207–208
  familial, 179
  secondary, 179–180
Dyspnea, in pregnancy, 305
  mitral valve prolapse syndrome and, 120t, 122t

E_1. See *Estrone (E_1)*.
E_2. See *Estradiol (E_2)*.
ECG. See *Electrocardiography (ECG)*.
Echocardiography, cardiac output measurement by, 312, 313
  exercise, 37
  in mitral valve prolapse diagnosis, 120–121, 123–124
  in peripartum cardiomyopathy, 345
  in pregnancy, 314, 320
  pulmonary hypertension and, 351
Eclampsia, 93–94, 337. See also *Toxemia*.
  late postpartum, 93
Economic factors. See *Socioeconomic factors*.
Ectasia, anuloaortic, 128, *129*
Edema, cerebral, in toxemia, 340
  peripheral, in pregnancy, 305, 338
Education status, risk and, 269–270
EE_2. See *Ethinyl estradiol (EE_2)*.
Eicosapentaenoic acid, in toxemia, 342
Eisenmenger's syndrome, in pregnancy, 330t, 335
Ejection fraction, diabetes and, 210
  exercise and, 37
  gender differences in, 108–110, *109*, *110*
  in pregnancy, 314
  postinfarction, 31–32
Elastin, hormones and, 108
Elderly. See also *Age*.
  hypertrophic cardiomyopathy of, 111–112
Electrocardiography (ECG), exercise, 36, 38
  in mitral valve prolapse diagnosis, 120–121
  in peripartum cardiomyopathy, 345

Electrocardiography (ECG) *(Continued)*
  in pregnancy, 319–320, 319t
Embolism, amniotic fluid, pulmonary hypertension and, 350–351
  pulmonary, in pregnancy, 239
Employment, 6–7, *7*
  after CABG surgery, 52
  after PTCA, 51–52
  cardiovascular risks from, 270–273
    by occupation, 271–272
    multiple roles and, 272–273
Endarterectomy, carotid, 140, 141–142
Endocarditis, infective, mitral valve involvement in, 127
  mitral valve prolapse and, 122–123, 123t
Endomyocardial biopsy, in peripartum cardiomyopathy, 346–347, 348–349
Endothelium, vascular, animal studies on, 295–296, 298
  coagulation and, 234–235, *234*, 234t
  fibrinolysis and, 233, *233*
  in pulmonary hypertension, 350
EPESE (Established Populations for Epidemiologic Study of the Elderly), on smoking, 219
Equine estrogens, 163
Erythromelalgia, 244
Essential hypertension, 68–69. See also *Hypertension*.
  management of, 91–92
Established Populations for Epidemiologic Study of the Elderly (EPESE), on smoking, 219
Estradiol (E_2), in hormonal replacement therapy, 163, 163t, *164*
  animal studies on, 295–296, *296*
  menopause and, 157, *157*
  menstrual cycle and, 156
  production of, 155–156
  synthetic, 159–160, *159*
Estrogen(s), animal studies on. See *Animal models*.
  aortic dissection and, 354
  cardiovascular effects of, 72, 107–108, 157–158, 167–169, *168–170*, 168t
    on blood pressure, 76, 77, 95, 164, *165*
    on carbohydrate intolerance, 164–165
    on coagulation, 165, *166*, 236–237, 236t
    on lipoproteins, 166–167, *166*, *167*, 168, 180–182
  in hormonal replacement therapy, 163–164, 163t, *164*, 237
    dosage of, 171
  menopause and, 156–158, *157*
  production of, 155–156
  prostacyclin and, 168–169, *169*
  synthetic, 159–160, *159*
  transdermal, 237
Estrogen replacement therapy. See *Hormonal replacement therapy*.
Estrone (E_1), 156
  in hormonal replacement therapy, 163, 163t, *164*
  menopause and, 157, *157*
Ethinyl estradiol (EE_2), 159–160, *159*
  animal studies of, 285–286
Ethynodiol diacetate, 160
  animal studies of, 285–286
European Working Party Study, on hypertension, 84t, 86
Evans County Study, on hypertension, 80
Exercise, 253–267
  adaptive hypertrophy and, 112, 255–256
  blood pressure and, 256–257
  body weight and, 257–258
  CHD and, 254
  diabetes and, 207, 211, 258–259

Exercise *(Continued)*
  during pregnancy, 314–318
    benefits of, 314, 314t
    cardiovascular effects of, 315–316
      on fetus, 316
    guidelines for, 317–318, 317t
    pregnancy outcome and, 317–318
    risks of, 315, 315t
  dynamic, 255
  gender differences in response to, 37, 253–254
  glucose tolerance and, 258–259
  injury from, 262–263
  lipoprotein levels and, 183, 259–261
  obesity and, 199, 257–258
  rehabilitative. See *Exercise therapy*.
  resistive, 255–256
  uterine blood flow and, 316
Exercise tests, 36–37, 38
  ECG, 36, 38
  echocardiographic, 37
  gender differences in, 37, 108–110, *110*
  in pregnancy, 320
  radionuclide, 36–37
  recommendations for, 38
Exercise therapy, 261–262
  after CABG surgery, 52
  after stroke, 261
  in congestive heart failure, 261
  in hypertension, 90
  in peripheral arterial disease, 261–262
  postinfarction, 30, 32–33, 56, 261

Factor X, estrogen and, 165, *166*
Familial lipoprotein disorders, 179, 180, 180t
Fasting glucose levels, 192t
  exercise and, 258
Fat, body, distribution of, animal studies of, 292, *293*, 299
    cardiovascular risk and, 197–198, *198*
    diabetes and, 207
    hyperinsulinemia and, 200–201, *200*
    hypertension and, 199
    lipoprotein levels and, 183, 200
    obesity definition and, 195, 197
  dietary, hypertension and, 91
Fetal loss, autoimmune disorders and, 243
  radiation exposure and, 323
  thrombocythemia and, 244
Fetus, aortic dissection and, 354
  drugs and, 331t, 334, 342–343
  exercise and, 315, 316–317
  radiation and, 322–323, 322t
Fibrillation, atrial, in pregnancy, 333
    stroke and, 141, 142
Fibrin, 232, *232*
Fibrinogen, 232, *232*, 241
  abnormalities and, 240
  in complicated pregnancy, 238
  in uncomplicated pregnancy, 235, 241
Fibrinolysis, 233–234, *233*, *234*
  defective, 241
  diabetes and, 209
  in pregnancy, 235, 238
  oral contraceptives and, 236
Fluoroscopy, in coronary artery calcification, 37–38
Foam cells, 180

Follicle-stimulating hormone, 154–156, *154*, *155*
  menopause and, 156, *157*
Follistatin, 154–155, *154*
Framingham Heart Study, on anger, 273
  on angina, 27
  on anxiety, 276
  on CHD, 26–27, 26t, 80
  on claudication, 144t
  on congestive heart failure, 78–79, 110
  on diabetes, 207, 208, 210
  on left ventricular mass, 105–106, *106*
  on mitral valve prolapse, 119
  on myocardial infarction, 28–29
  on obesity, *202*
  on risk factors, 158, 158t
  on smoking, 219, 220
  on stroke, 81
  on sudden death, 33
  on Type A behavior, 26–27
Furosemide, in pregnancy, 331t

Gender bias, in access, 33–35, 44–45, 57
  in referral for revascularization, 33–35, 44
  in research, 3, 10, 43–44
Gender differences, animal models of, 283–284, 284t
  cardiac, biochemical, 107–108
    in adaptation to overload, 110–112, *111*
    in size, 105–107, *106*
    in ventricular performance, 108–113, *109–111*
  in CABG surgery, 49–51, 49t, 51t
  in CHD, 3–4, 6t, 7, 25–27, 26t
  in compliance, 17, 17t
  in health care utilization, 8–9
  in health perceptions, 10–13
  in lipoprotein physiology, 180–182, *181*, 187
  in mitral valve prolapse, 119, 121–123, 122t, 123t
  in morbidity and mortality, 5–10, 8t, 25t
  in patient-physician relationship, 4–5, 13–14
  in PTCA, 46–49, 47t
  in peripheral vascular disease, 146–147
  in response to exercise, 37, 253–254
  in rheumatic heart disease, 125t
  in risk factors, 5–8
  in smoking cessation, 222–223
  in thrombolysis outcome, 52–54, 53t, 54t
  in treatment, 9
  in valvular heart disease, 118, 119, 121–123, 122t, 123t, 125t
Genetic factors, in diabetes, 206–207
  in hypertension, 69–70
  in lipoprotein disorders, 179, 180, 180t
  in mitral valve prolapse, 118–119
  in myopathies, 113
  in obesity, 199
  in thromboembolic disease, 239–240, 240t
Gestational diabetes, 194–195, 194t
Glucagon, 192–193, 193t
Glucocorticoid hormones, 192–193
Gluconeogenesis, 192–193, *192*, 192t, 193t
Glucose, 192–193, *192*, 192t
Glucose tolerance, estrogens and, 164–165
  exercise and, 258–259
  impaired, 194, 194t
    CHD and, 209
    epidemiology of, 206
    obesity and, 200–201, *200*

Glucose tolerance *(Continued)*
  oral contraceptives and, 161
Glyceryl trinitrate, in pulmonary hypertension of pregnancy, 352
Glycogenolysis, 192–193, *192*, 192t, 193t
Granulosa cells, 154–156
Growth factors, hypertension and, 71–72, *72*

HDFP (Hypertension Detection and Follow-up Program) Cooperative Group, 64, 83–85, 84t
  pooled results of, 88
HDL (high-density lipoprotein). See under *Lipoprotein(s)*.
Health, perception of, 10–13, *12*
Health Belief Model, 11, *12*
Health care services, access to, 33–35
  utilization of, 8–9
Health promotion and disease prevention, adherence to regimens in, 17–18, 18t
  emphasis on, 16–17, 17t
Health risk factors. See *Risk factors*.
Heart. See also *Cardiac* entries.
  diabetes and, 209–211
  exercise and, 255–256
  hormones and, 107–108
  in toxemia, 340
  obesity and, 203–205
  pregnancy and, 306–308, 307t, 311–314, 311t, *312*, *313*
  rupture of, 31, 112
  size of, 105–107, *106*
    in pregnancy, 313–314
Heart failure, congestive. See *Congestive heart failure*.
Heart rate, animal studies of, 291–292
  during labor, 318
  exercise and, 255
  fetal, exercise and, 316
  in pregnancy, 307
    with exercise, 315
  postpartum, 319
Heart sounds, in pregnancy, 306
Heart transplantation, in peripartum cardiomyopathy, 349
Heart valve disease. See *Valvular heart disease*.
HELLP (hemolysis, elevated liver enzymes, low platelets) syndrome, 93, 238, 340
Hemoglobinuria, paroxysmal nocturnal, in pregnancy, 239
Hemolysis, elevated liver enzymes, low platelets (HELLP) syndrome, 93, 238, 340
Hemoptysis, mitral stenosis and, 125
Hemorrhage, subarachnoid, in young women, 139
  smoking and, 221
  thrombolytic therapy and, 54
Hemostasis, 231–251
  abnormalities of, 241–245
    autoimmune, 242–244, 243t
    inherited, 239–240, 240t
    malignancy and, 244–245
    treatment of, 245–247
  fibrinolysis and, 233–234, *233*, *234*
    defective, 241
  hormonal replacement therapy and, 237
  in pregnancy, 235–237
    complicated, 237–239, 240, 340
  oral contraceptives and, 235–237, 236t
  primary, 232

Hemostasis *(Continued)*
  secondary, 232, *232*
  thromboembolic disease and, 239–240
  vascular endothelium and, 234–235, *234*, 234t
Heparin, 55, 247
  in pregnancy, 239, 331t, 334, 348
  in pulmonary hypertension of pregnancy, 351–352
High-density lipoprotein (HDL). See under *Lipoprotein(s)*.
Homemakers, cardiovascular risk factors among, 270–271, 276
Homocyst(e)ine, 242
Homocystinuria, 242
Hormonal replacement therapy, 45–46, 163–171
  animal studies on, 294–296, *296*, 299
  anticoagulants and, 247
  cardioprotection by, 167–169, *168–170*, 168t
  conflicting information on, 10
  diabetes and, 193
  dosage for, 171
  estrogen effects in, on blood pressure, 165, *165*
    on carbohydrate intolerance, 164–165
    on coagulation, 165, *166*, 237
    on lipoproteins, 166–167, *166*, *167*, 168, 185, 187, 237
    transdermal, 237
  pharmacokinetics of, 163–164, 163t, *164*
  progestins in, 169–171, 171t
  stroke and, 141
Hormones, 153–173. See also specific hormone.
  aortic dissection and, 354
  carbohydrate metabolism and, 192–193
  cardiovascular effects of, 157–158
  menopause and, 157, *157*
  ovary and, 153–156, *154*, *155*
  perimenopausal, 156
  therapeutic. See *Hormonal replacement therapy*; *Oral contraceptives*.
Hostility, 273–275
  stress and, 275
Hydralazine, in pregnancy, 331t
  in pregnancy complicated by cardiomyopathy, 348
  in toxemia of pregnancy, 94, 343
Hypercholesterolemia, familial, 179, 180t
  treatment of, 51, 185–187
  hypertension and, 80
Hyperinsulinemia, CHD and, 201
  hypertension and, 72–73, 200, 201
  obesity and, 200–201, *200*
Hypertension, 63–103
  age and, 63–66, *65*
  animal models of, 69, 73–77, *74*, *76*
  aortic dissection and, 353
  as risk factor, 77–83
    for CHD, 79–81
    for congestive heart failure, 78–79
    for death, 78, *78*
    for peripheral vascular disease, 82–83
    for renal failure, 79
    for stroke, 81–82, 140–141
  autonomic function and, 70
  cardiac hypertrophy and, 72, 110–111, *111*
  classification of, 64t
  diabetes and, 208
  diagnosis of, 88–89, 89t
    in pregnancy, 93
  economic impact of, 67–68
  epidemiology of, 63–66, *68*

Hypertension *(Continued)*
    essential, 68–69
        management of, 68–69, 91–92
    exercise and, 256–257
    genetic factors in, 69–70
    growth factors and, 71–72, *71*
    hemodynamics of, 70–71
    hormonal replacement therapy and, 95, 164, *165*
    in pregnancy, 92–95, 337, 344–345
        chronic, 94–95, 344–345
        coagulation abnormalities and, 237–238, 341–342
        toxemia and. See *Toxemia.*
        transient, 95
        treatment of, 94–95, 345
    incidence of, *67*
    insulin resistance and, 72–73
    isolated systolic, 64–65, 64t
    obesity and, 199–200, 201
    oncogenes and, 72
    oral contraceptives and, 92, 160
    prevalence of, *66*
    pulmonary, of pregnancy, 349–353
        clinical features of, 350
        pathophysiology of, 350–351
        prognosis in, 349, 352
        treatment of, 351–353
    renal sodium handling and, 70
    treatment of, 89–92
        clinical trials of, 83–88, 84t
        nonpharmacologic, 89–92
        other risk factors and, 95
        pharmacologic, 92
        quality of life and, 95–96
    trends in, 66–67
Hypertension Detection and Follow-up Program (HDFP) Cooperative Group, 64, 83–85, 84t
    pooled results of, 88
Hypertriglyceridemia, estrogen and, 167
    obesity and, 200
Hypertrophy, cardiac, concentric, exercise and, 255–256
    gender differences in, 110–113, *111*
    hypertension and, 72, 110–111, *111*
Hypotension, postexercise, 256
Hypoxia, right ventricular hypertrophy and, 112–113

Immunoglobulins, antibodies to, thrombosis and, 243
Immunosuppressive agents, in peripartum cardiomyopathy, 348–349
Impaired glucose tolerance, 194, 194t
    CHD and, 209
    epidemiology of, 206
    obesity and, 200–201, *200*
Impedance cardiography, cardiac output measurement by, 312–313
Infarction, myocardial. See *Myocardial infarction.*
Infective endocarditis, mitral valve in, 127
    mitral valve prolapse and, 122–123, 123t
Inheritance. See *Genetic factors.*
Inhibin, 154–155, *154*
    menopause and, 156
Inotropic agents, in peripartum cardiomyopathy, 348
    in pulmonary hypertension of pregnancy, 352
Insulin, carbohydrate metabolism and, 192–193, 193t
    exercise and, 258
    pregnancy and, 193
    resistance to, 193–194

Insulin *(Continued)*
    hypertension and, 72–73
    obesity and, 200–201, *200*
Insulin-dependent diabetes mellitus, 195, 206. See also *Diabetes mellitus.*
Intermittent claudication, 143–144, 144t
    exercise and, 262
    hypertension and, 82–83
Internal mammary artery grafts, in CABG surgery, 50
Ischemia, myocardial, 28
    silent, 33
        in diabetes, 209
ISIS-2 (Second International Study of Infarct Survival), 52–53
    on aspirin therapy, 55
Isoproterenol, in pregnancy, 331t
    in pulmonary hypertension of pregnancy, 352

Jogging, during pregnancy, 318
    lipoprotein levels and, 259

Ketoacidosis, 195
Kidney, blood flow to, in pregnancy, 309
    hypertension and, 70
    in pregnancy, 344
    in toxemia, 339–340
    sodium handling by, 70
Kidney failure, hypertension and, 79

Labetolol, in pregnancy, 331t
    complicated by aortic dissection, 354
    in toxemia of pregnancy, 342
Labor, anesthesia in, 318–319
    hemodynamic changes during, 318
    heparin and, 334
    mitral stenosis and, 333
    peripartum cardiomyopathy and, 348
    pulmonary hypertension and, 352
Lactation, blood flow and, 309
    cardiovascular drugs and, 331t
LDL (low-density lipoprotein). See under *Lipoprotein(s).*
Left ventricle, function of, diastolic, 32
    gender differences in, 108–111, *109*, *110*
    in pregnancy, 314
    peripartum cardiomyopathy and, 348
    postinfarction, 31–32
    hypertrophy of, adaptive, 112
        gender differences in, 110–112, *111*
    size of, 105–106, *106*
Leukemia, chronic myelogenous, 244
Levonorgestrel, 160, *287*
Lidocaine, in pregnancy, 331t
Life Change Event Study, on suppressed anger, 273–274
Lifestyle. See *Risk factors.*
Lipoprotein A, 182, 241–242
Lipoprotein(s), 175–189
    animal studies on, 296–298, *297*, *299*
    apoproteins in outer shell of, 175–176, 177t, 178–179
    atherogenesis and, 180, 182
    body fat distribution and, 183, 200
    classification of, 175–176, *176*
    diabetes and, 183–185, 207–208

Lipoprotein(s) *(Continued)*
　diet and, 182–183
　disorders of, 179–180, 180t
　　genetic, 179
　　secondary, 179–180
　　treatment of, 185–187, 186t
　estrogens and, 166–167, *166*, *167*, 168, 180–182
　exercise and, 183, 259–261
　function of, 175
　gender and, 180–182, *181*, 187
　high-density, 175, *176*
　　metabolism of, 178–179
　hormonal replacement therapy and, 166–167, *166*, *167*, 168, 185, 187, 237
　hostility and, 274–275
　hyperinsulinemia and, 201
　low-density, 175, *176*
　　metabolism of, 178
　menopause and, 158, *158*
　　animal studies of, 292, *293*, 294
　metabolism of, 176, *177*, 178–179
　normal levels of, 186t
　obesity and, 200
　oral contraceptives and, 162, *162*, 185
　　animal studies of, 285–286, *286*, *287*
　progestins and, 170–171, 171t
　remnant, metabolism of, 178
　smoking and, 221
　very low density, 175, *176*
　　remnant, metabolism of, 178
　weight loss and, 183
Lipoprotein lipase, exercise and, 259
Liver, glucose metabolism and, 192, *192*, 192t
　in toxemia, 340
　lipoproteins and, 176, *177*, 178–179
Low-density lipoprotein (LDL). See under *Lipoprotein(s)*.
Low-yield cigarettes, nicotine and carbon monoxide levels in, 220–221
Lung transplantation, in pulmonary hypertension, 352–353
Lupus anticoagulant, 243–244
Luteinizing hormone, 154, *154*, 155
　menopause and, *157*
Lysosomal enzymes, 107

Macaca fascicularis, 283–284. See also *Animal models*.
Magnesium sulfate, in toxemia, 94, 343
Magnesium supplementation, in hypertension, 91
Magnetic resonance imaging (MRI), in pregnancy, 320–321
Mammary souffles, 306–307
Marfan's syndrome, 128, 130–131
　management of, 131–132
　natural history of, 130
　pregnancy and, 130–131, 131t, 332–333, 353
Medical Research Council Trial, on hypertension, 86–87
　pooled results of, 88
Medications. See specific agents or classes.
Menopause, 156–157
　animal studies of, 289, *290*, 291, 292, *293*, 294
　average age at, 156
　blood pressure and, 65
　cardiovascular disease and, 27, 157–158
　hormonal changes at, 156–157, *157*
　lipoproteins and, 181

Menopause *(Continued)*
　transition to, 156
Menstrual cycle, 155–156, *155*
　lipoproteins and, 181
Methyldopa, in pregnancy, 94, 95, 342
Mexilitene, in pregnancy, 331t
Microangiopathy, thrombotic, in pregnancy, 239
MILIS (Multicenter Investigation of Limitation of Infarct Size) Study, 29–30, 32
　on diabetes, 210
Minnesota Heart Surveys, on hypertension, 67
Mitral valve, calcification of, 125–126
　anular, 127
　endocarditis involving, 127
　prolapse of, 118–124
　　age and, 119
　　complications of, 122–123, 123t
　　diagnosis of, 123–124
　　　erroneous, 120–121
　　gender and, 119, 121–123, 122t, 123t
　　inheritance of, 118–119
　　management of, 124, 124t
　　mitral regurgitation and, 122, 123t
　　syndrome of, 119–121, 120t
　rheumatic disease of, 125–126
　stenosis of, 125–126
　　in pregnancy, 333
　systemic lupus erythematosus and, 127
Morbidity, gender differences in, 5–10, 8t, 25t
　hypertension and, 85
　stroke and, 138–139
Mortality rates. See *Death rates*.
MRI (magnetic resonance imaging), in pregnancy, 320–321
Multicenter Investigation of Limitation of Infarct Size (MILIS) Study, 29–30, 32
　on diabetes, 210
Murmurs, in pregnancy, 306–307
Muscular dystrophies, 113
Musculoskeletal injury, exercise-induced, 262–263
　in pregnancy, 314–315
Myeloproliferative syndromes, 244
Myocardial infarction, 28–33
　absent coronary lesions, 30–31
　aspirin therapy and, 246–247
　by sex, 26t, 52
　cardiac rupture and, 31, 112
　depression after, 276
　diabetes and, 209–210
　hypertension and, 80
　in pregnancy, 329–330, 332
　mortality from, 29–30, 52
　non–Q wave, 29
　obesity and, 202–203, *203*, *204*
　oral contraceptives and, 32, 161–162
　prognosis after, 28–30, 38–39, 57
　psychosocial factors after, 32–33
　rehabilitation after, 56, 261
　silent, 29
　treatment after. See specific modality.
　Type A behavior and, 276
　ventricular arrhythmias and, 31
Myocardial ischemia, 28
　silent, 33
　　in diabetes, 209
Myocarditis, peripartum cardiomyopathy and, 346–347, 348–349
Myocytes, size differences and, 106

Myosin, 107

National Health and Nutrition Examination Survey
 (NHANES), on blood pressure, 63–64, 65, 67
 on body weight, 197t
 on hypertension mortality, 78, *78*
 on obesity, *198*
Necrosis, cystic medial, aortic dissection and, 354
Neurotransmitters, testosterone and, 74–75
NHANES (National Health and Nutrition Examination
 Survey), on blood pressure, 63–64, 65, 67
 on body weight, 197t
 on hypertension mortality, 78, *78*
 on obesity, *198*
Nicotine replacement therapy, 224–225
 effectiveness of, 223
 weight gain and, 224
Nifedipine, 343
 in pulmonary hypertension, 351
Nigeria, peripartum cardiomyopathy in, 346
Nitrates, 45
 in pregnancy, 331t, 343
  complicated by aortic dissection, 354
 in pulmonary hypertension of pregnancy, 352
Noninsulin-dependent diabetes mellitus, 195, *196*, 206.
 See also *Diabetes mellitus.*
 prevention and treatment of, 211
Noninvasive tests, recommendations for, 38
Norepinephrine, hypertension and, 75
Norethindrone, 160
Norethisterone, *287*
Norgestrel, animal studies of, 285–286
Nurses, cardiovascular risks among, 271–272
Nurses' Health Study, on aspirin therapy, 44, 246–247
 on diabetes, 207, 208
 on obesity, 203, *203, 204*, 207
 on smoking, 219, 220, 221

Obesity, 195, 197–205
 atherosclerosis and, 201–203
 body fat distribution and, 197–198, *198*
  animal studies of, 292, *293*, 299
 cardiac effects of, 203–205
 CHD and, 201–205, *202–204*
 defined, 195, 197, 197t
 diabetes and, 195, 197–198, 207
 diet and, 199
 exercise and, 199, 257–258
 genetic factors in, 199
 hypertension and, 199–200, 201
 insulin resistance and, 200–201, *200*
 lipoproteins and, 200
 prevalence of, 198, *198*
 prevention of, 205
 revascularization procedures and, 205
 syndrome X and, 201
 treatment of, 205
Occupation, multiple roles and, 272–273
 risk and, 271–272
Oncogenes, hypertension and, 72
Oral contraceptives, 158–162
 action of, 159–160
 animal studies on, 285–286, *286, 287*, 298
 carbohydrate intolerance and, 161

Oral contraceptives *(Continued)*
 composition of, 159–160, *159*
 hypertension and, 92, 160
 lipoprotein levels and, 162, *162*, 185
 myocardial infarction and, 32, 161–162
 smoking and, 162, *163*, 222, 236
 thrombosis and, 235–237, 236t
  arterial, 161–162
  venous, 142, 160–161
Ovary(ies), function of, 153–156, *154, 155*
 animal studies of, 289, *290*, 291
Oxygen therapy, in pulmonary hypertension, 352

Palmaz-Schatz intracoronary stent, 48
Palpitations, in pregnancy, 305
 mitral valve prolapse syndrome and, 120t, 121
Pancreas, glucagon production by, 193
 in toxemia, 340
Paroxysmal nocturnal hemoglobinuria, in pregnancy, 239
Partial thromboplastin time (PTT), heparin monitoring
 by, 334
Paternalism, 4–5
Patient Review, 15–16, 16t
Patient-physician relationship, 4–5, 13–16
 communication in, 14–15, 15t
 compliance and, 17–18, 18t
 patient's perspective on, 15–16, 16t
Percutaneous transluminal coronary angioplasty (PTCA),
 complications of, 46, 48
 coronary artery size and, 48
 emergency, 46–47, 56
 gender bias and, 33–35
 gender differences and, 46–49, 47t
 long-term outcome of, 48–49
 obesity and, 205
 rehabilitation after, 51–52
Perfusion studies, pharmacologic radionuclide, 37
Peripartum cardiomyopathy, 345–349
 clinical features of, 345–346
 pathophysiology of, 346–347
 treatment of, 347–349
Peripheral edema, in pregnancy, 305, 338
Peripheral vascular disease, 142–147
 arterial, 143–147
  economic implications of, 146
  isolated small-vessel, 146
  mortality from, 145, 145t
  natural history of, 144–145
  prevalence of, 143–144, *144*, 144t
  treatment of, 145–146
   exercise as, 262
 hypertension and, 82–83
 smoking and, 221
 venous, 142–143, 142t, *143*
  oral contraceptives and, 160–161
Personality factor(s), 273–277
 anxiety as, 275–276
 hostility as, 273–275
PET (positron emission tomography), in pregnancy, 322
Phenytoin, in pregnancy, 331t
Phospholipase C, 72
Physical activity. See *Exercise.*
Physical examination, cardiovascular, in pregnancy, 306–
 307, 311t
 in hypertension work-up, 88–89, 89t
Physician, female, 14

Physician (Continued)
    gender bias and, 9, 13
Physician-patient relationship, 4–5, 13–16
    communication in, 14–15, 15t
    compliance and, 17–18, 18t
    patient's perspective on, 15–16, 16t
Pigeons, research using, 284, 295
Pigs, research using, 284
Pitocin, hemodynamic effects of, 319
Pituitary hormones, menopause and, 157, *157*
Placenta, autoimmune disorders and, 243
    in toxemia, 339, 341
Plasma, in pregnancy, 308–309, *309*
Plasminogen, 233, *233*, *234*
    abnormalities of, 240
    lipoprotein A and, 241
    smoking and, 221
Plasminogen activators, 233–234
    in pregnancy, 235
    in pregnancy with complications, 238
    inhibitors of, 233, 241
Platelets, abnormalities of, 244
    activated, 234–235
    aspirin and, 245–246
    diabetes and, 209
    hemostasis and, 232–233
    in pregnancy, 235
    in pregnancy with complications, 238, 240
    smoking and, 221
    ticlopidine and, 246
Polycythemia vera, 244
Positron emission tomography (PET), in pregnancy, 322
Postpartum period. See also *Peripartum cardiomyopathy*.
    hemodynamics in, 319
Potassium supplementation, in hypertension, 91
Prazosin, in pregnancy, 343
Prednisone, in peripartum cardiomyopathy, 348
Preeclampsia. See *Toxemia*.
Pregnancy, animal studies of, 292, *293*, 299
    anticoagulants in, 247, 331t, 334–335
    aortic dissection in, 353–354
    arrhythmias in, 319, 320, 332
    autoimmune disorders and, 243
    carbohydrate metabolism in, 193
    cardiomyopathy of, 345–349
        clinical features of, 345–346
        pathophysiology of, 346–347
        treatment of, 347–349
    cardiovascular drugs in, 331t
    diabetes and, 194–195, 194t
    diagnostic testing in, 319–322
        cardiac catheterization for, 321–322
        echocardiographic, 320
        electrocardiographic, 319–320, 319t
        MRI for, 320–321
        radiographic, 321–322
        stress test for, 320
        systolic time interval on, 320
    exercise during, 314–318
        benefits of, 314, 314t
        cardiovascular effects of, 315–316
            on fetus, 316
        guidelines for, 317–318, 317t
        pregnancy outcome and, 316–317
        risks of, 315, 315t
        uterine blood flow and, 316
    hemostasis in, 235
        abnormalities of, 237–239

Pregnancy (Continued)
        factor deficiencies and, 240
    hypertension in, 92–95, 337, 344–345
        chronic, 94–95, 344–345
        coagulation abnormalities and, 237–238, 341–342
        pulmonary, 349–353
            clinical features of, 350
            pathophysiology of, 350–351
            prognosis in, 349, 352
            treatment of, 351–353
        toxemia and. See *Toxemia*.
        transient, 95
        treatment of, 94–95, 345
    lipoproteins and, 181–182
    Marfan's syndrome and, 130–131, 131t, 332–333, 353
    mitral stenosis in, 123, 333
    myocardial infarction in, 329–330, 332
    normal, 305–314
        blood pressure in, 307–308, *308*
            central, 311t
        blood volume in, 308–309, *309*
        cardiac output in, 311–313, *312*, *313*
        cardiovascular examination in, 306–307, 311t
        circulatory changes in, 307t
        heart rate in, 307
        heart size in, 313–314
        regional blood flow in, 309, *310*, 311
        symptoms and signs in, 305–306, 306t
        vascular resistance in, 311t, 313
    paroxysmal nocturnal hemoglobinuria in, 239
    prognosis of cardiac conditions in, 329, 330t
    prosthetic heart valves and, 334–335
    radiation exposure in, 322–323, 322t
    thrombocythemia in, 244
    thrombotic microangiopathy in, 239
    toxemia of. See *Toxemia*.
    valvular heart disease in, 239, 330t, 333
Preventive medicine, 16–18, 44
    compliance and, 17–18, 18t
    emphasis on, 16–17, 17t
    future of, 18–19
    in diabetes, 211
    in hypertension, 89–92
    in obesity, 205
    levels of, 17t
    research on, 44
Procainamide, in pregnancy, 331t
Prochaska Readiness for Change Model, smoking cessation and, 225, *226*
Progesterone, animal studies on, 295–296, *296*
    cardiovascular effects of, 170–171
    menstrual cycle and, *155*, 156
Progestin(s), cardiovascular effects of, 170–171, 171t
    in hormonal replacement therapy, 169–171, 171t
        dosage of, 171
    in oral contraceptives, 159–160, *159*
        animal studies of, 285–286
Prolactin, carbohydrate metabolism and, 193
    menopause and, 157, *157*
Prolapse, mitral valve. See *Mitral valve, prolapse of*.
Propranolol, in pregnancy, 331t
    postinfarction, 55
Prostacyclin, estrogen and, 168–169, *169*
    in pregnancy, 238
        complicated, 339, 340–341
    peripheral arterial disease and, 146
Prostaglandin(s), estrogen and, 169, *169*
    hemodynamic effects of, 319

Prostaglandin(s) *(Continued)*
  in pulmonary hypertension of pregnancy, 352
  toxemia and, 338–339, 340–341
Prosthetic heart valves, pregnancy and, 334–335
Protein C, 233, *233*, 234
  deficiency of, 240
Protein S, 236
  deficiency of, 240
  oral contraceptives and, 236–237
Prothrombin, 232, *232*
Psychoemotional factor(s), 273–277
  anxiety as, 275–276
  depression as, 275–276
  hostility as, 273–275
  in mitral valve prolapse syndrome, 119–121, 120t, 122t
  postinfarction, 32–33
PTCA. See *Percutaneous transluminal coronary angioplasty (PTCA)*.
PTT (partial thromboplastin time), heparin monitoring by, 334
Pulmonary embolism, in pregnancy, 239
Pulmonary hypertension, in pregnancy, clinical features of, 350
  pathophysiology of, 350–351
  prognosis in, 349, 352
  treatment of, 351–353
Pulmonary vascular resistance, in pregnancy, 311t, 313

Quality of life, antihypertensive agents and, 95–96
Quetelet index, CHD and, *203, 204*
Quinidine, in pregnancy, 331t

Rabbits, research using, 284, 285–286, *287*, 297, 298
Radiation exposure, in pregnancy, 321–323
Radiography, in pregnancy, 321–322
Radionuclide studies, exercise, 36, 38
  in pregnancy, 321–323
  pharmacologic perfusion, 37
  ventriculographic, exercise, 36–37
    in pregnancy, 321
Randomized Trial of Treatment of Hypertension in Elderly Patients in Primary Care, 84t, 86
Red blood cells, in pregnancy, 308–309, *309*
Regurgitation, aortic valve, 126–127
  mitral valve, in prolapse, 122, 123t
    in rheumatic disease, 126
  valvular, in pregnancy, 330t, 333
Rehabilitation. See also *Exercise therapy*.
  after CABG surgery, 52
  after myocardial infarction, 56
  after PTCA, 51–52
Relaxation techniques, hypertension and, 91
Renal. See *Kidney* entries.
Renin-angiotensin system, androgens and, 75–76, *76*
  in pregnancy, 308–309
  toxemia and, 338–339
Research. See also *Animal models*.
  gender bias in, 3, 10, 43–44
Restenosis, after PTCA, 48–49
Resuscitation, in pregnancy, 332
Rheumatic heart disease, 124–127
  aortic valve in, 126–127
  epidemiology of, 124–125
  gender predominances in, 125t

Rheumatic heart disease *(Continued)*
  in pregnancy, 333
  mitral valve in, 125–126
Right ventricle, hypertrophy of, 112–113
  pulmonary hypertension and, 350
Risk factors, cholesterol-lowering regimes and, 186
  employment status and, 270–271
  exercise and, 254
  for deep venous thrombosis, 142, 240t
  for peripheral arterial disease, 145–146
  for stroke, 140–141
  gender differences in, 35
  health differences and, 5–8
  hematologic, 240–241
  hypertension as. See *Hypertension*.
Running, during pregnancy, 318
  lipoprotein levels and, 259
Rupture, cardiac, 31, 112

Sales workers, cardiovascular risks among, 271
Salt restriction, in hypertension, 90, 345
SAVE (Survival and Ventricular Enlargement Study), 35, 45
  on diabetes, 210
Scintigraphya. See *Radionuclide studies*.
Second International Study of Infarct Survival (ISIS-2), 52–53
  on aspirin therapy, 55
Sex differences. See *Gender differences*.
Sex hormones. See *Hormones*.
Sexual function, antihypertensive agents and, 95–96
Shunts, in pregnancy, 330t, 335
Single photon emission computed tomography (SPECT), exercise, 36
Skeletal abnormalities, mitral valve prolapse syndome and, 120t, 121
Smoking, 217–229
  cessation of, 222–225
    CHD risk and, 220
    peripheral vascular disease and, 221
    readiness for, 225, *226*
    strategies for, 223, 224–225
    stroke risk and, 221
    trends in, 222–223
    weight gain and, 223–224
  CHD and, 219–220, 221–222
  employment status and, 270–271
  epidemiology of, 218–219, *218*, 218t
  hypertension and, 91
  noncigarette, 222
  of low-yield cigarettes, 220–221
  oral contraceptives and, 161, *163*, 222, 236
  peripheral vascular disease and, 221
  social factors and, 223, 225–226
  stroke and, 221
  weight and, 198–199, 223–224
Social factors, animal studies of, 286, 288–289, *288*, 289t, 291–292, *291*, 299
  health risks and, 6–8, *7*
  patient-physician communication on, 13
  smoking and, 223, 225–226
Social support, 277–279
  animal studies of, 291–292, *291*, 299
Socioeconomic factors, 269–270. See also *Employment*.
  health care utilization and, 8–9
Sodium, renal handling of, 70

Index **373**

Sodium nitroprusside, in pregnancy, 331t
  in pregnancy complicated by aortic dissection, 354
SPECT (single photon emission computed tomography), exercise, 36
Sphygmomanometry, 88–89
Stenosis, aortic, 128
  mitral, 125–126
  valvular, in pregnancy, 330t
Stent, intracoronary, 48
Streptokinase, 53
Stress, animal studies of, 286, 288–289, *288*, 289t, *290*, 291
  hostility and, 275
  hypertension and, 70, 91
  multiple roles and, 272–273
  occupational, 271–272
Stress tests. See *Exercise tests*.
Stroke, 137–142
  antiphospholipid syndrome and, 242–243
  aspirin therapy and, 246, 247
  autoimmune disorders and, 243
  carotid disease and, 139–140
  diagnosis of, 139
  disability from, 141
  economic impact of, 141
  epidemiology of, 137–139, *138–140*
  hemorrhagic, 141
  hypertension and, 81–82, 140–141
  ischemic, 140–141
  prevention of, 141–142
    exercise in, 261
  risk factors for, 140–141
    homocyst(e)ine levels as, 242
    smoking habits as, 221
  ticlopidine and, 246–247
Subarachnoid hemorrhage, in young women, 139
  smoking and, 221
Sudden death, 33
  by gender, 26t
  exercise and, 262
  mitral valve prolapse and, 122
  pulmonary hypertension of pregnancy and, 350
Survival and Ventricular Enlargement Study (SAVE), 35, 45
  on diabetes, 210
Swedish Trial in Old Patients with Hypertension, 84t, 87
Swimming, weight reduction and, 257
Syndrome X, 28, 46
  obesity and, 201
Systemic lupus erythematosus, thrombosis and, 242–243
  valvular heart disease and, 127
Systemic vascular resistance, in pregnancy, 311t, 313
Systolic Hypertension in the Elderly Program, 84t, 87
Systolic time interval recording, in pregnancy, 320

Tachycardias, in pregnancy, 332
TAMI (Thrombolysis and Angioplasty After Myocardial Infarction) trials, 54, 55t
Technetium, 321
Teratogenicity. See *Fetus*.
Testosterone, aspirin and, 246
  cardiac effects of, 107–108
  hypertension and, 73–77, *74*, *76*
  menopause and, 157, *157*
  menstrual cycle and, 156
Thallium scintigraphy, exercise, 36

Thallium scintigraphy *(Continued)*
  in pregnancy, 320, 321
Thiazides, in pregnancy, 331t
Thrombin, 232–234, *232*
Thrombocythemia, 244
Thrombocytopenia, heparin-induced, 247, 334
Thrombolysis and Angioplasty After Myocardial Infarction (TAMI) trials, 54, 55t
Thrombolysis in Myocardial Infarction (TIMI) trial, 54
Thrombolytic therapy, 30, 52–54
  age and, 53, 54, 55t
  complications of, 54
  in peripheral arterial disease, 146
  mortality and, 53–54, 53t, 54t
Thrombomodulin, 233–234, *234*
Thrombosis, 231–232, 239–240. See also *Hemostasis*.
  abnormal homocyst(e)ine metabolism and, 242
  autoimmune disorders and, 242–244, 243t
  deep venous, 142–143, *143*
    in pregnancy, 238–239
  endothelium and, 234–235, *234,* 234t
  factor deficiencies and, 239–240, 240t
  hormonal replacement therapy and, 237
  in pregnancy, 237–239, 240
    pulmonary hypertension and, 351
  lipoprotein A and, 241–242
  malignancy and, 244–245
  oral contraceptives and, 142, 161–162, 235–237
  plasminogen-activator inhibitors and, 241
  risk factors for, 240t
  treatment of, 245–247
Thrombotic microangiopathy, in pregnancy, 239
Ticlopidine therapy, 246–247
TIMI (Thrombolysis in Myocardial Infarction) trial, 54
Timolol, postinfarction, 30, 55
Timolol Myocardial Infarction Study, 55
Tissue plasminogen activators, 233
  complications with, 54
Toxemia, 93–94, 337–344
  clinical features of, 338
  coagulation abnormalities in, 237–238, 341–342
  eicosapentaenoic acid in, 342
  incidence of, 338
  multisystem involvement in, 339–340
  nontoxemic hypertension vs, 344
  ominous symptoms in, 93t
  pathophysiology of, 93, 338–339, 341
  placenta and, 339, 341
  prediction of, 238
  treatment of, 94, 341–344
  vasculopathy in, 339–340
Transdermal drug administration, estrogen, 237
  nicotine, 225
Transplantation, heart, in peripartum cardiomyopathy, 349
  lung, in pulmonary hypertension, 352–353
Triglycerides, 175–176, *177*, 178. See also *Lipoprotein(s)*.
  coronary risk and, 182
  diabetes and, 207–208
  disorders of, 179, 180, 180t
  estrogen and, 167
  gender and, 180–182
  lowering of, 186
  obesity and, 200
  transport of, *177*
Trophoblasts, in toxemia, 341
Trousseau's syndrome, 244–245

Type A behavior, 273–275, 276–277
　angina and, 277

Ultrasonography. See *Doppler* entries; *Echocardiography*.
Unstable angina, 33
U.S. Public Health Service Trial, of antihypertensive therapy, 83, 84t
Uterus, gravid, blood flow to, 309, *310*
　exercise and, 316

Valvular heart disease, 117–136
　aortic, 127–128
　　aortic root dilatation and, 128, *129*
　　bicuspid valve and, 127–128
　　stenotic, 128
　in pregnancy, 239, 330t, 333
　　prosthetic valve management in, 334–335
　incidence of, 117–118
　Marfan's syndrome and, 128, 130–131
　　in pregnancy, 130–131, 131t, 332–333, 353
　mitral, 118–126
　　anular calcification and, 127
　　endocarditis and, 122–123, 123t, 127
　　prolapse and, 118–124
　　　age in, 119
　　　complications of, 122–123, 123t
　　　diagnosis of, 120–121, 123–124
　　　gender in, 119, 121–123, 122t, 123t
　　　inheritance of, 118–119
　　　management of, 124, 124t
　　　regurgitation in, 122, 123t
　　　syndrome of, 119–121, 120t
　　rheumatic, 125–126
　rheumatic, 124–127
　　aortic, 126–127
　　epidemiology of, 124–125
　　gender predominances in, 125t
　　mitral, 125–126
　systemic lupus erythematosus and, 127
Valvuloplasty, in pregnancy, 333
Variant angina, 28
Varicose veins, 142, 142t
Vascular endothelium, animal studies on, 295–296, 298
　coagulation and, 234–235, *234,* 234t
　fibrinolysis and, 233, *233*
　in pulmonary hypertension, 350
Vascular resistance, in pregnancy, 311t, 313

Vasodilators, in pregnancy, 343
　in pulmonary hypertension of pregnancy, 352
　postinfarction, 30
Vasomotion, animal studies on, 298, *299*, 300
Venous thrombosis, 142–143, *143*. See also *Thrombosis*.
　in pregnancy, 238–239
　　factor deficiencies and, 240
　oral contraceptives and, 160–161, 236
Ventricle(s). See *Left ventricle; Right ventricle*.
Ventricular premature beats, postinfarction, 31
Ventriculography, radionuclide, exercise, 36–37
　in pregnancy, 321
Verapamil, in pregnancy, 331t
Very low density lipoprotein (VLDL). See under *Lipoprotein(s)*.
Video display terminals, cardiovascular risks associated with, 271
Viral infections, peripartum cardiomyopathy and, 347
VLDL (very low density lipoprotein). See under *Lipoprotein(s)*.
VO₂ max, 253–254, 255
　blood pressure and, 256–257
Volume, blood, in pregnancy, 308–309, *309*
　postpartum, 319

Walking, body fat percentage and, 257
　lipoprotein levels and, 260
Walnut Creek Contraceptive Study, on hypertension, 80
Warfarin, in pregnancy, 239, 331t, 334
Weight, body, 197, 197t. See also *Obesity*.
　exercise and, 257–258
　in mitral valve prolapse syndrome, 121
　smoking and, 198–199, 223–224
Weight lifting, 255
　blood pressure and, 257
　in pregnancy, 318
　lipoprotein levels and, 260–261
Weight reduction, 205
　in hypertension, 90
　in obesity, 204
　lipoprotein levels and, 183
WHO Monica Project, on blood pressure, 66, *68*
Women, physicians' attitudes toward, 13–14
Women's Health Initiative, 10
Workforce. See *Employment*.

X-linked cardiomyopathies, 113
X-rays, in pregnancy, 321